NURSING KEY TOPICS REVIEW

Pharmacology

ELSEVIER

ELSEVIER

3251 Riverport Lane
St. Louis, Missouri 63043

NURSING KEY TOPICS REVIEW: PHARMACOLOGY   ISBN: 978-0-323-44531-3

Notices

Practitioners and researchers must always rely on their own experience and knowledge in evaluating and using any information, methods, compounds or experiments described herein. Because of rapid advances in the medical sciences, in particular, independent verification of diagnoses and drug dosages should be made. To the fullest extent of the law, no responsibility is assumed by Elsevier, authors, editors or contributors for any injury and/or damage to persons or property as a matter of products liability, negligence or otherwise, or from any use or operation of any methods, products, instructions, or ideas contained in the material herein.

Although all advertising material is expected to conform to ethical (medical) standards, inclusion in this publication does not constitute a guarantee or endorsement of the quality or the value of such product or the claims made of it by its manufacturer.

International Standard Book Number: 978-0-323-44531-3

Senior Content Strategist: Jamie Blum
Senior Content Development Manager: Laurie Gower
Senior Content Development Specialist: Heather Bays
Publishing Services Manager: Julie Eddy
Project Manager: Abigail Bradberry
Design Direction: Margaret Reid

Printed in the United States of America

Last digit is the print number: 9 8 7 6 5 4 3 2

Reviewers

Melissa Bear, RN
Staff Nurse
DePaul Hospital
St. Louis, Missouri

Michelle Bonnheim
Nursing Student
California State University, Fresno
Fresno, California

Joanna Cain, BSN, BA, RN
Auctorial Pursuits, Inc.
President and Founder
Austin, Texas

Crystal Gallardo
CNA Nursing Assistant
Cypress College
Cypress, California

Rebecca Russo Hill, DNP, MSN, CNE
Assistant Professor
School of Nursing;
Chairperson
Admissions Committee
MGH Institute of Health Professions
Boston, Massachusetts

Carolyn M. Kruse, BS, DC
Educational Consultant/Owner
Kruisin Editorial
O'Fallon, Missouri

Katelynn Landers
Nursing Student
Brockton Hospital School of Nursing
Brockton, Massachusetts

Angela Lanzoni
Nursing Student
Brockton Hospital School of Nursing
Brockton, Massachusetts

Reagan Lizardi
Nursing Student
Polk State College
Lakeland, Florida

Michelle Luckett
Nursing Student
Polk State College
Winter Haven, Florida

Karla Psaros
Nursing Student
Brockton Hospital School of Nursing
Brockton, Massachusetts

Randolph E. Regal, PharmD
Clinical Associate Professor of Pharmacy
College of Pharmacy;
Clinical Pharmacist
UMH Hospital Pharmacy Services
University of Michigan
Ann Arbor, Michigan

Gina Rena
Nursing Student
Polk State College
Lakeland, Florida

Cianna Simpson
Nursing Student
Brockton Hospital School of Nursing
Brockton, Massachusetts

Briana Sundlie
Nursing Student
Cypress College
Cypress, California

Preface

The *Nursing Key Topics Review* book series was developed and designed with you, **the nursing student**, in mind. We know how difficult nursing school can be! How do you focus your study? How can you learn in the most time-efficient way possible? Where do you go when you need help?

We asked YOU and this is what we learned:

- You think textbooks are useful, but they can be overwhelming (also . . . heavy)
- You want quick and easy access to manageable levels of nursing information
- You like questions and rationales to challenge you and make sure you know what you need to know

Nursing Key Topics Review is your solution, whether you're looking for a textbook supplement or NCLEX® examination study aid. Review questions interspersed throughout the text make it easy to test your knowledge. The bulleted outline format allows for quick comprehension. A mobile app with key points lets you take your review with you anywhere you go!

In short, *Nursing Key Topics Review* helps you narrow down what's important and tells you what to focus on. Be sure to look for all the titles in the series to make your studies more effective . . . and your journey a little bit lighter!

Contents

Pharmacologic Principles 1

MEDICATION ADMINISTRATION

Definitions of Terms

- Desired effect (therapeutic effect): action for which drug is prescribed
- Adverse effect: harmful unintended reaction
- Toxic effect: serious adverse effect that occurs when plasma concentration of drug reaches dangerous, life-threatening level
- Side effect: response unrelated to desired action of drug; also an expected response based on known drug effects
- Chemical drug: a chemical substance found in a pharmaceutical drug used to treat, cure, prevent, or diagnose a disease or to promote well-being
- Cumulative action: when repeated doses of the drug accumulate in body and exert greater biologic effect than the initial dose
- Drug dependence: physical or psychologic reliance on chemical agent resulting from continued use, abuse, or addiction
- Generic drugs: copies of brand-name drugs that have exactly the same dosage intended use, effects, side effects, route of administration, risks, safety and strength of the original drug; generic drugs have the exact pharmacological effects as those of their brand-name counterparts
- Idiosyncratic response: individual's unique, unpredictable response
- Paradoxical reaction: response that contrasts sharply with usual, expected response
- Teratogen: an agent that can disturb the development of the embryo or fetus; teratogens halt pregnancy or produce a congenital malformation; classes of teratogens are radiation, maternal infections, chemicals, and drugs
- Trade/brand names: Name brand drugs that are usually under patent protection
- Tolerance: ability to endure ordinarily injurious amounts of drug or decreasing effect obtained from established dose; requires increasing dose to possibly toxic level to maintain same effect
- Hypersensitivity: excessive allergic reaction to exogenous agent (e.g., drug, food)
  - Anaphylaxis: life-threatening episode of bronchial constriction and edema that obstructs airway (leading to asphyxia) and causes generalized vasodilation, which depletes circulating blood volume; occurs when an allergen is administered to an individual who has antibodies produced by prior use of the drug or prior exposure to a substance
  - Urticaria: generalized pruritic skin eruptions or giant hives
  - Angioedema: fluid accumulation in periorbital, oral, and respiratory tissues
  - Delayed-reaction allergies: rash and fever occurring during drug therapy
- Drugs and food may interact and alter therapeutic effect adversely
  - Antagonistic/inhibiting effect: one drug diminishing the effect of another (e.g., pseudoephedrine decreases effectiveness of antihypertensives); these effects may be beneficial or harmful
  - Synergistic/potentiating effect: effect of two drugs is greater than either drug alone; often dose must be reduced; these effects may be beneficial or harmful

- Drug metabolism terms
  - Pharmacokinetics: the study of the action of drugs in the body, including absorption, distribution, metabolism, excretion, onset of action, duration of effect, biotransformation, and the effects and routes of excretion of the drug's metabolites
  - Pharmacodynamics: the study of how a drug acts on a living organism, including the response and duration and magnitude of response
  - Pharmacogenetics: the study of the effect of genetic factors of a group or individual on the response of the group or individual to certain drugs
- Ideal drug properties
  - Effectiveness: the most important ideal drug property; the drug's ability to elicit the response it was meant to
  - Safety: the drug's safety even at high concentrations and for long periods of administration
  - Selectivity: the drug's ability to elicit only the response for which it is given; selective for a specific reaction with no side effects
  - Reversible action: The drug's effect should be reversible and subside within a specified timeframe
  - Ease of administration: increases compliance and decreases errors; the number of dosages should be low and easy to administer
  - Predictability: knowing how the patient will respond to the drug
  - Freedom from drug interaction: the drug should not increase or decrease the action of other drugs; the drug should not have adverse combined effects
  - Low cost: easy to afford (especially in chronic illness)
  - Generic name ease: the drug's generic name should be easy to pronounce and remember
  - Chemical stability: the drug's potency or effectiveness is not decreased when the drug is stored

FACTORS INFLUENCING DOSAGE AND RESPONSE

Drug Factors

- Therapeutic index (TI): ratio between lethal dose and therapeutic dose; used as guide to safe dosing; a high TI is preferable to a low TI, which provides a narrow margin of safety (Fig. 1.1)
- Serum concentration of some drugs needs to be monitored; used as guide to safe dosing
  - Peak level: highest concentration of drug; usually within 1 to 2 hours after oral, 1 hour after intramuscular (IM), and 30 minutes after intravenous (IV) administration
  - Trough (residual) level: lowest concentration of drug; preferably within 15 minutes of next scheduled dose
- Concentration and duration of drug action are affected by the drug's characteristics (e.g., rate of absorption, distribution, biotransformation, and excretion)

Patient Factors

- Concentration and duration of drug action are also affected by
  - Individual factors (e.g., age, weight, gender, height, physiologic status, and genetic and environmental factors)
    - Pediatric factors: neonates higher surface area-to-mass ratio; less developed metabolism; liver is not fully developed until 1 year of age
    - Geriatric factors: slower renal and hepatic processing
  - Inability of body to metabolize or excrete drug effectively (e.g., drug affinity for particular tissues, ineffectiveness of enzymes required for metabolism of drug, depressed function of tissues naturally metabolizing (often liver) or excreting drug (often kidneys)

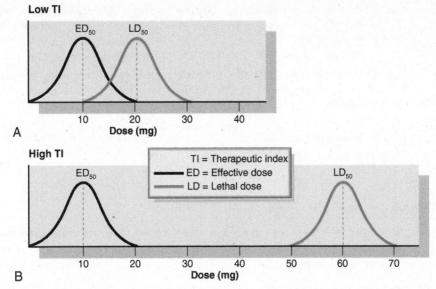

FIG. 1.1 A, Low therapeutic index drug has a narrow margin of safety, and the drug effect should be closely monitored. **B,** High therapeutic index drug has a wide margin of safety and carries less risk of drug toxicity. (From Kee, J.L., Hayes, E.R., McCuistion, L.E. [2015]. *Pharmacology: A patient-centered nursing process approach* [8th ed.]. St. Louis: Saunders.)

- Membrane barriers (e.g., placental, blood-brain) may block or selectively pass drug from circulating fluids to protected areas
- Genetic factors: different races respond differently to certain drugs; these biologic variations contribute to individual variations in response to drugs

APPLICATION AND REVIEW

1. A client is receiving an antihypertensive drug intravenously for control of severe hypertension. The client's blood pressure is unstable and 160/94 mm Hg before the infusion. Fifteen minutes after the infusion is started, the blood pressure increases to 180/100 mm Hg. Which type of response is the client demonstrating?
   1. Allergic
   2. Synergistic
   3. Paradoxical
   4. Hypersusceptibility
2. A client has an anaphylactic reaction after receiving intravenous penicillin. What does the nurse conclude is the cause of this reaction?
   1. An acquired atopic sensitization occurred.
   2. There was passive immunity to the penicillin allergen.
   3. Antibodies to penicillin developed after a previous exposure.
   4. Potent antibodies were produced when the infusion was instituted.
3. A client is brought to the emergency department after a bee sting. The client has a history of allergies to bees and is having difficulty breathing. What client reaction should cause a nurse the **most** concern?
   1. Ischemia
   2. Asphyxia
   3. Lactic acidosis
   4. Increased blood pressure

4. A client has been prescribed a medication and is now demonstrating unusual and unexpected effects. What term will the nurse use to document the client's current response?
   1. Toxic effect
   2. Therapeutic effect
   3. Cumulative action
   4. Paradoxical reaction

5. The nurse is concerned about the margin of safety for a newly prescribed medication. When reviewing medication information, which characteristic should the nurse focus on?
   1. Peak level
   2. Trough level
   3. Therapeutic index
   4. Serum concentration

See Answers on pages 8-11.

PATTERNS OF HEALTH CARE

- Adherence is the process in which a patient follows a prescription and recommendations for care
- Financial concerns (such as affordable health insurance) affect access to health care and adherence to treatment

Cultural Considerations

- Take into consideration how culture affects:
  - Health care practices and beliefs
  - Family roles, social organization, and social support
    - Consider legal and social aspects of consent by adults versus consent to treat minors
  - Patient-provider communication, including nonverbal behavior
  - Perceptions of time
- Nurses must consider their own cultural background and views about other cultures; education about other cultures is critical to providing culturally competent care
- Terminology
  - Transcultural nursing (Leininger): sensitivity to beliefs and practices about health and illness in various populations informs culturally competent care
  - Assimilation: the process in which a person or group from a different ethnic background become absorbed into a new culture
  - Ethnocentrism: a belief that one's beliefs and culture are better than those of others
  - Complementary health therapies are based on philosophies and techniques other than conventional Western medicine; often derived from those used by other cultures

NURSING RESPONSIBILITIES RELATED TO MEDICATION ADMINISTRATION

- Administration of medications is a dependent function requiring a legally written prescription that is not blindly followed
- Be aware of the patient's age, gender, socioeconomic status, ethnicity, medical history, and manifestations of common systemic and genetic disorders
- Make appropriate assessments before administering medications
  - Identify client: ensure that client is wearing identification bracelet; scan bar codes or use two identifiers such as client's name, birth date, and/or hospital number (these have reduced incidence of medication errors)
  - Identify medications client was taking before admission (including if generic or brand name drugs are prescribed/being taken) and compare list to medications prescribed after

admission to health care agency (medication reconciliation), before transfer to another facility, and upon discharge

- Question client regarding history of allergies and response to the allergen (rash, wheezing, etc.); ensure that client is wearing an allergy bracelet and allergy information is in all appropriate places in clinical record
- Determine whether client is taking any over-the-counter (OTC) medications, herbal products, or alcohol that may interact with prescribed medications
- Ensure ability to obtain and afford prescribed medications
- Establish whether drug is still appropriate based on client's status
  - Compatibility of medications with other medications or substances in diet
  - Untoward or toxic manifestations to earlier doses
  - Serum drug levels for attainment of therapeutic level, toxic level, and peak and trough levels
  - Be able to interpret a complete blood count
  - Final desired result is attained
- Other factors to assess
  - Patient's body for normal and abnormal manifestations
  - Mode of action of all classes of common drug therapy
  - If dosage is oral, topical, or intravenous
  - Drug interaction with diet and other drugs that could cause potential complications
  - Adverse effects of prescribed and OTC medication
- Know common symbols, equivalents, abbreviations, and calculation of dosage; The Joint Commission (TJC) recommends that the following should not be abbreviated: every day, every other day, right or left eye, both ears or eyes, units, cubic centimeters, morphine sulfate, and magnesium sulfate; subcutaneous can be indicated by the abbreviation Sub-Q or subQ; use a "0" before a decimal point for numbers less than 1; and no trailing "0" after a decimal
- Ensure traditional six rights of medication administration: right medication, right dose, right client, right route, right time, right documentation
- Ensure client rights related to medication administration: right client education, right to refuse medication, right client assessment, right to be advised of experimental nature of a medication and give consent, right to receive labeled medication safety, right to receive supportive therapy, right to not receive unnecessary medication, right documentation, right evaluation of client response
- Teach client about therapeutic effects, side/adverse effects, and any other pertinent information related to medication regimen, including the safety of medication and its effectiveness, and how treatment affect them throughout their lifespan for chronic conditions
- Respect client's right to refuse medication
- Know common routes
  - Oral
    - Most common, convenient, and least expensive
    - Absorption is slow; may be unpredictable; may cause GI irritation
    - Preparations include tablets, capsules, pills, powders, and liquids
      - Sustained-release or enteric-coated preparations should not be crushed or broken
      - Suspensions should be shaken well before pouring and can be used when a patient is having trouble swallowing a tablet, capsule or pill
  - Sublingual: placed under tongue; absorbed rapidly and directly into bloodstream
  - Parenteral: requires sterile technique
    - Intradermal: small volume (usually 0.1 mL) under epidermis; most commonly used for allergy and tuberculin testing

- Subcutaneous: 0.5 to 2 mL into tissues just below skin
- Intramuscular: up to 3 mL into muscle depending on site; sites include ventrogluteal, dorsogluteal (not generally recommended because of proximity to large blood vessels and sciatic nerve), vastus lateralis, rectus femoris, and deltoid
- Intravenous: given directly into vein by continuous infusion, intermittent infusion (intravenous piggy back [IVPB]), intravenous push
- Transdermal (through skin) preparations
- Inhalation: metered-dose inhaler or nebulizer; dry powdered inhalers
- Topical preparations: for localized effect on skin or in body cavities (e.g., bladder, eyes, ears, nose, vagina, oral cavity, and rectum); for systemic effect (e.g., rectal, nasal, sublingual)
- Calculate dosage of medications; use following formulas for ratio and proportion

$$\frac{\text{Desired}}{\text{Have}} \frac{\text{Ordered dose}}{\text{Available dose}} \times \frac{\text{Desired amount (e.g., tablets, mL)}}{\text{Available amount}}$$

- Calculate dosage for patients with a given body mass
  - Adults
  - Pediatric (infants and children): higher surface area to mass ratio; usually dosage calculation is based on weight for infants and children
  - Older adults: slower renal and hepatic metabolism
  - Pregnant and breastfeeding women: confirm provider and woman have considered risks/benefits to fetus/infant
- Evaluate client's response to medication
- Clearly and accurately record and report administration of medications and client's response
- Follow standard practice when counting, wasting, or documenting controlled substances; the wasting of controlled substances should be witnessed by two licensed personnel according to federal regulations; this can be done by an RN or LPN

APPLICATION AND REVIEW

6. Which client statement should cause the nurse most concern about the client's adherence to medication therapy?
   1. "How long will I need to take this medication?"
   2. "Should I take this medication with food?"
   3. "What should I do when I miss a dose?"
   4. "How much does this medication cost?"
7. Which assessment question demonstrates the nurse's understanding of the importance of determining the ongoing appropriateness on continuing a specific medication therapy?
   1. "Have you noticed any itching since starting this medication?"
   2. "Have you ever been prescribed this medication before?"
   3. "Would you rather take this medication with water or tea?"
   4. "When do you usually take bedtime medications?"
8. The nurse is caring for a client diagnosed with dysphagia. When a new medication is prescribed, what suggestion should the nurse make as to the form of medication to best address the client's needs?
   1. Sustained-release
   2. Enteric-coated
   3. Suspension
   4. Caplet

9. At the conclusion of visiting hours, the parent of a 14-year-old adolescent scheduled for orthopedic surgery the next day hands the nurse a bottle of capsules and says, "These are for my child's allergy. Will you be sure my child takes one about 9 tonight?" What is the nurse's **best** response?
   1. "I will give one capsule tonight before bedtime."
   2. "I will get a prescription so that the medicine can be taken."
   3. "Does your health care provider know about your child's allergy?"
   4. "Did you ask your health care provider if your child should have this tonight?"

10. A client is being admitted for a total hip replacement. When is it necessary for the nurse to ensure that a medication reconciliation is completed? **Select all that apply.**
    1. After reporting severe pain
    2. On admission to the hospital
    3. Upon entering the operating room
    4. Before transfer to a rehabilitation facility
    5. At time of scheduling for the surgical procedure

11. Based on the client's reported pain level, the nurse administers 8 mg of the prescribed morphine. The medication is available in a 10-mg syringe. Wasting of the remaining 2 mg of morphine should be done by the nurse and a witness. Who should be the witness?
    1. Nursing supervisor
    2. Licensed practical nurse
    3. Client's health care provider
    4. Designated nursing assistant

12. A nurse is supportive of a child receiving long-term rehabilitation in the home rather than in a health care facility. Why is living with the family so important to a child's emotional development?
    1. It provides rewards and punishment.
    2. The child's development is supported.
    3. It reflects the mores of a larger society.
    4. The child's identity and roles are learned.

13. A daughter of a Chinese-speaking client approaches a nurse and asks multiple questions while maintaining direct eye contact. What culturally related concept does the daughter's behavior reflect?
    1. Prejudice
    2. Stereotyping
    3. Assimilation
    4. Ethnocentrism

14. A nurse manager works on a unit where the nursing staff members are uncomfortable taking care of clients from cultures that are different from their own. How should the nurse manager address this situation?
    1. Assign articles about various cultures so that they can become more knowledgeable.
    2. Relocate the nurses to units where they will not have to care for clients from a variety of cultures.
    3. Rotate the nurses' assignments so they have an equal opportunity to care for clients from other cultures.
    4. Plan a workshop that offers opportunities to learn about the cultures they might encounter while at work.

15. A nurse in the health clinic is counseling a college student who was recently diagnosed with asthma. On what aspect of care should the nurse focus?
    1. Teaching how to make a room allergy-free
    2. Referring to a support group for individuals with asthma
    3. Arranging with the college to ensure a speedy return to classes
    4. Evaluating whether the necessary lifestyle changes are understood

16. A client is scheduled to receive phenytoin 100 mg orally at 6 PM but is having difficulty swallowing capsules. What method should the nurse use to help the client take the medication?
    1. Sprinkle the powder from the capsule into a cup of water.
    2. Insert a rectal suppository containing 100 mg of phenytoin.
    3. Administer 4 mL of phenytoin suspension containing 125 mg/5 mL.
    4. Obtain a change in the administration route to allow an IM injection.

17. Filgrastim 5 mcg/kg/day by injection is prescribed for a client who weighs 132 lb. The vial label reads "filgrastim 300 mcg/mL". How many milliliters should the nurse administer? **Record your answer using a whole number.**
    Answer: _____ mL

18. A child is to receive 60 mg of phenytoin. The medication is available as an oral suspension that contains 125 mg/5 mL. How many milliliters should the nurse administer? **Record your answer using one decimal place.**
    Answer: _____ mL

19. A health care provider prescribes an IV infusion ampicillin 375 mg every 6 hours. The drug is supplied as 500 mg of powder in a vial. The directions are to mix the powder with 1.8 mL of diluent, which yields 250 mg/mL. How much prepared solution should the nurse administer? **Record your answer using one decimal place.**
    Answer: _____ mL

20. A client with terminal cancer is to receive 2 mg of hydromorphone IV every 4 hours prn for severe breakthrough pain. The vial contains 10 mg/mL. When the client complains of severe pain, how much solution of hydromorphone should the nurse administer? **Record your answer using one decimal place.**
    Answer: _____ mL

See Answers on pages 8-11.

ANSWER KEY: REVIEW QUESTIONS

1. **3 A paradoxical response to a drug is directly opposite the desired therapeutic response.**
   1 An allergic response is an antigen-antibody reaction. **2** A synergistic response involves drug combinations that enhance each other. **4** A hypersusceptibility response to a drug is more pronounced than the common response.
   Client Need: Pharmacologic and Parenteral Therapies; **Cognitive Level:** Application; **Nursing Process:** Evaluation/Outcomes

2. **3 Hypersensitivity results from the production of antibodies in response to exposure to certain foreign substances (allergens). Earlier exposure is necessary for the development of these antibodies.**
   1 Acquired atopic sensitization is not a sensitivity reaction to penicillin; hay fever and asthma are atopic conditions. **2** An anaphylactic reaction is an active, not passive, immune response. **4** Antibodies developed when there was a prior, not current, exposure to penicillin.
   Client Need: Pharmacologic and Parenteral Therapies; **Cognitive Level:** Application; **Nursing Process:** Evaluation/Outcomes

3. **2 Hypersensitivity can produce an anaphylactic reaction with edema of the respiratory system, resulting in respiratory obstruction, respiratory arrest, and asphyxia.**
   1 Ischemia is unrelated to anaphylaxis. **3** Lactic acidosis is associated with excessive exercise. **4** In an anaphylactic reaction, the blood pressure decreases, not increases.
   Client Need: Physiologic Adaptation; **Cognitive Level:** Application; **Nursing Process:** Assessment/Analysis

4. **4 Paradoxical reaction is a response to a medication that contrasts sharply with the usual, expected response.**
   1 Toxic effect is a serious adverse effect that occurs when plasma concentration of drug reaches a dangerous, life-threatening level. **2** Therapeutic effect (desired effect) is a consequence of treatment that is deemed desired and beneficial. **3** Cumulative action occurs when repeated doses of the drug accumulate in the body and exert greater biologic effect than the initial dose.
   Client Need: Physiologic Adaptation; **Cognitive Level:** Application; Integrated Process: Communication/Documentation; **Nursing Process:** Assessment/Analysis

5. **3 Therapeutic index (TI) is the ratio between lethal dose and therapeutic dose; used as a guide to safe dosing; a high TI is preferable to a low TI, which provides a narrow margin of safety**
   1 Peak level is highest concentration of drug; usually within 1 to 2 hours after oral, 1 hour after IM, and 30 minutes after IV administration. **2** Trough (residual) level is the lowest concentration of drug; preferably within 15 minutes of next scheduled dose. **4** Serum concentration of some drugs is used to determine a guide to safe dosing.
   Client Need: Pharmacologic and Parenteral Therapies; **Cognitive Level:** Application; **Nursing Process:** Planning/Implementation

6. **4 Adherence is the process in which a patient follows a prescription and recommendations for care. Financial concerns, such as the cost of the medication, are often a major concern in a client's nonadherence to medication therapy.**
   1 Asking about how long the medication therapy will last is a question that relates to effective client education regarding the proper administration of the medication rather than to future adherence. **2** Asking about the appropriateness of taking the medication with food is a question that relates to effective client education regarding the proper administration of the medication rather than to future adherence. **3** Asking about how to manage a missed dose is a question that relates to effective client education regarding the proper administration of the medication rather than to future adherence.
   Client Need: Management of Care; **Cognitive Level:** Analysis; **Nursing Process:** Assessment/Analysis

7. **1 Determining the ongoing appropriateness of a specific medication therapy is dependent on the client's current status. Monitoring for side effects is an effective way to assess the client's status especially related to the introduction of medications.**
   2 Asking whether the client has even taken this medication before is an appropriate assessment question, but it does not address the client's current health condition but rather medication history. **3** Asking the client whether they prefer tea or water when swallowing the medication is an appropriate assessment question, but it does not address the client's current health condition but rather personal preference related to medication administration. **4** Asking the client when they prefer to take their bedtime medication is an appropriate assessment question, but it does not address the client's current health condition but rather personal preference related to medication administration.
   Client Need: Management of Care; **Cognitive Level:** Analysis; **Nursing Process:** Assessment/Analysis

8. **3 Suspensions can be used when a patient is having trouble swallowing.**
   1 Sustained released medications are formulated to be dissolved slowly and to release medication at specific intervals. They are not easier to swallow. **2** Enteric coated medications have an outer coating that prevents the medication from being broken down in the stomach but rather in the intestines. They are not easier to swallow. **4** A caplet is formed in an oval rather that round shape. Although it may be easier to swallow in some instances, it is not the best option for a client experiencing dysphagia.
   Client Need: Management of Care; **Cognitive Level:** Application; **Nursing Process:** Planning/Implementation

9. **2 Legally, a nurse cannot administer medications without a prescription from a legally licensed individual.**
   1 The nurse cannot give the medication without a current health care provider's prescription; this is a dependent function of the nurse. **3** The nurse should not ask if the health care provider is aware of the problem; it is the nurse's responsibility to document the client's health history. **4** It is the nurse's responsibility to review the health care provider's orders and question them when appropriate.

Client Need: Management of Care; **Cognitive Level:** Application; **Integrated Process:** Communication/Documentation; **Nursing Process:** Planning/Implementation

10. **Answers: 2, 4**

    2 Medication reconciliation involves the creation of a list of all medications the client is taking and comparing it to the health care provider's orders on admission. **4** Medication reconciliation involves the creation of a list of all medications the client is taking and comparing it to the health care provider's orders when there is a transfer to a different setting or service, and/or discharge.

    1 A change in status does not require medication reconciliation. **3** A medication reconciliation should be completed long before this time. **5** Total hip replacement is elective surgery, and scheduling takes place before admission; medication reconciliation takes place when the client is admitted and upon discharge.

    Client Need: Pharmacologic and Parenteral Therapies; **Cognitive Level:** Analysis; **Nursing Process:** Planning/Implementation

11. **2 The wasting of controlled substances should be witnessed by two licensed personnel according to federal regulations; this can be done by an RN or LPN.**

    1 Although the nursing supervisor is licensed and may perform this function, it is not an efficient use of this individual's expertise. **3** Federal regulations do not require the participation by the client's health care provider in this situation. **4** A nursing assistant is not a licensed person who can take responsibility for the wasting of controlled substances.

    Client Need: Pharmacologic and Parenteral Therapies; **Cognitive Level:** Application; **Nursing Process:** Planning/Implementation

> **Study Tip:** Because there is a legal concern about disposing of controlled substances, licensed personnel must witness it.

12. **4 Socialization, values, and role definition are learned within the family and help develop a sense of self. Once established in the family, the child can more easily move into society.**

    1 Reward and punishment is just one aspect of the family's influence; it is not as important as identity and roles in relation to emotional development. **2** Although important, the child's development is just one aspect of the family's influence; it is not as important as identity and roles in relation to emotional development. **3** Although important, reflection of social societal mores is just one aspect of the family's influence; it is not as important as identity and roles in relation to emotional development.

    Client Need: Psychosocial Integrity; **Cognitive Level:** Application; **Nursing Process:** Planning/Implementation

13. **3 Assimilation involves incorporating the behaviors of a dominant culture. Maintaining eye contact is characteristic of the American culture and not of Asian cultures.**

    1 Prejudice is a negative belief about another person or group and does not characterize this behavior. **2** Stereotyping is the perception that all members of a group are alike. **4** Ethnocentrism is the perception that one's beliefs are better than those of others.

    Client Need: Psychosocial Integrity; **Cognitive Level:** Application; **Nursing Process:** Planning/Implementation

14. **4 A workshop provides an opportunity to discuss cultural diversity; this should include identification of one's own feelings; also, it provides an opportunity for participants to ask questions.**

    1 Although reading articles will provide information, it does not promote a discussion about the topic. **2** Relocation is not feasible or desirable; clients from other cultures are found in all settings. **3** Rotation of nurse assignments probably will increase tension on the unit.

    Client Need: Psychosocial Integrity; **Cognitive Level:** Application; **Nursing Process:** Planning/Implementation

15. **4 Understanding the disorder and the details of care are essential for the client to be self-sufficient.**

    1 Although allergy-free is important, a perceived understanding of the need for specific interventions must be expressed before there is a readiness for learning. **2** Referral to a support group is premature; this may be done eventually. **3** Although a return to class is important, involving the college should be the client's decision.

    Client Need: Health Promotion and Maintenance; **Cognitive Level:** Application; **Nursing Process:** Planning/Implementation

16. **Answer: 3**

When an oral medication is available in a suspension form, the nurse can use it for clients who cannot swallow capsules. Use the "Desire over Have" formula to solve the problem.

$$\frac{\text{Desire}}{\text{Have}}\ \frac{100\,\text{mg}}{125\,\text{mg}} = \frac{x\,\text{mL}}{5\,\text{mL}}$$

$$125x = 500$$
$$x = 500 \div 125$$
$$x = 4\,\text{mL}$$

1 Because a palatable suspension is available, it is a better alternative than opening the capsule. **2** The route of administration cannot be altered without the health care provider's approval. **4** Intramuscular injections should be avoided because of risks for tissue injury and infection.

Client Need: Pharmacologic and Parenteral Therapies; **Cognitive Level:** Analysis; **Nursing Process:** Planning/Implementation

17. **Answer: 1 mL.**

When 132 pounds is converted to kilograms, it equals 60 kg.

The practitioner prescribed 5 mcg/kg; therefore, 5 × 60 = 300 mcg. This desired amount is contained in 1 mL, as indicated on the vial label.

Client Need: Pharmacologic and Parenteral Therapies; **Cognitive Level:** Application; **Nursing Process:** Planning/Implementation

18. **Answer: 2.4 mL.**

Use the "Desire over Have" formula to solve this problem.

$$\frac{\text{Desire}}{\text{Have}}\ \frac{60\,\text{mg}}{125\,\text{mg}} = \frac{x\,\text{mL}}{5\,\text{mL}}$$

$$125x = 300$$
$$x = 300 \div 125 = 2.4\,\text{mL}$$

Client Need: Pharmacologic and Parenteral Therapies; **Cognitive Level:** Application; **Nursing Process:** Planning/Implementation

19. **Answer: 1.5 mL.**

Use the "Desire over Have" formula to solve the problem.

$$\frac{\text{Desire}}{\text{Have}}\ \frac{375\,\text{mg}}{250\,\text{mg}} = \frac{x\,\text{mL}}{1\,\text{mL}}$$

$$250x = 375$$
$$x = 375 \div 250$$
$$x = 1.5\,\text{mL}$$

Client Need: Pharmacologic and Parenteral Therapies; **Cognitive Level:** Application; **Nursing Process:** Planning/Implementation

20. **Answer: 2 or 0.2**

Solve the problem using ratio and proportion.

$$\frac{\text{Desire}}{\text{Have}}\ \frac{2\,\text{mg}}{10\,\text{mg}} = \frac{x\,\text{mL}}{1\,\text{mL}}$$

$$10x = 2$$
$$x = 2 \div 10$$
$$x = 0.2\,\text{mL}$$

Client Need: Pharmacologic and Parenteral Therapies; **Cognitive Level:** Application; **Nursing Process:** Planning/Implementation

2 Analgesic Drugs, Muscle Relaxants, and Local Anesthetics

PAIN

Overview

- Definition: universally unpleasant emotional and sensory experience that occurs in response to actual or potential tissue trauma or inflammation
  - Referred to as fifth vital sign
  - Subjective; pain is whatever client says it is
  - Perception of client's pain is influenced by multiple factors (e.g., previous pain experience and emotional, physical, and psychologic status)

Types

By Duration

- Acute pain: mild to severe pain lasting less than 6 months; usually associated with specific injury; involves sympathetic nervous system response; leads to increased pulse rate and volume, rate, and depth of respirations, blood pressure (BP), and glucose level; urine production and peristalsis decrease
- Chronic pain: mild to severe pain lasting longer than 6 months; associated with parasympathetic nervous system; client may not exhibit signs and symptoms associated with acute pain; may lead to depression and decreased functional status

By Origin/Mechanism

- Nociceptive: normal function processes noxious stimuli
- Neuropathic: abnormal processing of stimuli; often supersensitivity
- Somatic: type of nociceptive pain; skin pain, tissue pain, muscle pain
- Visceral: pain that occurs in the organs
- Idiopathic: long-term pain with no detectable cause; also called *pain of unknown origin*

Terminology

- Pain threshold: minimum amount of stimulus required to cause sensation of pain
- Pain tolerance: maximum pain a client is willing or able to endure
- Referred pain: pain experienced in an area different from site of tissue trauma (Fig. 2.1)
- Intractable pain: pain not relieved by conventional treatment
- Neuropathic pain: pain caused by neurologic disturbance; may not be associated with tissue damage
- Phantom pain: pain experienced in missing body part
- Radiating pain: pain experienced at source and extending to other areas
- Psychogenic pain: physical pain that is caused, increased, or prolonged by mental, emotional, or behavioral factors; also called *psychalgia*

REVIEW OF PHYSIOLOGY

- Sensory neurons, nociceptors in peripheral nervous system, are stimulated by biochemical mediators (e.g., bradykinin, serotonin, histamine, potassium, and substance P) when there is

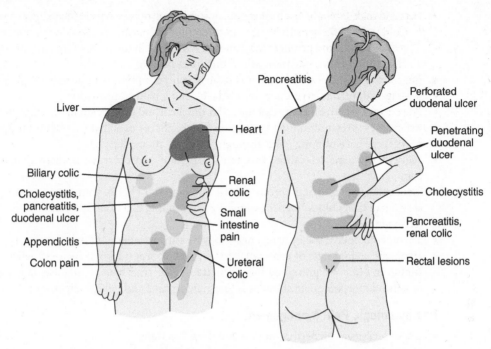

FIG. 2.1 Common sites of referred pain. Note that the location of the pain may not be directly over or even near the site of the organ. (From Monahan, F.D., Sands, J.K., Neighbors, M., Marek, J.F., Green, C. [2007]. *Phipps medical-surgical nursing: Health and illness perspectives* [8th ed.]. St. Louis: Mosby.)

mechanical, thermal, or chemical damage to tissue; viscera do not have special neurons for pain transmission; receptors respond to stretching, ischemia, and inflammation
- Pain impulses are transmitted to spinal column
  - A delta fibers: myelinated, large-diameter neurons
  - C fibers: unmyelinated, narrow-diameter neurons
- Impulse enters at dorsal horn and ascends spinothalamic tract to thalamus
- Impulse travels to basal areas of brain and to somatic sensory cortex
- Endogenous opioids, such as endorphins, are released and bind to receptors to modify pain transmission
- Gate-control theory (Melzack and Wall) suggests that stimulation of large-diameter fibers can block transmission of painful impulses through dorsal horn

TREATMENT OF PAIN

Nonpharmacologic Pain Management Strategies
- Acupuncture: insertion of disposable needles into meridians (energy pathways) to change energy flow; may use heat or electric stimulation
- Acupressure: finger pressure applied over meridians; less invasive but less effective than acupuncture
- Aromatherapy: plant oils applied topically or misted (e.g., lavender to reduce anxiety associated with pain) have shown benefit
- Biofeedback: provides information about changes in body function; clients can learn to use this to control a variety of body responses, including pain
- Distraction: focuses client's attention away from pain

- Heat and cold: diminishes pain experience by stimulation of large sensory fibers (gate-control theory)
  - Cold reduces the sensitivity of pain receptors and promotes vasoconstriction, which helps reduce edema and promote local anesthesia; can be in the form of ice pack or cold sitz bath
  - Heat promotes vasodilation, which enhances healing
- Imagery: calming, peaceful thoughts reduce pain perception (can be Guided Imagery)
- Massage: stimulates large-diameter fibers, blocking pain transmission
- Prayer: an alternative therapy that may relax the client and provide strength, solace, or acceptance.
- Reflexology: pressure applied to areas on feet, hands, or ears that correspond to specific body organ; may have calming effect through release of endorphins
- Sequential muscle relaxation: promotes relaxation and decreases anxiety, thereby reducing pain perception
- Transcutaneous or percutaneous electric stimulation (TENS): stimulation of peripheral sensory nerve fibers blocks transmission of pain impulse; dial is adjusted until patient no longer feels pain
- Therapeutic touch: use of hands near body to improve energy imbalances
- Hypnosis: altered state of consciousness in which concentration is focused; believed that pain stimuli in brain are prevented from penetrating the conscious mind; also, may cause release of natural morphine-like substances (e.g., endorphins and enkephalins)

Pharmacologic Pain Management

- Use of analgesia can permit motion and deep breathing
- Multimodal: use of two or more classes of analgesics
- Route of Administration: mainly oral, also IV and IM
- Around the Clock (ATC) Dosing: to maintain steady level of analgesia
- Patient-Controlled Analgesia (PCA): patient self-treats
- Three Groups of Pharmacologic Analgesics (Table 2.1)
  - Nonopioid Analgesics (includes acetaminophen and nonsteroidal antiinflammatory agents [NSAIDs])
  - Opioid Analgesics
  - Adjuvant Analgesics (includes drugs from different groups with variable mechanisms of action, e.g., some antidepressants, local anesthetics, muscle relaxants)

TABLE 2.1	The Three Analgesic Groups		
	Nonopioid Analgesics	**Opioid Analgesics**	**Adjuvant Analgesics**
Advantages	Versatile with multiple agents, formulations, and routes of administration available Flexible and useful for a wide variety of mild to moderate nociceptive-type pain conditions Identified as the foundation of a multimodal approach for nociceptive-type pain Can produce opioid dose-sparing effects Available in combination with opioids	Cornerstone of moderate to severe nociceptive-type pain Mu agonists have no ceiling on analgesia Opioid rotation can be initiated for development of tolerance With the exception of constipation, tolerance develops to side effects with regular daily doses over several days	Largest and most diverse analgesic group; wide variety of agents, formulations, and routes of administration available depending on agent Side effects often are responsive to dose reduction Tolerance develops to most of the adverse effects

TABLE 2.1 The Three Analgesic Groups—cont'd		
	Nonopioid Analgesics	**Opioid Analgesics**	**Adjuvant Analgesics**
Disadvantages	Wide interindividual differences in response Ineffective for neuropathic pain Acetaminophen adverse effects require careful consideration of patient's hepatic status before administration and care not to exceed recommended daily dose NSAID adverse effects prohibit use or suggest cautionary use in some patient populations, including older adults, patients with high CV and/or GI risk factors, and those with bleeding disorders All of the nonopioids and combination nonopioid/opioid formulations have a maximum daily dose that should not be exceeded	Constipation is an almost universal opioid side effect and the number-one reason people stop taking pain medication Although most side effects are manageable, undetected excessive sedation and respiratory depression are life threatening Close monitoring of sedation and respiratory status is indicated during at least the first 24 hours of opioid therapy Screening for appropriateness and ongoing monitoring via a therapeutic relationship between the patient and prescriber are required for safe and effective long-term opioid therapy Some opioids produce metabolites that can accumulate and produce toxicity, for example, morphine (morphine 3-glucuronide [M3G])	Contain the agents that are recommended for treatment of neuropathic pain Considerable variability among people in their response to agents used to treat chronic neuropathic pain, including to agents within the same class; a "trial and error" strategy must be used, and multiple analgesic trials are sometimes necessary Most require titration of dose over several weeks to evaluate effectiveness; patients must be forewarned of delayed onset of analgesia Most have a maximum daily dose Side effects can be significant and may limit dose escalation
Examples	Acetaminophen (Tylenol) Nonselective NSAIDs • Aspirin • Diclofenac • Ibuprofen • Ketoprofen • Ketorolac • Meloxicam • Naproxen COX-2-selective NSAIDs • Celecoxib	• Morphine • Fentanyl • Hydromorphone • Hydrocodone • Oxycodone • Oxymorphone • Methadone	Anticonvulsants • Gabapentin • Pregabalin Tricyclic antidepressants • Nortriptyline • Desipramine Serotonin-norepinephrine reuptake inhibitors (SNRIs) • Duloxetine • Venlafaxine Alpha$_2$-adrenergic agonists • Clonidine • Tizanidine Local anesthetics • Bupivacaine • Ropivacaine • Lidocaine injectable • Lidocaine patch 5% Muscle relaxants/antispasmodics • Baclofen • Cyclobenzaprine NMDA antagonists • Ketamine

CV, Cardiovascular; *NMDA*, N-methyl-D-aspartate.

Modified from Ignatavicius, D.D., Workman, L.M. (2016). *Medical-surgical nursing: Patient-centered collaborative care* (8th ed.). St. Louis: Elsevier.

APPLICATION AND REVIEW

1. A nurse applies an ice pack to a client's leg for 20 minutes. What clinical indicator helps the nurse determine the effectiveness of the treatment?
   1. Local anesthesia
   2. Peripheral vasodilation
   3. Depression of vital signs
   4. Decreased viscosity of blood

2. A client with an inflamed sciatic nerve is to have a conventional transcutaneous electrical nerve stimulation (TENS) device applied to the painful nerve pathway. When operating the TENS unit, which nursing action is appropriate?
   1. Maintain the settings programmed by the health care provider.
   2. Turn the machine on several times a day for 10 to 20 minutes.
   3. Adjust the dial on the unit until the client states the pain is relieved.
   4. Apply the color-coded electrodes on the client where they are most comfortable.

3. A health care provider performs a ligation of hemorrhoids with latex bands. What does the nurse expect to be prescribed for reduction of local discomfort?
   1. Sitz baths
   2. Water-soluble jelly
   3. Inflatable doughnut
   4. Medicated suppository

4. After abdominal surgery, a client refuses the nurse's request to cough and deep breathe, saying, "It's too painful." What action should the nurse take?
   1. Start administering pain medication regularly every 4 hours.
   2. Explain the consequences of not aerating the lungs after surgery.
   3. Substitute incentive spirometry for coughing and deep breathing.
   4. Medicate for pain before encouraging coughing and deep breathing.

5. Which alternative therapy may be beneficial for the nurse to discuss with a client who has terminal cancer?
   1. Biofeedback
   2. Radiotherapy
   3. Bariatric therapy
   4. Radioactive implants

6. Alternative therapy measures have become increasingly accepted within the past decade, especially in the relief of pain. Which methods qualify as alternative therapies for pain? **Select all that apply.**
   1. Prayer
   2. Hypnosis
   3. Medication
   4. Aromatherapy
   5. Guided imagery

See Answers on pages 31-35.

NONOPIOID ANALGESICS

- Weaker than opioid analgesics
- Includes acetaminophen; NSAIDs including aspirin, ibuprofen, and naproxen; and cyclooxygenase-2 (COX-2) inhibitors

Acetaminophen

- Analgesic and antipyretic (*not* an antiinflammatory); for mild to moderate pain
- Does not affect platelet aggregation
- Causes minimal to no gastric distress
- Included in many OTC preparations, which must be taken into consideration when calculating dose
- Hepatotoxicity may occur with regular use at doses as low as 3 grams/day

Mode of Action

- Inhibition of prostaglandin synthesis

Contraindications, Precautions, and Drug Interactions for Selected Nonopioid Analgesics*

Drug	Contraindications/Precautions	Drug Interaction
Acetaminophen	**Contraindications:** Hypersensitivity **Pregnancy:** No human studies available, but no adverse effects in animals	Alcohol, hepatotoxic drugs, hepatic enzyme inducers, barbiturates, hydantoins, NSAIDs, salicylates, anticholinergic drugs, beta blockers, oral contraceptives, warfarin, isoniazid, rifampin

*Pregnancy categories have been revised. See http://www.fda.gov/Drugs/DevelopmentApprovalProcess/DevelopmentResources/Labeling/ucm093307.htm for more information.

Side/Adverse Effects

- Hypersensitivity
- Oliguria
- Elevated hepatic enzymes
- Hepatotoxicity
- Hepatic dysfunction
- Hemolytic anemia
- Agranulocytosis
- Leukopenia
- Neutropenia
- Thrombocytopenia
- Pancytopenia
- Renal failure

Nonsteroidal Antiinflammatory Drugs (NSAIDs)

- Available in oral and parenteral (IM) preparations
- Analgesic, antiinflammatory, and antipyretic effects
- For mild to moderate pain

Mode of Action

- Acts on peripheral nerve endings and decreases inflammatory mediators by inhibiting prostaglandin synthesis
- NSAIDs inhibit COX-1 and COX-2 (both are isoforms of the enzyme cyclooxygenase), which inhibits the production of prostaglandins, thereby contributing to analgesia
- ASA causes irreversible inhibition of COX; this action is different from other NSAIDs

Contraindications, Precautions, and Drug Interactions for Pain Analgesia by NSAIDs*

Drug	Contraindications/Precautions	Drug Interaction
Aspirin (salicylate NSAID)	**Contraindications:** Hypersensitivity; pregnancy (especially 3rd trimester); breastfeeding; avoid in adolescents and children during fever and viral illnesses; GI bleeding; bleeding disorders; agranulocytosis; asthma **Pregnancy:** (third trimester) Definite fetal risks; may be given despite risks in life-threatening conditions	Alcohol, NSAIDs, ACE inhibitors, antacids, anticoagulants, diuretics, heparin, penicillins, oral hypoglycemics, sulfonamides, thrombolytic agents, urinary acidifiers
Ibuprofen (propionic acid NSAID)	**Contraindications:** Hypersensitivity, asthma, severe renal or hepatic disease, recent heart surgery **Precautions:** Breastfeeding, GI bleeding, cardiac disorders **Pregnancy:** Only given after risks to the fetus are considered	Alcohol, NSAIDs, anticoagulants, antidiabetics (oral), antihypertensives, antineoplastics, antiplatelet agents, corticosteroids, diuretics, salicylates, thrombolytics

Continued

Contraindications, Precautions, and Drug Interactions for Pain Analgesia by NSAIDs—cont'd

Drug	Contraindications/Precautions	Drug Interaction
Naproxen (propionic acid NSAID)	*Contraindications:* Hypersensitivity to NSAIDs or salicylates, recent heart surgery *Precautions:* Breastfeeding, GI bleeding, cardiac disorders, bleeding disorders, asthma, severe renal or hepatic disease *Pregnancy:* Only given after risks to the fetus are considered (second and third trimesters)	ACE inhibitors, alcohol, antacids, anticoagulants, antihypertensives, antineoplastics, aspirin, blood thinners, corticosteroids, diuretics, lithium; methotrexate; probenecid
Ketorolac (propionic acid NSAID)	*Contraindications:* Hypersensitivity, renal impairment, bleeding disorders, GI bleeding or ulceration, breastfeeding, recent heart surgery *Precautions:* GI bleeding, cardiac disorders *Pregnancy:* Only given after risks to the fetus are considered	ACE inhibitors, alcohol, anticoagulants, antidepressants (some), antihypertensives, aspirin, corticosteroids, diuretics, NSAIDs, salicylates, thrombolytics
Meloxicam (Oxicam NSAID; enolic acid derivative)	*Contraindications:* Hypersensitivity, cardiac conditions, sulfa allergy, before or after coronary artery bypass graft surgery, breastfeeding *Pregnancy:* (third trimester) Definite fetal risks; may be given despite risks in life-threatening conditions; (second trimester) only given after risks to the fetus are considered;	ACE inhibitors, alcohol, aspirin, blood thinners, cyclosporine, lithium
Celecoxib (Cyclo-oxygenase-2 inhibitor)	*Contraindications:* Hypersensitivity to it or other NSAIDs, sulfa allergy, salicylate allergy, before or after coronary artery bypass graft surgery, hepatic impairment, bleeding disorders, breastfeeding, GI bleeding/ulcers, myocardial infarction, stroke *Precautions:* Severe hepatic or renal disease *Pregnancy:* (third trimester) Definite fetal risks; may be given despite risks in life-threatening conditions; (first and second trimesters) only given after risks to the fetus are considered	ACE inhibitors, angiotensin II antagonists, anticoagulants, antineoplastics, antiplatelets, aspirin, bisphosphonates, fluconazole, glucocorticoids, lithium, NSAIDs, salicylates, SSRIs, thiazide diuretics, thrombolytics, warfarin
Indomethacin	*Contraindications:* Hypersensitivity to NSAIDs or salicylates, before or after coronary artery bypass graft surgery, aortic coarctation, asthma, hepatic impairment, GI bleeding, stroke, myocardial infarction *Pregnancy:* Only given after risks to the fetus are considered	Aminoglycosides, anticoagulants, antihypertensives, diuretics (potassium sparing), SNRIs, SSRIs, thrombolytics

*Pregnancy categories have been revised. See http://www.fda.gov/Drugs/DevelopmentApprovalProcess/DevelopmentResources/Labeling/ucm093307.htm for more information.

Side/Adverse Effects
- Reye's syndrome (aspirin)
- Gastrointestinal (GI) distress, ulceration and bleeding
- Peptic ulcer disease (PUD)
- Blood dyscrasias: thrombocytopenia, agranulocytosis, leukopenia, neutropenia, hemolytic anemia
- Bone marrow depression and impaired coagulation

- Central nervous system (CNS) and genitourinary (GU) disturbances
- CNS disturbances: dizziness, drowsiness, tremors, confusion, seizures, headache, coma
- Constipation or diarrhea
- Dysrhythmias
- Hepatotoxicity, hepatitis
- Hypertension and fluid retention, especially with older adults
- Hyperkalemia
- Kidney and liver impairment
- Increased liver enzymes
- Non-viral hepatitis (Tylenol)
- Myocardial infarction (increased risk)
- Cerebrovascular accident (increased risk)
- Nausea and vomiting
- Potentially fatal cardiovascular thrombolytic events increase with duration of use (COX-2 inhibitors)
- Skin rash (hypersensitivity)
- Stroke increased risk
- Tarry stools (melena)
- Tinnitus (especially with aspirin), hearing loss
- Vertigo
- Visual disturbances

Nursing Care
- Monitor for side effects
- Administer with meals or milk to reduce GI irritation
- Administer enteric coated preparation to reduce GI irritation
- Monitor complete blood count (CBC)
- Monitor aspartate transaminase (AST)
- Monitor alanine transaminase (ALT)
- Monitor coagulation and liver profiles
- Monitor liver and kidney function
- Assess vital signs; may increase BP
- Instruct to report side effects such as bleeding or hearing disturbance; aspirin toxicity affects cranial nerve VIII causing tinnitus
- Encourage diet rich in nutrient-dense foods (e.g., fruits, vegetables, whole grains, and legumes) to improve and maintain nutritional status and prevent drug-induced nutrient deficiencies; restrict sodium intake to limit fluid retention
- Teach patient:
  - To drink six to eight glasses of water daily
  - To avoid alcohol, smoking, and aspirin when taking other NSAIDs
  - Not to crush extended-relief products
  - To avoid alcohol and other over-the-counter (OTC) products that contain acetaminophen (avoid exceeding maximum dose of 3 g daily)
  - That acetaminophen can be taken concurrently with anticoagulants
  - To ensure availability of antidote for acetaminophen if there is a risk for toxicity (e.g., acetylcysteine [Acetadote]); must administer antidote within 24 hours of acetaminophen ingestion

APPLICATION AND REVIEW

7. What are the desired outcomes that the nurse expects when administering a nonsteroidal antiinflammatory drug (NSAID)? **Select all that apply.**
   1. Diuresis
   2. Pain relief
   3. Antipyresis
   4. Bronchodilation
   5. Anticoagulation
   6. Reduced inflammation

8. Aspirin is prescribed for a client with rheumatoid arthritis. Which clinical indicators of aspirin toxicity should the nurse teach the client to report? **Select all that apply.**
   1. Nausea
   2. Joint pain
   3. Blood in the stool
   4. Ringing in the ears
   5. Increased urine output

9. A client with arthritis increases the dose of ibuprofen (Motrin, Advil) to abate joint discomfort. After several weeks, the client becomes increasingly weak. The health care provider determines that the client is severely anemic and admits the client to the hospital. What clinical indicators does the nurse expect to identify when performing an admission assessment? **Select all that apply.**
   1. Melena
   2. Tachycardia
   3. Constipation
   4. Clay-colored stools
   5. Painful bowel movements

10. A health care provider prescribes acetylsalicylic acid (aspirin) therapy for a client with arthritis, and the nurse provides teaching about the undesirable side effects of this medication. What responses should the client identify as reasons to notify the health care provider? **Select all that apply.**
    1. Nausea
    2. Constipation
    3. Easy bruising
    4. Decreased pulse
    5. Ringing in the ears

11. A nurse is teaching an older adult client about managing chronic pain with acetaminophen (Tylenol). Which client statement indicates that the teaching is effective?
    1. "I need to limit my intake of acetaminophen to 650 mg a day."
    2. "I can take oxycodone with the acetaminophen if it is ineffective."
    3. "I should take an emetic if I accidentally overdose on the acetaminophen."
    4. "I have to be careful about which over-the-counter cold preparations I take when I have a cold."

See Answers on pages 31-35.

OPIOID ANALGESICS

- For moderate to severe pain; act mainly on the CNS
- Examples: morphine (drug of choice for myocardial infarction), codeine, meperidine, hydromorphone, fentanyl, tapentadol, hydrocodone
- Administered via oral, buccal, nasal spray, intramuscular (IM), subcutaneous, IV, transdermal, epidural, or rectal routes, depending on drug
- Reduce pain and anxiety that limits the response of the sympathetic nervous system, ultimately decreasing cardiac preload and the workload of the heart—an intentional effect; side effects can include decreasing respiratory rate and potentially depressing level of consciousness
- High abuse potential
- Naloxone is antidote

- Methadone is for opiate agonist dependence and withdrawal
- Suboxone is opiate agonist for opiod dependence and withdrawal

Mode of Action

- Bind to opiate receptors in CNS
- Result in diminished transmission and perception of pain impulse

Contraindications, Precautions, and Drug Interactions of Opioid Analgesics*

Drug	Contraindications/Precautions	Drug Interaction
codeine	**Contraindications:** Hypersensitivity, severe respiratory disorders including asthma and hyperventilation, paralytic ileus, to a child after tonsillectomy or adenoidectomy, breastfeeding, increased intracranial pressure (ICP), seizure disorders **Precautions:** Geriatric dosing should start at lower end of range; concurrent medications for depression, mental illness, Parkinson's disease, migraine headaches, serious infections, or prevention of nausea and vomiting; cardiac dysrhythmias; prostatic hypertrophy **Pregnancy:** Only given after risks to the fetus are considered	Alcohol, central nervous system (CNS) depressants, sedatives, hypnotics, antipsychotics, CYP2D6, opiates, skeletal muscle relaxants, monoamine oxidase inhibitors (MAOIs)
fentanyl	**Contraindications:** Hypersensitivity to opiates, myasthenia gravis, severe hepatic or renal disease **Precautions:** Breastfeeding, geriatric, increased ICP, seizure disorders, cardiac dysrhythmias, severe respiratory disorders, history of head injury, moderate hepatic/renal disease, concurrent sedative or MAOI use; patches can cause overdose **Pregnancy:** Only given after risks to the fetus are considered	Alcohol, antipsychotics, CNS depressants, CYP3A4 inducers, opioids, skeletal muscle relaxants
hydrocodone	**Contraindications:** Hypersensitivity, acne rosacea/vulgaris, Cushing's, measles, perioral dermatitis, varicella **Precautions:** Breastfeeding, geriatric, increased ICP, seizure disorders, cardiac dysrhythmias, severe respiratory disorders, history of head injury, hepatic or renal disease, concurrent sedative or MAOI use **Pregnancy:** Only given after risks to the fetus are considered	Alcohol, CNS depressants, MAOIs, sedative-hypnotics, skeletal muscle relaxants, tricyclics
meperidine	**Contraindications:** Hypersensitivity, severe respiratory disease **Precautions:** Breastfeeding, geriatric, increased ICP, seizure disorders, cardiac disorders, respiratory disorders, gastrointestinal (GI) disorders, hepatic or renal disease, history of head injury **Pregnancy:** Definite fetal risks; may be given despite risks in life-threatening conditions; only given after risks to the fetus are considered	Alcohol, antipsychotics, CNS depressants, opioids, MAOIs, phenytoin, procarbazine, protease inhibitor antiretrovirals, sedative-hypnotics, skeletal muscle relaxants, SSRIs, SNRIs
methadone	**Contraindications:** Hypersensitivity, severe asthma, paralytic ileus **Precautions:** Breastfeeding; increased ICP; seizures; respiratory disorders; heart disorders; electrolyte imbalances; renal or hepatic diseases; history of head injury; gallbladder, pancreas, or thyroid problems; urination problems **Pregnancy:** Only given after risks to the fetus are considered	Alcohol, antipsychotic drugs, classes I and III antidysrrhythmics, CNS depressants, CYP3A4 inducers and inhibitors, MAOIs, skeletal muscle relaxants, sedative-hypnotics
morphine	**Contraindications:** Hypersensitivity, addiction, CNS or respiratory depression, hemorrhage, status asthmaticus, increased intracranial pressure, shock, alcoholism, GI obstruction, hypovolemia, severe renal/hepatic disease, concurrent MAOI therapy **Precautions:** Seizures, respiratory insufficiency, renal or hepatic diseases; breastfeeding, urinary retention; bowel impaction, older adults; do not discontinue abruptly **Pregnancy:** Only given after risks to the fetus are considered	Alcohol, antipsychotic drugs, CNS depressants, MAOIs, muscle relaxants sedative-hypnotics

Continued

Contraindications, Precautions, and Drug Interactions of Opioid Analgesics—cont'd

Drug	Contraindications/Precautions	Drug Interaction
oxycodone	**Contraindications:** Hypersensitivity, addiction, asthma, ileus **Precautions:** Breastfeeding; children; increased ICP; lung, heart, renal, adrenal gland, gallbladder, pancreas, thyroid, or liver disease; bowel impaction; history of brain injury **Pregnancy:** No human studies available, but no adverse effects in animals	Alcohol, antipsychotic drugs, cimetidine, CNS depressants, CYP3A4 inhibitors, MAOIs, muscle relaxants sedative-hypnotics

*Pregnancy categories have been revised. See http://www.fda.gov/Drugs/DevelopmentApprovalProcess/DevelopmentResources/Labeling/ucm093307.htm for more information.

Side/Adverse Effects

- Respiratory depression
- Allergic reaction
- Bradycardia
- Cardiac arrest
- Constipation
- Drowsiness
- Dysrrhythmias
- Euphoria
- Hypotension
- Lethargy
- Mental cloudiness
- Nausea and vomiting
- Pruritus
- Psychologic dependence
- Sedation
- Seizures
- Urinary retention
- Urticaria

Nursing Care

- Monitor for side effects, especially for respiratory depression (e.g., decreased respiratory rate and depth, decreased oxygen saturation) and level of consciousness; monitor vital signs
- Institute measures to support respiratory function (e.g., encourage frequent turning, coughing, and deep breathing)
- Ensure availability of opioid antagonist (e.g., naloxone, naltrexone) in case of overdose
- Administer naloxone via IM, IV, SUBQ, nasal, via ET tube
- Ensure medications are renewed at required intervals
- Keep accurate count of opioids
- Use measures to promote elimination (e.g., provide fluids, roughage; encourage upright position)
- Monitor and maintain therapeutic levels of medication; may take 24 hours to achieve when using transdermal route
- Administer before pain becomes severe because analgesics are less effective when pain is severe
- Realize that tolerance will develop, so larger doses will be needed for pain management the longer the therapy continues
- Teach how to use patient-controlled analgesia (PCA) pump for management of severe pain; first, determine the integrity of the intravenous delivery system; program infusion pump for continuous basal dose, client-controlled bolus dose, and lockout time interval that allow client to control administration without overdose; may be IV, subcutaneous, or epidural
- Maintain safety after administration of opioid analgesia
- Instruct to keep medication in secure environment; dispose of excess doses by returning to pharmacy
- Monitor liver enzymes (AST, ALT)
- Teach patient to avoid other sedatives while taking this product, use sugarless gum for dry mouth, that confusion and dizziness are common, and that physical dependence may occur if used for long periods

ADJUVANT ANALGESICS

- Usually used along with a nonopioid and opioid medication
- The combination approach (nonopioid + opioid + adjuvant analgesic) means that dosages can often be decreased to reduce adverse effects.
- Include some anticonvulsants (see Chapter 4), some antidepressants, alpha-adrenergic agonists (see Chapter 6), corticosteroids (see Chapter 13), local anesthetics, skeletal muscle relaxants, and an NMDA antagonist (a general anesthetic).

Antidepressants Used in Analgesia

- Tricyclics and Serotonin-Norepinephrine Reuptake Inhibitors (SNRIs) are the antidepressants most commonly used in analgesia.
- See Chapter 5 for more information on antidepressants.
- Tricyclics should be decreased gradually when discontinuing in order to avoid withdrawal symptoms, including nausea, vomiting, anxiety, and akathisia.

Mode of Action

- SNRIs inhibit the reuptake of the neurotransmitters serotonin (5-HT) and norepinephrine by blocking it from the fibers; because more is circulating, more is available to the cells.
- Tricyclics inhibit the reuptake of the neurotransmitters serotonin (5-HT) and/or norepinephrine by blocking it from the fibers; because more is circulating, more is available to the cells.
- Tricyclics also cause direct blockade of receptors for histamine and acetylcholine.

Contraindications, Precautions, and Drug Interactions of Antidepressants used in Analgesia*†

Drug	Contraindications/Precautions	Drug Interaction
Tricyclic Antidepressants		
Amitriptyline	***Contraindications:*** Hypersensitivity, concurrent carbamazepine or MAOI, narrow-angle glaucoma, recovery from myocardial infarction (MI) ***Precautions:*** Breastfeeding, geriatric, cardiac/renal/hepatic disease, hyperthyroidism, seizures, prostatic hypertrophy, psychosis, urinary retention, abrupt discontinuation ***Pregnancy:*** Only given after risks to the fetus are considered	Alcohol, anticholinergics, antithyroid medications, barbiturates, Class IA/III dysrrhythmics, CNS depressants, hypnotics, MAOIs, sedatives, sympathomimetics
Nortriptyline	***Contraindications:*** Hypersensitivity, concurrent MAOI, recent MI, seizure disorders, prostatic hypertrophy, narrow-angle glaucoma ***Precautions:*** Breastfeeding; abrupt discontinuation, suicide ideation, cardiac/hepatic disease, hyperthyroidism, urinary retention ***Pregnancy:*** Only given after risks to the fetus are considered	Alcohol, anticholinergics, barbiturates, Class IA/III dysrrhythmics, CNS depressants, CYP3A4 inhibitors, hypnotics, MAOIs, sedatives, SSRIs, SNRIs, sympathomimetics
Imipramine	***Contraindications:*** Hypersensitivity, recent MI, concurrent MAOI or linezolid, narrow-angle glaucoma ***Precautions:*** History of irregular heartbeat, enlarged prostate, geriatric, renal/hepatic/cardiac problems, thyroid problems, diabetes, seizures, porphyria, or difficulty urinating, suicide ideation, abrupt discontinuation ***Pregnancy:*** Fetal risk is unknown	Alcohol, anticholinergics, barbiturates, CNS depressants, hypnotics, MAOIs, sedatives, sympathomimetics, thyroid medication

Continued

Contraindications, Precautions, and Drug Interactions of Antidepressants used in Analgesia—cont'd

Drug	Contraindications/Precautions	Drug Interaction
Tricyclic Antidepressants		
Desipramine	*Contraindications:* Hypersensitivity, breastfeeding, recent MI, concurrent MAOI or linezolid, narrow-angle glaucoma *Precautions:* History of irregular heartbeat, enlarged prostate, geriatric, renal/hepatic/cardiac problems, diabetes, problems urinating, stroke, seizures, suicidal ideation, thyroid problems, or porphyria, urinary retention, abrupt discontinuation *Pregnancy:* Only given after risks to the fetus are considered	Alcohol, anticholinergics, barbiturates, Class IA/III dysrrhythmics, CNS depressants, hypnotics, MAOIs, sedatives, SSRIs, SNRIs, tricyclics
Serotonin-Norepinephrine Reuptake Inhibitors (SNRIs)		
Duloxetine	*Contraindications:* Hypersensitivity, severe kidney or liver disorders, concurrent MAOI, thioridazine or linezolid, closed-angle glaucoma, alcoholism, hepatitis or liver disease, jaundice *Precautions:* Discontinue gradually; breastfeeding, geriatric, mania, hypertension, cardiac/renal/hepatic disease, seizures, increased intraocular pressure, anorexia nervosa, bleeding, dehydration, diabetes, hyponatremia, hypotension, hypovolemia, orthostatic hypotension *Pregnancy:* Only given after risks to the fetus are considered	Alcohol, anticholinergics, benzodiazepines, CNS depressants (including opiates and sedative-hypnotics), CYP1A2 inhibitors, CYP2D6 metabolized drugs, antihistamines, MAOIs, anticoagulants, NSAIDs, salicylates, SSRIs, sympathomimetics
Venlafaxine	*Contraindications:* Hypersensitivity, simultaneous MAOIs *Precautions:* CNS depression, SIADH, breastfeeding, in children, mania, geriatric, suicidal ideation, seizure disorder, hypertension, cardiac/renal/hepatic disease, bleeding, narrow-angle glaucoma, malnourishment, MI, hypovolemia, hypokalemia, hyponatremia, hyperthyroidism, eosinophilic pneumonia, labile hypertension *Pregnancy:* Only given after risks to the fetus are considered	Alcohol, anticoagulants, antihistamines, CNS depressants, MAOIs, anticoagulants, aspirin, cimetidine, haloperidol, NSAIDs, platelet inhibitors, salicylates, sedative-hypnotics, SNRIs, SSRIs, serotonin receptor agonists (triptans), amphetamines

*Pregnancy categories have been revised. See http://www.fda.gov/Drugs/DevelopmentApprovalProcess/DevelopmentResources/Labeling/ucm093307.htm for more information.

†Additional information on antidepressants is presented in Chapter 5.

Side/Adverse Effects: Tricyclics

- Blurred vision
- Changes to CBC and differential: agranulocytosis, thrombocytopenia, eosinophilia, leukopenia, aplastic anemia
- Dizziness
- Drowsiness
- ECG changes, dysrhythmias
- Fatigue
- Headache
- Hypertension
- Neuroleptic malignant syndrome
- Orthostatic hypotension
- Seizures
- Serotonin syndrome
- Suicidal ideation
- Tachycardia

Side/Adverse Effects: SNRIs

- Anxiety
- Diarrhea
- Dry mouth, nausea

- Edema, angioedema
- Headache
- Insomnia
- Neuroleptic malignant syndrome
- Serotonin syndrome: confusion, coma, agitation, tachycardia, BP changes, nausea, myoclonus, hyperreflexia, tremors, ataxia, hyperpyrexia
- Seizures
- Sexual dysfunction
- Stevens-Johnson syndrome
- Suicide ideation
- Thrombophlebitis

Nursing Care
- See *General Nursing Care of Clients in Pain*
- Remind patients not to discontinue tricyclics abruptly
- Monitor CBC and differential

Local Anesthetics
- Used for obstetric, dental, and minor surgical procedures; used for postoperative pain control when administered subcutaneously on a continuous basis (e.g., on Q Pain Buster pump)
- Available in topical, spinal, regional, and nerve block preparations; epinephrine may be added to enhance duration of local anesthetic effect and to decrease regional bleeding
- Advantage over general anesthetics is that patient usually avoids systemic effects
- Forms
  - Topical: local infiltration of tissue (e.g., benzocaine, lidocaine); nerve block (e.g., tetracaine, also used for spinal anesthesia)
  - Spinal: injected into subarachnoid space (e.g., lidocaine, procaine); also used for nerve block; causes vascular dilation and can drop BP
  - Epidural: injected into epidural space of spinal column (e.g., bupivacaine, lidocaine)
  - Nerve block: injected at perineural site distant from desired anesthesia site (e.g., bupivacaine, chloroprocaine, mepivacaine, ropivacaine)

Mode of Action
- Block nerve impulse conduction in sensory, motor, and autonomic nerve cells by decreasing nerve membrane permeability to sodium ion influx; used for pain control without loss of consciousness

Contraindications, Precautions, and Drug Interactions of Local Anesthetics for Analgesia*

Drug	Contraindications/Precautions	Drug Interaction
Bupivacaine	**Contraindications:** Hypersensitivity, severe bleeding, low blood pressure, infection at site, blood infection, irregular heartbeat, breastfeeding **Precautions:** Can have systemic effects; cardiac/hepatic/renal/nervous disorders, pernicious anemia, polio, syphilis, tumors in the brain or spine, blood or bleeding problems, blood pressure problems, persistent backache, psychosis **Pregnancy:** Only given after risks to the fetus are considered	Anticoagulants, antihypertensives, barbiturates, beta-blockers, digoxin

Continued

Contraindications, Precautions, and Drug Interactions of Local Anesthetics for Analgesia—cont'd

Drug	Contraindications/Precautions	Drug Interaction
Ropivacaine	*Contraindications:* Hypersensitivity *Precautions:* Can have systemic effects; cardiac/hepatic disorders, low blood pressure, low blood volume, hyperthyroidism *Pregnancy:* No human studies available, but no adverse effects in animals	Azole antifungals, Class III antiarrhythmics, MAOIs, phenothiazines, theophylline, tricyclic antidepressants
Lidocaine injectable	*Contraindications:* Hypersensitivity, heart block, some dysrrhythmias *Precautions:* Can have systemic effects; breastfeeding, cardiac/renal/hepatic disease, coronary artery disease, history of malignant hyperthermia; patch form can have local skin reactions as well *Pregnancy:* No human studies available, but no adverse effects in animals	Analgesics, antihypertensives, barbiturates, β-blockers, MAOIs, neuromuscular blockers, protease inhibitors, bupropion

*Pregnancy categories have been revised. See http://www.fda.gov/Drugs/DevelopmentApprovalProcess/DevelopmentResources/Labeling/ucm093307.htm for more information.

Side/Adverse Effects
- Allergic reactions; anaphylaxis (hypersensitivity), local skin reactions from patches
- Respiratory arrest (depression of medullary respiratory center)
- Dysrhythmias, cardiac arrest (depression of cardiovascular system)
- Seizures (depression of CNS)
- Hypotension (depression of cardiovascular system)

Nursing Care of Patients Receiving Local Anesthetics
- Assess for allergies and medical problems that could alter response to anesthetic agent
- Have oxygen and emergency resuscitative equipment available
- Assess vital signs before, during, and after anesthetic administration
- Protect anesthetized body parts from mechanical and/or thermal injury
- If spinal anesthetic is administered, keep flat for specified period of time (usually 6–12 hours) to prevent severe headache; avoid pillows; monitor for hypotension; monitor return of motor and sensory function to lower extremities
- If local anesthetic is administered along a nerve via a pump for pain control, teach how to use pump; monitor for local anesthetic toxicity
- Also see *General Nursing Care of Clients in Pain*

Skeletal Muscle Relaxants
- Relieve muscle spasms
- Available in oral and parenteral (IM, IV) preparations
- Examples: carisoprodol; cyclobenzaprine; diazepam; methocarbamol; baclofen, metaxalone tizanidine, chlorzoxazone

Mode of Action
- Central agents: depress CNS to promote relaxation of voluntary muscles
- Peripheral agents: block nerve impulse conduction at the myoneural junction

Contraindications, Precautions, and Drug Interactions of Muscle Relaxants Used for Analgesia*

Drug	Contraindications/Precautions	Drug Interaction
Baclofen	*Contraindications:* Hypersensitivity *Precautions:* Overdose may cause CNS depression; breastfeeding, diabetes mellitus, geriatric, peptic ulcer, renal/hepatic disease, stroke, seizure disorder, abrupt withdrawal *Pregnancy:* Only given after risks to the fetus are considered	Alcohol, antidepressants, antihypertensives, barbiturates, CNS depressants, opioids, sedative-hypnotics
Cyclobenzaprine	*Contraindications:* Hypersensitivity, dysrhythmias, cerebral palsy, diabetes mellitus, heart failure, thyroid disorder, hypertension, hypokalemia, paralytic ileus, concurrent use of MAOI therapy *Precautions:* Overdose may cause CNS depression; seizure disorder, alcohol, CNS depressants, glaucoma, prostatic hypertrophy, urinary retention, hepatic disease, breastfeeding, driving or operating machinery, morbidity in geriatric patients, sunlight UV exposure, urinary disorders *Pregnancy:* No human studies available, but no adverse effects in animals	Alcohol, barbiturates, anticholinergics, CNS depressants, MAOIs, tricyclics
Carisoprodol	*Contraindications:* Hypersensitivity, intermittent porphyria *Precautions:* breastfeeding, geriatric patients, Asian patients, renal/hepatic disease, substance abuse, CNS depression, seizure disorder, abrupt discontinuation *Pregnancy:* only given after risks to the fetus are considered; animal studies have shown adverse reactions; no human studies available	Alcohol, barbiturates, CYP 219 inducers/inhibitors, hypnotics, meprobamate, sedatives, tricyclics
Methocarbamol	*Contraindications:* Hypersensitivity *Precautions:* breastfeeding, renal disease, myasthenia gravis *Pregnancy:* only given after risks to the fetus are considered; animal studies have shown adverse reactions; no human studies available	Alcohol, barbiturates, CNS depressants, hypnotics, sedatives
Chlorzoxazone	*Contraindications:* Hypersensitivity *Precautions:* breastfeeding, liver disease *Pregnancy:* only given after risks to the fetus are considered; animal studies have shown adverse reactions; no human studies available	Alcohol, barbiturates, CNS depressants, hypnotics, sedatives
Metaxalone tizanidine	*Contraindications:* Hypersensitivity *Precautions:* breastfeeding, hepatic/liver disease, anemia *Pregnancy:* only given after risks to the fetus are considered; animal studies have shown adverse reactions; no human studies available	Alcohol, barbiturates, CNS depressants, hypnotics, sedatives, sodium oxybate (GHB)

*Pregnancy categories have been revised. See http://www.fda.gov/Drugs/DevelopmentApprovalProcess/DevelopmentResources/Labeling/ucm093307.htm for more information.

Side/Adverse Effects

- Dizziness, drowsiness (CNS depression)
- Nausea (irritation of gastric mucosa)
- Headache (central antimuscarinic effect)
- Ileus
- Myocardial infarction
- Seizures
- Tachycardia (brainstem stimulation)
- Angioedema

Nursing Care

- See *General Nursing Care of Clients in Pain*

- Encourage diet rich in nutrient-dense foods (e.g., fruits, vegetables, whole grains, and legumes) to improve and maintain nutritional status and prevent drug-induced nutrient deficiencies
- Teach client receiving central agents to use safety precautions during initial therapy and to avoid engaging in potentially hazardous activities or using alcohol and other CNS depressants

GENERAL NURSING CARE OF CLIENTS IN PAIN

Assessment
- Client's description of pain: location; intensity as measured by numeric rating scale of 0 to 10, Wong-Baker FACES Pain Rating Scale, FLACC Scale (Face, Legs, Activity, Cry, Consolability); character; onset; duration; and aggravating and alleviating factors
- Associated signs and symptoms: increased vital signs (may be decreased with visceral pain), nausea, vomiting, diarrhea, diaphoresis
- Nonverbal cues: distraught facial expression, rigid or self-splinting body posture
- Assess for nonverbal cues even when the patient denies pain.
- Contributing factors: age (older adults may expect pain or may fear addiction, so they may not complain), culture, past experience, anxiety, fear, uncertainty (lack of information), fatigue
- Effect of pain on ability to perform activities of daily living (ADLs)

Planning/Implementation
- Individualize pain management based on client's needs and not on own personal experiences, biases, or cultural beliefs regarding pain
- Monitor and document client's pain, associated symptoms, and response to pain management interventions
- Use nonpharmacologic techniques
- Administer prescribed analgesics and local anesthetics
- Teach client to use PRN (as needed) pain medication as soon as discomfort begins
- Institute measures to counteract side effects of medications (e.g., increase fiber and fluids to prevent constipation associated with opioids)
- Provide preoperative and postoperative care for clients requiring surgical intervention for pain management
  - Rhizotomy: posterior spinal nerve root is resected between ganglion and spinal cord, resulting in permanent loss of sensation; anterior root may be cut to alleviate pain usually associated with lung cancer
  - Cordotomy: alleviates intractable pain in trunk or lower extremities; transmission of pain and temperature sensation is interrupted by creation of lesion in ascending tract; performed percutaneously using an electrode or surgically via laminectomy
  - Sympathectomy: controls ischemic and phantom limb pain
  - Dorsal column stimulator and peripheral nerve implant: direct attachment of electrode to sensory nerve; electrode is attached to a transmitter that is carried by client so electric stimulation can be administered as needed

Evaluation/Outcomes
- Reports a reduction in pain of equal to or less than 4 on numeric rating scale
- Participates actively in ADLs

12. What is a nurse's responsibility when administering prescribed opioid analgesics? **Select all that apply.**
    1. Count the client's respirations.
    2. Document the intensity of the client's pain.
    3. Withhold the medication if the client reports pruritus.
    4. Verify the number of doses in the locked cabinet before administering the prescribed dose.
    5. Discard the medication in the client's toilet before leaving the room if the medication is refused.

13. A client who had abdominal surgery is receiving patient-controlled analgesia (PCA) intravenously to manage pain. The pump is programmed to deliver a basal dose and bolus doses that can be accessed by the client with a lock-out time frame of 10 minutes. The nurse assesses use of the pump during the last hour and identifies that the client attempted to self-administer the analgesic 10 times. Further assessment reveals that the client is still experiencing pain. What should the nurse do **first?**
    1. Monitor the client's pain level for another hour.
    2. Determine the integrity of the intravenous delivery system.
    3. Reprogram the pump to deliver a bolus dose every 8 minutes.
    4. Arrange for the client to be evaluated by the health care provider.

14. In the postanesthesia care unit, it is reported that the client received intrathecal morphine intraoperatively to control pain. Considering the administration of this medication, what should the nurse include as part of the client's **initial** 24-hour postoperative care?
    1. Assessing the client for tachycardia
    2. Monitoring of respiratory rate hourly
    3. Administering naloxone every 3 to 4 hours
    4. Observing the client for signs of CNS excitement

15. A terminally ill client in a hospice unit for several weeks is receiving a morphine drip. The dose is now above the typical recommended dosage. The client's spouse tells the nurse that the client is again uncomfortable and needs the morphine increased. The prescription states to titrate the morphine to comfort level. What should the nurse do?
    1. Add a placebo to the morphine to appease the spouse.
    2. Discuss with the spouse the risk for morphine addiction.
    3. Assess the client's pain before increasing the dose of morphine.
    4. Check the client's heart rate before increasing the morphine to the next level.

16. Morphine via an epidural catheter is prescribed for a client after abdominal surgery. The client asks the nurse why this medicine is necessary. What **primary** rationale does the nurse give for the administration of an opioid analgesic after abdominal surgery?
    1. Facilitates oxygen use
    2. Relieves abdominal pain
    3. Decreases anxiety and restlessness
    4. Dilates coronary and peripheral blood vessels

17. The nurse is caring for a client who just had a myocardial infarction. Which analgesic does the nurse expect the health care provider to prescribe?
    1. Diazepam   3. Flurazepam
    2. Meperidine   4. Morphine

18. A nurse is giving discharge instructions to a client with a recently applied long leg cast. When should the client be advised to take the prescribed prn analgesic for pain management?
    1. Just as a last resort
    2. Before going to sleep
    3. When the discomfort begins
    4. As the pain becomes intense

19. When a nurse requests that a client's pain intensity be rated on a scale of 0–10, the client states that the pain is "99." The nurse concludes that the client:
    1. needs the instructions to be repeated.
    2. requires an intervention immediately.
    3. does not understand the numeric scale.
    4. is using humor to get the nurse's attention.

20. A client is receiving oxycodone postoperatively for pain. The health care provider's prescription indicates that the dose should be administered every 3 hours for eight doses. What should the nurse assess before administering each dose of oxycodone?
    1. Respiratory rate and level of consciousness
    2. Color, character, and amount of urine output
    3. Intravenous site and patency of the intravenous catheter
    4. Amount and character of drainage in the portable drainage system

21. A health care provider prescribed 10 mg of morphine immediately and then every 4 hours for a client who had a myocardial infarction. What clinical response will be reduced if the client experiences the intended therapeutic effect of morphine?
    1. Respiratory rate
    2. Workload of the heart
    3. Size of the clot blocking the coronary artery
    4. Metabolites within the ischemic heart muscle

22. Immediately after receiving spinal anesthesia a client develops hypotension. To what physiologic change does the nurse attribute the decreased blood pressure?
    1. Dilation of blood vessels
    2. Decreased response of chemoreceptors
    3. Decreased strength of cardiac contractions
    4. Disruption of cardiac accelerator pathways

23. A client who had a total hip replacement asks the nurse about the continuous regional analgesia being used. What information should the nurse include when explaining the benefits of this treatment over conventional methods to control pain?
    1. Adjusting the dose is easily done.
    2. Neuropathic pain can be relieved.
    3. Systemic side effects are minimal.
    4. The need for parenteral medication is avoided.

24. A woman in the 28 weeks of pregnancy is experiencing a health issue that would ordinarily be treated with a muscle relaxant. When the client asks why cyclobenzaprine has been specifically prescribed, what response should the nurse provide to best support this choice in medication?
    1. "Research has shown no adverse reaction to this medication in animal studies."
    2. "This medication is one muscle relaxant that will not make you sleepy."
    3. "Cyclobenzaprine wouldn't interfere with your desire to breastfeed."
    4. "Cyclobenzaprine carries a very low risk for overdose."

25. Which assessment finding observed in a client prescribed a tricyclic antidepressant should be considered the priority adverse reaction?
    1. Orthostatic hypotension
    2. Suicidal ideation
    3. Dysrhythmia
    4. Leukopenia

See Answers on pages 31–35.

ANSWER KEY: REVIEW QUESTIONS

1. **1 Cold reduces the sensitivity of pain receptors in the skin. In addition, local blood vessels constrict, limiting the amount of edema and its related pressure and discomfort.**

   2 Local blood vessels constrict. **3** Local cold applications do not depress vital signs. **4** Local cold applications do not directly affect blood viscosity. This is not a clinical indicator that a nurse can observe.
   Client Need: Basic Care and Comfort; **Cognitive Level:** Application; **Nursing Process:** Evaluation/Outcomes

2. **3 The voltage or current is adjusted on the basis of the degree of pain relief experienced by the client.**

   1 Maintaining the health care provider's settings may provide too little or too much stimulation to achieve the desired response. **2** A pain suppressor transcutaneous electrical nerve stimulation (TENS) unit should be turned on several times a day for 10 to 20 minutes, not the conventional unit. **4** The electrodes should be applied either on the painful area or immediately below or above the area.
   Client Need: Basic Care and Comfort; **Cognitive Level:** Application; **Nursing Process:** Planning/Implementation

3. **1 Sitz baths may be cool or warm. Warm baths dilate blood vessels and promote circulation, relieving local inflammation and itching. Cool sitz baths constrict blood vessels, limiting bleeding and edema.**

   2 Water-soluble jelly will not alleviate pain. **3** Inflatable doughnuts separate the buttocks, putting tension on the area, which increases discomfort. **4** Local applications of medications are rarely prescribed post-procedure; if systemic analgesia is prescribed, aspirin or acetaminophen is most effective in reducing pain after this procedure.
   Client Needs: Basic Care and Comfort; **Cognitive Level:** Application; **Nursing Process:** Planning/Implementation

4. **4 Analgesics limit pain, thereby facilitating effective coughing and deep breathing.**

   1 Regular administration of pain medication may or may not be necessary. **2** Explaining the consequences of not aerating the lungs after surgery can cause anxiety and guilt; the client should not have to suffer when coughing and deep breathing. **3** Incentive spirometry will cause pain, and the client may not cooperate if pain is not relieved.
   Client Needs: Basic Care and Comfort; **Cognitive Level:** Application; **Nursing Process:** Planning/Implementation

5. **1 Biofeedback provides information about changes in body function; clients can learn to use this to control a variety of body responses, including pain.**

   2 Radiotherapy is a part of standard medical regimens. **3** Bariatrics is a type of therapy that focuses on the correction of obesity; it encompasses prevention, control, and treatment of the problem, which involves medications and surgery. **4** Placement of radioactive sources into or in contact with tissues (brachytherapy) is part of standard medical treatment for cancer.
   Client Needs: Basic Care and Comfort; **Cognitive Level:** Application; **Nursing Process:** Planning/Implementation

6. **Answers: 1, 2, 4, 5**

   1 Prayer is an alternative therapy that may relax the client and provide strength, solace, or acceptance. **2** The relief of pain through hypnosis is based on suggestion; also, it focuses attention away from the pain. Some clients learn to hypnotize themselves. **4** Aromatherapy can help relax and distract the individual and thus increase tolerance for pain, as well as relieve pain. **5** Guided imagery can help relax and distract the individual and thus increase tolerance for pain, as well as relieve pain.
   3 Analgesics, both opioid and nonopioid, long have been part of the standard medical regimen for pain relief, so they are not considered an alternative therapy.
   Client Needs: Basic Care and Comfort; **Cognitive Level:** Analysis; **Nursing Process:** Planning/Implementation

7. **Answers: 2, 3, 6**

   2 Prostaglandins accumulate at the site of an injury, causing pain; NSAIDs inhibit COX-1 and COX-2 (both are isoforms of the enzyme cyclooxygenase), which inhibit the production of prostaglandins, thereby contributing to analgesia. **3** NSAIDs inhibit COX-2, which is associated with fever, thereby causing antipyresis. **6** NSAIDs inhibit COX-2, which is associated with inflammation, thereby reducing inflammation.
   1 NSAIDs do not cause diuresis; reversible renal ischemia and renal insufficiency in clients with heart failure, cirrhosis, or hypovolemia can be potential adverse effects of NSAIDs. **4** NSAIDs do not cause

bronchodilation. **5** Anticoagulation is an adverse effect, not a desired outcome; NSAIDs can impair platelet function by inhibiting thromboxane, an aggregating agent, resulting in bleeding.
Client Need: Pharmacologic and Parenteral Therapies; **Cognitive Level:** Analysis; **Nursing Process:** Evaluation/ Outcomes

> **Study Tip:** To remember that NSAID antiinflammatories help—not just with pain relief and inflammation—but also with antipyresis, think what a pyromaniac likes: fire! The word part *pyr/o* means fire. The word antiinflammatory has "flam(e)" in it. Anti- means against, so antiinflammatories work against fire/fever.

8. **Answers: 3, 4**

    3 Blood in the stool indicates gastrointestinal irritation; it also may have resulted from aspirin's anticoagulant effect. **4** Salicylates, such as aspirin, can cause ototoxicity (affects eighth cranial nerve), which may manifest as ringing in the ears (tinnitus) or muffled hearing; it should be reported.

    1 Nausea is a common side effect; it can be diminished by administering the drug with food or using an enteric-coated product. **2** Joint pain is not a symptom of salicylate toxicity; it is related to the disease process and should be minimized by the administration of aspirin. **5** Increased urine output (polyuria) is not an indication of salicylate toxicity.
    Client Need: Pharmacologic and Parenteral Therapies; **Cognitive Level:** Analysis; **Integrated Process:** Teaching/ Learning; **Nursing Process:** Planning/Implementation

9. **Answers: 1, 2**

    1 Ibuprofen (Motrin, Advil) irritates the gastrointestinal (GI) mucosa and can cause mucosal erosion, resulting in bleeding; blood in the stool (melena) occurs as the digestive process acts on the blood in the upper GI tract. **2** Hemoglobin, which carries oxygen to body cells, is decreased with anemia; the heart rate increases as a compensatory response to increase oxygen to body cells.

    3 Constipation usually is related to immobility, a low-fiber diet, and inadequate fluid intake, not the data listed in this situation. **4** Clay-colored stools are related to biliary problems, not GI bleeding. **5** Painful bowel movements are related to hemorrhoids, not GI bleeding.
    Client Need: Pharmacologic and Parenteral Therapies; **Cognitive Level:** Analysis; **Nursing Process:** Evaluation/ Outcomes

10. **Answers: 1, 3, 5**

    1 Aspirin is a gastrointestinal irritant that can cause nausea, vomiting, and gastrointestinal bleeding. **3** Salicylates decrease platelet aggregation, resulting in easy bruising and gastrointestinal bleeding. **5** Tinnitus and hearing loss can occur as a result of the effects of the drug on the eighth cranial nerve.

    2 Salicylates may cause diarrhea, not constipation, because of gastrointestinal irritation. **4** Salicylates may increase, not decrease, the heart rate.
    Client Needs: Pharmacologic and Parenteral Therapies; **Cognitive Level:** Analysis; **Nursing Process:** Evaluation/ Outcomes

> **Study Tip:** Here's a *sssss*illy mnemonic. To link salicylates with hearing loss, tinnitus, and ototoxicity, think of those adverse effects with alternate spellings: hearing lo*sss*, tinnitu*sss*, and ototox*sssis*ssity; then say salicylates and draw out all the *ss*'s: "*sss*ali*sss*cylate*sss*" so you can "hear" that they may cause the problems that each have *ss*'s: hearing lo*sss*, tinnitu*sss*, and ototox*sssis*ssity. Just a few repetitions and you'll remember these!

11. **4** Many over-the-counter cold preparations contain acetaminophen (Tylenol); the amount of acetaminophen in cold preparations must be taken into consideration when the total amount of acetaminophen taken daily is calculated.

    1 650 mg/day amount is a typical single dose for adults. Acetaminophen should not exceed 3 to 4 g a day, with a lower dose preferred in older adults. **2** Taking oxycodone with acetaminophen may result in an overdose. Oxycodone (Percocet) contains 325 to 650 mg of acetaminophen per dose, which should be calculated into the total grams of acetaminophen permitted daily. **3** An emetic is contraindicated because it may reduce the client's ability to tolerate oral acetylcysteine, the antidote for acetaminophen toxicity.

Client Needs: Pharmacologic and Parenteral Therapies; **Cognitive Level:** Analysis; **Nursing Process:** Evaluation/Outcomes

12. **Answers: 1, 2, 4**

    1 Opioid analgesics can cause respiratory depression; the nurse must monitor respirations. **2** The intensity of pain must be documented before and after administering an analgesic to evaluate its effectiveness. **3** Pruritus is a common side effect that can be managed with antihistamines. It is not an allergic response, so it does not preclude administration. **4** Because of the potential for abuse, the nurse is legally required to verify an accurate count of doses before taking a dose from the locked source and at the change of the shift.

    5 The nurse should not discard an opioid in a client's room. Any waste of an opioid must be witnessed by another nurse.

    Client Need: Pharmacologic and Parenteral Therapies; **Cognitive Level:** Analysis; **Nursing Process:** Planning/Implementation

13. **2 Initially, integrity of the intravenous system should be verified to ensure that the client is receiving medication. The intravenous tubing may be kinked or compressed, or the catheter may be dislodged.**

    1 Continued monitoring will result in the client experiencing unnecessary pain. **3** The nurse may not reprogram the pump to deliver larger or more frequent doses of medication without a health care provider's prescription. **4** The health care provider should be notified if the system is intact and the client is not obtaining relief from pain. The prescription may have to be revised; the basal dose may be increased, the length of the delay may be reduced, or another medication or mode of delivery may be prescribed.

    Client Need: Pharmacologic and Parenteral Therapies; **Cognitive Level:** Application; **Nursing Process:** Evaluation/Outcomes

14. **2 Intrathecal morphine can depress respiratory function depending on the level it reaches within the spinal column; hourly assessments during the first 12 to 24 hours will allow for early intervention with an antidote if respiratory depression needs to be corrected.**

    1 Bradycardia and hypotension occur. **3** Administration of naloxone every 3 to 4 hours between doses is too long if the client's respirations are depressed. The recommended adult dosage usually is 0.4 to 2 mg every 2 to 3 minutes, if indicated. **4** Central nervous system depression occurs secondary to hypoxia.

    Client Need: Pharmacologic and Parenteral Therapies; **Cognitive Level:** Application; **Nursing Process:** Evaluation/Outcomes

15. **3 Over time, clients receiving morphine develop tolerance and require increasing doses to relieve pain, thus requiring continuing reassessments.**

    1 A placebo will not meet client's need for relief from pain. **2** The client is terminal and the risk for addiction is of no concern. **4** The respiratory, not heart, rate is the significant vital sign to be monitored; morphine depresses the CNS, specifically the respiratory center in the brain.

    Client Need: Pharmacologic and Parenteral Therapies; **Cognitive Level:** Application; **Nursing Process:** Assessment/Analysis

16. **2 Analgesics alleviate pain by binding with opioid receptors in the brain, thus altering the perception of and response to pain; patient-controlled analgesia (PCA) via an epidural catheter gives the client control over medication administration and usually results in the client using less medication.**

    1 Opioids do not facilitate oxygen use; they decrease the respiratory rate, and less oxygen is used; the client should be monitored. **3** Although these may be responses to an opioid, they are not the primary reason why opioids are used after abdominal surgery. **4** Opioids are not given to dilate blood vessels; antianginal medications and vasodilators are used for this purpose.

    Client Needs: Pharmacologic and Parenteral Therapies; **Cognitive Level:** Application; **Nursing Process:** Planning/Implementation

17. **4 For a severe myocardial infarction, morphine is the drug of choice because it relieves pain quickly and reduces anxiety.**

    1 Diazepam is a muscle relaxant that may be used for its sedative effect; it is not effective for the pain of a myocardial infarction. **2** Although effective, meperidine is not the drug of choice. **3** Flurazepam is a hypnotic that may be used to reduce fear and restlessness; it is not effective for the pain of a myocardial infarction.

    Client Needs: Pharmacologic and Parenteral Therapies; **Cognitive Level:** Comprehension; **Nursing Process:** Planning/Implementation

18. **3 Pain is relieved most effectively when the analgesic is administered at the onset of pain, before it becomes intense; this prevents a pain cycle from occurring.**

    1 Analgesics are least effective when administered as pain reaches its peak. **2** The medication should be taken when the client begins to feel uncomfortable within the parameters specified by the prescription; this may or may not happen before going to sleep. **4** Analgesics are least effective when administered as pain reaches its peak.

    Client Needs: Pharmacologic and Parenteral Therapies; **Cognitive Level:** Application; **Nursing Process:** Planning/Implementation

19. **2 When numbers above 10 are identified, clients are communicating that the pain is excessive; immediate nursing action is indicated.**

    1, 3 It is not likely that the client misunderstood the instructions; the client reported a number as instructed but chose a number beyond the stated intensity scale. **4** The client has the nurse's attention; the use of humor is not commonly associated with clients in pain.

    Client Needs: Basic Care and Comfort; **Cognitive Level:** Application; **Nursing Process:** Assessment/Analysis

20. **1 Oxycodone is an opioid that depresses the central nervous system, resulting in a decreased level of consciousness and depressed respirations. The medication should be administered, delayed, or held, depending on the client's status.**

    2 Although urinary output of postoperative clients should be assessed, urinary output is not related directly to the administration of opioid medications. **3** Oxycodone is administered via tablets, not intravenously. **4** Wound drainage is unrelated to the administration of oxycodone.

    Client Needs: Pharmacologic and Parenteral Therapies; **Cognitive Level:** Application; **Nursing Process:** Evaluation/Outcomes

21. **2 Morphine reduces pain and anxiety that limits the response of the sympathetic nervous system, ultimately decreasing cardiac preload and the workload of the heart.**

    1 Reduced respiratory rate is a side effect of morphine; if the respiratory rate drops to below 10 breaths per minute, the dose of morphine may have to be adjusted. **3** Reduction of the clot blocking the coronary artery is the action of antithrombolytic therapy. **4** Metabolite reduction within the ischemic heart muscle is not the action of morphine.

    Client Needs: Pharmacologic and Parenteral Therapies; **Cognitive Level:** Comprehension; **Nursing Process:** Planning/Implementation

22. **1 Paralysis of the sympathetic vasomotor nerves after administration of a spinal anesthetic results in dilation of blood vessels, which causes a subsequent decrease in blood pressure.**

    2 These receptors are sensitive to pH, oxygen, and carbon dioxide tension; they are not related to hypotension and are not affected by spinal anesthesia. **3** The strength of cardiac contractions is not affected by spinal anesthesia. **4** The cardiac accelerator center neurons in the medulla regulate heart rate; they are not related to hypotension and are not affected by spinal anesthesia.

    Client Need: Reduction of Risk Potential; **Cognitive Level:** Comprehension; **Nursing Process:** Evaluation/Outcomes

23. **3 Regional analgesia uses a local anesthetic to control pain; the local effect avoids systemic reactions.**

    1 The dose adjustment involves the same level of complexity as conventional methods. **2** The hip replacement involves somatic, not neuropathic, pain. **4** Parenteral medication is used in conjunction with regional analgesia.

    Client Need: Physiologic Adaptation; **Cognitive Level:** Comprehension; **Integrated Process:** Teaching/Learning; **Nursing Process:** Planning/Implementation

24. **1 Considering the client's pregnancy, the response should focus on the safety associated with the medication. While no human studies are available, there has been no adverse effects noted in animals.**

    2 Muscle relaxants generally cause sleepiness and cyclobenzaprine is no exception. 3 There is a stated precaution concerning cyclobenzaprine's effect on breastfeeding so there is concern about it being prescribed to a woman who is interested in breastfeeding. 4 There is a stated precaution concerning cyclobenzaprine's risk for overdose and so it is incorrect to state there is little risk.

    Client Need: Reduction of Risk Potential; **Cognitive Level:** Analysis; **Nursing Process:** Evaluation/Outcomes

25. **3 A cardiac dysrhythmia can have acute, fatal consequences and so is the priority concern regarding this client.**

    1, 2, 4 While considered an adverse reaction and a risk to the client's safety, orthostatic hypertension, suicidal ideation, and leukopenia do not carry the same acute, fatality risk that exists with a physiologic disorder like a cardiac dysrhythmia.

    Client Need: Reduction of Risk Potential; **Cognitive Level:** Analysis; **Nursing Process:** Assessment/Analysis

3 Central Nervous System Depressants

- Central nervous system (CNS) depressants are used to manage insomnia, for sedation induction, to manage anxiety (see Chapter 5), and a few are used for seizure control (see Chapter 4).
- This chapter reviews CNS depressants called sedatives-hypnotics that used to manage insomnia: benzodiazepines, nonbenzodiazepines, and a melatonin agonist; barbiturates are reviewed for historic consideration.

INTRODUCTION TO SLEEP DISORDERS

Basic Information

- Sleep disorders are a common problem in adults, rarely treated in an inpatient psychiatric setting, and can present as a symptom of depressive, manic, or anxiety disorders.
- Sleep consists of two distinct states: REM (rapid eye movement), also called dream sleep, and NREM (non-REM) sleep, which is divided into four stages.
- Sleep is a cyclic phenomenon with restorative qualities.
- Sleep disorders are conditions that repeatedly disrupt the pattern of sleep, leading to diminished performance.

Etiologic Factors

- The sleep cycle evolves throughout the life cycle and decreases with age.
- It is a disorder from which the client usually recovers, because the changes may be reversible and temporary if treated.
- Neuroendocrine arousal system is thought to release corticosteroids by the hypothalamic-pituitary-adrenal axis, as well as stimulate the neurotransmitter system, producing norepinephrine and serotonin.
- Genetic factors show a biologic tendency that may be inherited (e.g., light sleepers in a family); no single gene has been identified.
- Environmental factors are thought to contribute to sleep disturbances, such as jet lag, shift work, fast pace of life, stress, and noise.
- Biologic factors such as cardiovascular, endocrine, psychiatric, infections, cough related to pulmonary disease, pain, use of stimulants including caffeine, and side effects or drug interactions of many medications contribute to sleep-related problems.
- Impaired function results from sleep deprivation.

Types of Sleep Disorders

Primary

- Insomnia: disorder of initiating or maintaining sleep not caused by physical or mental illness
- Parasomnias: disorders associated with sleep stages (e.g., sleepwalking, night terrors, nightmares, restless leg syndrome, and enuresis); most common in children
- Narcolepsy: disorder of repeated uncontrollable brief episodes of sleep while engaging in meaningful activities

Secondary

- Sleep disorders related to mental disorders: noted in this category are anxiety-related disorders, depressive disorders, and manic episodes
- Substance-induced sleep disorders: included in this subclass are conditions related to intoxication, periods of withdrawal, use of stimulants, and side effects of many medications
- Sleep disorders related to general medical condition: included in this category is sleep apnea; etiology must be established through history, physical examination, or laboratory findings in this subclass
  - Can include hypersomnia
  - Sleep studies, including EEG, are used to establish sleep apnea and other sleep disorders

Behavioral/Clinical Findings

- Onset usually in young adulthood; more prevalent with increasing age
- Difficulty initiating or maintaining sleep, or nonrestorative sleep, for at least 1 month
- Depression usually associated with fragmented sleep patterns
- Sleeplessness as a cardinal feature noted in manic disorders; an early sign of impending mania in bipolar disorders
- Abuse of alcohol or stimulants, heavy smoking, and use of over-the-counter (OTC) cold remedies cause decreased total sleep time (Box 3.1)
- Insomnia precipitated by anxiety

Therapeutic Interventions

- Relaxation techniques
- Sleep hygiene practices (interventions that enhance sleep; See General Nursing Care of Clients with Sleep Disorders)
- Sedative/hypnotic agents (the focus of the remainder of the chapter)

BOX 3.1 Common Factors Affecting Sleep

Common Conditions that Affect Sleep

- Alzheimer's disease
- Anxiety
- Arthritis
- Asthma
- Cancer
- Chronic obstructive pulmonary disease
- Chronic kidney disease
- Depression
- Diabetes
- Epilepsy
- Febrile conditions
- Fibromyalgia
- Gastroesophageal reflux disease
- Heart failure
- Hyperthyroidism
- Menopause
- Pain
- Parkinson's disease
- Stroke

Pharmaceutical Categories that Impair Sleep

- Corticosteroids
- Diuretics
- Nicotine products
- Selective serotonin reuptake inhibitors
- Stimulants
- Theophylline

From Giddens, J.F. (2017). *Concepts for nursing practice* (2nd ed.). St. Louis: Elsevier.

General Nursing Care of Clients with Sleep Disorders

- Assessment/Analysis
  - History of onset, duration, and sleep patterns
  - Daily routines, night rituals
  - Diet and physical activity
  - Stressors
  - Level of daytime alertness, nap patterns
  - Restless leg movement, snoring
  - Drug, alcohol, caffeine, nicotine use
  - Pharmacologic or herbal remedies
  - Sleep journal
  - Mental status and alertness
- Planning/Implementation
  - Assist with ruling out medical conditions that contribute to sleep-related problems
  - Obtain a diet diary to assess food/liquid intake and caffeine consumption
  - Control physical disturbances at night; provide a private room if necessary
  - Administer prescribed hypnotic
  - Teach sleep hygiene practices
    - Establish a daily exercise regimen during the day hours to reduce stress
    - Engage in diversional activities during the day to avoid napping
    - Eat a larger meal at noon rather than at dinner
    - Avoid stimulants (e.g., coffee, tea, chocolate, nicotine, and OTC cold remedies) at least 3 hours before bedtime
    - Perform relaxation techniques
    - Establish set sleep patterns (bedtime and awakening schedule)
    - Ensure a quiet, restful environment at bedtime
    - Avoid physical exercise or mental stimulation just before bedtime
    - Limit bedroom activities to sleep and sex; leave the bedroom if unable to sleep
    - Avoid use of electronic products before bed
- Evaluation/Outcomes
  - Copes with anxiety-producing situations effectively
  - Uses relaxation techniques
  - Limits use of stimulants
  - Reports restorative sleep
  - Reports improved sense of well-being

APPLICATION AND REVIEW

1. A client tells a nurse, "I have been having trouble sleeping and feel wide awake as soon as I get into bed." Which strategies should the nurse teach the client that will promote sleep? **Select all that apply.**
   1. Eat a heavy snack near bedtime.
   2. Read in bed before shutting out the light.
   3. Leave the bedroom if you are unable to sleep.
   4. Drink a cup of warm tea with milk at bedtime.
   5. Exercise in the afternoon rather than in the evening.
   6. Count backward from 100 to 0 when your mind is racing.

2. A nurse is assessing a client with a diagnosis of primary insomnia. Which findings from the client's history may be the cause of this disorder? **Select all that apply**.
   1. Chronic stress
   2. Severe anxiety
   3. Generalized pain
   4. Excessive caffeine
   5. Chronic depression
   6. Environmental noise
3. A client who is in a four-bed room since admission becomes extremely anxious and is having difficulty sleeping. What is the nurse's **best** response?
   1. "You seem unable to sleep at night."
   2. "I'm going to move you to a private room."
   3. "I'll get you the sedative that was prescribed."
   4. "You'll be able to fall asleep when you're tired."
4. Which assessment question should the nurse ask to determine the effect a client's insomnia is having on their function?
   1. "How many hours do you usually sleep each night?"
   2. "When did you first notice you weren't sleeping well?"
   3. "Do you ever get sleepy and fall asleep during the day?"
   4. "Do you experience nightmares when you are able to sleep?"
5. Which assessment question should the nurse ask a client being evaluated for a diagnosis of secondary sleep disorder?
   1. "Do you have any rituals that help you fall asleep?"
   2. "Have you ever been told that you walk in your sleep?"
   3. "Do you ever fall asleep will engaging in some activities?"
   4. "What medications both prescribed and over-the-counter do you take regularly?"
6. An older adult client shares that, "I don't sleep as well as I did when I was younger." What fact about sleep disorders should the nurse use to base the response to this specific client's statement?
   1. Sleep cycles are affected by age.
   2. Sleep disorders are common among adults.
   3. Sleep is very important to restoring the body.
   4. Sleep disorders are usually reversible with appropriate treatment.

See Answers on pages 48-51.

SEDATIVE AND HYPNOTIC AGENTS

Overview
- Benzodiazepines have almost entirely replaced barbiturates in the treatment of anxiety and sleep disorders; sedative and hypnotic agents are primarily used in general medicine rather than psychiatry.
- Sedative-hypnotic preparations are generally intended for either occasional or short-term use.
- Insomnia, hypersomnia, narcolepsy, parasomnias, periodic leg movements (nocturnal myoclonus), and sleep apnea are among the disorders that are responsive to these agents; specific psychiatric conditions predispose clients to insomnia (mood disorders, anxiety, and dementias).
- CNS depressants have antianxiety effects in low dosages, produce sleep in high dosages, and have general anesthetic-like states in very high dosages.
- Sedatives reduce nervousness, excitability, and irritability without inducing sleep, but a sedative can become a hypnotic in large doses.
- All hypnotic drugs (with the probable exception of the melatonin agonist) probably alter either the character or the duration of rapid eye movement (REM) sleep.

- Hypnotics cause sleep and have a more potent effect on the CNS than sedatives.
- Sedative-hypnotics are classified chemically into three groups: barbiturates, benzodiazepines, and nonbenzodiazepines.
- Tolerance to the sedative and hypnotic effects develops eventually with all these drugs, although it develops more slowly with the benzodiazepines than other drugs; tolerance can contribute to self-medication and dosage escalation.

Types

- Barbiturates, such as pentobarbital (see Chapter 4 for use as antiseizure drug)
- Benzodiazepines
- Nonbenzodiazepine hypnotics
- Antidepressant: trazodone (see Chapter 5)
- Antihistamines: diphenhydramine; hydroxyzine (see Chapter 15)
- Beta-adrenergic blocker: propranolol (see Chapter 8)
- Anxiolytic: buspirone (see Chapter 5)

Precautions

- The sedative-hypnotics are CNS depressants.
- General adverse effects:
  - Hypnotic drugs have undesirable effects (e.g., physiologic addiction, fatal overdose potential, and dangerous interactions with other drugs and alcohol [Table 3.1]).
  - Barbiturate sedatives increase the metabolism of anticoagulants because they induce liver enzyme synthesis.
- Tolerance develops to sedative and hypnotic agents; therefore, the client in the outpatient setting may resort to increasing doses to produce the desired effect.
- Physical and emotional dependence occurs if taken in large dosages or for a long time period.
- Once physical dependence develops, abrupt discontinuation of sedative-hypnotics leads to withdrawal.
  - Withdrawal characteristics: insomnia, weakness, muscle tremors, anxiety, irritability, sweating, anorexia, fever, nausea and vomiting, headache, incoordination, and restlessness
  - After several days, severe symptoms of withdrawal may develop: postural hypotension, tinnitus, incoherence, delirium, psychosis, seizures, status epilepticus, cardiovascular collapse, loss of temperature regulation, and/or death.
- To avoid severe withdrawal that could result in death, it is important to slowly and gradually taper the dose with the same drug or one that is cross-tolerant.
- Treatment for overdose: removal of the drug from the stomach by aspiration, resuscitative measures (e.g., assisted ventilation, cardiac massage), hemodialysis of diffusible drug, vasopressor administration to counteract vascular collapse, and correction of acidosis
- Follow-up drug supervision is needed to avoid repetition of the problem.
- Psychotherapy may be required for depressed clients.

Barbiturates

- Have been replaced by benzodiazepines and nonbenzodiazepines as treatments of choice for insomnia
- Classified as long-acting (to control seizures), short-to-intermediate-acting (used to sustain sleep for long periods and for procedural sedation), and ultrashort-acting (sedation)

TABLE 3.1 Common Side Effects and Adverse Reactions of Sedative-Hypnotics

Side Effects and Adverse Reactions	Explanation of the Effects
Hangover	A hangover is residual drowsiness resulting in impaired reaction time. The intermediate- and long-acting hypnotics are frequently the cause of drug hangover. The liver biotransforms these drugs into active metabolites that persist in the body, causing drowsiness.
REM rebound	REM rebound, which results in vivid dreams and nightmares, frequently occurs after taking a hypnotic for a prolonged period then abruptly stopping. However, it may occur after taking only one hypnotic dose.
Dependence	Dependence is the result of chronic hypnotic use. Physical and psychologic dependence can result. Physical dependence results in the appearance of specific withdrawal symptoms when a drug is discontinued after prolonged use. The severity of withdrawal symptoms depends on the drug and dosage. Symptoms may include muscular twitching and tremors, dizziness, orthostatic hypotension, delusions, hallucinations, delirium, and seizures. Withdrawal symptoms start within 24 hours and can last for several days.
Tolerance	Tolerance results when there is a need to increase the dosage over time to obtain the desired effect. It is mostly caused by an increase in drug metabolism by liver enzymes. The barbiturate drug category can cause tolerance after prolonged use. Tolerance is reversible when the drug is discontinued.
Excessive depression	Long-term use of a hypnotic may result in CNS depression, which is characterized by lethargy, sleepiness, lack of concentration, confusion, and psychologic depression.
Respiratory depression	High doses of sedative-hypnotics can suppress the respiratory center in the medulla.
Hypersensitivity	Skin rashes and urticaria can result when taking barbiturates. Such reactions are rare.

From McCuistion, L., Vuljoin-DiMaggio, K., Winton, M.B., Yeager, J.J. (2018). *Pharmacology: A patient-centered nursing process approach* (9th ed.). St. Louis: Elsevier.

- Should be restricted to short-term use
- Overdose can cause death
- Except for phenobarbital (used to control seizures), they are nonselective CNS depressants
- Can result in tolerance and physical dependence; popular drugs of abuse
- Acute toxicity:
  - Remove barbiturate from body
  - Maintain oxygenation to brain
  - No specific antidote available; naloxone is NOT effective in barbiturate poisoning

Mode of Action
- Mimic the inhibitor neurotransmitter GABA and enhance the inhibitory actions of GABA

Contraindications, Precautions, and Drug Interactions for Barbiturates*

Drug	Contraindications/Precautions	Drug Interaction
Short-Acting Secobarbital	*Contraindications:* Hypersensitivity, suicide ideation, porphyria, liver dysfunction, respiratory disease, concomitant sodium oxybate *Precautions:* Monitor vital signs closely; lowest effective dose to be used, particularly in older adults *Pregnancy:* Definite fetal risks, may be given despite risks in life-threatening conditions	CNS depressants, alcohol; more than 1,000 drugs are known to interact with secobarbital
Intermediate-Acting Butabarbital	*Contraindications:* Hypersensitivity, porphyria, suicide ideation *Pregnancy:* Definite fetal risks, may be given despite risks in life-threatening conditions	CNS depressants, alcohol; nearly 1,000 drugs are known to interact with secobarbital
Long-Acting Phenobarbital	Seizure prevention and treatment: see Chapter 4 *Note: Phenobarbital (long-acting) is different from pentobarbital (ultrashort-acting)* *Pregnancy:* Definite fetal risks, may be given despite risks in life-threatening conditions	Seizure prevention and treatment: see Chapter 4

*Pregnancy categories have been revised. See http://www.fda.gov/Drugs/DevelopmentApprovalProcess/DevelopmentResources/Labeling/ucm093307.htm for more information.

Side/Adverse Effects
- Abuse
- Agitation
- Angioedema
- Ataxia
- Bradycardia
- Confusion
- Constipation
- Depression
- Drowsiness
- Headache
- Hypotension
- Nightmares
- Respiratory depression
- Sleep-related behaviors
- Suicide, suicide ideation
- Withdrawal

Nursing Care
- See General Nursing Care of Clients with Sleep Disorders
- See General Nursing Care of Clients Receiving Sedative and Hypnotic Agents
- Teach patients:
  - Do not increase your dosage
  - Do not stop taking suddenly

Benzodiazepines
- Used to decrease insomnia, anxiety and panic disorders, anesthesia induction, as well as some for treatment of status epilepticus
- Antagonist, Flumazenil, is used for benzodiazepine overdose
- Use raises the seizure threshold

Mode of Action
- Enhance the action of GABA

Contraindications, Precautions, and Drug Interactions for Benzodiazepines*

Drug	Contraindications/Precautions	Drug Interaction
Estazolam	*Contraindications:* Pregnancy, breastfeeding *Precautions:* Should not be used longer than 6 weeks *Pregnancy:* Definite fetal abnormalities; do not use during pregnancy	Alcohol, CNS depressants
Flurazepam	*Contraindications:* Pregnancy, breastfeeding, hypersensitivity *Pregnancy:* Only given after risks to the fetus are considered	Alcohol, CNS depressants
Lorazepam	*Contraindications:* Hypersensitivity, narrow-angle glaucoma, myasthentia gravis, COPD, sleep apnea *Pregnancy:* Definite fetal risks, may be given despite risks in life-threatening conditions	Alcohol, CNS depressants, disulfiram, oral contraceptives, valproic acid
Temazepam	*Contraindications:* Pregnancy, breastfeeding, hypersensitivity *Precautions:* Habit-forming *Pregnancy:* Definite fetal abnormalities; do not use during pregnancy	Alcohol, CNS depressants, cimetidine, disulfiram, probenecid, rifampin, theophylline
Triazolam	*Contraindications:* Pregnancy, breastfeeding, hypersensitivity, angle-closure glaucoma, severe liver disease or mental disorder; concomitant use of indinavir, itraconazole, ketoconazole, lopinavir, nefazodone, nelfinavir, ritonavir, or saquinavir *Precautions:* Habit-forming; should not be used longer than 7–10 days *Pregnancy:* Definite fetal abnormalities; do not use during pregnancy	Alcohol, CNS depressants, antacids, contraceptives, CYP3A4 inhibitors, protease inhibitors, probenecid, rifampin, theophylline

*Pregnancy categories have been revised. See http://www.fda.gov/Drugs/DevelopmentApprovalProcess/DevelopmentResources/Labeling/ucm093307.htm for more information.

Side/Adverse Effects
- Agitation
- Anterograde amnesia
- Anxiety
- Apnea
- Blurred vision
- Cardiac arrest
- Confusion
- Dependence
- Depression
- Dizziness
- Drowsiness
- Dry mouth
- ECG changes
- Headache
- Hepatic injury
- Hypotension
- Memory impairment
- Nausea
- Nightmares
- Sleep-related behaviors
- Suicidal ideation
- Tachycardia
- Unpleasant taste
- Visual impairment
- Withdrawal

Nursing Care
- See General Nursing Care of Clients with Sleep Disorders
- See General Nursing Care of Clients Receiving Sedative and Hypnotic Agents
- Teach patient:
  - Not to drive or perform activities that require alertness
  - For short-term use only (especially triazolam, estazolam)
  - Do not take more than prescribed
  - Take right before you get into bed
  - Do not take if you cannot get a full night's sleep
  - Do not take if you drink alcohol

- Do not take with other medications that make you sleepy
- Do not discontinue suddenly
- Benzodiazepines help treat, but do not cure, insomnia
- Benzodiazepines should only be used for 7–10 days (they can lose effectiveness in as little as 3–14 days)
- Difficulty sleeping for longer than 2 weeks warrants provider evaluation

Nonbenzodiazepines

- Short-term treatment of insomnia
- Short-to-intermediate-acting

Mode of Action

- Enhance the depressant actions of GABA

Contraindications, Precautions, and Drug Interactions for Nonbenzodiazepines*

Drug	Contraindications/Precautions	Drug Interaction
Eszopiclone	**Contraindications:** Hypersensitivity **Precautions:** Pregnancy, breastfeeding, severe hepatic disease, do not discontinue abruptly, depression, CNS depression, suicide ideation **Pregnancy:** Only given after risks to the fetus are considered	Alcohol, CNS depressants, azole antifungals, rifamycins, anticonvulsants
Zaleplon	**Contraindications:** Hypersensitivity, severe hepatic disease **Precautions:** Pregnancy, breastfeeding, children 14 years or younger, renal or hepatic disease, concomitant use of sodium oxybate, respiratory disease, psychosis, depression **Pregnancy:** Only given after risks to the fetus are considered	Alcohol, CNS depressants, carbamazepine, cimetidine, phenobarbital, phenytoin, rifampin
Zolpidem	**Contraindications:** Hypersensitivity, respiratory depression, breastfeeding **Precautions:** Pregnancy, breastfeeding, renal or hepatic disease, mental depression, suicide ideation, children **Pregnancy:** Only given after risks to the fetus are considered	Alcohol, CNS depressants, anticonvulsants, azole antifungals, rifamycins

*Pregnancy categories have been revised. See http://www.fda.gov/Drugs/DevelopmentApprovalProcess/DevelopmentResources/Labeling/ucm093307.htm for more information.

Side/Adverse Effects

- Dizziness
- Daytime drowsiness
- Headache
- Suicidal ideation
- Pulmonary edema
- Renal failure
- Performing activities while not fully awake and not aware of doing them (sleep-related complex behaviors, such as sleep-driving)
- Severe allergic reaction
- Memory loss
- Abnormal thoughts and behavior
- Anxiety, depression
- Leukopenia, granulocytopenia

- Nausea
- Tolerance, psychologic or physical dependence, withdrawal symptoms

Nursing Care

- See General Nursing Care of Clients with Sleep Disorders
- See Nursing Care of Clients Receiving Sedative and Hypnotic Agents
- Teach patients:
  - For short-term use only (zaleplon, zolpidem)
  - Do not drive or perform other tasks that require alertness
  - Do not take more than prescribed
  - Take right before you get into bed, not sooner
  - Do not take if you cannot get a full night's sleep
  - Do not take if you drink alcohol
  - Do not eat a high-fat meal before taking
  - Do not take with other medications that make you sleepy
  - Do not discontinue suddenly

Melatonin Agonist

- Melatonin regulates circadian clock (Fig. 3.1)
- An increase in melatonin (a hormone produced by the pineal gland) levels is associated with the onset of sleep and a decreased level leads to awakening.
- Ramelteon has not been shown to decrease REM sleep
- Only drug for insomnia that is not a controlled substance
- Has a rapid onset, but short duration: used to induce sleep, but not to maintain it
- Note: no rebound insomnia reported

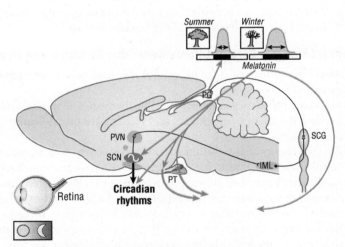

The clock is localized in the suprachiasmatic nucleus.
The clock controls nocturnal melatonin secretion.
Melatonin distributes photoperiodic day/night and circadian message.
Melatonin synchronizes circadian and seasonal function.

FIG. 3.1 Melatonin: A circadian and seasonal regulator of the suprachiasmatic nucleus. (From Kryger, M.H., Roth, T., Dement, W.C. [2011]. *Principles and practice of sleep medicine* [5th ed.]. St. Louis: Saunders.)

Mode of Action

- Ramelteon (only drug in this category) activates receptors for melatonin to regulate circadian rhythms and treat sleep-onset insomnia

Contraindications, Precautions, and Drug Interactions for Melatonin Agonists*

Drug	Contraindications/Precautions	Drug Interaction
ramelteon	**Precautions:** Use with caution by patients with moderate hepatic impairment; should be avoided in those with severe hepatic impairment **Contraindications:** Hypersensitivity, severe hepatic impairment, sleep apnea, concurrent use of fluvoxamine, breastfeeding, infants, children **Pregnancy:** Only given after risks to the fetus are considered	• Fluvoxamine, can increase levels of ramelteon more than 50-fold; avoid concomitant use • Alcohol and CNS depressants can intensify sedation; avoid concomitant use • Azole antifungals (such as fluconazole or ketoconazole) may increase the risk of side effects • Rifampin may decrease ramelteon's effectiveness

*Pregnancy categories have been revised. See http://www.fda.gov/Drugs/DevelopmentApprovalProcess/DevelopmentResources/Labeling/ucm09 3307.htm for more information.

Side/Adverse Effects

- Angioedema
- Dizziness
- Drowsiness
- Fatigue
- Headache
- Nausea
- Severe allergic reactions
- Suicidal thoughts/behaviors

Nursing Care

- See General Nursing Care of Clients with Sleep Disorders
- Teach Patients:
  - Avoid alcohol and other CNS depressants
  - Avoid dangerous activities, such as driving or operating heavy machinery
  - Report adverse effects, especially suicide ideation

General Nursing Care of Clients Receiving Sedative and Hypnotic Agents

- Assess for history of drug or alcohol abuse or suicide attempts by overdose because of the increased risk for abuse
- Assess for pregnancy and breastfeeding, because safe use has not been established
- Explore the client's perceptions and feelings about medications; clarify any misinformation and concerns
- Plan for client teaching about specific sedative-hypnotic agents; institute safety precautions
- Supplement verbal teaching with appropriate written or audiovisual materials
- Administer controlled substances according to schedule restrictions
- Evaluate client's response to medication and understanding of teaching
- Assess for undesired effects (e.g., respiratory depression, increased sedation, and hypotension)
- Review methods to improve sleep (e.g., minimizing daytime napping, increasing physical activity except just before bedtime, eliminating caffeine intake after dinner, establishing bedtime routines, maintaining a regular sleep schedule)
- Patient Education
  - Proper nutrition
  - Avoid alcohol intake
  - Avoid the use of controlled substances, such as marijuana, that are also CNS depressants

- Avoid operating a motor vehicle or heavy equipment
- Maintain normal gas exchange
- Report any injury or unusual dizziness

APPLICATION AND REVIEW

7. A nurse is caring for a client who abruptly withdrew from barbiturate use. What should the nurse anticipate that the client may experience?
   1. Ataxia
   2. Seizures
   3. Diarrhea
   4. Urticaria
8. A client is scheduled for a 6-week electroconvulsive therapy (ECT) treatment program. What intervention is important during the 6-week course of treatment?
   1. Provision of tyramine-free meals
   2. Avoidance of exposure to the sun
   3. Maintenance of a steady sodium intake
   4. Elimination of benzodiazepines for nighttime sedation
9. What medication should the nurse expect to administer to actively reverse the overdose sedative effects of benzodiazepines?
   1. Lithium
   2. Flumazenil
   3. Methadone
   4. Chlorpromazine
10. A client is treated with lorazepam for status epilepticus. What effect of lorazepam does the nurse consider therapeutic?
    1. Slows cardiac contractions
    2. Dilates tracheobronchial structures
    3. Depresses the central nervous system
    4. Provides amnesia for the convulsive episode
11. A client newly prescribed a sedative-hypnotic medication asks the nurse, "How long will I be expected to take this medication?" Considering client safety, what fact about this classification of medications should the nurse base the response to the client's question?
    1. Duration of treatment depends on the nature of the sleep disorder.
    2. This type of medication is generally prescribed for short-term or occasional use.
    3. Hypnotic medications alter the character or duration of rapid eye movement sleep.
    4. This classification's tendency to cause the development of tolerance limits its long-term usefulness.
12. What principle should the nurse rely upon when responding to a client who inquires about "feeling hung-over" after taking their prescribed sedative?
    1. Long-term use of such medications can result in depression
    2. The body is demonstrating a need for additional medication
    3. Abruptly stopping the medication after taking it for an extended period of time
    4. The liver causes the medication to persist in the body causing a hangover effect
13. Which statements should the nurse rely upon when preparing information to discuss with a client who has been prescribed a CNS depressant/sedative? **Select all that apply.**
    1. Causes a general anesthetic effect with very large doses
    2. Produces no hypnotic effect with any dosage
    3. Helps relieve anxiety with low doses
    4. Reduces excitability
    5. Causes insomnia

14. When considering client safety, which statements should the nurse stress most when discussing medication instructions with a client who has been recently prescribed a hypnotic sedative?
    1. "I need to share with you the signs and symptoms of drug tolerance."
    2. "This medication will affect your rapid eye movement (REM) sleep."
    3. "This medication has more effect on sleep than sedatives do."
    4. "A barbiturate is a type of sedative-hypnotic."

15. Which statement made by a nurse preparing to care for an unconscious client just admitted with a diagnosis of acute barbiturate poisoning demonstrates a need for further instructions on the appropriate treatment?
    1. "We'll need to support brain function."
    2. "I'll prepare for the client's intubation."
    3. "Naloxone needs to be placed at the bedside."
    4. "Flushing the system of the barbiturate is a priority."

16. Which clients have considerations that contraindicate the use of the melatonin agonist, ramelteon? **Select all that apply.**
    1. The woman who is breastfeeding
    2. The toddler diagnosed with asthma
    3. The man diagnosed with sleep apnea
    4. The woman who is 30 weeks pregnant
    5. The man diagnosed with cirrhosis of the liver

17. Which statement made by a client, who has developed a physical dependence on a hypnotic drug, demonstrates effective learning concerning the withdrawal process? **Select all that apply.**
    1. "The symptoms of withdrawal will occur as soon as I stop the medication."
    2. "I understand I might need to taper off from a cross-tolerant drug."
    3. "There is a risk that I might become delirious doing withdrawal."
    4. "At least this drug doesn't make you emotionally dependent."
    5. "I will have to gradually come off of the medication."

18. An adult client is prescribed zalephlon 15 mg at bed time for a sleep disorder. The nurse provides medication education that the medication may be dispensed in a variety of mg doses. The nurse asks the client to calculate the appropriate dosage when given 5 mg tablets. The nurse determines that the client can accurately administer the medication when selecting how many tablets? Record your answer using whole numbers. Answer: _____ 5 mg tablets

See Answers on pages 48-51.

ANSWER KEY: REVIEW QUESTIONS

1. **Answers: 3, 5, 6**

    3 Lying in bed when one is unable to sleep increases frustration and anxiety, which further impede sleep; other activities, such as reading or watching television, should not be conducted in bed. **5** Exercise during the day uses energy that promotes sleep at night; exercise too close to bedtime is stimulating and may interfere with sleep. **6** Counting backward requires minimal concentration, but it is enough to interfere with thoughts that distract a person from falling asleep.

    1 A heavy meal places pressure against the diaphragm that may be uncomfortable, and the body is expending energy to digest the food. A light, not heavy, snack is preferred before bedtime. **2** The bed should be used exclusively for sleep so that the expectation when getting into bed is that sleep will be the outcome. **4** Although milk may promote sleep, tea contains caffeine, which is a stimulant that should be avoided after the midafternoon; otherwise, it may interfere with sleep.

Client Need: Basic Care and Comfort; **Cognitive Level:** Analysis; **Integrated Process:** Teaching/Learning; **Nursing Process:** Planning/Implementation

2. **Answers: 1, 4, 6**

   1 Acute or primary insomnia is caused by emotional or physical stress not related to the direct physiologic effects of a substance or illness. **4** Excessive caffeine intake can cause disruptive sleep hygiene; caffeine is a stimulant that inhibits sleep. **6** Environmental noise causes physical and/or emotional discomfort and therefore is related to primary insomnia.

   2 Severe anxiety usually is related to a psychiatric disorder and therefore causes a secondary insomnia. **3** Generalized pain usually is related to a medical or neurologic problem and therefore causes a secondary insomnia. **5** Chronic depression usually is related to a psychiatric disorder and therefore causes a secondary insomnia.

   Client Need: Basic Care and Comfort; **Cognitive Level:** Analysis; **Nursing Process:** Assessment/Analysis

3. **2 The client is too anxious to sleep in a four-bed room and should be moved to a private room.**

   1 Just talking about the problem will not improve it; moving the client to a private room is a better intervention at this time. **3** Offering a sedative does not address the problem at its inception. **4** The nurse is providing false reassurance by stating the client will fall asleep when tired.

   Client Need: Management of Care; **Cognitive Level:** Application; **Integrated Process:** Caring; **Nursing Process:** Planning/Implementation

   Test-Taking Tip: Did you notice that the statement "Select all that apply" does NOT appear for this question? This means there is only ONE correct answer. This is NOT a multiple response question. Be alert for the presence or absence of that statement.

4. **3 Sleep disorders are conditions that repeatedly disrupt the pattern of sleep, leading to diminished performance in accomplishing daily work and self-care functions.**

   1 Although asking the client to share how many hours of sleep they typically get each night is an appropriate assessment question, it does not provide insight to how the client's insomnia is affecting their ability to function. **2** Although asking the client when they first noticed a sleep problem is an appropriate assessment question, it does not provide insight to how the client's insomnia is affecting their ability to function. **4** Although asking the client whether they experience nightmares is an appropriate assessment question, it does not provide insight to how the client's insomnia is affecting their ability to function.

   Client Need: Basic Care and Comfort; **Cognitive Level:** Analysis; **Nursing Process:** Assessment/Analysis

5. **4 Secondary sleep disorders are outcomes of another condition. Substance-induced sleep disorders are included as a subclass secondary sleep disorders and are related to intoxication, periods of withdrawal, use of stimulants, and side effects of many medications.**

   1 Asking about sleep routines and rituals is an appropriate assessment question related to primary sleep disorders but it does not focus on factors associated with secondary sleep disorders. **2** Sleep walking is considered a parasomnia which is a category of disorders that are associated with a disruption in the sleep stages. These disorders are related to primary sleep disorders. **3** Narcolepsy is a disorder that involves repeated uncontrollable brief episodes of sleep while engaging in meaningful activities. Narcolepsy is a primary sleep disorder

   Client Need: Basic Care and Comfort; **Cognitive Level:** Analysis; **Nursing Process:** Assessment/Analysis

6. **1 Because the sleep cycle evolves throughout the life cycle and decreases with age, it is most appropriate to explain that age affects sleep.**

   2 Sleep disorders are common amongst adults, but providing this information would not address the client's concern about changes in sleep with age. **3** Sleep is important to restore the body, but providing this information would not address the client's concern about changes in sleep with age. **4** Sleep disorders may be reversible and temporary if treated, but providing this information would not address the client's concern about changes in sleep with age.

    Client Need: Basic Care and Comfort; **Cognitive Level:** Application; **Integrated Process:** Teaching/Learning; **Nursing Process:** Planning/Implementation

7. **2 Seizure is a serious side effect that may occur with abrupt withdrawal from barbiturates.**

    1, 3, 4. Ataxia, diarrhea, and urticaria are not associated with barbiturate withdrawal.

    Client Need: Pharmacologic and Parenteral Therapies; **Cognitive Level:** Application; **Nursing Process:** Evaluation/Outcomes

8. **4 The use of benzodiazepine can raise the seizure threshold, which is counterproductive.**

    1 A tyramine-free diet is required with MAOI therapy, not after electroconvulsive therapy. **2** Photosensitivity is not a side effect of electroconvulsive therapy. **3** A stable sodium level is necessary with lithium, not electroconvulsive, therapy.

    Client Need: Pharmacologic and Parenteral Therapies; **Cognitive Level:** Analysis; **Nursing Process:** Planning/Implementation

9. **2 Flumazenil (Romazicon) is the drug of choice in the management of overdose when a benzodiazepine is the only agent ingested by a client not at risk for seizure activity. This medication competitively inhibits activity at benzodiazepine recognition sites on GABA/benzodiazepine receptor complexes.**

    1 Lithium is used in the treatment of mood disorders. **3** Methadone is used for narcotic addiction withdrawal. **4** Chlorpromazine is contraindicated in the presence of central nervous system depressants.

    Client Need: Pharmacologic and Parenteral Therapies; **Cognitive Level:** Comprehension; **Nursing Process:** Planning/Implementation

10. **3 Lorazepam, an anxiolytic and sedative, is used to treat status epilepticus because it depresses the CNS.**

    1 Slowed cardiac contractions is not an effect of lorazepam. **2** Dilation of tracheobronchial structures is not an effect of lorazepam. **4** Amnesia is not an effect of lorazepam.

    Client Needs: Pharmacologic and Parenteral Therapies; **Cognitive Level:** Application; **Nursing Process:** Planning/Implementation

11. **2 Sedative-hypnotic preparations are generally intended for either occasional or short-term use. Here are a variety of reasons for this limitation that includes physiologic addiction, overdose potential, and dangerous interactions with other drugs and alcohol.**

    1 Although it is true that the duration of the medication therapy will depend on the nature of the sleep disorder, that is not the basis for the nurse's response because the greatest issue is client safety. **3** Although it is true that this classification of medications alters the character or duration of rapid eye movement sleep, that is not the basis for the nurse's response because the greatest issue is client safety. **4** Although it is true that this classification of medications has a high tendency for the development of drug tolerance, that is not the basis for the nurse's response because the greatest issue is client safety.

    Client Need: Pharmacologic and Parenteral Therapies; **Cognitive Level:** Analysis; **Integrated Process:** Teaching/Learning; **Nursing Process:** Planning/Implementation

12. **4 A hangover is residual drowsiness resulting in impaired reaction time. The intermediate- and long-acting hypnotics are frequently the cause of drug hangover. The liver biotransforms these drugs into active metabolites that persist in the body, causing drowsiness.**

    1 Long-term use of a hypnotic may result in CNS depression, which is characterized by lethargy, sleepiness, lack of concentration, confusion, and psychologic depression but this is not the basis for a hang-over effect. **2** Tolerance results when there is a need to increase the dosage over time to obtain the desired effect. **3** REM rebound, which results in vivid dreams and nightmares, frequently occurs after taking a hypnotic for a prolonged period then abruptly stopping.

    Client Need: Pharmacologic and Parenteral Therapies; **Cognitive Level:** Application; **Integrated Process:** Teaching/Learning; **Nursing Process:** Planning/Implementation

13. **Answers: 1, 3, 4**

    CNS depressants have antianxiety effects in low dosages, produce sleep in high dosages, and have general anesthetic-like states in very high dosages. This type of sedative reduces nervousness, excitability, and irritability.

    2 A CNS depressant/sedative can become a hypnotic in large doses. **5** A CNS depressant/sedative reduces nervousness, excitability, irritability, and impaired sleep. CNS depressants do not cause insomnia.

14. **1 Tolerance to the sedative and hypnotic effects develops eventually with all these drugs, although it develops more slowly with the benzodiazepines than other drugs; tolerance can contribute to self-medication and dosage escalation.**

    2 Although REM sleep may be affected, it is not a safety concern. **3** Although it is true that hypnotic sedatives have more effect on sleep than sedative, it is not a safety concern. **4** Although it is true that barbiturates are a form of sedative-hypnotics, this statement doesn't address a safety issue.

    Client Need: Pharmacologic and Parenteral Therapies; **Cognitive Level:** Analysis; **Integrated Process:** Teaching/Learning; **Nursing Process:** Planning/Implementation

15. **3 This item asks you to identify the incorrect statement. No specific antidote is available and so naloxone is NOT effective in reversing barbiturate poisoning.**

    1 It is true that supporting brain function is a priority when caring for an unconscious client just admitted with a diagnosis of acute barbiturate poisoning. **2** It is true that supporting brain function with effective oxygenation is a priority when caring for an unconscious client just admitted with a diagnosis of acute barbiturate poisoning. **4** It is true that removing the barbiturate from the body is a priority when caring for an unconscious client just admitted with a diagnosis of acute barbiturate poisoning.

    Client Need: Pharmacologic and Parenteral Therapies; **Cognitive Level:** Analysis; **Integrated Process:** Teaching/Learning; **Nursing Process:** Evaluation/Outcomes

16. **Answers: 1, 2, 3, 5**

    Ramelteon is contraindicated in clients with hypersensitivity, severe hepatic impairment, sleep apnea, concurrent use of fluvoxamine, breastfeeding, infants, children.

    4 Ramelteon is prescribed during pregnancy only after risks to the fetus are considered.

    Client Need: Pharmacologic and Parenteral Therapies; **Cognitive Level:** Analysis; **Integrated Nursing Process:** Assessment/Analysis

17. **Answers: 2, 3, 5**

    Once physical dependence develops, abrupt discontinuation of sedative-hypnotics leads to withdrawal. Severe symptoms of withdrawal may develop that include delirium. To avoid severe withdrawal that could result in death, it is important to slowly and gradually taper the dose with the same drug or one that is cross-tolerant.

    1 After several days, severe symptoms of withdrawal may develop. **4** Physical and emotional dependence occurs if taken in large dosages or for a long time period.

    Client Need: Pharmacologic and Parenteral Therapies; **Cognitive Level:** Analysis; **Integrated Process:** Teaching/Learning; **Nursing Process:** Evaluation/Outcomes

18. **Answer: 3**

    Use the "Mass for Mass" formula to solve this problem.

    Dosage ordered = Tablets required

    Dosage available

    15 mg = 3 (5 mg) tablets

    5 mg/tablet

    Client Need: Pharmacologic and Parenteral Therapies; **Cognitive Level:** Application; **Integrated Process:** Teaching/Learning; **Nursing Process:** Evaluation/Outcomes

4 Antiepileptic Drugs

INTRODUCTION TO EPILEPSY

Etiology and Pathophysiology
- Abnormal discharge of electric impulses by nerve cells in brain from idiopathic or secondary causes, resulting in loss of consciousness; seizures; motor, sensory, behavioral changes
- Onset of idiopathic epilepsy generally before age 30; seizures can be associated with brain tumor, brain attack, Alzheimer disease, hypoglycemia, head trauma, fluid shifts in the brain
- Types of seizures
  - Partial seizures (seizures beginning locally)
    - Simple: focal motor or sensory effect; no loss of consciousness
    - Complex: cognitive, psychosensory, psychomotor, or affective effect; brief loss of consciousness
  - Generalized seizures (bilaterally symmetric and without local onset)
    - Absence (petit mal): brief transient loss of consciousness with or without minor motor movements of eyes, head, or extremities; most common in childhood and adolescence
    - Myoclonic: brief, transient rigidity or jerking of extremities, singly or in groups
    - Tonic-clonic (grand mal): aura, loss of consciousness, rigidity followed by tonic-clonic movements, interruption of respirations, loss of bladder and bowel control; may last 2 to 5 minutes (Fig. 4.1)
    - Atonic: loss of muscle control; loss of consciousness may be brief
  - Status epilepticus: prolonged repetitive seizures without recovery between attacks; may result in complete exhaustion, cerebral injury, or death; status epilepticus is a medical emergency

Clinical Findings (Tonic-Clonic Seizures)
- Subjective: often preceded by an aura or warning sensation such as seeing spots or feeling dizzy; lethargy following return to consciousness (postictal phase)
- Objective
  - Shrill cry as seizure begins and air is forcefully exhaled
  - Loss of consciousness during seizure
  - Tonic-clonic movement of muscles
  - Incontinence
  - Abnormal EEG, MRI

Therapeutic Interventions
- Anticonvulsant therapy usually continued throughout life
- Diazepam or lorazepam (see Chapters 3 and 5) given IV to treat status epilepticus
- Sedatives used to reduce emotional stress
- Neurosurgery is sometimes indicated if source of seizures is localized; vagal nerve stimulation, which involves implantation of an electrical impulse generator, is a palliative treatment if therapy has been unsuccessful

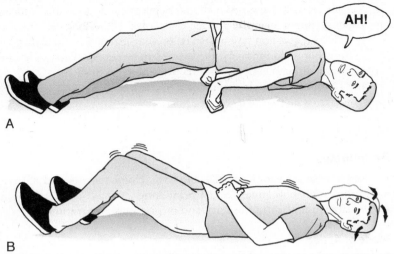

FIG. 4.1 A, This man in the tonic phase of a tonic-clonic seizure arches his torso and extends his arms and legs. He assumes this position because of the relatively greater strength of the extensor muscles compared with the flexor muscles. Simultaneous diaphragm, chest wall, and laryngeal muscle contractions force air through his tightened larynx to produce the shrill "epileptic cry." During this phase, he may also bite his tongue and lose control of his urine. **B,** In the clonic phase, his head, neck, and legs contract symmetrically and forcefully for about 10 to 20 seconds. Saliva, aerated and often blood-tinged from tongue lacerations, froths from his mouth. His pupils dilate and he sweats profusely. Finally, his muscular contractions lose strength. The seizure usually ends with stertorous breathing. In the immediate postictal period, he remains unresponsive. Before regaining consciousness, he often passes through a state of confusion and agitation, loosely termed "postictal psychosis." (From Kaufman, D.M., Milstein, M.J. [2013]. *Kaufman's clinical neurology for psychiatrists* [7th ed.]. Philadelphia: Saunders.)

APPLICATION AND REVIEW

1. When entering a room on a medical unit, the nurse identifies that a client is having a seizure. What should the nurse do in addition to protecting the client from self-injury?
   1. Insert an oral airway.
   2. Monitor the seizure activity.
   3. Turn the client on the left side.
   4. Begin oxygen by mask at 8 L/min.
2. What is the **primary** responsibility of a nurse during a client's generalized motor seizure?
   1. Inserting a plastic airway between the teeth
   2. Determining whether an aura was experienced
   3. Administering the prescribed prn anticonvulsant
   4. Clearing the immediate environment for client safety
3. A client who has a history of seizures is scheduled for an arteriogram at 10 AM and is to have nothing by mouth before the test. The client is scheduled to receive an anticonvulsant medication at 9 AM. What should the nurse do?
   1. Omit the 9 AM dose of the drug.
   2. Give the same dosage of the drug rectally.
   3. Administer the drug with 30 mL of water at 9 AM.
   4. Ask the health care provider if the drug can be given IV.

4. A client, recently diagnosed with status epilepticus, is prescribed anticonvulsant therapy. What response should the nurse provide when asked, "How long will I need to take this medicine?"
   1. "That's a question best answered by your primary health care provider."
   2. "It is not uncommon for the therapy to be necessary for a lifetime."
   3. "It is a difficult situation but try your best not to worry."
   4. "That decision varies from client to client."

See Answers on pages 63-66.

ANTIEPILEPTIC AGENTS

Barbiturates

- Used to treat myoclonic, partial, and tonic-clonic seizures and status epilepticus
- Examples: phenobarbital CSS IV, primidone
- Available in oral, intramuscular, and intravenous preparations

Mode of Action

- Causes enhancement of the activity of GABA, resulting in a reduction of seizures.

Contraindications, Precautions, and Drug Interactions of Barbituates*

Drug	Contraindications/Precautions	Drug Interaction
Phenobarbital CSS IV	**Contraindications:** Hypersensitivity to barbiturates, hepatic/respiratory disease, porphyria **Precautions:** Anemia, breastfeeding, geriatric, pregnancy, renal disease **Pregnancy:** Evidence of fetal risk, but benefits outweigh risks	Alcohol, anticoagulants, chloramphenicol, central nervous system depressants, disulfiram, doxycycline, estrogens, furosemide, glucocorticoids, hormonal contraceptives, MAOIs, metronidazole, quinidine, skeletal muscle relaxants (nondepolarizing), sulfonamides, theophylline, valproic acid
Primidone	**Contraindications:** Breastfeeding, hypersensitivity primidone or barbiturates, porphyria **Precautions:** Chronic obstructive pulmonary disease, hepatic encephalopathy, hyperactive children, pregnancy, renal/hepatic disease, sleep apnea, suicidal ideation **Pregnancy:** Evidence of fetal risk, but benefits outweigh risks	Acebutolol, acetazolamide, alcohol, antidepressants (tricyclic), carbamazepine, CNS depressants, CYP3A4 inducers, CYP3A4 inhibitors, heparin, isoniazid, lamotrigine, MAOIs, metoprolol, nicotinamide, oral contraceptives, phenothiazines, phenytoin, phenytoins, propranolol, succinimides

MAOI, monoamine oxidase inhibitor.
*Pregnancy categories have been revised. See http://www.fda.gov/Drugs/DevelopmentApprovalProcess/DevelopmentResources/Labeling/ucm093307.htm for more information.

Adverse/Side Effects

- Agranulocytosis
- Angioedema
- Ataxia
- Bradycardia
- Coma
- Confusion
- Constipation
- Dependence
- Depression
- Dizziness
- Drowsiness
- Erectile dysfunction
- GI distress
- Hypotension
- Megaloblastic anemia
- Respiratory depression
- Seizures
- Stevens-Johnson syndrome
- Suicidal ideation
- Thrombocytopenia
- Thrombophlebitis

Nursing Care

- Assess for barbiturate toxicity
- Assess for blood dyscrasias
- Assess for pain in postop patients
- Assess for withdrawal insomnia after short-term use
- Assess mental status, respiratory dysfunction and seizure activity
- Teach patient not to discontinue medication quickly after long-term use; taper over 1 week
- Teach patient that medication may take up to 4 weeks to reach therapeutic levels
- Teach patient that physical dependency may result when used for extended time
- Teach patient to avoid alcohol and CNS depressants
- Teach patient to avoid driving and other activities requiring alertness
- Teach patient to immediately report suicidal thoughts or behavior
- Teach patient to notify prescriber immediately if unexplained bruising or bleeding occurs
- Teach patient to tell all prescribers about prescribed barbiturates
- Teach the patient to change positions slowly

Hydantoins

- Used to prevent tonic-clonic and partial seizures and status epilepticus
- Examples: fosphenytoin, phenytoin
- Available in oral and intravenous preparations

Mode of Action

- Causes a reduction in motor cortex activity by changing ion transport
- Controls the amount of sodium that is let into the nerve cell, which regulates the amount of action potentials

Contraindications, Precautions, and Drug Interactions of Hydantoins*

Drug	Contraindications/Precautions	Drug Interaction
Fosphenytoin	*Contraindications:* Bradycardia, hypersensitivity, SA and AV block, Stokes-Adams syndrome *Precautions:* Abrupt discontinuation, agranulocytosis, alcoholism, allergies, Asian patients positive for HLA-B 1502, bone marrow suppression, breastfeeding, CAD, geriatrics, hemolytic anemia, hypersensitivity to carbamazepine or barbiturates, hypoalbuminemia, hyponatremia, hypothyroidism, methemoglobinemia, myasthenia gravis, myocardial insufficiency, psychosis, renal/hepatic disease, suicidal ideation *Pregnancy:* Evidence of fetal risk, but benefits outweigh risks	Alcohol, amiodarone, antacids, antihistamines, antineoplastics, carbamazepine, chloramphenicol, cimetidine, CYP1A2 inhibitors, delavirdine, estrogens, folic acid, H_2-receptor antagonists, phenothiazines, rifampin, salicylates, sulfonamides, theophylline, tramadol
Phenytoin	*Contraindications:* Adams-Stokes syndrome, bradycardia, heart block, hypersensitivity *Precautions:* Alcoholism, Asian, diabetes, hypoglycemia, hyponatremia, hypotension, IV use, Suicidal ideation, myasthenia gravis, thyroid disease, mellitus, renal and hepatic impairment *Pregnancy:* Evidence of fetal risk, but benefits outweigh risks	Antacids, anticoagulants, antihistamines, calcium, cimetidine, cisplatin, corticosteroids, cyclosporine, dopamine, folic acid, isoniazid, chloramphenicol, metronidazole, oral contraceptives, quinidine, rifampin, sucralfate, theophylline, vinblastine

*Pregnancy categories have been revised. See http://www.fda.gov/Drugs/DevelopmentApprovalProcess/DevelopmentResources/Labeling/ucm093307.htm for more information.

Adverse/Side Effects

- Agranulocytosis
- Anorexia
- Aplastic anemia
- Ataxia
- Bradycardia
- Confusion
- Depression
- Diplopia
- Dizziness
- Drowsiness
- Fatigue
- Gingival hyperplasia
- Headache
- Hepatic impairment
- Hirsutism
- Hyperglycemia
- Hypotension
- Insomnia
- Leukopenia
- Nausea
- Nystagmus
- Peripheral neuropathy
- Pink-red/brown discoloration of urine
- Purple glove syndrome
- Rash
- Stevens-Johnson syndrome
- Suicidal ideation
- Thrombocytopenia
- Tremor
- Ventricular fibrillation
- Vomiting

Nursing Care

- Assess for rash, allergic reaction and toxicity
- Assess drug level
- Assess for blood dyscrasias
- Assess mental status
- Assess renal and hepatic studies
- Assess seizure activity
- Monitor blood studies
- Administer phenytoin at least 1-2 hours before or after tube feedings
- Teach patient not to use machinery or engage in hazardous activity; drowsiness, dizziness may occur
- Teach patient to wear emergency ID
- Teach patient to notify prescriber of rash, bleeding, bruising, slurred speech, jaundice of skin or eyes, joint pain, nausea, vomiting, severe headache, depression, suicidal ideation
- Teach patient to use contraception and to notify prescriber if pregnancy is planned or suspected

APPLICATION AND REVIEW

5. A client who is receiving phenytoin to control a seizure disorder questions the nurse regarding this medication after discharge. The nurse's **best** response is "This medication:
   1. will probably be continued for life."
   2. prevents the occurrence of seizures."
   3. needs to be taken during periods of emotional stress."
   4. can usually be stopped after a year's absence of seizures."
6. A client with a history of seizures is admitted with a partial occlusion of the left common carotid artery. The client has been taking phenytoin for 10 years. When planning care for this client, what should the nurse do **first**?
   1. Place an airway and restraints at the bedside.
   2. Obtain a history of seizure type and incidence.
   3. Ask the client to remove any dentures and eyeglasses.
   4. Observe the client for increased restlessness and agitation.

7. Phenytoin suspension 200 mg is prescribed for a client with epilepsy. The suspension contains 125 mg/5 mL. How much solution should the nurse administer? **Record your answer using a whole number.**
   Answer: _____ mL

8. A nurse is providing instructions for a client who is receiving phenytoin but has limited access to health care. What side effect is the basis for the nurse's emphasis on meticulous oral hygiene?
   1. Hyperplasia of the gums
   2. Alkalinity of the oral secretions
   3. Irritation of the gingiva and destruction of tooth enamel
   4. Promotion of plaque and bacterial growth at the gum lines

9. A client who is receiving phenytoin asks why folic acid was prescribed. What is the **best** explanation by the nurse?
   1. Absorption from foods is inhibited.
   2. The action of phenytoin is potentiated.
   3. Absorption of iron from foods is improved.
   4. Neuropathy caused by phenytoin is prevented.

10. A client is receiving phenytoin for a seizure disorder and heparin for a deep vein thrombosis. Warfarin is added in preparation for discontinuing the heparin. Why must the nurse observe the client closely during the **initial** days of treatment with warfarin?
    1. Warfarin affects the metabolism of phenytoin.
    2. Phenytoin decreases warfarin's anticoagulant effect.
    3. Warfarin's action is greater in clients with seizure disorders.
    4. Seizures increase the metabolic degradation rate of warfarin.

11. A child is to receive 60 mg of phenytoin. The medication is available as an oral suspension that contains 125 mg/5 mL. How many milliliters should the nurse administer? **Record your answer using one decimal place.**
    Answer: _____ mL

12. A child with a seizure disorder is to be discharged with a prescription for phenytoin 140 mg a day to be divided into two doses. The hospital pharmacy prepares an oral suspension at a concentration of 125 mg/5 mL. What amount of solution should the nurse teach the parents to give for each dose? **Record your answer using one decimal place.**
    Answer: _____ mL

13. A client is scheduled to receive phenytoin 100 mg orally at 6 PM but is having difficulty swallowing capsules. What method should the nurse use to help the client take the medication?
    1. Sprinkle the powder from the capsule into a cup of water.
    2. Insert a rectal suppository containing 100 mg of phenytoin.
    3. Administer 4 mL of phenytoin suspension containing 125 mg/5 mL.
    4. Obtain a change in the administration route to allow an IM injection.

See Answers on pages 63-66.

Iminostilbenes

- Used to control tonic-clonic and partial seizures
- Examples: carbamazepine, oxcarbazepine
- Available in oral preparations

Mode of Action
- Causes a decrease in nerve impulses that cause seizures and pain

Contraindications, Precautions, and Drug Interactions of Iminostilbenes*

Drug	Contraindications/Precautions	Drug Interaction
Carbamazepine	**Contraindications:** Hypersensitivity to carbamazepine or tricyclics **Precautions:** Alcoholism, breastfeeding, cardiac disease, child <6 yr, hepatic porphyria, AV or bundle branch block, glaucoma, pregnancy, psychosis, renal/hepatic disease **Pregnancy:** Evidence of fetal risk, but benefits outweigh risks	Benzodiazepines, cimetidine, cisplatin, clarithromycin, CYP3A4 inducers, CYP3A4 inhibitors, danzol, darunavir, delavirdine, desmopressin, diltiazem, doxorubicin, doxycycline, erythromycin, felbamate, fluoxetine, fluvoxamine, grapefruit juice, haloperidol, hypressin, isoniazid, lithium, MAOIs, nefazodone, NNRTIs, oral contraceptives, oxcarbazepine, phenobarbitol, phenytoin, primidone, propoxyphene, rifampin, theophylline, thyroid hormones, valproic acid, vasopressin, verapamil, voriconazole, warfarin
Oxcarbazepine	**Contraindications:** Hypersensitivity **Precautions:** Abrupt discontinuation, breastfeeding, children <4 yr, fluid restriction, hypersensitivity to carbamazepine, hyponatremia, pregnancy, renal disease, suicidal ideation **Pregnancy:** Only given after risks to the fetus are considered	Alcohol, carbamazepine, felpdipine, MAOIs, nisoldipine, oral contraceptives, phenobarbital, phenytoin

MAOI, monoamine oxidase inhibitor; *NNRTI*, nonnucleoside reverse-transcriptase inhibitor.
*Pregnancy categories have been revised. See http://www.fda.gov/Drugs/DevelopmentApprovalProcess/DevelopmentResources/Labeling/ucm093307.htm for more information.

Adverse/Side Effects
- Agranulocytosis
- Alopecia
- Anemia
- Aplastic anemia
- Ataxia
- AV block
- Blurred vision
- Confusion
- Congestive heart failure
- Depression
- Diplopia
- Dizziness
- Drowsiness
- Eosinophilia
- Hallucinations
- Headache
- Hepatic porphyria
- Hepatitis
- Hypercholesterolemia
- Hypertension
- Increased protime
- Infection
- Leukocytosis
- Leukopenia
- Lymphadenopathy
- Nausea
- Neuroleptic malignant syndrome (when used with psychotropics)
- Pancreatitis
- Paralysis
- Photosensitivity
- Rash
- Speech Disturbances
- Stevens-Johnson syndrome
- Suicidal ideation
- Thrombocytopenia
- Toxic epidermal necrolysis

- Unsteadiness
- Urticaria
- Vomiting
- Weakness
- Worsening of seizures

Nursing Care

- Assess eye problems, hypersensitivity, and serious skin reactions
- Assess mental status
- Assess seizure activity
- Teach patient to avoid alcohol
- Teach patient to avoid driving or activities requiring alertness
- Teach patient to immediately report skin rashes
- Teach patient to immediately report signs and symptoms of infection
- Teach patient to report suicidal thoughts/behavior immediately
- Teach patient to take as directed and not to discontinue medication quickly after long-term use
- Teach patient to use alternative contraception if using hormonal method, report if pregnancy is planned or suspected

APPLICATION AND REVIEW

14. What should the nurse monitor to evaluate the effectiveness of carbamazepine in the management of a client's trigeminal neuralgia?
    1. Pain intensity
    2. Liver function
    3. Cardiac output
    4. Seizure activity
15. A client diagnosed with tonic-clonic seizures is being considered for iminostilbene therapy. Which situation would likely prevent the client from safely being prescribed either carbamazepine or oxcarbazepine?
    1. Currently prescribed warfarin
    2. Has a history of bundle branch block
    3. Currently on MAOI antidepressant therapy
    4. Admits to having frequent suicidal ideations
16. The client has been prescribed oxcarbazepine. Which adverse reaction requires the nurse's priority attention to best assure client safety?
    1. Ataxia
    2. Depression
    3. Blurred vision
    4. Agranulocytosis
17. The client has been prescribed oxcarbazepine. Which nursing assessments are of particular importance to a client prescribed iminostilbene therapy for a seizure disorder? **Select all that apply.**
    1. Eye
    2. Skin
    3. Hearing
    4. Hematologic
    5. Gastrointestinal

See Answers on pages 63-66.

Other Antiepileptic Agents

- Used to control seizures
- Examples: valproate, gabapentin, lamotrigine, levetiracetam, tiagabine, topiramate, zonisamide, pregabalin, lacosamide, ezogabine, perampanel
- Available in oral preparations

Mode of Action

- Various modes of action; they work by affecting chemicals or nerves involved in the cause of seizures.

Contraindications, Precautions, and Drug Interactions of Other Antiepileptic Agents*

Drug	Contraindications/Precautions	Drug Interaction
Valproate, valproic acid	*Contraindications:* Hepatic disease, hypersensitivity, pancreatitis, urea cycle disorders *Precautions:* Breastfeeding, children <2 yr, geriatric, pregnancy *Pregnancy:* Evidence of fetal risk, but benefits outweigh risks.	Abciximab, alcohol, antidepressants, antihistamines, barbituates, cefoperazone, cefotetan, cimetidine, chlorpromazine, eptifibatide, erythromycin, felbamate, heparin, MAOIs, opiods, phenytoin, sedatives/hypnotics, tirofiban, tricyclics, warfarin
Gabapentin	*Contraindications:* Hypersensitivity to gabapentin *Precautions:* Breastfeeding, children <3 yr, depression, geriatric, hemodialysis, renal disease, pregnancy, suicidal thoughts *Pregnancy:* Only given after risks to the fetus are considered	Alcohol, antacids, antihistamines, cimetidine, CNS depressants, hydrocodone, morphine, sedatives, sevelamer
Lamotrigine	*Contraindications:* Hypersensitivity *Precautions:* Blood dyscrasias, breastfeeding, children <16 yr, depression, geriatric, renal/hepatic/cardiac disease, pregnancy, serious rash, suicidal thoughts *Pregnancy:* Only given after risks to the fetus are considered	Acetaminophen, carbamazepine, CYP3A4 inhibitors, estrogens, oral contraceptives, oxcarbazepine, phenobarbital, phenytoin, primidone, rifamycins, succinimides, valproic acid
Levetiracetam	*Contraindications:* Breastfeeding, hypersensitivity *Precautions:* Breastfeeding, cardiac/renal disease, geriatric, pregnancy, psychosis *Pregnancy:* Only given after risks to the fetus are considered	Alcohol, carbamazepine, sevelamer
Tiagabine	*Contraindications:* Hypersensitivity *Precautions:* Abrupt discontinuation, bipolar disorder, breastfeeding, child <12 yr, depression, geriatric, mania, pregnancy, renal/hepatic disease, status epilepticus, suicidal ideation/behavior *Pregnancy:* Only given after risks to the fetus are considered	Alcohol, carbamazepine, CNS depressants, phenobarbital, phenytoin, primidone, sevelamer, valproate
Topiramate	*Contraindications:* Hypersensitivity, metabolic acidosis, pregnancy *Precautions:* Acute myopia, behavioral disorders, breastfeeding, children, COPD, dialysis, glaucoma, maculopathy, nephrolithiasis, renal/hepatic disease, secondary closed-angle encephalopathy, status asthmaticus, status epilepticus, surgery, paresthesias *Pregnancy:* Evidence of fetal risk, but benefits outweigh risks	Acute myopia, behavioral disorders, breastfeeding, children, COPD, dialysis, encephalopathy, maculopathy, nephrolithiasis, paresthesias, renal/hepatic disease, secondary closed-angle glaucoma, status asthmaticus, status epilepticus, surgery
Zonisamide	*Contraindications:* Hypersensitivity to zonisamide or sulfonamides *Precautions:* Allergies, breastfeeding, children <16 yr, geriatric, hepatic failure, pregnancy, psychiatric condition, renal/hepatic disease *Pregnancy:* Only given after risks to the fetus are considered	Alcohol, carbamazepine, CYP3A4 inducers, CYP3A4 inhibitors, grapefruit juice, phenobarbital, phenytoin

Contraindications, Precautions, and Drug Interactions of Other Antiepileptic Agents—cont'd

Drug	Contraindications/Precautions	Drug Interaction
Pregabalin	*Contraindications:* Hypersensitivity to pregabalin or gabapentin *Precautions:* Angioedema history, breastfeeding, children <12 yr, creatine kinase elevations, congestive heart failure (class III, IV), decreased platelets, dependence, drug abuse, geriatric, glaucoma, myopathy, PR interval prolongation, pregnancy, renal disease, suicidal behavior *Pregnancy:* Only given after risks to the fetus are considered	Angioedema history, breastfeeding, children <12 yr, congestive heart failure (class III, IV), creatine kinase elevations, decreased platelets, dependence, drug abuse, geriatric, glaucoma, myopathy, PR interval prolongation, pregnancy, renal disease, suicidal behavior
Lacosamide	*Contraindications:* Hypersensitivity *Precautions:* Acute MI, allergies, atrial fibrillation/flutter, AV block, bradycardia, breastfeeding, cardiac disease, child <17 yr, congenital heart disease, dehydration, depression, dialysis, electrolyte imbalance, geriatric patients, hazardous activity, heart failure, labor, PR prolongation, pregnancy, renal/hepatic disease, sick sinus syndrome, substance abuse, suicidal ideation, syncope, torsades de pointes *Pregnancy:* Only given after risks to the fetus are considered	Atazanavir, beta blockers, calcium-channel blockers, CYP2C19 inhibitors, dronedarone, digoxin, lopinavir, ritonavir
Ezogabine	*Contraindications:* Hypersensitivity *Precautions:* Abrupt discontinuation, adolescents, breastfeeding, children, congestive heart failure, dementia, geriatrics, hepatic disease, hypokalemia, hypomagnesemia, infants, neonates, pregnancy, prostatic hypertrophy, psychotic disorders, QT prolongation, renal impairment, suicidal ideation/behavior, ventricular hypertrophy *Pregnancy:* Only given after risks to the fetus are considered	Amantadine, antimuscarinics, anxiolytics, arsenic trioxide, buprenorphine, butorphanol, carbamazepine, chloroquine, chlorpromazine, clarithromycin, Class IA antiarrhythmics, Class III antiarrhythmics, dextromethorphan, digoxin, dronabinol, dronedarone, droperidol, erythromycin, ethanol, grepafloxacin, H1-blockers, halofantrine, hypnotics, levomethadyl, mesoridazine, methadone, mirtazapine, nabilone, nalbuphine, opiate agonists, pentamidine, pentazocine, phenytoin, pimozide, posaconazole, pregabalin, probucol, propafenone, quinidine, saquinavir, sedatives, skeletal muscle relaxants, sparfloxacin, terfenadine, thioridazine, tramadol, trazodone, troleandomycin, ziprasidone
Perampanel	*Contraindications:* Hypersensitivity *Precautions:* Abrupt discontinuation, bipolar disorder, breastfeeding, children <12 yr, depression, driving or operating machinery, geriatric patients, kidney disease, liver disease, pregnancy, psychosis, schizophrenia, substance abuse, suicidal ideation *Pregnancy:* Only given after risks to the fetus are considered	Alcohol, antihistamines, benzodiazepines, CNS depressants, CYP3A4 inducers, CYP3A4 inhibitors, oral/implant contraceptives with levonorgestrel/estrogen, sedatives

COPD, chronic obstructive pulmonary disease; *CNS*, central nervous system; *MAOI*, monoamine oxidase inhibitor; *yr*, year.
*Pregnancy categories have been revised. See http://www.fda.gov/Drugs/DevelopmentApprovalProcess/DevelopmentResources/Labeling/ucm093307.htm for more information.

Adverse/Side Effects

- Agranulocytosis
- Anemia
- Angioedema
- Aplastic anemia
- Atrial fibrillation
- Atrial flutter
- AV block
- Coma
- Confusion
- Constipation
- DIC
- Dizziness
- DRESS syndrome
- Drowsiness
- Granulocytopenia
- Headache
- Hepatic failure
- Hepatitis
- Hepatotoxicity
- Leukopenia
- Lymphocytosis
- Nausea
- Neutropenia
- Pancreatitis
- Pancytopenia
- PR prolongation
- Rash
- Sedation
- Seizures
- Status epilepticus
- Stevens-Johnson syndrome
- Suicidal ideation
- Thrombocytopenia
- Toxic epidermal necrolysis
- Toxic hepatitis
- Vomiting

Nursing Care

- Assess for cardiovascular status
- Assess for hypersensitive reactions
- Assess for rash; product should be discontinued at first sign of rash
- Assess for seizure activity
- Assess mental status; assess for suicidal thoughts or behaviors
- Assess renal function
- Assess urine function
- Teach patient not to breastfeed
- Teach patient not to discontinue product abruptly
- Teach patient to avoid driving or hazardous activities until stabilized on medication
- Teach patient to avoid grapefruit juice
- Teach patient to notify prescriber immediately of suicidal thoughts or behaviors
- Teach patient to notify prescriber of skin rash or increased seizure activity
- Teach patient to report to prescriber if pregnancy is suspected or planned and to avoid breastfeeding
- Teach patient to use nonhormonal contraception
- Teach patient to use sunscreen and protective clothing
- Teach patient to wear emergency ID

APPLICATION AND REVIEW

18. A nurse is evaluating the medication regimens of a group of clients to determine whether the therapeutic level has been achieved. For which medication should the nurse review the client's serum blood level?
    1. Sertraline
    2. Lorazepam
    3. Olanzapine
    4. Valproic acid

See Answers on pages 63-66.

ANSWER KEY: REVIEW QUESTIONS

1. **2 Monitoring of the seizure activity, the body parts involved, the area of its progression, and the length of the episode, as well as the activity of the head and eyes, characteristics of the respiration, and alteration in consciousness provides information that assists in the identification of the type of seizure and, thus, its treatment.**

   1 Inserting an oral airway is contraindicated. Attempting to insert an oral airway may injure the client and/or the nurse. **3** Turning the client on the side should be done after the tonic-clonic phase of the seizure subsides. **4** Beginning oxygen is unnecessary because breathing does not occur during a seizure; this may be done after the seizure.

   Client Need: Safety and Infection Control; **Cognitive Level:** Application; **Nursing Process:** Assessment/Analysis

2. **4 A seizure is generally self-limiting; the nurse's responsibilities include protecting the client from injury and assessing the characteristics of the seizure.**

   1 Nothing should be forced into the client's mouth when the teeth are clenched during a seizure; this may damage the teeth or cause an airway occlusion if improperly placed. **2** During a seizure the client loses consciousness and will be unable to discuss any aura experienced. **3** Anticonvulsants are given on a regular basis, not prn, to achieve therapeutic levels.

   Client Need: Safety and Infection Control; **Cognitive Level:** Application; **Nursing Process:** Planning/Implementation

3. **4 To achieve the anticonvulsant effect, therapeutic blood levels must be maintained. If the client is not able to take the prescribed oral preparation, the health care provider should be questioned about alternate routes of administration.**

   1 Omission will result in lowered blood levels, possibly to less than the necessary therapeutic level to prevent a seizure. **2** The route of administration cannot be altered without health care provider approval. **3** The client is being kept NPO.

   Client Need: Management of Care; **Cognitive Level:** Application; **Nursing Process:** Planning/Implementation

4. **2 Anticonvulsant therapy is usually continued throughout one's life.**

   1 The question about how long the therapy might last is a question the nurse can and should answer. It is not appropriate to refer such questions to another health care provider. **3.** Encouraging the client, "not to worry" is a nontherapeutic response that minimizes the client's concerns; something the nurse should never do. **4** Although there is some truth to that statement, that the length of treatment is client specific, in this situation there is reason to believe the treatment will last a lifetime.

   Client Need: Pharmacologic and Parenteral Therapies; **Cognitive Level:** Analysis; **Integrated Process:** Teaching/Learning; **Nursing Process:** Planning and Implementation

5. **1 Seizure disorders usually are associated with marked changes in the electrical activity of the cerebral cortex, requiring prolonged or lifelong therapy.**

   2 Seizures may occur despite drug therapy; the dosage may need to be adjusted. **3** A therapeutic blood level must be maintained through consistent administration of the drug irrespective of emotional stress. **4** Absence of seizures will probably result from medication effectiveness rather than from correction of the pathophysiologic condition.

   Client Need: Pharmacologic and Parenteral Therapies; **Cognitive Level:** Application; **Integrated Process:** Teaching/Learning; **Nursing Process:** Planning/Implementation

6. **2 Phenytoin is an anticonvulsant most effective in controlling tonic-clonic seizures. Data collection before planning nursing care for a client with a seizure disorder should always include a history of the seizures (e.g., type and incidence).**

   1 Although protection is important, the use of restraints and insertion of an object into the mouth during a seizure often causes injury as a result of tonic-clonic muscle contractions and should not be used.

3 Although dentures and eyeglasses may be removed during a seizure, the client's normal routines should be respected. **4** Increased restlessness may be evidence of the prodromal phase of a seizure in some individuals, but signs and symptoms vary so widely that the client's history should be obtained.

Client Need: Pharmacologic and Parenteral Therapies; **Cognitive Level:** Application; **Nursing Process:** Assessment/Analysis

7. **Answer: 8 mL**

Use the "Desire over Have" formula of ratio and proportion to solve this problem.

$$\frac{\text{Desire}}{\text{Have}} \frac{200 \text{ mg}}{125 \text{ mg}} = \frac{x \text{ ml}}{5 \text{ mL}}$$

$$125x = 200 \times 5$$

$$125x = 1,000$$

$$x = 1,000 \div 125$$

$$x = 8 \text{ mL}$$

Client Need: Pharmacologic and Parenteral Therapies; **Cognitive Level:** Application; **Nursing Process:** Planning/Implementation

8. **1 Gingival hyperplasia is an adverse effect of long-term phenytoin therapy; incidence can be decreased by maintaining therapeutic blood levels and meticulous oral hygiene.**

2 Alkalinity is not related to phenytoin or to gingival hyperplasia caused by phenytoin. **3** Irritation of the gingiva and destruction of tooth enamel are not direct effects of phenytoin. **4** Plaque and bacterial growth at gum line are unrelated to phenytoin or to hyperplasia caused by it.

Client Need: Pharmacologic and Parenteral Therapies; **Cognitive Level:** Application; **Integrated Process:** Teaching/Learning; **Nursing Process:** Planning/Implementation

9. **1 Phenytoin inhibits folic acid absorption and potentiates the effects of folic acid antagonists. Folic acid is helpful in correcting certain anemias that can result from administration of phenytoin. The dosage must be carefully adjusted because folic acid diminishes the effects of phenytoin.**

2, 3, 4 These are not effects of folic acid. Folic acid does not potentiate phenytoin, improve absorption of iron from foods, or prevent neuropathy caused by phenytoin.

Client Need: Pharmacologic and Parenteral Therapies; **Cognitive Level:** Comprehension; **Integrated Process:** Communication/Documentation; **Nursing Process:** Assessment/Analysis

10. **1 Warfarin has been shown to inhibit metabolism of phenytoin, which results in an accumulation of phenytoin in the body. Additionally, phenytoin can substantially increase the rate at which warfarin is metabolized.**

2 Warfarin potentiates the anticoagulant effect of heparin. **3** 'Warfarin's action is greater in clients with seizure disorders': this is true only if the client is receiving phenytoin to control the seizure disorder. **4** Seizures do not have a significant effect on the metabolism of warfarin.

Client Need: Pharmacologic and Parenteral Therapies; **Cognitive Level:** Analysis; **Nursing Process:** Assessment/Analysis

---

Study Tip: To recall that the formula is "Desire over Have", write Desire, a line underneath it, and Have beneath the line, like this:

$$\frac{\text{Desire}}{\text{Have}}$$

Post this on your mirror or somewhere you will see it daily. Also consider that D comes before H in the alphabet, so write D first.

---

11. **Answer: 2.4 mL**

Use the "Desire over Have" formula of ratio and proportion to solve this problem.

$$\frac{\text{Desire}}{\text{Have}} \quad \frac{60 \text{ mg}}{125 \text{ mg}} = \frac{x \text{ ml}}{5 \text{ mL}}$$

$$125x = 300$$

$$x = 300 \div 125$$

$$x = 2.4 \text{ mL}$$

Client Need: Pharmacologic and Parenteral Therapies; **Cognitive Level:** Application; **Nursing Process:** Planning/Implementation

12. **Answer: 2.8**

Use the "Desire over Have" formula of ratio and proportion to solve this problem.

If 140 mg is divided into two doses, 70 mg will be given per dose. Use ratio and proportion to calculate the amount to be administered.

$$\frac{\text{Desire}}{\text{Have}} \quad \frac{70 \text{ mg}}{125 \text{ mg}} = \frac{x \text{ ml}}{5 \text{ mL}}$$

$$125x = 300$$

$$x = 300 \div 125$$

$$x = 2.8 \text{ mL}$$

Client Need: Pharmacologic and Parenteral Therapies; **Cognitive Level:** Application; **Nursing Process:** Planning/Implementation

13. **Answer: 3**

When an oral medication is available in a suspension form, the nurse can use it for clients who cannot swallow capsules. Use the "Desire over Have" formula to solve the problem.

$$\frac{\text{Desire}}{\text{Have}} \quad \frac{100 \text{ mg}}{125 \text{ mg}} = \frac{x \text{ ml}}{5 \text{ mL}}$$

$$125x = 500$$

$$x = 500 \div 125$$

$$x = 4 \text{ mL}$$

1 Because a palatable suspension is available, it is a better alternative than opening the capsule. **2** The route of administration cannot be altered without the health care provider's approval. **4** Intramuscular injections should be avoided because of risks for tissue injury and infection.

Client Need: Pharmacologic and Parenteral Therapies; **Cognitive Level:** Application; **Nursing Process:** Planning/Implementation

14. **1 Carbamazepine is administered to control pain by reducing transmission of nerve impulses in clients with trigeminal neuralgia.**

2 Liver function is monitored to detect adverse reactions to carbamazepine, not to determine therapeutic effectiveness. **3** Carbamazepine is not given to influence cardiac output. **4** Carbamazepine is not administered to clients with trigeminal neuralgia (tic douloureux) for its anticonvulsant properties because seizures are not present with this disorder.

Client Need: Pharmacologic and Parenteral Therapies; **Cognitive Level:** Application; **Nursing Process:** Evaluation/Outcomes

> **Study Tip:** If you were having trouble recalling that trigeminal neuralgia is painful, remember to look for common medical word parts within terms: -algia is a suffix meaning pain; neuralgia is neur/o + -algia, so neuralgia means nerve pain.

15. **3 MAOI antidepressants produce a drug interaction when administered with both carbamazepine and oxcarbazepine. This situation would prevent either medication from being prescribed.**
    1 Warfarin produces a drug interaction when administered with carbamazepine. **2** A bundle branch block is a precautionary risk to be seriously considered when prescribing carbamazepine. **4** Suicidal ideations are precautionary risks to be seriously considered when prescribing oxcarbazepine.
    Client Need: Pharmacologic and Parenteral Therapies; **Cognitive Level:** Application; **Nursing Process:** Planning and Implementation

16. **4 Agranulocytosis is a deficiency of granulocytes in the blood, causing increased vulnerability to infection. The risk for infection is a safety issue that requires priority attention by the nurse regarding the implementation of appropriate interventions.**
    1 Ataxia, a lack of muscle control, does produce a potential risk for injuries especially related to falls. The risk for falls, although serious, does not have the same priority as a systemic risk like infection. **2** Depression does produce a potential risk for injuries especially related to suicide, The risk for suicide, although serious, does not have the same priority as a systemic risk like infection. **3** Blurred vision does produce a potential risk for injuries, especially related to falls. The risk for falls, although serious, does not have the same priority as a systemic risk like infection.
    Client Need: Pharmacologic and Parenteral Therapies; **Cognitive Level:** Analysis; **Nursing Process:** Assessment/Analysis

17. **Answers: 1, 2, 4**
    Iminostilbene therapy increases the client's risk for the development of eye-related problems like diplopia, blurred vision, photosensitivity, and the exacerbation of glaucoma. Iminostilbene therapy also raises the risk for rashes and urticaria making a skin assessment a priority. Finally, the client is at risk for thrombocytopenia, leukopenia, leukocytosis, eosinophilia, agranulocytosis, and anemia.
    3 Iminostilbene therapy is not known to pose a significant risk to hearing. **5** Although vomiting (GI related) may occur, generally all clients have a gastrointestinal assessment.
    Client Need: Pharmacologic and Parenteral Therapies; **Cognitive Level:** Application; **Integrated Process:** Teaching/Learning; **Nursing Process:** Assessment/Analysis

18. **4 Valproic acid must reach a therapeutic level to be effective, and the serum level must be monitored for therapeutic and toxic levels of the drug.**
    1, 2, 3 The serum drug levels are not monitored with Sertraline, Lorazepam, or Olanzapine.
    Client Need: Pharmacologic and Parenteral Therapies; **Cognitive Level:** Analysis; **Nursing Process:** Planning/Implementation

Psychotherapeutic Drugs   5

INTRODUCTION TO MENTAL HEALTH DISORDERS

Affective Disorders

Overview of Anxiety

- Description of anxiety
  - Diffuse feeling of uneasiness, uncertainty, and helplessness that occurs as a result of a threat to an individual's self-concept, esteem, identity, or safety
  - Usual response to a real or perceived threat
  - Different from fear, which has a specific source or object that can be identified and described
  - An emotion that is subjective in nature and without a specific object
  - Related to one's culture, because culture influences one's values
  - Causes are uncertain, but research indicates a combination of physical, psychosocial, and environmental factors
  - Activates the fight-or-flight response in the autonomic nervous system
- Levels of anxiety
  - Mild—alertness level: automatic response of the central nervous system (CNS) that prepares the body for danger by regulating internal processes and concentrating all energies for internal activity; perceptual field is increased; may enhance learning
    - Moderate—apprehension level: response to anticipation of short-term threat that prepares the individual for efficient performance; perceptual field is narrowed, because focus is on the immediate concern
    - Severe—high anxiety level: focus is on a specific detail, and behavior is aimed at relieving anxiety; needs direction by others to focus on another detail or area; marked reduction in the perceptual field limits cognitive abilities
    - Panic—extreme level: involves disorganization of the personality and is associated with dread and terror; communication abilities and problem solving are nonexistent; has great difficulty following commands even with direction; perceptual field is distorted; prolonged period of panic results in exhaustion and death; intervention is essential
- Common defense mechanisms against anxiety
  - Compensation: the individual makes up for a perceived lack in one area by emphasizing capabilities in another
  - Identification: the individual internalizes characteristics of an idealized person
  - Rationalization: the individual makes acceptable excuses for behavior, feelings, outcomes; attempts to explain behavior by logical reasoning but does not address underlying feelings
  - Sublimation: the individual substitutes a socially acceptable behavior for an unacceptable instinct
    - Substitution: the individual replaces an unacceptable emotion or goal by another that is more acceptable
  - Conversion: emotional conflict is unconsciously changed into a physical symptom that can be expressed openly and without anxiety

- Denial: emotional conflict is blocked from the conscious mind, and the individual cannot recognize its existence
- Displacement: emotions related to an emotionally charged situation or object are shifted to a relatively safe substitute situation or object
- Dissociation: separation of any group of mental or behavioral processes from the rest of the individual's consciousness or identity
- Fantasy: conscious distortion of unconscious wishes and needs to obtain gratification and satisfaction
- Intellectualization: use of thinking, ideas, or intellect to avoid emotions
- Introjection: acceptance of another's opinions and values as one's own
- Projection: unconscious denial of unacceptable feelings and emotions in oneself while attributing them to others
- Reaction formation: unconscious prevention of unacceptable thoughts or behaviors from being expressed by exaggerating opposite thoughts or behaviors
- Regression: return to an earlier stage of behavior when stress is overwhelming at the present stage of development
- Repression: involuntary exclusion from consciousness of those ideas, feelings, and situations that are creating conflict and causing discomfort
- Splitting: viewing others or situations as either all good or all bad; failure to integrate the positive and negative qualities in oneself
- Suppression: voluntary exclusion from consciousness of those ideas, feelings, and situations that are creating conflict and causing discomfort
  - Undoing: act or communication that attempts to compensate for or negate a previous one

Generalized Anxiety Disorder (GAD)

- Etiologic factors
  - Psychologic, behavioral, and neurobiologic theories are postulated; the latter is most promising
  - Functions to permit some measure of social adjustment
  - Commonly begins in early adulthood as a result of environmental factors and pressures of decision making; early life is rigid and orderly
  - Excessive anxiety and worry involves at least two life situations
  - Unrelated to physiologic effects of substances or a medical condition
- Behavioral/clinical findings
  - Persistent anxiety (longer than 6 months) and excessive worry associated with three or more of the following symptoms: restlessness (akathisia) or feeling on-edge, becomes easily fatigued, difficulty concentrating, irritability, muscle tension, and sleep disturbance
    - Inability to control the anxiety
    - Impairment in social or occupational relationships
  - Symptoms of autonomic hyperarousal (e.g., tachycardia, tachypnea, dizziness, and dilated pupils); however, they are less prominent than in other anxiety disorders
- Therapeutic interventions
  - Provide an environment that limits demands and permits attention to resolution of conflicts; establish a trusting relationship
  - Identify precipitating stressors and limit them if possible
  - Intervene to protect from acting out on impulses that may be harmful to self or others
  - Accept symptoms as real to client; do not emphasize or call attention to them

- Attempt to limit client's use of negative defenses, but do not try to stop them until ready to give them up
- Help to develop appropriate ways of managing anxiety-producing situations through problem solving and cognitive/behavioral therapies; assist to expand supportive network; assist significant others to understand the client's situation
- Plan a routine schedule of activities
- Manage aggressive behavior progressively (e.g., diversion, limit setting, medication administration, seclusion, restraints)
- Collect and document information to assist with determining presence of both an anxiety disorder and depression (comorbidity)
- Encourage to develop a balance between work and relaxation

Overview of Bipolar Disorder

- Description of bipolar disorder
  - Characterized by a cyclical disturbance of mood, encompassing emotional extremes: episodes of vehement energy of mania, despair and lethargy of depression, or a mixture of both
  - Presence of one or more manic or hypomanic episodes with a history of depressive episodes; predominant mood is elevated or irritable, accompanied by one or more of these symptoms: hyperactivity, lack of judgment with no regard for consequences, pressured speech, flight of ideas, distractibility, inflated self-esteem, risky behavior, and hypersexuality
    - Hypomanic: mood elation with higher than usual activity and social interaction, but not as expansive as full mania; a distinct period of elevated or irritable mood that is different from mania; duration of at least 4 days
    - Mania: elevated, expansive, or irritable mood accompanied by hyperactivity, grandiosity, and loss of reality
- Etiologic factors
  - Neurotransmitters, or certain chemicals in the brain that regulate mood, have been identified (e.g., serotonin, dopamine, norepinephrine, and gamma-aminobutyric acid [GABA])
    - Increased levels of norepinephrine, dopamine, and serotonin in acute mania
      - Decreased levels of norepinephrine, dopamine, and serotonin in depression
  - Family and twin studies suggest a genetic component, but no gene has been identified except in rare, familial forms of the disorder
  - Biologic rhythms and physiology related to depression show abnormal sleep electroencephalogram (EEG), sensitivity to absence of sunlight, and circadian rhythm disturbance
  - Drugs associated with depressive status: alcohol, sedative-hypnotics, amphetamine withdrawal, glucocorticoids, propranolol, risperidone, and steroid contraceptives
  - Drugs associated with manic status: cocaine, MAOIs, tricyclic antidepressants, steroids, and levodopa
  - Physical illness, such as brain attack (cerebrovascular accident) and some endocrine disorders (e.g., Cushing disease and hypothyroidism) can lead to depressive episodes
  - Obesity is a related factor to depression
- May be response to loss (dysfunctional grieving), increased stress, or change in life events, role, and sleeping and/or eating patterns; overreaction to stress may lead to suicide
- Generally occurs between 20 and 40 years of age; however, reported in clients older than 50 years, and increasingly in children and adolescents

Depressive Episode of Bipolar Disorder

- Behavioral/clinical findings of depressive episode
  - Either a depressed mood or loss of interest or pleasure, occurring during a 2-week period, with a change in level of functioning, plus five or more of the following:
    - Change in weight
    - Insomnia (especially early morning awakening)
    - Psychomotor agitation or retardation
    - Fatigue
    - Worthless feelings or inappropriate guilt
    - Somatic complaints
    - Diminished hygiene
    - Concentration difficulties
    - Inability to make decisions
    - Social withdrawal
      - Pessimism
      - Suicidal behavior progresses from suicidal ideation, suicide threats, suicide gestures, suicide attempts, to successful suicides; presuicidal behaviors include no interest in the future, giving away personal possessions
  - Orientation and logic unaffected
  - Sex drive (libido) decreased
  - Constipation and urinary retention
  - Anniversary reaction: depression and suicidal gestures may increase as anniversary of loss of loved object nears
- Therapeutic interventions
  - Antidepressant medications that increase the level of norepinephrine and serotonin
  - Cognitive and behavioral psychotherapy
  - High-protein, high-carbohydrate diet; dietary supplements if necessary
  - Electroconvulsive therapy (ECT)

Manic Episode of Bipolar Disorder

- Behavioral/clinical findings
  - Persistently elevated, expansive, or irritable mood for a duration of 1 week, plus three or more of the following:
    - Grandiosity
    - Insomnia
    - Verbosity (pressured speech)
    - Flight of ideas
    - Hypersexuality
    - Distractibility
    - Social intrusiveness
    - Psychomotor agitation
    - Excessive involvement in pleasurable activities without regard for consequences (e.g., shopping, gambling, sexual activity)
  - Marked impairment in daily functioning, occupational and social activities, and relationships
  - Excessive overactivity requiring hospitalization to prevent harm to self or others
  - Symptoms are unrelated to physical illness or physiologic effects of a substance

- Therapeutic interventions
  - High-protein, high-carbohydrate diet; handheld foods should be available; adequate fluids
  - Behavioral and cognitive therapy when medication has decreased mania
  - Pharmacologic approach: improves productivity by decreasing psychomotor activity or response to environmental stimuli

Major Depressive Disorder (MDD)

- Etiologic factors
  - See information under Bipolar Disorder and Depressive Episode of a Bipolar Disorder
  - Neurotransmitter dysregulation includes serotonin, norepinephrine, dopamine, acetylcholine, and GABA systems; altered neuropeptides include corticotropin-releasing hormones
  - Individuals with chronic or severe medical conditions are at increased risk
  - Psychosocial stressors associated with a major loss play a significant role in first or second depressive onset
  - Familial history among close biologic relatives increases risk for disorder
  - Onset usually in late 20s, but may occur across life span
- Behavioral/clinical findings
  - Recurrent pessimistic thoughts; suicidal ideation with or without a plan
  - Interruption in thinking and concentration that may interfere with occupational and social functioning; difficulty making decisions
  - Diminished interest or pleasure in all activities (anhedonia); apathy
  - Decreased appetite with weight loss or overeating with weight gain
  - Psychomotor retardation; anergia; constipation
  - Anxiety, somatic ailments, tearfulness, fearfulness, and hopelessness
  - Insomnia or hypersomnia
  - Feelings of worthlessness
  - Inappropriate guilt
- Therapeutic interventions
  - See Depressive Episode of a Bipolar Disorder

PSYCHOTIC DISORDERS

Schizophrenia

- Etiologic factors
  - Foremost etiology is the biologic perspective (e.g., neuroanatomy, genetics, endocrinology, and immunology all produce symptoms; trauma and disease as causation continue to be researched)
  - Biologic components
    - Heredity and genetics
    - Neuroanatomic differences and neurochemicals (e.g., dopamine hyperactivity or over-production)
      - Structure and function of nervous system
      - Teratogenic drug exposure
      - Neuroanatomic differences in brain (e.g., enlarged ventricles)
    - Neurotransmitter function: abnormal neurotransmitter-endocrine interactions
    - Immunologic factors: viral exposure during pregnancy

- High arousal levels from stress, disease, drugs, and trauma
  - Stress such as bombardment of stimuli from life events may contribute to relapse and return of symptoms
  - Diseases such as encephalitis
  - Trauma from birth complications, head trauma
  - Drugs such as cannabis and cocaine
- Psychosocial considerations are significant; causative models postulate that biologic vulnerability interacts with stressful environmental influences
- Onset in men usually between ages 18 and 25 years; later onset for women, between 25 and 35 years; incidence slightly higher in men
- Chronic insecurity and failure in interpersonal relationships impair functioning
- Disturbed relationship with environment and family is an almost universal characteristic regardless of the etiology
- Course of disease is either acute or chronic; some demonstrate almost normal functioning with intermittent psychotic episodes; others have diminished functioning with intermittent psychotic episodes; about 10% to 25% demonstrate severely diminished functioning with ongoing psychotic symptoms
- Types
  - Classification of types is not static; there is overlapping symptomatology; individuals diagnosed in one classification frequently are diagnosed at a later time in another classification
  - Paranoid: delusions of persecution and/or grandiosity; less often noted are delusional themes of jealousy, religiosity, or somatization
  - Disorganized: disorganized speech and behavior; childlike affect and uninhibited sexual behaviors; socially inept
  - Catatonic type: marked psychomotor disturbance that may involve motor immobility (waxy flexibility), excessive motor activity, extreme negativism, mutism, posturing, echolalia, or echopraxia
  - Undifferentiated: delusions, hallucinations, disorganized speech, disorganized behavior; excludes behaviors observed in paranoid, disorganized, or catatonic types
  - Residual: criteria for schizophrenia subtypes previously listed are not met; there is continuing evidence of negative symptoms and two or more of these characteristic symptoms (e.g., delusions, hallucinations, disorganized speech, and gross disorganization); develops later in the course of the disease
- Behavioral/clinical findings
  - Characteristic symptoms generally fall into two broad categories
    - Positive symptoms (additional behaviors)
      - Disorganized or bizarre alterations in thinking, speech, perception (e.g., altered reality testing, hallucinations, delusions), behavior, and mood
      - More apparent during acute relapses
      - More responsive to medication and interactive therapies
    - Negative symptoms (deficits of behaviors)
      - Flat affect, apathy/avolition, anhedonia, and attention deficit
      - More apparent during nonacute periods
      - Less responsive to therapy; more complex and difficult to treat
  - Problems in cognitive functioning: attention deficits, abstract concept formation, decision making, and problem solving
  - Alterations in mood: dysphoria, suicidality, and hopelessness; approximately 15% commit suicide
  - Ability to test reality is distorted by psychopathology

- Social and occupational role dysfunction
- Duration of at least 6 months
- Therapeutic interventions
  - Psychotherapy (e.g., individual, family, group)
  - Motivational therapy
  - Occupational and vocational therapy
  - Daycare treatment programs in community settings that foster interpersonal relationships
  - Pharmacologic therapy
    - Positive symptoms: traditional antipsychotic drugs
    - Negative symptoms: atypical antipsychotic drugs
  - Paranoid schizophrenia is most responsive to treatment compared with other subtypes; clients appear to function at a higher level

Delusional/Paranoia Disorders

- Etiologic factors
  - Neurobiologic perspective
    - Exact physiologic disruption is not well-defined
    - Psychotic disorders thought to involve: neurochemicals such as dopamine, serotonin, and norepinephrine; abnormal transmission of neural impulses; and difficulties at the synaptic level
    - Neurologic and cognitive impairments are fewer and prognosis seems better than other subtypes of schizophrenia
    - See Biologic components under Schizophrenic Disorders
  - Paranoid defenses considered by some to be a protective mechanism against unconscious homosexuality or overt hostility
  - Premorbid personality used the compensatory mechanisms of the projective pattern of behavior
  - Cultural and religious background variations
  - Course varies but is more hopeful than other psychotic disorders, because they are most responsive to treatment
- Behavioral/clinical findings
  - Elaborate, highly organized paranoid delusional system while preserving other functions of the personality
  - Delusions (fixed false beliefs) draw from real-life situations and have a coherent theme; delusions are not bizarre; usually limited to specific areas in client's life; predominant theme determines type of paranoia (e.g., grandiose, jealous, persecutory)
  - Suspiciousness and delusions do not exhibit the thinking and behavioral disorganization or the personality disintegration found in the other psychoses
  - Hallucinations usually are auditory and relate to the delusional theme
  - Intellectual and occupational functioning less impaired than social or marital relationships
- Types
  - Erotomanic: belief that another person is in love with client; idealized, romantic love or spiritual union, rather than sexual attraction
  - Grandiose: belief that client has some great (but unrecognized) talent or insight or has made an important discovery; less commonly, claims a special relationship with a prominent person or is a prominent person
  - Jealous: belief of unfaithfulness by one's spouse or lover based on incorrect inferences

- Persecutory: belief that client is being conspired against, spied upon, cheated, followed, poisoned or drugged, maligned, harassed, or obstructed in the pursuit of long-term goals
- Somatic: belief that something abnormal or dangerous is happening to the body
- Therapeutic interventions
  - Pharmacotherapy with antipsychotic agents
  - Individual psychotherapy

Schizoaffective Disorder

- Etiologic factors
  - Unrelated to direct physiologic effects of a substance or medication or a general medical condition
  - Uninterrupted period of illness including a major depressive episode or manic episode concurrent with symptoms of schizophrenia (e.g., delusions or hallucinations, disorganized speech or behavior, and negative symptoms)
  - Onset in early adulthood
- Behavioral/clinical findings
  - Mixture of symptoms associated with both schizophrenia and mood disorders (mania or depression)
  - Thought processes and bizarre behavior appear schizophrenic in conjunction with alterations in mood (e.g., marked elation, depression)
- Therapeutic interventions
  - Antipsychotic and/or mood stabilizers; antidepressants may be used to treat symptoms
  - Therapy depends on type and severity of symptoms

PARKINSON'S DISEASE

Parkinson's Disease

- Etiologic factors
  - Mostly unknown
  - Possible exposure to toxins: manganese dust, carbon monoxide, permethrin, maneb, beta-hexachlorocyclohexane, Agent Orange
  - Affects extrapyramidal system of corpus striatum, globus pallidus, substantia nigra
  - Dopamine deficiency in basal ganglia that connects the substantia nigra to the corpus striatum
  - Reduction of dopamine in corpus striatum impedes normal balance of dopamine and acetylcholine
- Behavioral/clinical findings
  - Pseudoparkinsonism (extrapyramidal syndrome)
    - Akinesia
    - Muscle rigidity
    - "Pill rolling" tremor
    - Dysarthria
    - Dysphagia
    - Mood changes
- Therapeutic interventions
  - Antiparkinsonian agents
  - Deep brain stimulation
  - Physical therapy
  - Cognitive behavioral therapy

APPLICATION AND REVIEW

1. A client is scheduled for a 6-week electroconvulsive therapy (ECT) treatment program. What intervention is important during the 6-week course of treatment?
    1. Provision of tyramine-free meals
    2. Avoidance of exposure to the sun
    3. Maintenance of a steady sodium intake
    4. Elimination of benzodiazepines for nighttime sedation
2. Antipsychotic drugs can cause extrapyramidal side effects. Which responses should the nurse document as indicating pseudoparkinsonism? **Select all that apply.**
    1. Rigidity
    2. Tremors
    3. Mydriasis
    4. Photophobia
    5. Bradykinesia

See Answers on pages 99-102.

DRUGS USED TO TREAT AFFECTIVE DISORDERS

Anxiolytics

- Used in the treatment of anxiety
- Examples include alprazolam, chlordiazepoxide, chlorpromazine, clonazepam, diazepam, buspirone, hydroxyzine, paroxetine
- Available in PO, IM, IV, rectal preparations

Mode of Action

- Potentiates brain chemicals that help decrease anxiety

Contraindications, Precautions, and Drug Interactions of Anxiolytics*

Drug	Contraindications/Precautions	Drug Interaction
alprazolam	*Contraindications:* Hypersensitivity to benzodiazepines, breastfeeding, addiction, closed angle glaucoma, psychosis *Precautions:* Geriatric patients, debilitated patients, hepatic disease, obesity, severe pulmonary disease *Pregnancy:* Definite fetal risks, may be given in spite of risks if needed in life-threatening conditions	CYP3A4 inhibitors, CYP3A4 inducers, alcohol, anticonvulsants, opioids, antihistamines, sedative/hypnotics, xanthines, levopoda, cigarette smoking
chlordiazepoxide	*Contraindications:* Hypersensitivity to benzodiazepines, breastfeeding, children <6 yr, psychosis, closed angle glaucoma *Precautions:* Geriatric patients, debilitated patients, hepatic/renal disease, abrupt discontinuation, respiratory depression, suicidal ideation, myasthenia gravis, Parkinson's disease *Pregnancy:* Definite fetal risks, may be given in spite of risks if needed in life-threatening conditions	Alcohol, CNS, CYP450 inducers, depressants, cimetidine, disulfiram, fluoxetine, isoniazid, ketoconazole, metoprolol, oral contraceptives, propranolol, valproic acid, levodopa, CYP3A4 inhibitors

Continued

Contraindications, Precautions, and Drug Interactions of Anxiolytics—cont'd

Drug	Contraindications/Precautions	Drug Interaction
chlorpromazine	**Contraindications:** Hypersensitivity, children <6 months, cerebral arteriosclerosis, coronary disease, coma, circulatory collapse, liver damage **Precautions:** Breastfeeding, geriatric patients, renal/hepatic/cardiac disease, closed-angle glaucoma, hypertension, seizure disorder, pulmonary disease, Parkinson's disease, prostatic enlargement, severe hypo/hypertension, brain damage, blood dyscrasias, alcohol/barbiturate withdrawal, bone marrow depression **Pregnancy:** Only given after risks to the fetus are considered; animal studies have shown adverse reactions; no human studies available	Alcohol, CNS depressants, antidepressants, sedatives/hypnotics, barbiturates, antihistamines, epinephrine, beta blockers, thyroid agents, anticholinergics, antiparkinsonian agents, MAOIs, valproic acid, anticonvulsants, cimetidine, antacids, levodopa, cromocriptine, lithium, warfarin
clonazepam	**Contraindications:** Hypersensitivity to benzodiazepines, acute closed-angle glaucoma, psychosis, severe hepatic disease **Precautions:** Breastfeeding, geriatric patients, renal/hepatic/respiratory disease, open-angle glaucoma **Pregnancy:** Definite fetal risks, may be given in spite of risks if needed in life-threatening conditions	Oral contraceptives, CYP3A4 inhibitors, CYP3A4 inducers, alcohol, barbiturates, opiates, antidepressants, anticonvulsants, sedatives, hypnotics, general anesthetics
diazepam	**Contraindications:** Hypersensitivity to benzodiazepines, closed-angle glaucoma, sleep apnea, hepatic disease, ethanol intoxication, myasthenia gravis, coma **Precautions:** Breastfeeding, children <6 months, geriatric patients, debilitated patients, substance abuse, smoking, asthma, bipolar disorder, renal disease, asthma, COPD, CNS depression, labor, psychosis, seizures, Parkinson's disease, neutropenia **Pregnancy:** Definite fetal risks, may be given in spite of risks if needed in life-threatening conditions	Barbiturates, CNS depressants, cimetidine, SSRIs, CYP3A4 inhibitors, CYP450 inducers, valproic acid, alcohol, amiodarone, diltiazem, protease inhibitors, amiodarone, clarithromycin, disulfiram, erythromycin, fluconazole, nicardipine, verapamil, ketoconazole
buspirone	**Contraindications:** Hypersensitivity, children <18 yr **Precautions:** Breastfeeding, geriatric patients, impaired hepatic/renal function **Pregnancy:** No adverse effects in animals; no human studies available	CYP3A4 inducers, MAOIs, procarbazine, alcohol, psychotropic products, SSRIs, SNRIs, serotonin receptor agonists, rifampin
hydroxyzine	**Contraindications:** Hypersensitivity to hydroxyzine/cetirizine, pregnancy first trimester, acute asthma **Precautions:** Breastfeeding, pregnancy second/third trimester, geriatric patients, debilitated patients, asthma, renal/hepatic disease, closed-angle glaucoma, COPD, prostatic hypertrophy **Pregnancy:** Only given after risks to the fetus are considered; animal studies have shown adverse reactions; no human studies available	Alcohol, analgesics, barbiturates, opioids, sedatives, hypnotics, CNS depressants, antidepressants, MAOIs, atropine, haloperidol, phenothiazines, quinidine, disopyramide

Contraindications, Precautions, and Drug Interactions of Anxiolytics—cont'd

Drug	Contraindications/Precautions	Drug Interaction
paroxetine	**Contraindications:** Hypersensitivity **Precautions:** Breastfeeding, geriatric patients, renal/hepatic disease, history of mania, seizure **Pregnancy:** Definite fetal risks, may be given in spite of risks if needed in life-threatening conditions	MAOIs, alcohol, SSRIs, SNRIs, atypical psychotics, tricyclics, amphetamines, tramadol, sertotonin receptor agonists, methylphenidate, digoxin, pimozide, thioridazine, NSAIDs, salicylates, thrombolytics, anticoagulants, platelet inhibitors, cimetidine, theophylline, CYP2D6 inhibitors, phenytoin, phenobarbital

*Pregnancy categories have been revised. See http://www.fda.gov/Drugs/DevelopmentApprovalProcess/DevelopmentResources/Labeling/ucm093307.htm for more information.

Adverse/Side Effects

- Headache
- Confusion
- Dizziness
- Drowsiness
- Fatigue
- Anxiety
- Depression
- Insomnia
- Hallucinations
- Memory impairment
- Poor coordination
- Suicide
- Neuroleptic malignant syndrome
- Angioedema
- Laryngospasm
- Respiratory depression
- Dyspnea
- CVA
- CHF
- MI
- Hypotension
- Orthostatic hypotension
- ECG changes
- Cardiac arrest
- Tachycardia
- Mydriasis
- Blurred vision
- Tinnitus
- Nausea
- Vomiting
- Constipation
- Diarrhea
- Dry mouth
- Weight gain/loss
- Increased appetite
- Ileus perforation
- Ischemic colitis
- Jaundice
- Agranulocytosis
- Leukopenia
- Leukocytosis
- Decreased libido
- Rash
- Dermatitis
- Pruritus
- Death in geriatric patients with dementia

Nursing Care

- Monitor for suicidal ideation
- Monitor for mental status/CNS changes
- Monitor for BP changes
- Monitor blood studies
- Monitor for infection
- Monitor renal/hepatic status
- Monitor for dependency/withdrawal/toxicity

- Teach patient to take medication exactly as prescribed
- Teach patient not to abruptly discontinue medication
- Teach patient not to use for more than 4 months unless prescriber approves
- Teach patient that drug may be habit forming and affect CNS functioning
- Teach patient to avoid OTC products unless prescriber approves
- Teach patient not to drive or engage in other hazardous activities
- Teach patient to avoid alcohol, other psychotropic medications
- Teach patient to change positions slowly
- Teach patient to report signs and symptoms of infection

APPLICATION AND REVIEW

3. A nurse is teaching clients in a medication education group about side effects of medications. Which drug will cause a heightened skin reaction to sunlight?
   1. Lithium   3. Methylphenidate
   2. Sertraline   4. ChlorproMAZINE

See Answers on pages 99-102.

Mood Stabilizers

- Used in the prevention and treatment of mania
- Example includes lithium
- Available in PO preparations

Mode of Action

- Increases norepinephrine and serotonin uptake

Contraindications, Precautions, and Drug Interactions of Mood Stabilizers*

Drug	Contraindications/Precautions	Drug Interaction
lithium	**Contraindications:** Hypersensitivity, breastfeeding, children <12 yr, hepatic/renal/cardiac disease, schizophrenia, severe dehydration, brain trauma, organic brain syndrome **Precautions:** Geriatric patients, QT prolongation, thyroid disease, seizures, urinary retention, systemic infection, diabetes mellitus **Pregnancy:** Definite fetal risks, may be given in spite of risks if needed in life-threatening conditions	Haloperidol, thioridazine, neuromuscular blocking agents, phenothiazines, thyroid agents, calcium iodide, potassium iodide, iodinated glycerol, sodium bicarbonate, mannitol, acetazolamide, aminophylline, beta blockers, indomethacin, diuretics, losartan, NSAIDs, probenecid, methyldopa, thiazide diuretics, carbamazepine, fluoxetine, urea, theophyllines, urinary alkalinizers

*Pregnancy categories have been revised. See http://www.fda.gov/Drugs/DevelopmentApprovalProcess/DevelopmentResources/Labeling/ucm093307.htm for more information.

Adverse/Side Effects

- Headache
- Confusion
- Drowsiness
- Fatigue
- Dizziness
- Tremors
- Twitching
- Restlessness
- Slurred speech
- Stupor
- Ataxia
- Seizure
- Memory loss
- Clonic movements
- Hypotension

- Dysrhythmias
- ECG changes
- QT prolongation
- Circulatory collapse
- Edema
- Bragada syndrome
- Blurred vision
- Tinnitus
- Nausea

- Vomiting
- Diarrhea
- Abdominal pain
- Anorexia
- Dry mouth
- Metallic taste
- Incontinence
- Polyuria
- Glycosuria

- Albuminuria
- Proteinuria
- Polydipsia
- Leukocytosis
- Rash
- Pruritus
- Muscle weakness

Nursing Care
- Weigh patient daily
- Assess skin turgor daily
- Monitor I&O
- Monitor electrolyte status (especially sodium)
- Monitor mental status/CNS changes
- Monitor ECG in patients with history of CV disease
- Monitor for lithium toxicity
- Teach patient to report signs and symptoms of lithium toxicity (Table 5.1)
- Teach patient not to drive or engage in other hazardous activities

TABLE 5.1 Lithium	
Drug Class	**Dosage**
Mood stabilizer Trade Names: Eskalith, Lithane, Lithonate, Lithobid, Carbolith, Lithizine Pregnancy Category: D	A: PO: initially 600 mg t.i.d.; maint: 300 mg t.i.d./q.i.d.; max: 2.4 g/d C: PO: 15–20 mg/kg/d in 3–4 divided doses Therapeutic drug range: 0.5–1.5 mEq/L
Contraindications	**Drug-Laboratory-Food Interactions**
Liver and renal disease, pregnancy, lactation, severe cardiovascular disease, severe dehydration, hyponatremia, children <12 yr of age Caution: Thyroid disease, seizure disorder	Drug: May increase lithium level with thiazide diuretics, methyldopa, haloperidol, NSAIDs, antidepressants, carbamazepine, calcium channel blockers, spironolactone, ACE inhibitors, sodium bicarbonate, phenothiazines May increase lithium excretion with theophylline, aminophylline May increase risk of serotonin syndrome with SSRIs and SNRIs May increase hyperglycemia with antidiabetics Caffeine may decrease lithium levels Amphetamines may increase risk of mania Laboratory: Increase urine and blood glucose, protein; decrease serum sodium level Food: Increase sodium intake; lithium may cause sodium depletion Herbs: Use of St. John's wort, kava kava, and valerian may lead to neurotoxicity
Pharmacokinetics	**Pharmacodynamics**
Absorption: PO: well absorbed Distribution: PB: UK Metabolism: t½: 21–30 h Excretion: 98% in urine, mostly unchanged	PO: Onset: UK Peak: 2–4 h Duration: 24 h

Continued

TABLE 5.1 Lithium—cont'd	
Therapeutic Effects/Uses	
To treat bipolar psychosis, manic episodes	
Mode of Action: alteration of ion transport in muscle and nerve cells; increased receptor sensitivity to serotonin	
Side Effects	**Adverse Reactions**
Headache, memory impairment, blurred vision, metallic taste, dental caries, lethargy, drowsiness, dizziness, tremors, slurred speech, dry mouth, anorexia, vomiting, diarrhea, polyuria, dehydration, hypotension, abdominal pain, muscle weakness, restlessness	Urinary and fecal incontinence, hyperglycemia, hyponatremia, proteinuria, polyuria, leukocytosis, nephrotoxicity Life-threatening: Cardiac dysrhythmias, seizures, cardiac arrest, serotonin syndrome, neuroleptic malignant syndrome

A, Adult; *C,* child; *d,* day; *h,* hour; *max,* maximum; *NSAIDs,* nonsteroidal antiinflammatory drugs; *PB,* protein-binding; *PO,* by mouth; *q.i.d.,* four times a day; *SR,* sustained release; *t.i.d.,* three times a day; *t½,* half-life; *UK,* unknown; <, less than; >, greater than. From Kee, J.L., Hayes, E.R., McCuistion, L.E. (2015). *Pharmacology: A patient-centered nursing process approach* (8th ed.). St. Louis: Saunders.

- Teach patient that drug takes 1 to 3 weeks to reach therapeutic level
- Encourage fluid, sodium intake
- Teach patient not to use OTC products unless prescriber approves

APPLICATION AND REVIEW

4. A client is receiving lithium. What is an important nursing intervention while this medication is being administered?
   1. Restrict the client's daily sodium intake.
   2. Test the client's urine specific gravity weekly.
   3. Monitor the client's drug blood level regularly.
   4. Withhold the client's other medications for several days.
5. A client in the hyperactive phase of a mood disorder, bipolar type, is receiving lithium. A nurse identifies that the client's lithium blood level is 1.8 mEq/L. What is the most appropriate nursing action?
   1. Continue the usual dose of lithium and note any adverse reactions.
   2. Discontinue the drug until the lithium serum level drops to 0.5 mEq/L.
   3. Ask the health care provider to increase the dose of lithium because the blood lithium level is too low.
   4. Hold the drug and notify the health care provider immediately because the blood lithium level may be toxic.

See Answers on pages 99-102.

Tricyclic Antidepressants (TCAs)

- Used in the prevention and treatment of depression
- Examples include amitriptyline, doxepin, clomipramine, desipramine, imipramine
- Available in PO preparations

Mode of Action

- Increases amount of norepinephrine and serotonin in nerve cells by preventing their reuptake

Contraindications, Precautions, and Drug Interactions of Tricyclic Antidepressants*

Drug	Contraindications/Precautions	Drug Interaction
amitriptyline	**Contraindications:** Hypersensitivity to tricyclics, MI recovery **Precautions:** Breastfeeding, geriatric patients, cardiac/hepatic/renal disease, schizophrenia, prostatic hypertrophy, seizures, psychosis, severe depression, hyperthyroidism, urinary retention, electroshock therapy, elective surgery, increased intraocular pressure, closed-angle glaucoma **Pregnancy:** Only given after risks to the fetus are considered; animal studies have shown adverse reactions; no human studies available	MAOIs, procainamide, antithyroid agents, quinidine, tricyclics, amiodarone, class IA/IC/III antidysrhythmics, oral contraceptives, cimetidine, phenothiazines, fluoxetine, antidepressants, carbamazepine, sympathomimetics, barbiturates, alcohol, CNS depressants, benzodiazepines, opioids, sedatives, hypnotics, clonidine
doxepin	**Contraindications:** Hypersensitivity to tricyclics, MI recovery, urinary retention, prostatic hypertrophy, closed-angle glaucoma **Precautions:** Breastfeeding, geriatric patients, seizures **Pregnancy:** Only given after risks to the fetus are considered; animal studies have shown adverse reactions; no human studies available	MAOIs, clonidine, epinephrine, norepinephrine, anticholinergics, SSRIs, SNRIs, serotonin-receptor agonists, class IC/III antidysrhythmics, alcohol, other CNS depressants, sedatives/hypnotics, barbiturates, benzodiazepines, cimetidine, fluoxetine, fluvoxamine, paroxetine, sertraline
clomipramine	**Contraindications:** Hypersensitivity to clomipramine/tricyclics/carbamazepine, MI recovery, MAOI therapy **Precautions:** Breastfeeding, geriatric patients, seizures, glaucoma, cardiac disease, prostatic hypertrophy, urinary retention **Pregnancy:** Only given after risks to the fetus are considered; animal studies have shown adverse reactions; no human studies available	MAOIs, SSRIs, SNRIs, serotonin syndrome, tricyclics, linezolid, cimetidine, fluoxetine, fluvoxamine, sertraline, clonidine, epinephrine, norepinephrine, CYP1A2, CYP2D6, CNS depressants, alcohol, general anesthetics, phenothiazines, quinolones, antidysrhythmics, droperidol, mefloquine, mesoridazine, moxifloxacin, pentamidine, pimozide, tacrolimus, ziprasidone, levodopa, haloperidol, opiates, barbiturates, carbamazepine, phenytoin
desipramine	**Contraindications:** Hypersensitivity to tricyclics/carbamazepine, acute MI, MAOI therapy, closed-angle glaucoma **Precautions:** Breastfeeding, geriatric patients, seizures, severe depression, increased intraocular pressure, cardiac disease, prostatic hypertrophy, urinary retention, thyroid disease, dysrhythmias **Pregnancy:** Only given after risks to the fetus are considered; animal studies have shown adverse reactions; no human studies available	MAOIs, SSRIs, SNRIs, serotonin receptor agonists, tricyclics, barbiturates, alcohol, opioids, CNS depressants, skeletal muscle relaxants, cimetidine, fluoxetine, fluvoxamine, sertraline, clonidine, verapamil, dilitiazem, paroxetine, epinephrine, norepinephrine, sunitinib, vorinostat, ziprasidone, gatifloxacin, levofloxacin, moxifloxacin, sparfloxacin, class IA/III antidysrhythmics
imipramine	**Contraindications:** Hypersensitivity to tricyclics/carbamazepine, acute MI **Precautions:** Breastfeeding, geriatric patients, suicidal patients, severe depression, seizures, glaucoma, hepatic/renal/cardiac disease, prostatic hypertrophy, urinary retention, increased intraocular pressure, closed-angle glaucoma, hyperthyroidism, ECT, MI, AV block, QT prolongation **Pregnancy:** Definite fetal risks, may be given in spite of risks if needed in life-threatening conditions	MAOIs, clonidine, SSRIs, SNRIs, serotonin-receptor agonists, linezolid, class IA/III antidysrhythmics, tricyclics, gatifloxacin, levofloxacin, moxifloxacin, ziprasidone, sympathomimetics, alcohol, CNS depressants, barbiturates, benzodiazepines

*Pregnancy categories have been revised. See http://www.fda.gov/Drugs/DevelopmentApprovalProcess/DevelopmentResources/Labeling/ucm093307.htm for more information.

Adverse/Side Effects

- Headache
- Confusion
- Drowsiness
- Weakness
- Dizziness
- Tremors
- Sweating
- Insomnia
- Nightmares
- EPS
- Increased psychiatric symptoms
- Anxiety
- Seizure
- Suicidal ideation
- Asthma
- Orthostatic hypotension
- Hypertension
- ECG changes
- Dysrhythmias
- Tachycardia
- Blurred vision
- Photosensitivity
- Tinnitus
- Nausea
- Vomiting
- Constipation
- Increased appetite
- Weight gain
- Dry mouth
- Paralytic ileus
- Jaundice
- Hepatitis
- Acute renal failure
- Urinary retention
- Sexual dysfunction
- Agranulocytosis
- Thrombocytopenia
- Leukopenia
- Eosinophilia
- Aplastic anemia
- Rash
- Pruritus
- Urticaria
- Neuroleptic malignant syndrome
- Serotonin syndrome

Nursing Care

- Monitor mental status/CNS changes
- Monitor ECG in patients with history of CV disease
- Monitor blood studies
- Monitor renal/hepatic function
- Monitor for withdrawal
- Monitor for chronic pain
- Teach patient to report suicidal ideation, behavior
- Teach patient to take medication as prescribed
- Teach patient not to drive or engage in other hazardous activities
- Teach patient to report signs and symptoms of serotonin syndrome
- Teach patient to avoid alcohol, other CNS depressants
- Teach patient not use OTC products unless prescriber approves
- Teach patient to wear sunscreen, protective clothing, sunglasses
- Teach patient that reaching therapeutic levels may take 2 to 3 weeks
- Teach patient not to abruptly discontinue medication

Monamine Oxidase Inhibitors (MAOIs)

- Used in the prevention and treatment of depression
- Examples include isocarboxazid, phenelzine, selegiline, tranylcypromine
- Available in PO, transdermal preparations

Mode of Action

- Inhibits MAO, thus increasing norepinephrine, dopamine, serotonin at receptor sites

Contraindications, Precautions, and Drug Interactions of MAOIs*

Drug	Contraindications/Precautions	Drug Interaction
isocarboxazid	*Contraindications:* Hypersensitivity to MAOIs *Precautions:* Breastfeeding *Pregnancy:* Only given after risks to the fetus are considered; animal studies have shown adverse reactions; no human studies available	SSRIs, SNRIs, apraclonidine, bupropion, buspirone, carbamazepine, cyclobenzaprine, dextromethorphan, guanethidine, methyldopa, beta blockers, diuretics, MAOIs, epinephrine, sumatriptan, rizatriptan, tramadol, tyrosine, tryptophan
phenelzine	*Contraindications:* Hypersensitivity to MAOIs *Precautions:* Breastfeeding *Pregnancy:* Only given after risks to the fetus are considered; animal studies have shown adverse reactions; no human studies available	Amphetamines, methylphenidate, levodopa, sympathomimetics, appetite suppressants, fluoxetine, tricyclics, citalopram, clomipramine, trazodone, sertraline, paroxetine, fluvoxamine, doxapram, meperidine
selegiline	*Contraindications:* Hypersensitivity to MAOIs, breastfeeding, children, adolescents *Precautions:* Pregnancy *Pregnancy:* Only given after risks to the fetus are considered; animal studies have shown adverse reactions; no human studies available	Tricyclics, opioids, fluoxetine, paroxetine, sertraline, fluvoxamine, levodopa, carbidopa, dextromethorphan, antihypertensives
tranylcypromine	*Contraindications:* Hypersensitivity to MAOIs *Pregnancy:* Only given after risks to the fetus are considered; animal studies have shown adverse reactions; no human studies available *Precautions:* Breastfeeding	Amphetamines, methylphenidate, levodopa, sympathomimetics, appetite suppressants, fluoxetine, tricyclics, citalopram, clomipramine, trazodone, sertraline, paroxetine, fluvoxamine, doxapram, meperidine

*Pregnancy categories have been revised. See http://www.fda.gov/Drugs/DevelopmentApprovalProcess/DevelopmentResources/Labeling/ucm093307.htm for more information.

Adverse/Side Effects

- Headache
- Confusion
- Dizziness
- Lethargy
- Apathy
- Sweating
- Insomnia
- Nightmares
- Hallucinations
- Tremors
- Restlessness
- Bradykinesia
- Tardive dyskinesia
- Dystonic symptoms
- Apraxia
- Involuntary movement
- Anxiety
- Suicidal ideation
- Mood/personality changes
- Asthma
- Orthostatic hypotension
- Hypo/hypertension
- Dysrhythmias
- Tachycardia
- Hypertensive crisis (children)
- Blurred vision
- Diplopia
- Photosensitivity
- Tinnitus
- Nausea
- Vomiting
- Constipation
- Anorexia
- Weight loss
- Dry mouth
- Nocturia
- Urinary hesitation
- Retention
- Sexual dysfunction
- Rash
- Alopecia

Nursing Care

- Administer during the day to prevent insomnia
- Monitor mental status
- Monitor for CNS/mood/personality changes
- Monitor for Parkinson's symptoms
- Monitor cardiac status
- Monitor renal/hepatic function
- Teach patient to report suicidal ideation, behavior
- Teach patient to take medication as prescribed
- Teach patient to avoid high tyramine foods: aged cheese, sauerkraut, cured meats, draft beer, fermented soy products
- Teach patient to change positions slowly
- Teach patient not to abruptly discontinue medication
- Teach patient to avoid driving and other hazardous activities
- Teach patient to report signs and symptoms of serotonin syndrome
- Teach patient to report signs and symptoms of hypertensive crisis

Selective Serotonin Reuptake Inhibitors (SSRIs)

- Used in the treatment of depression
- Examples include citalopram, escitalopram, fluoxetine, fluvoxamine, paroxetine, sertraline
- Available in PO preparations

Mode of Action

- Inhibit neuronal reuptake of serotonin (Fig. 5.1)

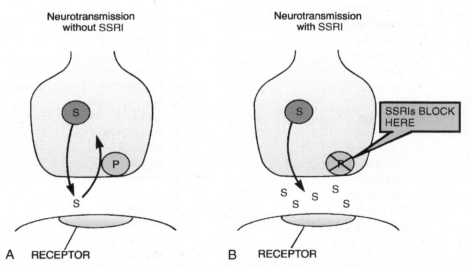

FIG. 5.1 Mechanism of action of selective serotonin reuptake inhibitors. **A,** Under drug-free conditions, the actions of serotonin are terminated by active uptake of the transmitter back into the nerve terminals from which it was released. **B,** By inhibiting the reuptake pump for serotonin, the SSRIs cause the transmitter to accumulate in the synaptic space, thereby intensifying transmission. (From Burchum, J.R., Rosenthal, L.D. [2016]. *Lehne's pharmacology for nursing* [9th ed.]. St. Louis: Saunders.)

Contraindications, Precautions, and Drug Interactions of SSRIs*

Drug	Contraindications/Precautions	Drug Interaction
citalopram	**Contraindications:** Hypersensitivity **Precautions:** Breastfeeding, geriatric patients, renal/hepatic disease, seizures, bradycardia, recent MI, QT prolongation **Pregnancy:** Only given after risks to the fetus are considered; animal studies have shown adverse reactions; no human studies available	MAOIs, tricyclics, SSRIs, SNRIs, serotonin receptor agonists, escitalopram, dofetilide, halofantrine, probucol, pimoside, quinolones, ziprasidone, tramadol, lithium, trazadone, NSAIDs, salicylates, thrombolytics, anticoagulants, antiplatelets, barbiturates, CNS depressants, sedative/hypnotics, macrolides, azole antifungals, beta blockers, carbamazepine, clonidine
escitalopram	**Contraindications:** Hypersensitivity to escitalopram/MAOIs/citalopram **Precautions:** Breastfeeding, geriatric patients, renal/hepatic disease, seizures, anticoagulants, bleeding **Pregnancy:** Only given after risks to the fetus are considered; animal studies have shown adverse reactions; no human studies available	MAOIs, tricyclics, SSRIs, SNRIs, serotonin receptor agonists, buspirone, CNS depressants, sedative/hypnotics, tryptophan, amphetamines, lithium, amantadine, bromocriptine, tramadol, alcohol, antidepressants, opioids, sedatives, warfarin, phenytoin, antipsychotics, antidysrhythmics, phenothiazines, haloperidol, diazepam, NSAIDs, salicylates, anticoagulants, platelet inhibitors, cyproheptadine
fluoxetine	**Contraindications:** Hypersensitivity **Precautions:** Breastfeeding, geriatric patients, QT prolongation, osteoporosis, diabetes mellitus, narrow-angle glaucoma **Pregnancy:** Only given after risks to the fetus are considered; animal studies have shown adverse reactions; no human studies available	MAOIs, SSRIs, SNRIs, serotonin receptor agonists, tricyclics, buspirone, CNS depressants, sedatives, tryptophan, alcohol, phenothiazines, antidepressants, opioids, sedatives, warfarin, phenytoin, antipsychotics, antidysrhythmics, phenothiazines, haloperidol, diazepam, NSAIDs, salicylates, anticoagulants, platelet inhibitors, cyproheptadine
fluvoxamine	**Contraindications:** Hypersensitivity to MAOIs **Precautions:** Breastfeeding, geriatric patients, bipolar disorder, seizures, hepatic/cardiac disease, dehydration, ECT, hyponatremia, hypovolemia **Pregnancy:** Only given after risks to the fetus are considered; animal studies have shown adverse reactions; no human studies available	MAOIs, alcohol, barbiturates, benzodiazepines, pimozide, tricyclics, clozapine, tizanidine, SSRIs, SNRIs, serotonin-receptor agonists, atypical antipsychotics, tramadol, anticoagulants, NSAIDs, salicylates, thrombolytics, clopidogrel
paroxetine	**Contraindications:** Hypersensitivity, MAOI use, alcohol use **Precautions:** Breastfeeding, geriatric patients, renal/hepatic disease, seizure history, history of mania **Pregnancy:** Definite fetal risks, may be given in spite of risks if needed in life-threatening conditions	SSRIs, SNRIs, MAOIs, atypical antipsychotics, serotonin-receptor agonists, tricyclics, amphetamines, methylphenidate, tramadol, digoxin, pimozide, thioridazine, NSAIDs, thrombolytics, salicylates, platelet inhibitors, anticoagulants, cimetidine, theophylline, CYP2D6 inhibitors, phenobarbital, phenytoin
sertraline	**Contraindications:** Hypersensitivity to sertraline/SSRIs **Precautions:** Breastfeeding, geriatric patients, renal/hepatic disease, seizure history, recent MI, epilepsy, latex sensitivity **Pregnancy:** Only given after risks to the fetus are considered; animal studies have shown adverse reactions; no human studies available	MAOIs, SSRIs, SNRIs, serotonin-receptor agonists, pimozide, lithium, sibutramine, trazadone, buspirone, linezolid, tramadol, disulfiram, warfarin, cimetidine, tricyclics, diazepam, tolbutamide, benzodiazepines, sumatriptan, phenytoin, clozapine, anticoagulants, NSAIDs, thrombolytics, platelet inhibitors, salicylates

*Pregnancy categories have been revised. See http://www.fda.gov/Drugs/DevelopmentApprovalProcess/DevelopmentResources/Labeling/ucm093307.htm for more information.

Adverse/Side Effects

- Headache
- Dizziness
- Drowsiness
- Sedation
- Fatigue
- Nervousness
- Apathy
- Insomnia
- Delusions
- Hallucinations
- Abnormal dreams
- Poor concentration
- Tremors
- Agitation
- Euphoria
- Psychosis
- Suicidal attempts
- Neuroleptic malignant-like syndrome reaction
- Hot flashes
- Fever
- Chills
- Asthma
- Dyspnea
- Bronchitis
- Orthostatic hypotension
- Hypertension
- Bradycardia
- MI
- Vision changes
- Photophobia
- Tinnitus
- Nausea
- Vomiting
- Diarrhea
- Constipation
- Anorexia
- Dry mouth
- Thrombophlebitis
- Hemorrhage
- Hepatitis
- Urinary frequency
- Impotence
- Myalgia
- Rash
- Alopecia
- Urticaria
- Serotonin syndrome
- Neonatal abstinence syndrome

Nursing Care

- Administer with food or milk to prevent GI distress
- Administer at night if oversedation occurs during day
- Do not administer within 14 days of MAOIs
- Weigh patient weekly
- Monitor mental status
- Monitor for CNS/mood/personality changes
- Monitor for serotonin syndrome
- Monitor cardiac status
- Monitor heart rhythm
- Monitor blood studies
- Monitor renal/hepatic function
- Teach patient to report suicidal ideation, behavior
- Teach patient to take medication as prescribed
- Teach patient not to abruptly discontinue medication
- Teach patient to avoid driving and other hazardous activities
- Teach patient to report signs and symptoms of serotonin syndrome
- Teach patient to avoid alcohol, CNS depressants

APPLICATION AND REVIEW

6. A depressed client has been prescribed a tricyclic antidepressant. How long should the nurse inform the client it will take before noticing a significant change in the depression?
   1. 4 to 6 days
   2. 2 to 4 weeks
   3. 5 to 6 weeks
   4. 12 to 16 hours

7. A nurse is teaching clients about dietary restrictions when taking a monoamine oxidase inhibitor (MAOI). What response does the nurse tell them to anticipate if they do not follow these restrictions?
   1. Occipital headaches
   2. Generalized urticaria
   3. Severe muscle spasms
   4. Sudden drop in blood pressure
8. A monoamine oxidase inhibitor (MAOI) is prescribed. What should the nurse include in the teaching plan about what to avoid when taking this drug?
   1. Ingesting aged cheeses
   2. Prolonged exposure to the sun
   3. Engaging in active physical exercise
   4. Over-the-counter antihistamine drugs
9. Imipramine 75 mg three times per day, is prescribed for a client. What nursing action is appropriate when administering this medication?
   1. Tell the client that barbiturates and steroids will not be prescribed.
   2. Warn the client not to eat cheese, fermenting products, and chicken liver.
   3. Monitor the client for increased tolerance and report if the dosage is no longer effective.
   4. Monitor the client for signs and symptoms of glaucoma.
10. A client with depression is to receive fluoxetine (Prozac). What precaution should the nurse consider when initiating treatment with this drug?
    1. It must be given with milk and crackers to avoid hyperacidity and discomfort.
    2. Eating cheese or pickled herring or drinking wine may cause a hypertensive crisis.
    3. Blood levels may not be sufficient to cause noticeable improvement for 2–4 weeks.
    4. Blood levels should be obtained weekly for 3 months to monitor for appropriate levels.
11. A client has been receiving escitalopram for treatment of a major depressive episode. On the fifth day of therapy, the client refuses the medication stating, "It doesn't help, so what's the use of taking it?" What is the nurse's best response?
    1. "Sometimes it takes 1 to 4 weeks to see an improvement."
    2. "It takes 6 to 8 weeks for this medication to have an effect."
    3. "I'll talk to your health care provider about increasing the dose. That may help."
    4. "You should have felt a response by now. I'll notify your health care provider immediately."

See Answers on pages 99-102.

Serotonin Norepinephrine Reuptake Inhibitors (SNRIs)

- Used in the treatment of depression
- Examples include duloxetine, desvenlafaxine, venlafaxine
- Available in PO preparations

Mode of Action
- Inhibits neuronal reuptake of serotonin and norepinephrine

Contraindications, Precautions, and Drug Interactions of SNRIs*

Drug	Contraindications/Precautions	Drug Interaction
duloxetine	**Contraindications:** Hypersensitivity, alcoholism, closed-angle glaucoma, hepatic disease, hepatitis, jaundice **Precautions:** Breastfeeding, geriatric patients, renal/cardiac disease, hypertension, seizures, mania, anorexia nervosa, increased intra-ocular pressure, bleeding, dehydration, diabetes, hypotension, orthostatic hypotension, hyponatremia, hypovolemia **Pregnancy:** Only given after risks to the fetus are considered; animal studies have shown adverse reactions; no human studies available	CYP2D6 inhibitors, CYP1A2 inhibitors, MAOIs, alcohol, linezolid, methylene blue IV, antihistamines, opioids, sedative/hypnotics, SSRIs, serotonin receptor agonists, anticoagulants, antiplatelets, NSAIDs, salicylates,

Continued

Contraindications, Precautions, and Drug Interactions of SNRIs—cont'd

Drug	Contraindications/Precautions	Drug Interaction
desvenlafaxine	**Contraindications:** Hypersensitivity to desvenlafaxine **Precautions:** Breastfeeding, geriatric patients, labor and delivery, angina, bleeding, CNS depression, hypertension, MI, stroke, hepatic/renal disease, hyponatremia, dysrhythmias, mania, hypovolemia, dehydration, intraocular pressure, venlafaxine, MAOIs **Pregnancy:** Only given after risks to the fetus are considered; animal studies have shown adverse reactions; no human studies available	SSRIs, SNRIs, serotonin receptor agonists, MAOIs, tricyclics, trazodone, lithium, ergots, sumatriptan, sibutramine, nefazodone, meperidine, phentermine, dextromethorphan, linezolid, promethazine, methylphenidate, tryptophan, salicylates, NSAIDs, thrombolytics, platelet inhibitors, anticoagulants, alcohol, opioids, antihistamines, sedatives/hypnotics, zolpidem
venlafaxine	**Contraindications:** Hypersensitivity **Precautions:** Breastfeeding, geriatric patients, bipolar disorder, interstitial lung disease, mania, hypertension, seizure, MI, renal/hepatic/cardiac disease, eosinophilic pneumonia **Pregnancy:** Only given after risks to the fetus are considered; animal studies have shown adverse reactions; no human studies available	MAOIs, salicylates, NSAIDs, anticoagulants, platelet inhibitors, cimetidine, alcohol, opioids, antihistamines, sedative/hypnotics, clozapine, haloperidol, warfarin, sumatriptan, trazodone, tramadol, SSRIs, serotonin receptor agonists, tryptophan, cyproheptadine

*Pregnancy categories have been revised. See http://www.fda.gov/Drugs/DevelopmentApprovalProcess/DevelopmentResources/Labeling/ucm093307.htm for more information.

Adverse/Side Effects

- Headache
- Dizziness
- Drowsiness
- Sedation
- Fatigue
- Insomnia
- Anxiety
- Tremor
- Agitation
- Hallucinations
- Aggression
- Seizures
- Abnormal dreams
- Suicidal ideation
- Neuroleptic malignant-like syndrome reaction
- Hot flashes
- Flushing
- Chills
- Anaphylaxis
- Angioedema
- Orthostatic hypotension
- Hypertension
- Peripheral edema
- Supraventricular dysrhythmia
- Vision changes
- Photosensitivity
- Hypo/hyperglycemia
- SIADH
- Nausea
- Vomiting
- Diarrhea
- Constipation
- Anorexia
- Dry mouth
- Thrombophlebitis
- Hepatic failure
- Urinary frequency/hesitancy/retention
- Impotence
- Myalgia
- Serotonin syndrome
- Stevens-Johnson syndrome
- Toxic epidermal necrolysis

Nursing Care

- Weigh patient weekly
- Monitor mental status
- Monitor for CNS/mood/personality changes
- Monitor for serotonin syndrome
- Monitor cardiac status
- Monitor heart rhythm
- Monitor blood studies
- Monitor renal/hepatic function
- Teach patient to report suicidal ideation, behavior
- Teach patient to take medication as prescribed
- Teach patient not to abruptly discontinue medication
- Teach patient to avoid driving and other hazardous activities
- Teach patient to report signs and symptoms of serotonin syndrome
- Teach patient to avoid alcohol, CNS depressants, MAOIs
- Teach patient to report urinary retention

Miscellaneous Antidepressants

- Used in the treatment of depression
- Examples include bupropion, trazadone
- Available in PO preparations

Mode of Action

- Various effects on brain chemistry

Contraindications, Precautions, and Drug Interactions of Miscellaneous Antidepressants*

Drug	Contraindications/Precautions	Drug Interaction
bupropion	**Contraindications:** Hypersensitivity, head trauma, stroke, eating disorders, seizure disorders, intracranial mass **Precautions:** Breastfeeding, geriatric patients, renal/hepatic/cardiac disease, cranial trauma, recent MI, seizures, substance abuse, heart failure, smoking, glaucoma **Pregnancy:** Only given after risks to the fetus are considered; animal studies have shown adverse reactions; no human studies available	MAOIs, phenothiazines, levodopa, benzodiazepines, antidepressants, alcohol, theophylline, systemic steroids, ritonavir, cimetidine, CYP2D6/CYP2B6 inhibitors, CYP2B6 inducer, tamoxifen, carbamazepine, cimetidine, phenobarbital, phenytoin
trazadone	**Contraindications:** Hypersensitivity to tricyclics **Precautions:** Breastfeeding, suicidal patients, severe depression, glaucoma, cardiac/renal/hepatic disease, ECT, hyperthyroidism, bleeding, bipolar disorder, dehydration, MI recovery, seizures **Pregnancy:** Only given after risks to the fetus are considered; animal studies have shown adverse reactions; no human studies available	MAOIs, SSRIs, SNRIs, fluoxetine, nefazodone, linezolid, methylene blue (IV) sympathomimetics, alcohol, barbiturates, benzodiazepines, CNS depressants, digoxin, phenytoin, carbamazepine, CYP3A4/2D6 inhibitors, warfarin, clonidine

*Pregnancy categories have been revised. See http://www.fda.gov/Drugs/DevelopmentApprovalProcess/DevelopmentResources/Labeling/ucm093307.htm for more information.

Adverse/Side Effects

- Headache
- Dizziness
- Confusion
- Agitation
- Bradykinesia
- Delusions
- Aggression
- Insomnia
- Sedation
- Seizures
- Mania
- Suicidal ideation
- Hot flashes
- Flushing
- Hypo/Hypertension
- Tachycardia
- AV block
- QRS prolongation
- Vision changes
- Auditory disturbances
- Nausea
- Vomiting
- Diarrhea
- Constipation
- Anorexia
- Dry mouth
- Paralytic ileus
- Hepatitis
- Agranulocytosis
- Thrombocytopenia
- Leukopenia
- Eosinophilia
- Impotence
- Acute renal failure
- Urinary frequency/retention
- Altered libido
- Rash
- Pruritus
- Stevens-Johnson syndrome

Nursing Care

- Monitor weight regularly
- Monitor mental status
- Monitor for CNS/mood/personality changes
- Monitor renal/hepatic function
- Teach patient to report suicidal ideation, behavior
- Teach patient to take medication as prescribed
- Teach patient not to abruptly discontinue medication
- Teach patient to avoid driving and other hazardous activities
- Teach patient to avoid alcohol, CNS depressants, MAOIs
- Teach patient therapeutic dose of drug may take 2 to 4 weeks to reach
- Teach patient to report auditory, visual, CNS changes
- Teach patient to notify prescriber if urinary retention occurs
- Teach patient to report signs and symptoms of serotonin syndrome

DRUGS USED TO TREAT PSYCHOTIC DISORDERS

Phenothiazines

- Used to treat symptoms of psychosis
- Examples include chlorpromazine, fluphenazine, prochlorperazine
- Available in PO, IM, IV SUBCUT preparations

Mode of Action

- Depresses limbic system to decrease aggression

Contraindications, Precautions, and Drug Interactions of Phenothiazines*

Drug	Contraindications/Precautions	Drug Interaction
chlorpromazine	**Contraindications:** Hypersensitivity, children <6 months, coma, coronary disease, liver damage, cerebral arteriosclerosis, circulatory collapse **Precautions:** Breastfeeding, geriatric patients, renal/hepatic/cardiac disease, seizures, Parkinson's disease, hypertension, prostatic enlargement, pulmonary disease, blood dyscrasias, brain damage, bone marrow suppression, alcohol/barbiturate withdrawal, closed-angle glaucoma **Pregnancy:** Only given after risks to the fetus are considered; animal studies have shown adverse reactions; no human studies available	CNS depressants, alcohol, barbiturate anesthetics, antihistamines, sedatives/hypnotics, antidepressants, epinephrine, antithyroid agents, beta-adrenergic blockers, anticholinergics, antidepressants, antiparkinsonian agents, MAOIs, valproic acid, anticonvulsants, cimetidine, antacids, lithium, barbiturates, warfarin
fluphenazine	**Contraindications:** Hypersensitivity, blood dyscrasias, bone marrow depression, coma **Precautions:** Breastfeeding, children <12 yr, geriatric patients, cardiac/renal/pulmonary disease, hypertension, seizures, agranulocytosis, angina, QT prolongation, suicidal ideation, Parkinson's disease, prostatic hypertrophy, infection, breast cancer, chemotherapy **Pregnancy:** Only given after risks to the fetus are considered; animal studies have shown adverse reactions; no human studies available	Amiodarone, arsenic trioxide, astemizole, aripiprazole, antidepressants, haloperidol, CNS depressants, alcohol, risperidone, epinephrine, anticholinergics, levodopa, lithium, barbiturates, smoking
prochlorperazine	**Contraindications:** Hypersensitivity to phenothiazines, infants, neonates, children <2 yr or 20 lb, coma, surgery **Precautions:** Breastfeeding, geriatric patients, seizures, encephalopathy, hepatic disease, glaucoma, BPH, Parkinson's disease **Pregnancy:** only given after risks to the fetus are considered; animal studies have shown adverse reactions; no human studies available	Antidepressants, anticholinergics, antiparkinsonian products, CNS depressants, SSRIs, SNRIs, barbiturates, lithium, antacids

*Pregnancy categories have been revised. See http://www.fda.gov/Drugs/DevelopmentApprovalProcess/DevelopmentResources/Labeling/ucm093307.htm for more information.

Adverse/Side Effects

- Seizures
- Drowsiness
- Pseudoparkinsonism
- Dystonia
- Tardive dyskinesia
- Depression
- Neuroleptic malignant syndrome
- Laryngospasm
- Respiratory depression
- Orthostatic hypotension
- Hypertension
- Tachycardia
- Cardiac arrest
- Circulatory failure
- Vision changes
- Nausea
- Vomiting
- Diarrhea
- Constipation
- Anorexia
- Dry mouth
- Paralytic ileus
- Hepatitis
- Jaundice
- Agranulocytosis
- Thrombocytopenia
- Leukopenia
- Leukocytosis
- Aplastic anemia
- Urinary frequency/retention
- Impotence
- Rash
- Neuroleptic malignant syndrome
- Death in geriatric patients with dementia

Nursing Care

- Administer with food, milk, or full glass of water to prevent GI distress
- Monitor mental status
- Monitor for CNS/mood/personality changes
- Monitor renal/hepatic function
- Monitor for hypo/hypertension
- Monitor I&O
- Monitor for neuroleptic malignant syndrome
- Teach patient to report suicidal ideation, behavior
- Teach patient to take medication as prescribed
- Teach patient not to abruptly discontinue medication
- Teach patient to avoid driving and other hazardous activities
- Teach patient to avoid alcohol, CNS depressants
- Teach patient to change positions slowly
- Teach patient to wear sunscreen, protective clothing, sunglasses
- Teach patient to avoid OTC products unless prescriber permission
- Teach patient to report signs and symptoms of infection

Nonphenothiazines

- Used to treat symptoms of psychosis
- Examples include haloperidol, thiothixene, pimozide
- Available in PO, IM, IV, SUBCUT preparations

Mode of Action

- Depresses cerebral cortex, hypothalamus, limbic system to decrease aggression

Contraindications, Precautions, and Drug Interactions of Nonphenothiazines*

Drug	Contraindications/Precautions	Drug Interaction
haloperidol	***Contraindications:*** Hypersensitivity, coma, Parkinson's disease ***Precautions:*** Breastfeeding, geriatric patients, children, cardiac/hepatic/pulmonary disease, alcohol/barbiturate withdrawal, closed-angle glaucoma, angina, CNS depression, blood dyscrasias, bone marrow depression, brain damage, epilepsy, urinary retention, seizures, QT prolongation, hypertension, torsades de pointes, prostatic hypertrophy, thyrotoxicosis, hyperthyroidism ***Pregnancy:*** Only given after risks to the fetus are considered; animal studies have shown adverse reactions; no human studies available	SSRIs, SNRIs, tricyclics, class IA/III antidysrhythmics, amoxapine, pimozide, maprotiline, phenothiazines, risperidone, droperidol, beta blockers, methadone, erythromycin, vardenafil, CNS depressants, alcohol, barbiturate anesthetics, lithium, epinephrine, anticholinergics, beta adrenergic blockers, phenobarbital, carbamazepine, levodopa
thiothixene	***Contraindications:*** Hypersensitivity, blood dyscrasias, bone marrow depression ***Precautions:*** Breastfeeding, geriatric patients, children, cardiac/hepatic/pulmonary disease, alcohol/barbiturate withdrawal, closed-angle glaucoma, angina, CNS depression, blood dyscrasias, bone marrow depression, urinary retention, seizures, hypertension, prostatic hypertrophy ***Pregnancy:*** Only given after risks to the fetus are considered; animal studies have shown adverse reactions; no human studies available	Anticholinergics, antispasmodics, levodopa, alpha blockers, carbamazepine, alcohol, antihistamines, CNS depressants, SSRIs, SNRIs, phenothiazines, tricyclics, tramadol

Contraindications, Precautions, and Drug Interactions of Nonphenothiazines—cont'd

Drug	Contraindications/Precautions	Drug Interaction
pimozide	**Contraindications:** Hypersensitivity **Precautions:** Breastfeeding, geriatric patients, children, cardiac/hepatic/pulmonary disease, alcohol/barbiturate withdrawal, closed-angle glaucoma, angina, CNS depression, blood dyscrasias, bone marrow depression, urinary retention, seizures, hypertension, prostatic hypertrophy, thyrotoxicosis, hyperthyroidism **Pregnancy:** Only given after risks to the fetus are considered; animal studies have shown adverse reactions; no human studies available	Azithromycin, CNS depressants, alcohol, SSRIs, SNRIs, tricyclics, phenothiazines

*Pregnancy categories have been revised. See http://www.fda.gov/Drugs/DevelopmentApprovalProcess/DevelopmentResources/Labeling/ucm093307.htm for more information.

Adverse/Side Effects

- Headache
- Drowsiness
- Confusion
- Seizures
- Akathisia
- Pseudoparkinsonism
- Dystonia
- Tardive dyskinesia
- Neuroleptic malignant syndrome
- Laryngospasm
- Respiratory depression
- Orthostatic hypotension
- Hypertension
- Tachycardia
- Cardiac arrest
- QT prolongation
- Torsades de pointes
- Sudden death
- Vision changes
- Dry eyes
- Nausea
- Vomiting
- Diarrhea
- Constipation
- Anorexia
- Dry mouth
- Weight gain
- Paralytic ileus
- Hepatitis
- Jaundice
- Urinary frequency/retention
- Impotence
- Rash
- Neuroleptic malignant syndrome
- Death in geriatric patients with dementia

Nursing Care

- Monitor mental status
- Monitor for CNS/mood/personality changes
- Monitor renal/hepatic/cardiac function
- Monitor for hypo/hypertension
- Monitor ECG in patients with CV disease
- Monitor I&O
- Monitor for neuroleptic malignant syndrome
- Teach patient to report suicidal ideation, behavior
- Teach patient to take medication as prescribed
- Teach patient not to abruptly discontinue medication
- Teach patient to avoid driving and other hazardous activities

- Teach patient to avoid alcohol, CNS depressants
- Teach patient to change positions slowly
- Teach patient to avoid OTC products unless prescriber permission

Atypical Antipsychotics

- Used to treat schizophrenia, bipolar disorder, mania, treatment-resistant depression
- Examples include aripiprazole, clozapine, olanzapine, quetiapine, risperidone, ziprasidone
- Available in PO, IM preparations

Mode of Action

- Blocks dopamine and serotonin receptor activity

Contraindications, Precautions, and Drug Interactions of Atypical Antipsychotics*

Drug	Contraindications/Precautions	Drug Interaction
aripiprazole	*Contraindications:* Hypersensitivity, breastfeeding, seizures *Precautions:* Geriatric patients, cardiac/hepatic/renal disease, neutropenia *Pregnancy:* Only given after risks to the fetus are considered; animal studies have shown adverse reactions; no human studies available	CYP3A4/CYP2D6 inhibitors, CYP3A4 inducers, alcohol, CNS depressants, lithium, antipsychotics, famotidine, valproate
clozapine	*Contraindications:* Hypersensitivity, coma, severe granulocytopenia *Precautions:* Breastfeeding, children, cardiac/hepatic/pulmonary/renal disease, closed-angle glaucoma, prostatic hypertrophy, stroke, seizures *Pregnancy:* No adverse effects in animals; no human studies available	Alcohol, CNS depressants, psychoactives, warfarin, digoxin, caffeine, citalopram, CYP1A2/CYP3A4 inhibitors, CYP1A2 inducers, sertraline, fluoxetine, ritonavir, risperidone, beta blockers, class IA/III antidysrhythmics, benzodiazepines, phenobarbital
olanzapine	*Contraindications:* Hypersensitivity *Precautions:* Breastfeeding, geriatric patients, Asian patients, cardiac/hepatic/renal disease, suicidal ideation, closed-angle glaucoma, hypertension, diabetes, agranulocytosis, leucopenia, coma, QT prolongation, tardive dyskinesia, torsades de pointes, TIA, stroke *Pregnancy:* Only given after risks to the fetus are considered; animal studies have shown adverse reactions; no human studies available	SSRIs, SNRIs, alcohol, CNS depressants, antidepressants, barbiturate anesthetics, antihistamines, sedatives/hypnotics, CYP1A2 inhibitors/inducers, antihypertensives, diazepam, anticholinergics, rifampin, omeprazole, carbamazepine, levodopa, bromocriptine, dopamine agonists
quetiapine	*Contraindications:* Hypersensitivity *Precautions:* Breastfeeding, geriatric patients, Asian patients, cardiac/hepatic/renal disease, suicidal ideation, closed-angle glaucoma, hypertension, diabetes, agranulocytosis, leucopenia, coma, QT prolongation, tardive dyskinesia, torsades de pointes, TIA, stroke *Pregnancy:* Only given after risks to the fetus are considered; animal studies have shown adverse reactions; no human studies available	Alcohol, opioids, antihistamines, sedatives/hypnotics, antihypertensives, class IA/III antidysrhythmics, lithium, phenothiazines, beta agonists, tricyclics, haloperidol, methadone, chloroquine, droperidol, clarithromycin, erythromycin, pentamidine, phenytoin, thioridazine, barbiturates, glucocorticoids, rifampin, carbamazepine, CYP3A4 inhibitors, cimetidine, dopamine agonists

Contraindications, Precautions, and Drug Interactions of Atypical Antipsychotics —cont'd

Drug	Contraindications/Precautions	Drug Interaction
risperidone	**Contraindications:** Hypersensitivity, breastfeeding **Precautions:** Breastfeeding, children, geriatric patients, cardiac/hepatic/renal/hematologic disease, Parkinson's disease, suicidal ideation, breast cancer, diabetes, CNS depression, brain tumor, dehydration, seizures, phenylketonuria **Pregnancy:** Only given after risks to the fetus are considered; animal studies have shown adverse reactions; no human studies available	Furosemide, tramadol, alcohol, CNS depressants, antipsychotics, carbamazepine, CYP2D6 inducers/inhibitors, levodopa, class IA/III antidysrhythmics, phenothiazines, tricyclics, beta agonists, local anesthetics, haloperidol, clarithromycin, erythromycin, acetylcholinesterase inhibitors
ziprasidone	**Contraindications:** Hypersensitivity, breastfeeding, acute MI, heart failure, QT prolongation **Precautions:** Children, geriatric patients, cardiac/hepatic/renal disease, CNS depression, seizures, AV block, agranulocytosis, suicidal ideation, strenuous exercise, torsades de pointes **Pregnancy:** Only given after risks to the fetus are considered; animal studies have shown adverse reactions; no human studies available	CNS depressants, alcohol, lithium, antipsychotics, class IA/III antidysrhythmics, phenothiazines, beta agonists, tricyclics, haloperidol, methadone, pentamidine, barbiturates, carbamazepine, antihypertensives, SSRIs, SNRIs

*Pregnancy categories have been revised. See http://www.fda.gov/Drugs/DevelopmentApprovalProcess/DevelopmentResources/Labeling/ucm093307.htm for more information.

Adverse/Side Effects

- Headache
- Drowsiness
- Insomnia
- Akathisia
- Tremor
- Dystonia
- Seizures
- Agitation
- Anxiety
- Anaphylaxis
- Fatal pneumonia (geriatric patients)
- Neuroleptic malignant syndrome
- Orthostatic hypotension
- Hypertension
- Tachycardia
- QT prolongation
- Heart failure
- Peripheral edema
- Blurred vision
- Nausea
- Vomiting
- Constipation
- Weight gain
- Hepatitis
- Jaundice
- Hyperglycemia
- Dyslipidemia
- Leukopenia
- Agranulocytosis
- Eosinophilia
- Neutropenia
- Myalgia
- Rhabdomyolysis
- Death in geriatric patients with dementia
- Stevens-Johnson syndrome

Nursing Care

- Monitor mental status
- Monitor for CNS/neurologic/mood/personality changes
- Monitor renal/hepatic/cardiac function
- Monitor blood studies

- Monitor for infection
- Monitor for hypotension
- Monitor I&O
- Monitor for neuroleptic malignant syndrome
- Monitor geriatric patients closely for serious reactions
- Teach patient to report suicidal ideation, behavior
- Teach patient to take medication as prescribed
- Teach patient not to abruptly discontinue medication
- Teach patient to avoid driving and other hazardous activities
- Teach patient to avoid alcohol, CNS depressants
- Teach patient to change positions slowly
- Teach patient to avoid OTC products unless prescriber permission
- Teach patient to avoid activities/conditions that cause hypotension (hot tubs, hot showers, heat stroke)
- Teach patient to report signs and symptoms of infection

APPLICATION AND REVIEW

12. A nurse administers an antipsychotic to a client. For which **common** manageable side effect should the nurse assess the client?
    1. Jaundice
    2. Melanocytosis
    3. Drooping eyelids
    4. Unintentional tremors

13. A primary nurse observes that a client has become jaundiced after 2 weeks of antipsychotic drug therapy. The primary nurse continues to administer the antipsychotic until the health care provider can be consulted. What does the nurse manager conclude concerning this situation?
    1. Jaundice is sufficient reason to discontinue the antipsychotic.
    2. The blood level of antipsychotics must be maintained once established.
    3. Jaundice is a benign side effect of antipsychotics that has little significance.
    4. The prescribed dose for the antipsychotic should have been reduced by the nurse.

14. A client with chronic undifferentiated schizophrenia is receiving an antipsychotic medication. For which potentially irreversible extrapyramidal side effect should a nurse monitor the client?
    1. Torticollis
    2. Oculogyric crisis
    3. Tardive dyskinesia
    4. Pseudoparkinsonism

15. Neuroleptic malignant syndrome is a potentially fatal reaction to antipsychotic therapy. What signs and symptoms of this syndrome should the nurse identify? **Select all that apply**.
    1. Jaundice
    2. Diaphoresis
    3. Hyperrigidity
    4. Hyperthermia
    5. Photosensitivity

16. A client with a diagnosis of schizophrenia is discharged from the hospital. At home the client forgets to take the medication, is unable to function, and must be rehospitalized. What medication may be prescribed that can be administered on an outpatient basis every 2 to 3 weeks?
    1. Lithium
    2. Diazepam
    3. Fluvoxamine
    4. Fluphenazine

17. A client has been receiving fluphenazine for several months. For which side effects should the nurse assess the client? **Select all that apply.**
    1. Tremors
    2. Excess salivation
    3. Rambling speech
    4. Reluctance to converse
    5. Minimal use of nonverbal expression
    6. Uncoordinated movement of extremities

18. A health care provider prescribes haloperidol (Haldol) for a client. What should the nurse teach the client to avoid while taking this medication?
    1. Driving at night
    2. Staying in the sun
    3. Ingesting aged cheeses
    4. Taking medications containing aspirin

19. A client with type 1 diabetes is diagnosed with a psychosis and is to receive haloperidol (Haldol). Which response should a nurse anticipate with this drug combination?
    1. Depressed respirations
    2. Intensified action of both drugs
    3. Decreased control of the diabetes
    4. Intensified action of both drugs

20. A nurse is educating a client who is taking clozapine (Clozaril) for paranoid schizophrenia. What should the nurse emphasize about the side effects of clozapine?
    1. Risk for falls
    2. Inability to sit still
    3. Increase in temperature
    4. Dizziness upon standing

21. Olanzapine (Zyprexa) is prescribed for a client with bipolar disorder, manic episode. What cautionary advice should the nurse give the client?
    1. Sit up slowly.
    2. Report double vision.
    3. Expect increased salivation.
    4. Take the medication on an empty stomach.

22. Olanzapine (Zyprexa) is prescribed for a client who experienced agranulocytosis from Clozapine (Clozaril). Which statements indicate that the nurse's teaching about olanzapine has been effective? **Select all that apply.**
    1. "I need to be careful that I do not gain too much weight."
    2. "I should be careful so I don't nick myself when I shave."
    3. "This medication should help me enjoy pleasurable activities."
    4. "I will have to remember to take my benztropine (Cogentin)."
    5. "Restlessness can occur when I am taking this medication."

DRUGS USED TO TREAT PARKINSON'S DISEASE

Dopaminergics

- Used to treat Parkinson's disease
- Examples include amantadine, bromocriptine, levodopa-carbidopa, pramipexole, rasagiline, ropinirole, selegiline
- Available in PO preparations

Mode of Action

- Increases dopamine at receptor sites

Contraindications, Precautions, and Drug Interactions of Dopaminergics*

Drug	Contraindications/Precautions	Drug Interaction
amantadine	*Contraindications:* Hypersensitivity, breastfeeding, children <1 yr, rash *Precautions:* Geriatric patients, cardiac/hepatic/renal disease, epilepsy, CHF, orthostatic hypotension, peripheral edema, psychiatric disorders *Pregnancy:* Only given after risks to the fetus are considered; animal studies have shown adverse reactions; no human studies available	Anticholinergic drugs, atropine, CNS stimulants, phenothiazines, metoclopramide, triamterene, hydrochlorothiazide, H1N1 influenza A vaccine

Continued

Contraindications, Precautions, and Drug Interactions of Dopaminergics—cont'd

Drug	Contraindications/Precautions	Drug Interaction
bromocriptine	**Contraindications:** Hypersensitivity to bromocriptine/ergots, severe ischemic disease, severe peripheral vascular disease, uncontrolled hypertension **Precautions:** Breastfeeding, children, hepatic/renal disease, peptic ulcer disease, GI bleed, dementia, pulmonary fibrosis, bipolar disorder, pituitary tumors, sulfite hypersensitivity **Pregnancy:** No adverse effects in animals; no human studies available	Alcohol, antihypertensives, levodopa, sulfonamides, chloramphenicol, salicylates, probenecid, phenothiazines, progestins, oral contraceptives, estrogens, MAOIs, haloperidol, loxapine, methyldopa, metoclopramide, reserpine, CYP3A4 inducers/inhibitors, thioxanthenes
levodopa-carbidopa	**Contraindications:** Hypersensitivity, malignant melanoma **Precautions:** Breastfeeding, cardiac/hepatic/renal/pulmonary disease, closed-angle glaucoma, diabetes, depression, peptic ulcer disease, seizures, MI **Pregnancy:** Only given after risks to the fetus are considered; animal studies have shown adverse reactions; no human studies available	CNS depressants, metoclopramide, antacids, nonselective MAOIs, dopamine, tricyclics, epinephrine, norepinephrine, antipsychotics, anticholinergics, benzodiazepines
pramipexole	**Contraindications:** Hypersensitivity **Precautions:** Cardiac/renal disease, psychosis, MI, anxiety, depression, bipolar disease, preexisting dyskineisias **Pregnancy:** Only given after risks to the fetus are considered; animal studies have shown adverse reactions; no human studies available	Dopamine antagonists, phenothiazines, butyrophenones, levodopa, ranitidine, cimetidine, verapamil, quinidine
rasagiline	**Contraindications:** Hypersensitivity to rasagiline/MAOIs, breastfeeding, pheochromocytoma **Precautions:** Children, hepatic disease, psychiatric disorders **Pregnancy:** Only given after risks to the fetus are considered; animal studies have shown adverse reactions; no human studies available	Analgesics, meperidine, sympathomimetics, CYP1A2 inhibitors, ciprofloxacin, SSRIs, SNRIs, tricyclics, MAOIs
ropinirole	**Contraindications:** Hypersensitivity **Precautions:** Cardiac/hepatic/renal disease, dysrhythmias, psychosis, affective disorders **Pregnancy:** Only given after risks to the fetus are considered; animal studies have shown adverse reactions; no human studies available	Cimetidine, ciprofloxacin, digoxin, diltiazem, enoxacin, erythromycin, fluvoxamine, levodopa, mexiletine, norfloxacin, tacrine, theophylline, phenothiazines, butyrophenones, thioxanthenes
selegiline	**Contraindications:** Hypersensitivity, breastfeeding, children, adolescents **Precautions:** Pregnancy **Pregnancy:** Only given after risks to the fetus are considered; animal studies have shown adverse reactions; no human studies available	Opioids, fluoxetine, fluvoxamine, paroxetine, sertraline, tricyclics, antihypertensives, dextromethorphan, levodopa/carbidopa

*Pregnancy categories have been revised. See http://www.fda.gov/Drugs/DevelopmentApprovalProcess/DevelopmentResources/Labeling/ucm093307.htm for more information.

Adverse/Side Effects

- Headache
- Drowsiness
- Sudden sleep onset
- Dizziness
- Fatigue
- Confusion
- Insomnia
- Anxiety
- Depression
- Restlessness
- Hallucinations
- Psychosis

- Tremor
- Seizures
- Shock
- MI
- Orthostatic hypotension
- CHF
- Tachycardia
- Sinus bradycardia
- Blurred vision
- Nausea
- Vomiting
- Constipation

- Anorexia
- Dry mouth
- GI hemorrhage
- Urinary frequency/ retention
- Leukopenia
- Agranulocytosis
- Anemia
- Photosensitivity
- Dermatitis
- Skin cancer

Nursing Care

- Monitor mental status
- Monitor for CNS/neurologic changes
- Monitor renal/hepatic/cardiac function
- Monitor blood studies
- Monitor for infection
- Monitor for hypotension/hypertension
- Monitor for changes in skin/melanomas
- Monitor for neuroleptic malignant syndrome
- Teach patient to report suicidal ideation, behavior
- Teach patient to take medication as prescribed
- Teach patient not to abruptly discontinue medication
- Teach patient to avoid driving and other hazardous activities
- Teach patient to avoid alcohol, CNS depressants
- Teach patient to change positions slowly
- Teach patient to avoid OTC products unless prescriber permission
- Teach patient to avoid activities/conditions that cause hypotension (hot tubs, hot showers, heat stroke)
- Teach patient to report signs and symptoms of infection
- Teach patient to reports signs and symptoms of MI
- Teach patient to report signs and symptoms of neuroleptic malignant syndrome
- Teach patient to use contraception during treatment
- Teach patient that sudden sleep may occur with pramipexole and to avoid driving/hazardous activities
- Teach patient to avoid sun exposure
- Teach patient to avoid tyramine foods that may lead to hypertensive crisis

ANSWER KEY: REVIEW QUESTIONS

1. **4 The use of benzodiazepines can raise the seizure threshold, which is counterproductive.**
   1 A tyramine-free diet is required with MAOI therapy, not after electroconvulsive therapy. **2** Photosensitivity is not a side effect of electroconvulsive therapy. **3** A stable sodium level is necessary with lithium, not electroconvulsive, therapy.
   Client Need: Pharmacologic and Parenteral Therapies; **Cognitive Level:** Analysis; **Nursing Process:** Planning/ Implementation

2. **Answers: 1, 2, 5**

   Rigidity, tremors, and bradykinesia may occur because of the effect of the antipsychotic on the postsynaptic dopamine receptors in the brain.

   3, 4 Mydriasis and photophobiside are side effects of anticholinergic, not antipsychotic, drugs.

   Client Need: Pharmacologic and Parenteral Therapies; **Cognitive Level:** Analysis; **Integrated Process:** Communication/Documentation; **Nursing Process:** Evaluation/Outcomes

3. **4 Clients taking chlorproMAZINE should be instructed to stay out of the sun. Photosensitivity makes the skin more susceptible to burning.**

   1, 2, 3 Photosensitivity is not a side effect of this medication.

   Client Need: Pharmacologic and Parenteral Therapies; **Cognitive Level:** Comprehension; **Integrated Process:** Teaching/Learning; **Nursing Process:** Planning/Implementation

4. **3 Lithium alters sodium transport in nerve and muscle cells and causes a shift toward intraneuronal metabolism of catecholamines. Because the range between therapeutic and toxic levels is very small, the client's serum lithium level should be monitored closely.**

   1 Sodium restriction may cause electrolyte imbalance and lithium toxicity. **2** It is not necessary or useful to test the client's urine specific gravity weekly. **4** It may or may not be necessary to withhold the client's other medications for several days; it depends on what the client is receiving. Also, it requires a health care provider's order.

   Client Need: Pharmacologic and Parenteral Therapies; **Cognitive Level:** Application; **Nursing Process:** Planning/Implementation

> **Study Tip:** Write the words lithium and monitor using just one *m:* lithiumonitor! Say it to yourself several times, emphasizing the *mmmmm*. Because toxic levels of lithium are an ever-present danger, it is vital that you associate these two words together.

5. **4 The lithium level should be maintained between 0.5 and 1.5 mEq/L.**

   1, 3 1.8 mEq/L is an unsafe level of lithium in the blood; it should not be increased. **2** The lithium level is currently unsafe, but it does not need to drop to 0.5 mEq/L before being resumed.

   Client Need: Pharmacologic and Parenteral Therapies; **Cognitive Level:** Analysis; **Nursing Process:** Planning/Implementation

6. **2 It takes 2 to 4 weeks for the drug to reach a therapeutic blood level.**

   1, 4 Less than 2 weeks is too short a time for a therapeutic blood level of the drug to be achieved. **3** Improvement in depression should be demonstrated earlier than 5 weeks.

   Client Need: Pharmacologic and Parenteral Therapies; **Cognitive Level:** Comprehension; **Integrated Process:** Teaching/Learning; **Nursing Process:** Planning/Implementation

> **Study Tip:** *Tri* in tricyclic means three, just like a tricycle has three wheels. Three is about how many weeks it takes for tricyclics to reach therapeutic blood level.

7. **1 Occipital headaches are the beginning of a hypertensive crisis that results from excessive tyramine.**

   2 Generalized urticaria is unrelated to the ingestion of tyramine. **3** Severe muscle spasms are unrelated to the ingestion of tyramine. **4** Excessive tyramine causes an increase, not a decrease, in blood pressure.

   Client Need: Pharmacologic and Parenteral Therapies; **Cognitive Level:** Application; **Integrated Process:** Teaching/Learning; **Nursing Process:** Evaluation/Outcomes

8. **1 The monoamine oxidase inhibitors can cause a hypertensive crisis if food or beverages that are high in tyramine are ingested.**

   2 Monitoring sun exposure is important for clients taking one of the phenothiazines. **3** Physical exercise is not contraindicated. **4** Antihistamines are not prohibited with MAOI medications.

Client Need: Pharmacologic and Parenteral Therapies; **Cognitive Level:** Application; **Integrated Process:** Teaching/Learning; **Nursing Process:** Planning/Implementation

9. **4 The development of glaucoma is one of the side effects of imipramine, and the client should be taught the symptoms.**

   1, 2 With monoamine oxidase inhibitors (MAOIs), barbiturates and steroids will not be prescribed and clients are warned not to eat cheese, fermenting products, and chicken liver. Imipramine is not an MAOI. **3** Tolerance is not an issue with tricyclic antidepressants such as imipramine.

   Client Need: Pharmacologic and Parenteral Therapies; **Cognitive Level:** Analysis; **Nursing Process:** Planning/Implementation

10. **3 Fluoxetine does not produce an immediate effect; nursing measures must be continued to decrease the risk for suicide.**

    1 It is not necessary for fluoxetine to be given with milk and crackers to avoid hyperacidity and discomfort. Eating cheese or pickled herring or drinking wine may cause a hypertensive crisis when taking MAO inhibitors. **4** Obtaining blood levels weekly for 3 months to monitor for appropriate levels is not necessary with fluoxetine (Prozac).

    Client Need: Pharmacologic and Parenteral Therapies; **Cognitive Level:** Application; **Nursing Process:** Planning/Implementation

11. **1 It usually takes 1 to 4 weeks to attain a therapeutic blood level of this monoamine oxidase inhibitor (MAOI).**

    2, 3 Escitalopram works within 1 to 4 weeks. **4** The client needs longer than 5 days to see an effect from escitalopram.

    Client Need: Pharmacologic and Parenteral Therapies; **Cognitive Level:** Application; **Integrated Process:** Teaching/Learning; **Nursing Process:** Planning/Implementation

12. **4 Unintentional tremors are one of the extrapyramidal side effects of the antipsychotics and are considered common and manageable.**

    1 Jaundice is a severe but not a common occurrence; periodic liver function tests should be performed. **2** An excessive number of melanocytes is not a side effect of antipsychotics. **3** Dropping eyelids is not a common side effect.

    Client Need: Pharmacologic and Parenteral Therapies; **Cognitive Level:** Application; **Nursing Process:** Evaluation/Outcomes

13. **1 Liver damage is a well-documented toxic side effect of antipsychotics. By continuing to administer the drug, the nurse failed to use professional knowledge in the performance of responsibilities as outlined in the Nurse Practice Act.**

    2 Blood levels must be reduced when signs of liver damage are present. **3** Liver damage, indicated by jaundice, is a well-documented side effect. **4** The antipsychotic should be stopped, not reduced; liver damage is a well-documented toxic side effect.

    Client Need: Management of Care; **Cognitive Level:** Analysis; **Nursing Process:** Evaluation/Outcomes

14. **3 Tardive dyskinesia occurs as a late and persistent extrapyramidal complication of long-term antipsychotic therapy. It is most often manifested by abnormal movements of the lips, tongue, and mouth.**

    1, 2, 4 Torticollis, oculogyric crisis, and pseudoparkinsonism are reversible with administration of an anticholinergic (e.g., benztropine [Cogentin]) or an antihistamine (e.g., diphenhydramine [Benadryl]) or by stopping the medication.

    Client Need: Pharmacologic and Parenteral Therapies; **Cognitive Level:** Application; **Nursing Process:** Evaluation/Outcomes

15. **Answers: 2, 3, 4**

    Diaphoresis, Hyperrigidity, and Hyperthermia occur with neuroleptic malignant syndrome as a result of dopamine blockade in the hypothalamus.

    1, 5 Jaundice and photosensitivity are not associated with neuroleptic malignant syndrome.

    Client Need: Pharmacologic and Parenteral Therapies; **Cognitive Level:** Analysis; **Nursing Process:** Evaluation/Outcomes

16. **4 Fluphenazine can be given IM every 2 to 3 weeks for clients who are unreliable in taking oral medications; it allows them to live in the community while keeping the disorder under control.**

    1 Lithium is a mood stabilizing medication that is given to clients with bipolar disorder. This drug is not given for schizophrenia. **2** Diazepam (Valium) is an antianxiety/anticonvulsant/skeletal muscle relaxant that is not given for schizophrenia. **3** Fluvoxamine (Luvox) is a selective serotonin reuptake inhibitor (SSRI); it is administered for depression, not schizophrenia.

    Client Need: Pharmacologic and Parenteral Therapies; **Cognitive Level:** Analysis; **Nursing Process:** Planning/Implementation

17. **Answers: 1, 6**

    1 Acute dystonic reactions, such as tremors, dyskinesia, and akathisia, are observable side effects of fluphenazine therapy. **6** Acute dystonic reactions, including uncoordinated movement of extremities, are observable side effects of fluphenazine therapy.

    2 There is a decrease, not an increase, in salivation. **3** Rambling speech is not a side effect of fluphenazine therapy. **4** Reluctance to converse is not a side effect of fluphenazine therapy. **5** Minimal use of nonverbal expression is not a side effect of fluphenazine therapy.

    Client Need: Pharmacologic and Parenteral Therapies; **Cognitive Level:** Analysis; **Nursing Process:** Evaluation/Outcomes

18. **2 Haloperidol (Haldol) causes photosensitivity. Severe sunburn can occur on exposure to the sun.**

    1 There is no known side effect that affects night driving. **3** A client would be advised against eating aged cheeses if the client were taking an MAO inhibitor. However, people taking psychotropic medications should avoid alcohol. **4** Aspirin is not contraindicated.

    Client Need: Pharmacologic and Parenteral Therapies; **Cognitive Level:** Application; **Integrated Process:** Teaching/Learning; **Nursing Process:** Planning/Implementation

19. **3 Haloperidol (Haldol) alters the effectiveness of exogenous insulin, and the combination of haloperidol and insulin must be used with caution.**

    1 The occurrence of respiratory depression is more likely with a combination of antipsychotics and barbiturates. **2** Intensified action of both drugs would be more likely to occur if the antipsychotic were fluoxetine (Prozac). **4** There are no data to support that there is an intensified action of both drugs.

    Client Need: Pharmacologic and Parenteral Therapies; **Cognitive Level:** Analysis; **Nursing Process:** Evaluation/Outcomes

20. **3 Clozapine (Clozaril) may cause agranulocytosis, which can result in acquiring an infection.**

    1 Risk for falls is more common with typical antipsychotic medications because they may cause orthostatic hypotension and extrapyramidal side effects. **2** An inability to sit still (akathisia) is more common with typical antipsychotics because they may cause extrapyramidal side effects. **4** Dizziness upon standing (orthostatic hypotension) is more common with typical antipsychotics because they may cause extrapyramidal side effects.

    Client Need: Pharmacologic and Parenteral Therapies; **Cognitive Level:** Analysis; **Integrated Process:** Teaching/Learning; **Nursing Process:** Planning/Implementation

21. **1 Olanzapine (Zyprexa), a thienobenzodiazepine, can cause orthostatic hypotension.**

    2 Blurred, not double, vision may occur. **3** An anticholinergic effect of olanzapine is decreased salivation. **4** Olanzapine may cause nausea and other GI upsets; it should be taken with fluid or food.

    Client Need: Pharmacologic and Parenteral Therapies; **Cognitive Level:** Application; **Integrated Process:** Teaching/Learning; **Nursing Process:** Planning/Implementation

22. **Answers: 1, 3**

    1 Weight gain is a common side effect of olanzapine. **3** Olanzapine, being an atypical antipsychotic, affects the negative symptoms of schizophrenia, one of which is lack of pleasure (anhedonia).

    2 Olanzapine (Zyprexa) has no significant effect on blood clotting time. **4** Olanzapine, being an atypical antipsychotic, has a decreased chance of extra pyramidal side effects. **5** Olanzapine, being an atypical antipsychotic, has a significantly reduced chance of akathisia.

    Client Need: Pharmacologic and Parenteral Therapies; **Cognitive Level:** Analysis; **Integrated Process:** Teaching/Learning; **Nursing Process:** Evaluation/Outcomes

    Client Need: Pharmacologic and Parenteral Therapies; **Cognitive Level:** Analysis; **Nursing Process:** Planning/Implementation

Adrenergic and Adrenergic Blocking Drugs $\quad$ 6

INTRODUCTION TO ADRENERGIC & ADRENERGIC BLOCKING DRUGS

Adrenal Glands

- Two closely associated structures, adrenal medulla and adrenal cortex, positioned at each kidney's superior border

Adrenal Hormones

- Adrenal medulla: produces two catecholamines, epinephrine and norepinephrine
  - Stimulate liver and skeletal muscle to break down glycogen to produce glucose
  - Increase oxygen use and carbon dioxide production
  - Increase blood concentration of free fatty acids through stimulation of lipolysis in adipose tissue
  - Cause constriction of most blood vessels of body, thus increasing total peripheral resistance and arterial pressure to shunt blood to vital organs
  - Increase heart rate and force of contraction, thus increasing cardiac output
  - Inhibit contractions of gastrointestinal and uterine smooth muscle
  - Epinephrine significantly dilates bronchial smooth muscle
- Adrenal cortex: secretes the mineralocorticoid aldosterone and the glucocorticoids cortisol and corticosterone
  - Aldosterone
    - Markedly accelerates sodium and water reabsorption by kidney tubules
    - Markedly accelerates potassium excretion by kidney tubules
  - Secretion increases as sodium ions decrease or potassium ions increase
  - Cortisol and corticosterone
    - Accelerate mobilization and catabolism of tissue protein and fats
    - Accelerate liver gluconeogenesis (hyperglycemic effect)
    - Decrease antibody formation (immunosuppressive, antiallergic effect)
    - Slow proliferation of fibroblasts characteristic of inflammation (antiinflammatory effect)
    - Decrease adrenocorticotropic hormone (ACTH) secretion
    - Mildly accelerate sodium and water reabsorption and potassium excretion by kidney tubules
    - Increase release of coagulation factors

AUTONOMIC NERVOUS SYSTEM

- Conducts impulses from brainstem or cord out to visceral effectors (e.g., cardiac muscle, smooth muscle, and glands)
- Consists of two divisions:
  - Sympathetic division (adrenergic fibers) secretes norepinephrine: influences heart, smooth muscle of blood vessels and bronchioles, and glandular secretion
  - Parasympathetic division (cholinergic fibers) secretes acetylcholine: influences digestive tract and smooth muscle to promote digestive gland secretion, peristalsis, and defecation; influences heart to decrease rate and contractility

- Autonomic antagonism and summation: sympathetic and parasympathetic impulses tend to produce opposite effects
- Under conditions of stress, sympathetic impulses to visceral effectors dominate over parasympathetic impulses; however, in some individuals under stress, parasympathetic impulses via the vagus nerve increase to glands and smooth muscle of the stomach, stimulating hydrochloric acid secretion and gastric motility.

Adrenergic Drugs

- Adrenergic agonists (also called adrenergics, sympathomimetics): act on adrenergic receptor sites in effector cells of muscles
- The main receptors include (Fig. 6.1):
    - Alpha$_1$ receptors are in the bladder, blood vessels, eyes, prostate: when stimulated, they control vasomotor tone by constricting arteriole and venules, causing increased peripheral

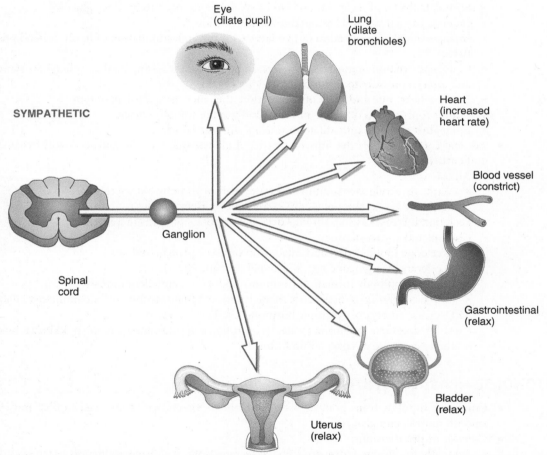

FIG. 6.1 Sympathetic responses. Stimulation of the sympathetic nervous system or use of sympathomimetic (adrenergic agonist) drugs can cause the pupils and bronchioles to dilate; heart rate to increase; blood vessels to constrict; and muscles of the gastrointestinal tract, bladder, and uterus to relax, thereby decreasing contractions. (From Kee, J.L., Hayes, E.R., McCuistion, L.E. [2015]. *Pharmacology: A patient-centered nursing process approach* [8th ed.]. St. Louis: Saunders.)

- resistance and improved circulation. If stimulated too much, blood flow to vital organs is reduced.
  - Alpha$_2$ receptors are in the postganglionic sympathetic nerve endings: when stimulated, they inhibit the release of norepinephrine, resulting in vasodilation and decreased blood pressure.
  - Beta$_1$ receptors are in the heart and kidneys: when stimulated, they increase myocardial contractility and increase heart rate.
  - Beta$_2$ receptors are in the lungs, liver, gastrointestinal tract and uterus in the smooth muscle: when stimulated, they relax the smooth muscle of the lungs and uterus, decrease gastrointestinal tone and motility, and activate glycogenolysis in the liver and increase blood glucose.
  - Dopaminergic receptors are in the cerebral, coronary, mesenteric and renal arteries: when stimulated by dopamine, they cause blood vessels to dilate and increase blood flow.
- Adrenergic agonists can be selective or nonselective.
  - Nonselective adrenergic agonists activate more than one receptor site (e.g., epinephrine acts on alpha$_1$, beta$_1$, and beta$_2$ receptors).
- Inactivating the action of a neurotransmitter
  - Neurotransmitters such as norepinephrine may be inactivated by reuptake back into the neuron, enzymatic transformation/degradation, or diffusion.
  - L-monoamine oxidase and catechol-O-methyltransferase are enzymes that inactivate neurotransmitters.
  - Once a neurotransmitter has performed its function, inactivation prevents a prolonged effect.
- Prolonging the action of a neurotransmitter
  - Neurotransmitters may be prolonged with the use of drugs that inhibit reuptake or enzymatic degradation.
- Classes of adrenergic agonists (sympathomimetics) include:
  - Direct (e.g., epinephrine, norepinephrine)
  - Indirect (e.g., amphetamine)
  - Mixed: direct and indirect (e.g., ephedrine, pseudoephedrine)
- Catecholamines produce sympathomimetic response and include two types:
  - Endogenous (e.g., dopamine, epinephrine, norepinephrine)
  - Synthetic (e.g., dobutamine, isoproterenol)
- Inhibitors of catecholamine reuptake
  - Cocaine, tricyclic antidepressants (TCAs) are examples of drugs that inhibit catecholamine reuptake
  - More information on these drugs can be found in Chapters 2 and 5
- Inhibitors of catecholamine metabolism
  - Monoamine oxidase inhibitors (MAOIs) are drugs that inhibit catecholamine metabolism
    - Tyramine is an amine that comes from tyrosine (an amino acid). It occurs naturally in plants and animals, particularly in aged food. In conjunction with MAOIs, it can cause hypertensive crisis.
- Noncatecholamines activate adrenergic receptors (e.g., albuterol, metaproterenol, phenylephrine).
- Adrenergic antagonists (also called adrenergic blockers or sympatholytics): prevent the action of agonists by blocking alpha and beta receptor sites. This action may be direct (by binding to the receptor) or indirect (by inhibiting norepinephrine and epinephrine).
  - Alpha-adrenergic antagonists (also called alpha blockers) promote vasodilation and decrease blood pressure. They may be selective (blocking only alpha$_1$ receptors) or nonselective (blocking alpha$_1$ and alpha$_2$ receptors).

- Beta-adrenergic antagonists (also called beta blockers) decrease heart rate, usually resulting in decreased blood pressure. They may be selective (blocking only beta$_1$ receptors) or nonselective (blocking both beta$_1$ and beta$_2$ receptors).
- Some beta blockers possess intrinsic sympathomimetic activity (also called intrinsic sympathomimetic effect). They can act as partial agonists while blocking endogenous catecholamines from the receptor site. Examples include acebutolol (selective) and carvedilol, penbutolol, and pindolol (nonselective).
- Adrenergic neuron antagonists (also called adrenergic neuron blockers) block norepinephrine release from the sympathetic terminal neurons (e.g., reserpine).

APPLICATION AND REVIEW

1. A nurse identifies which clinical indicator of parasympathetic dominance in a client under stress?
   1. Constipation
   2. Goose bumps
   3. Excess epinephrine secretion
   4. Increased gastrointestinal secretions
2. Damage or dysfunction of what organ increases the client's need for adrenergic medication therapy?
   1. Adrenal glands
   2. Cerebral cortex
   3. Lungs
   4. Liver
3. An adrenergic agonist targets which receptors to improve circulation in the eyes, prostate, and blood vessels?
   1. Dopaminergic
   2. Alpha$_1$
   3. Beta$_1$
   4. Beta$_2$
4. What is an example of a direct adrenergic agonistic drug?
   1. Ephedrine
   2. Epinephrine
   3. Amphetamine
   4. Pseudoephedrine
5. A client is being treated for depression. Which question is directed at assessing the client's ability to metabolize catecholamines?
   1. "What chronic physical conditions are you being treated for?"
   2. "What antidepressant medication are you prescribed?"
   3. "Are you adhering to any specific diet restrictions?"
   4. "Do you exercise regularly?"
6. By what process do alpha blockers decrease blood pressure?
   1. Decreasing heart rate
   2. Blocking beta$_1$ receptors
   3. Blocking beta$_2$ receptors
   4. Fostering vasodilation

See Answers on pages 117-120.

Nonselective Adrenergic Agonists

- Used to treat allergic reaction, anaphylaxis, angioedema, asthma, bronchospasm, cardiogenic shock, heart failure, hypotension, nasal congestion, septic shock, status asthmaticus
- Categories include direct, indirect, and mixed action
- Examples: epinephrine, norepinephrine, dopamine, amphetamine, ephedrine, pseudoephedrine
- Available in intravenous, injectable, and inhalation preparations

Mode of Action

- Acts primarily on beta receptors with some alpha receptor interaction to improve coronary output and constrict blood vessels.

Contraindications, Precautions, and Drug Interactions of Nonselective Adrenergic Agonists*

Drug	Contraindications/Precautions	Major Drug Interactions
Direct Action		
Epinephrine *alpha₁, beta₁,* *beta₂*	***Contraindications:*** Cardiac tachydysrhythmias, cerebral arteriosclerosis, closed-angle glaucoma, hypersensitivity ***Precautions:*** Diabetes mellitus, hypertension, hyperthyroidism, pregnancy, prostatic hypertrophy ***Pregnancy:*** Only given after risks to the fetus are considered	Antidepressants, beta-adrenergic blockers, MAOIs, other sympathomimetics
Norepinephrine *alpha₁, beta₁*	***Contraindications:*** Cardiac disease, hypersensitivity to norepinephrine or cyclopropane/halothane anesthesia, hypovolemia, hyperthyroidism, pheochromocytoma, tachydysrhythmias, ventricular fibrillation ***Precautions:*** Arterial embolism, breastfeeding, cardiac disease, geriatric, hypertension, hyperthyroidism, peripheral vascular disease, pregnancy ***Pregnancy:*** Only given after risks to the fetus are considered	Alpha blockers, antihistamines, ergots, guanethidine, MAOIs, methyldopa, oxytocics, sodium bicarbonate, tricyclics
Dopamine *alpha₁, beta₁*	***Contraindications:*** Hypersensitivity, hypovolemia, pheochromocytoma, tachydysrhythmias, ventricular fibrillation ***Precautions:*** Acute MI, arterial embolism, breastfeeding, geriatric, peripheral vascular disease, pregnancy, sulfite hypersensitivity, ***Pregnancy:*** Only given after risks to the fetus are considered	Alpha-adrenergic blockers, beta adrenergic blockers, ergots, general anesthetics, tricyclic antidepressants, MAOIs, oxytocics
Indirect Action		
Amphetamine	***Contraindications:*** <6 yr, congenital heart defect, coronary heart disease, heart disease, high blood pressure, history of drug or alcohol addiction, history of heart disease or sudden death, overactive thyroid, severe anxiety ***Precautions:*** Abnormal EEG, compromised circulation, depression, epilepsy, mental illness, motor tics, Tourette's syndrome, thyroid disorder, seizures ***Pregnancy:*** Only given after risks to the fetus are considered	Alcohol, antihypertensives, monoamine oxidase inhibitors (MAOIs), many selective serotonin and norepinephrine reuptake inhibitors (SNRIs; SSNRIs) bupropion, some contrast agents, furazolidone, pimozide, procarbazine, sibutramine, tapentadol, tramadol, vortioxetine
Mixed Action		
Ephedrine *alpha₁, beta₁,* *beta₂*	***Contraindications:*** Diabetes, heart disease, high blood pressure, irregular heartbeat, hypersensitivity, thyroid disease, severe heart problems ***Precautions:*** Drug resistance with long-term use ***Pregnancy:*** Only given after risks to the fetus are considered	Beta-blockers, MAOIs, oxytocics, tricyclics, catechol-O-methyltransferase inhibitors, ergot alkaloids, bromocriptine, cocaine, digoxin, guanadrel, guanethidine, indomethacin, linezolid, mecamylamine, methyldopa, reserpine

Continued

Contraindications, Precautions, and Drug Interactions of Nonselective Adrenergic Agonists—cont'd

Drug	Contraindications/Precautions	Major Drug Interactions
Mixed Action		
Pseudoephedrine $alpha_1$, $alpha_2$, $beta_1$	**Contraindications:** Hypersensitivity, closed-angle glaucoma **Precautions:** Diabetes, heart disease, high blood pressure, thyroid disorder **Pregnancy:** Only given after risks to the fetus are considered	Alkalinizing agents, alpha$_1$ blockers, sympathomimetics, MAOIs, serotonin/norepinephrine reuptake inhibitors, urinary acidifying agents, carbonic anhydrase inhibitors, ergot derivatives, atomoxetine, benzylpenicilloyl polylysine, cocaine, dihydroergotamine, doxofylline, ergonovine, ergotamine, fentanyl, furazolidone, Iobenguane I 123, linezoid, methylene blue, methylergonovine, methysergide maleate, phenelzine, procarbazine, spironolactone, tedizolid

MAOI, monoamine oxidase inhibitor.
*Pregnancy categories have been revised. See http://www.fda.gov/Drugs/DevelopmentApprovalProcess/DevelopmentResources/Labeling/ucm093307.htm for more information.

Adverse/Side Effects

- Agitation
- Angina
- Anorexia
- Bradycardia
- Cerebral hemorrhage
- Dizziness
- Dyspnea
- Dysrhythmia
- Ectopic beats
- Gastrointestinal distress
- Headache
- Hyperglycemia
- Hypertension
- Insomnia
- Mental changes
- Nausea/vomiting/diarrhea
- Pallor
- Palpitations
- Peripheral edema
- Pulmonary edema
- Restlessness
- Sweating
- Tachycardia
- Tissue necrosis/gangrene
- Ventricular fibrillation
- Weakness
- Wide QRS complex

Nursing Care

- Assess blood pressure, heart rhythm during infusion
- Assess for sensitivity to sulfite
- Assess I&O, peripheral blood flow; assess for infiltration/extravasation at the injection site
- Teach patient/family to report adverse effects

APPLICATION AND REVIEW

7. A client who is obtund has a blood pressure of 80/35 mm Hg after a blood transfusion. In an effort to support renal perfusion, the nurse administers dopamine at 2 mcg/kg/min as prescribed. What is the **most** relevant outcome indicating effectiveness of the medication for this client?

   1. A decrease in blood pressure   3. A decrease in core temperature
   2. An increase in urinary output   4. An increase in level of consciousness

8. What is the primary desired outcome of nonselective adrenergic agonist medication therapy? **Select all that apply.**
   1. Improved coronary output
   2. Decreased nasal congestion
   3. Relaxation of bronchial tree
   4. Vasoconstriction of blood vessels
   5. Management of anaphylactic shock

9. For which client diagnosis would epinephrine therapy be contraindicated? **Select all that apply.**
   1. Closed angle glaucoma
   2. Hyperthyroidism
   3. Hypotension
   4. Tachycardia
   5. Lactation

10. A client is being considered for a prescription for pseudoephedrine. After assessing the client's current medication history, which medication poses a major drug interaction?
    1. A serotonin/norepinephrine reuptake inhibitor
    2. Tricyclic antidepressant
    3. A beta-blocker
    4. Digoxin

11. The nurse should stress to a client prescribed a nonselective adrenergic agonist the importance of reporting which potential side effect of the therapy? **Select all that apply.**
    1. Dizziness
    2. Anorexia
    3. Insomnia
    4. Constipation
    5. Restlessness

12. Considering client safety, which component of medication education has the most importance for a client prescribed a nonselective adrenergic agonists?
    1. Recognizing and reporting adverse effects
    2. Administering the medication as prescribed
    3. Protocol for scheduling missed medication doses
    4. The need to stop smoking any tobacco-based product

See Answers on pages 117-120.

Inhibitors of Catecholamine Metabolism

Monoamine Oxidase Inhibitors (MAOIs)

- Used to treat symptoms of depression (see Chapter 5)
- Examples: phenelzine, tranylcypromine
- Available in oral preparations
- Multiple MAOI-drug interactions

Mode of Action

- Increases certain chemicals in the brain

Adverse/Side Effects and Nursing Care

- See Chapter 5

Selected Receptor Agonists

- Used to treat hypertension, benign prostatic hyperplasia, nasal decongestion, bronchospasm, and certain dysrhythmias

- Categories are alpha-adrenergic antagonists and beta-adrenergic antagonists
- Examples: phenylephrine, tetrahydrozoline, clonidine, guanabenz, guanfacine, isoproterenol, dobutamine, terbutaline, albuterol, salmeterol, formoterol, levalbuterol
- Available in oral, injectable, inhaled, intravenous, topical eye drop, and transdermal preparations

Mode of Action
- Binds to a receptor to cause an action.

Contraindications, Precautions, and Drug Interactions of Receptor Agonists*

Drug	Contraindications/Precautions	Major Drug Interaction
Alpha₁–Adrenergic Agonists		
Phenylephrine	**Contraindications:** Closed-angle glaucoma, hypersensitivity, pheochromocytoma, tachydysrhythmias, severe hypertension, ventricular fibrillation **Precautions:** A embolism, bradycardia, breastfeeding, geriatric, hyperthyroidism, myocardial disease, partial heart block, peripheral vascular disease, pregnancy, severe arteriosclerosis **Pregnancy:** Only given after risks to the fetus are considered	Alpha-blockers, antidepressants, digoxin, general anesthetics, MAOIs, oxytocics
tetrahydrozoline	**Contraindications:** Hypersensitivity **Precautions:** Diabetes, glaucoma, heart problems, high blood pressure, pregnancy, thyroid problems **Pregnancy:** Only given after risks to the fetus are considered	Bromocriptine, cocaine, furazolidone, MAOIs, tricyclic antidepressants
Alpha₂–Adrenergic Agonists		
Clonidine	**Contraindications:** Anticoagulants, bleeding disorders, hypersensitivity **Precautions:** Asthma, breastfeeding, child <12 yr (transdermal), chronic renal failure, COPD, depression, diabetes mellitus, geriatric, MI (recent), pregnancy, Raynaud's disease, thyroid disease **Pregnancy:** Only given after risks to the fetus are considered	Alcohol, amphetamines, anesthetics, antidepressants (tricyclic), appetite suppressants, diltiazem, diuretics, hypnotics, levodopa, MAOIs, nitrates, opiates, prazosin, tricyclics, sedatives
Guanabenz	**Contraindications:** Hypersensitivity **Precautions:** Hepatic impairment, sedation, renal impairment, vascular insufficiency **Pregnancy:** Only given after risks to the fetus are considered	CNS depressants, tizanidine
Dexmedetomidine	**Contraindications:** Dysrhythmias, hypersensitivity **Precautions:** AV block, breastfeeding, depression, dehydration, diabetes mellitus, glaucoma, liver disease, hypertension **Pregnancy:** Only given after risks to the fetus are considered	Alcohol, buprenorphine, propoxyphene, sodium oxybate, tizanidine

Contraindications, Precautions, and Drug Interactions of Receptor Agonists—cont'd

Drug	Contraindications/Precautions	Major Drug Interaction
Beta-Adrenergic Agonists		
Isoproterenol	*Contraindications:* Angina, cardiac glycoside intoxication, tachydysrhythmias, ventricular dysrhythmias *Precautions:* Cardiovascular disease, diabetes mellitus, distributive shock, geriatric, hyperthyroidism *Pregnancy:* Only given after risks to the fetus are considered	Similar interactions to epinephrine: Antidepressants, beta-adrenergic blockers, MAOIs, other sympathomimetics
Dobutamine	*Contraindications:* Hypersensitivity, idiopathic hypertrophic subaortic stenosis *Precautions:* Breastfeeding, CAD, children, dysrhythmias, geriatric, hypertension, hypersensitivity to sulfite, hypovolemia, myocardial infarction, pregnancy, renal failure *Pregnancy:* No human studies available, but no adverse effects in animals	Antidepressants, atomoxetine, beta-blockers, bretylium, COMT inhibitors, MAOIs, oxytocin, oxytocics, general anesthetics
Terbutaline	*Contraindications:* Hypersensitivity to sympathomimetics, closed-angle glaucoma, tachydysrhythmias *Precautions:* Breastfeeding, cardiac disorders, diabetes mellitus, geriatric, hyperthyroidism, prostatic hypertension, hypertension, seizure disorder *Pregnancy:* No human studies available, but no adverse effects in animals	Arsenic trioxide, beta agonists, beta-adrenergic blockers, chloroquine, class IA/III antidysrhythmics, CYP3A4 inhibiters, droperidol, haloperidol, levomethadyl, MAOIs, pentamidine, sympathomimetics
Albuterol	*Contraindications:* Hypersensitivity to albuterol or milk protein *Precautions:* Cardiac dysrhythmia, coronary artery disease, diabetes mellitus, hypertension, hyperthyroidism, geriatric, MAOI therapy, pregnancy, renal dysfunction, seizures, severe cardiac disease *Pregnancy:* Only given after risks to the fetus are considered	Beta blockers, MAOIs, other sympathomimetics, TCAs
Salmeterol	*Contraindications:* Hypersensitivity to sympathomimetics, monotherapy treatment of asthma, severe cardiac disease, tachydysrythmias *Precautions:* Acute asthma, breastfeeding, cardiac disorders, closed-angle glaucoma, diabetes mellitus, hypertension, hyperthyroidism, prostatic hypertrophy, QT prolongation, seizures *Pregnancy:* Only given after risks to the fetus are considered	Aerosol bronchodilators, antidepressants, beta-adrenergic blockers, CYP3A4 inhibitors, MAOIs
Levalbuterol	*Contraindications:* Hypersensitivity to sympathomimetics/levalbuterol/albuterol *Precautions*: Angle-closure glaucoma breastfeeding, children, diabetes mellitus, hypertension, hypokalemia, hypotension, hyperthyroidism, prostatic hypertrophy, QT prolongation, renal disease, seizures, severe cardiac disease, tachydysrhythmias, *Pregnancy:* Only given after risks to the fetus are considered; animal studies have shown adverse reactions; no human studies available	Adrenergics, aerosol bronchodilators, class IA/III antidysrhythmics, beta blockers, loop/thiazide diuretics, MAOIs, tricyclics

Continued

Contraindications, Precautions, and Drug Interactions of Receptor Agonists—cont'd

Drug	Contraindications/Precautions	Major Drug Interaction
Beta-Adrenergic Agonists		
Formoterol	**Contraindications:** Hypersensitivity to sympathomimetics, COPD, monotherapy treatment of asthma, status asthmaticus **Precautions:** African descent, aneurysm, cardiac disorders, diabetes mellitus, geriatric patients, hypertension, hyperthyroidism, prostatic hypertrophy **Pregnancy:** Only given after risks to the fetus are considered; animal studies have shown adverse reactions; no human studies available	Clarithromycin, class IA/III antiarrythmics, haloperidol, loop/thiazide diuretics, MAOIs, sympathomimetics, thyroid hormones, tricyclics

MAOI, monoamine oxidase inhibitor; *TCA,* tricyclic antidepressants; *yr,* years.
*Pregnancy categories have been revised. See http://www.fda.gov/Drugs/DevelopmentApprovalProcess/DevelopmentResources/Labeling/ucm093307.htm for more information.

Adverse/Side Effects

- Anaphylaxis
- Angina
- Angioedema
- Anxiety
- Bronchospasm
- Congestive heart failure
- Cough
- Diarrhea
- Dizziness
- Dyspnea
- Dysrhythmias
- Gangrene
- Headache
- Hyperglycemia
- Hypertension
- Hypokalemia
- Hypotension
- Infection
- Insomnia
- Irritability
- Irritation of nose/throat
- Nausea
- Orthostatic hypertension
- Palpitations
- QT prolongation
- Rash
- Restlessness
- Stevens-Johnson syndrome
- Tachycardia
- Tremors
- Vomiting
- Weakness

Nursing Care

- Assess for paradoxical bronchospasm, paresthesias, and coldness of extremities.
- Assess for allergic reaction, angioedema, anaphylaxis.
- Assess respiratory function; monitor I&O, monitor ECG during administration, monitor blood pressure/pulse.
- Teach patient not to use OTC medications, except as directed by a prescriber.
- Teach patient to administer inhalation medication correctly and to use medication before other medications and allow at least 1 minute between each.
- Teach patient to report adverse effects and stop drug immediately if adverse effects occur.

Selected Receptor Antagonists

- Used to treat hypertension and dysrhythmias
- Categories are alpha-adrenergic antagonists and beta-adrenergic antagonists

- Examples: phenoxybenzamine, phentolamine, prazosin, terazosin, doxazosin, tamsulosin, propranolol, nadolol, labetalol, acebutolol, esmolol, atenolol, carvedilol, metoprolol
- Available in oral, injectable, and intravenous preparations

Mode of Action
- Blocks agonist-mediated responses.

Contraindications, Precautions, and Drug Interactions of Receptor Antagonists*

Drug	Contraindications/Precautions	Major Drug Interaction
Alpha-Adrenergic Antagonists		
Phenoxybenzamine	*Contraindications:* Allergy to phenoxybenzamine *Precautions:* Cerebral or coronary arteriosclerosis, renal damage, respiratory infection *Pregnancy:* Only given after risks to the fetus are considered	Alcohol, tizanidine
Phentolamine	*Contraindications:* Angina, coronary insufficiency, hypersensitivity, hypotension, myocardial infarction *Precautions:* Breastfeeding, dysrhythmia, peptic ulcer disease, pregnancy *Pregnancy:* Only given after risks to the fetus are considered	Antihypertensives, epinephrine, sildenafil, tadalafil
Prazosin	*Contraindications:* Hypersensitivity *Precautions:* Breastfeeding, children, eye surgery, geriatric, orthostatic hypertension, pregnancy, prostate cancer *Pregnancy:* Only given after risks to the fetus are considered	Alcohol, antihypertensives, beta-adrenergic blockers, clonidine, diuretics, MAOIs, nitroglycerin, NSAIDs, phosphodiesterase inhibitors
Terazosin	*Contraindications:* Hypersensitivity *Precautions:* Breastfeeding, children, pregnancy, prostate cancer, renal disease, syncope *Pregnancy:* Only given after risks to the fetus are considered	Alcohol, antihypertensives, beta blockers, estrogens, nitroglycerin, NSAIDs, salicylates, sympathomimetics, verapamil
Doxazosin	*Contraindications:* Hypersensitivity to quinazolines *Precautions:* Breastfeeding, children, hepatic disease, geriatric, pregnancy *Pregnancy:* Only given after risks to the fetus are considered	Alcohol, clonidine, nitrates, other antihypertensives, PDE-5 inhibitors
Tamsulosin	*Contraindications:* Hypersensitivity *Precautions:* Breastfeeding, children, CAD, cataract surgery, pregnancy, prostate cancer, severe renal disease *Pregnancy:* No human studies available, but no adverse effects in animals	Alpha-blockers, cimetidine, doxazosin
Beta-Adrenergic Antagonists		
Propranolol	*Contraindications:* Asthma, atrioventricular heart block, bronchospasm, bronchospastic disease, hydrochloride, hypersensitivity to propranolol, cardiogenic shock, sinus bradycardia *Precautions:* Breastfeeding, cardiac failure, children, chronic obstructive pulmonary disease, diabetes mellitus, hyperthyroidism, hypotension, myasthenia gravis, peripheral vascular disease, pregnancy, renal/hepatic disease, Raynaud's disease, sick sinus syndrome, smoking, thyrotoxicosis, vasospastic angina, Wolff-Parkinson-White syndrome *Pregnancy:* Only given after risks to the fetus are considered	Barbiturates, calcium channel blockers, cimetidine, disopyramide, haloperidol, propafenone, phenothiazines, smoking

Continued

Contraindications, Precautions, and Drug Interactions of Receptor Antagonists—cont'd

Drug	Contraindications/Precautions	Major Drug Interaction
Beta-Adrenergic Antagonists		
Nadolol	***Contraindications:*** Bronchospastic disease, cardiac failure, cardiogenic shock, heart block (second and third degree), hypersensitivity to nadolol, sinus bradycardia, chronic obstructive pulmonary disease, congestive heart failure ***Precautions:*** Breastfeeding, COPD, diabetes mellitus, hyperthyroidism, myasthenia gravis, major surgery, nonallergic bronchospasm, peripheral vascular disease, pregnancy, renal disease ***Pregnancy:*** Only given after risks to the fetus are considered	Antihypertensives, clonidine, epinephrine, ergots, digoxin, MAOIs, NSAIDs, phenothiazines, thyroid
Labetalol	***Contraindications:*** Congestive heart failure, bronchial asthma, hypersensitivity to beta blockers, cardiogenic shock, heart block, sinus bradycardia ***Precautions:*** Breastfeeding, CAD, COPD, diabetes mellitus, geriatric, major surgery, nonallergic bronchospasm, peripheral vascular disease, pregnancy, well-compensated heart failure ***Pregnancy:*** Only given after risks to the fetus are considered	Alcohol, antidiabetics, antidepressants, antihypertensives, beta blockers, bronchodilators, lidocaine, verapamil
Acebutolol	***Contraindications:*** Bronchospastic disease, cardiac failure, cardiogenic shock, second- and third-degree heart block, severe bradycardia ***Precautions:*** Allergies, impaired renal or hepatic function ***Pregnancy:*** No human studies available, but no adverse effects in animals	Animophylline, arbutamine, atazanavir, catecholamine-depleting medications, diltiazem, disopyramide, dolasetron, dyphylline, fingolimod, methacholine, NSAIDS, oxtriphylline, ritodrine, saquinavir, theophylline, tizanidine, verapamil
Esmolol	***Contraindications:*** Acute heart failure, bradycardia, cardiogenic shock, heart block ***Precautions:*** Atrial fibrillation, breastfeeding, bronchospasms, diabetes, geriatric patients, myasthenia gravis, hyperthyroidism, hypoglycemia, hypotension, thyrotoxicosis, renal disease, peripheral vascular disease, pregnancy ***Pregnancy:*** Only given after risks to the fetus are considered	Amphetamine, digoxin, ephedrine, epinephrine, general anesthetics, MAOIs, thyroid hormones
Atenolol	***Contraindications:*** Cardiac failure, cardiogenic shock, hypersensitivity to β-blockers, heart block (second-and third-degree), sinus bradycardia, pregnancy ***Precautions:*** Asthma, breastfeeding, diabetes mellitus, major surgery, renal disease, thyroid disease, congestive heart failure, chronic obstructive pulmonary disease, asthma, well-compensated heart failure, dialysis, myasthenia gravis, Raynaud's disease, pulmonary edema ***Pregnancy:*** Evidence of fetal risk, but benefits outweigh risks	Amphetamines, anticholinergics, antihypertensives, antidiabetic agents, digoxin, diltiazem, dopamine, ephedrine, hydralazine, insulin, methyldopa, prazosin, pseudoephedrine, reserpine, sympathomimetics, theophylline, verapamil

Contraindications, Precautions, and Drug Interactions of Receptor Antagonists—cont'd

Drug	Contraindications/Precautions	Major Drug Interaction
Beta-Adrenergic Antagonists		
Carvedilol	***Contraindications:*** Asthma, cardiogenic shock, class IV decompensated cardiac failure, hypersensitivity, pulmonary edema, second- or third-degree heart block, severe bradycardia, severe hepatic disease, sick sinus symptoms ***Precautions:*** Anesthesia, breastfeeding, cardiac failure, children, chronic bronchitis, diabetes mellitus, emphysema, geriatric patients, hepatic injury, major surgery, peripheral vascular disease, renal disease, thyrotoxicosis ***Pregnancy:*** Only given after risks to the fetus are considered; animal studies have shown adverse reactions; no human studies available	Acute alcohol ingestion, antidiabetic agents, calcium channel blockers, cimetidine, clonidine, cyclosporine, CYP2D6 inhibitors, digoxin, levodopa, MAOIs, nitrates, NSAIDs, reserpine, rifampin, thyroid medications
Metoprolol	***Contraindications:*** Hypersensitivity to beta blockers, cardiogenic shock, second- or third-degree heart block, pheochromocytoma, sick sinus symptoms, sinus bradycardia ***Precautions:*** Bronchial asthma, breastfeeding, CAD, children, COPD, CVA, depression, diabetes mellitus, geriatric patients, hepatic/renal/thyroid disease, major surgery, nonallergic bronchospasm, vasospastic angina ***Pregnancy:*** Only given after risks to the fetus are considered; animal studies have shown adverse reactions; no human studies available	Amphetamines, barbiturates, benzodiazepines, calcium channel blockers, cimetidine, epinephrine, H2 antagonists, hydralazine, insulin, MAOIs, methyldopa, NSAIDs, oral antidiabetics, prazosin, respirine, salicylates, xanthines
Adrenergic Neuron Antagonists		
Reserpine	***Contraindications:*** Depression, electroconvulsive therapy, hypersensitivity, ulcer, ulcerative colitis ***Precautions:*** History of gallstones, history of peptic ulcer, renal insufficiency, history of ulcerative colitis ***Pregnancy:*** Only given after risks to the fetus are considered	Alcohol, amphetamine, digitalis, digoxin, direct-acting amines, furazolidone, isoproterenol, MOAI inhibitors, other antihypertensive agents, quinidine, phenylephrine, sympathomimetics, tetrabenazine, tizanidine, tricyclic antidepressants

COPD, chronic obstructive pulmonary disease; *MAOI,* monoamine oxidase inhibitor; *NSAID,* nonsteroidal antiinflammatory drug.
*Pregnancy categories have been revised. See http://www.fda.gov/Drugs/DevelopmentApprovalProcess/DevelopmentResources/Labeling/ucm093307.htm for more information.

Adverse/Side Effects
- Agranulocytosis
- AV block
- Bradycardia
- Bronchospasm
- Chest pain
- Congestive heart failure
- Depression
- Diarrhea
- Dizziness
- Fatigue
- Headache
- Hyperglycemia

- Hypotension
- Insomnia
- Ischemic colitis
- Lung edema
- Mental changes
- Mesenteric arterial thrombosis

- Nausea
- Postural hypotension
- Pulmonary edema
- Purpura
- Shortness of breath
- Thrombocytopenia

Nursing Care

- Assess baselines in renal and liver function tests before beginning therapy.
- Assess for hypertension, congestive heart failure, hypoglycemia, and allergic reactions.
- Assess for lower extremity edema daily.
- Monitor daily weights
- Teach patient not to use OTC products unless directed by prescriber.
- Teach patient that product may mask symptoms of hypoglycemia in diabetic patients.
- Teach patient to avoid hazardous activities if dizzy or drowsy.
- Teach patient to change positions slowly.
- Teach patient to comply with weight control, dietary adjustments such as limiting caffeine and avoiding alcohol, modified exercise program.
- Teach patient to limit alcohol, smoking; to limit sodium intake as prescribed.
- Teach patient to monitor blood pressure at home.
- Teach patient to notify prescriber of mouth sores, sore throat, fever, swelling of hands or feet, irregular heartbeat, chest pain, cold extremities, bleeding, bruising, weight gain.
- Teach patient to report symptoms of congestive heart failure.
- Teach patient to take product as prescribed; not to discontinue product abruptly; taper as directed; take at same time each day.
- Teach patient to use contraception while taking this product and avoid breastfeeding.
- Teach patient to wear emergency ID for medications, allergies, conditions being treated.

APPLICATION AND REVIEW

13. A health care provider in the emergency department identifies that a client is in mild hypovolemic shock. Which type of drug should the nurse anticipate will be prescribed?
    1. Loop diuretic
    2. Cardiac glycoside
    3. Sympathomimetic
    4. Alpha-adrenergic blocker
14. A client who is receiving atenolol for hypertension frequently reports feeling dizzy. What effect of atenolol should the nurse consider may be responsible this response?
    1. Depleting acetylcholine
    2. Stimulating histamine release
    3. Blocking the adrenergic response
    4. Decreasing adrenal release of epinephrine
15. A client with a history of coronary artery disease is admitted with pneumonia. The health care provider prescribes atenolol. What should the nurse monitor to determine the therapeutic effect of atenolol?
    1. Heart rate
    2. Respirations
    3. Temperature
    4. Pulse oximetry

16. Propranolol is prescribed for a client with hypertension. For which side effect should the nurse monitor the client?
    1. Hirsutism
    2. Bradycardia
    3. Restlessness
    4. Hypertension
17. A client diagnosed with depression is likely to be prescribed which medication to inhibit catecholamine metabolism?
    1. A beta-blocker
    2. An alpha-blocker
    3. Monoamine oxidase inhibitors
    4. A selective adrenergic agonist
18. Which client diagnosis would be a contraindication to the prescription of the receptor antagonist, phentolamine?
    1. Angina
    2. Pneumonia
    3. Kidney disease
    4. Cerebral arteriosclerosis

See Answers on pages 117-120.

ANSWER KEY: REVIEW QUESTIONS

1. **4 Parasympathetic nerves increase peristalsis and GI secretion.**
   1 The parasympathetic nervous system increases intestinal motility, which may cause diarrhea. **2** Goose bumps (piloerection), caused by contraction of the musculi arrectores pilorum, are under sympathetic control; vasoconstriction is also under sympathetic control. **3** Epinephrine is a sympathomimetic.
   Client Need: Physiologic Adaptation; **Cognitive Level:** Comprehension; **Nursing Process:** Assessment/Analysis

2. **1 The adrenal glands produce and secrete substances that help regulate metabolism, blood glucose levels and blood pressure. A dysfunction would require either adrenergic or adrenergic blocking medications.**
   2 A dysfunctional cerebral cortex would not generally require adrenergic medication therapy. **3** A lung disorder would not generally require adrenergic medication therapy. **4** A liver disorder will not generally require adrenergic medication therapy.
   Client Need: Pharmacologic and Parenteral Therapies; **Cognitive Level:** Analysis; **Nursing Process:** Assessment/Analysis

3. **2 Alpha1 receptors are in the bladder, blood vessels, eyes, prostate: when stimulated, they control vasomotor tone by constricting arteriole and venules, causing increased peripheral resistance and improved circulation.**
   1 Dopaminergic receptors are in the cerebral, coronary, mesenteric, and renal arteries: when stimulated by dopamine, they cause blood vessels to dilate and increase blood flow. **3** $Beta_1$ receptors are in the heart and kidneys: when stimulated, they increase myocardial contractility and increase heart rate. **4** $Beta_2$ receptors are in the lungs, liver, gastrointestinal tract, and uterus in the smooth muscle: when stimulated, they relax the smooth muscle of the lungs and uterus, decrease gastrointestinal tone and motility, and activate glycogenolysis in the liver and increase blood glucose.
   Client Need: Pharmacologic and Parenteral Therapies; **Cognitive Level:** Comprehension; **Nursing Process:** Assessment/Analysis

4. **2 Epinephrine and norepinephrine are direct agonistic drugs.**
   1 Ephedrine is a mixed agonistic drug. **3** Amphetamine is an indirect agonistic drug. **4** Pseudoephedrine is a mixed agonistic drug.
   Client Need: Pharmacologic and Parenteral Therapies; **Cognitive Level:** Comprehension; **Nursing Process:** Assessment/Analysis

5. **2 Monoamine oxidase inhibitors (MAOIs), sometimes prescribed for the management of depression, are drugs that inhibit catecholamine metabolism.**
   1 Although assessing the history of chronic illness is appropriate, it does not have a direct bearing on catecholamine metabolism. **3** Although assessing dietary restrictions is appropriate, it does not have a

direct bearing on catecholamine metabolism. **4** Although assessing for regular physical activity is appropriate, it does not have a direct bearing on catecholamine metabolism.

Client Need: Pharmacologic and Parenteral Therapies; **Cognitive Level:** Analysis; **Nursing Process:** Assessment/Analysis

6. **4 Alpha-adrenergic antagonists (also called alpha blockers) promote vasodilation and decrease blood pressure.**

1 Beta-adrenergic antagonists (also called beta blockers) decrease heart rate, usually resulting in decreased blood pressure. **2** Beta-adrenergic antagonists may be selective (blocking only beta$_1$ receptors) or nonselective (blocking both beta$_1$ and beta$_2$ receptors). **3** Beta-adrenergic antagonists may be selective (blocking only beta$_1$ receptors) or nonselective (blocking both beta$_1$ and beta$_2$ receptors).

Client Need: Pharmacologic and Parenteral Therapies; **Cognitive Level:** Analysis; **Nursing Process:** Assessment/Analysis

7. **2 As renal perfusion increases, urinary output also should increase; doses greater than 10 mcg/kg/min can cause renal vasoconstriction and decreased urinary output.**

1 A change in blood pressure is not a direct predictor of the effectiveness of dopamine given at a level of 2 mcg/kg/min; at 10 mcg/kg/min a client will experience an increased cardiac output and an increased blood pressure. **3** Body temperature does not indicate improved renal perfusion. **4** In this situation, improvement of renal perfusion is not directly related to the client's level of consciousness.

Client Need: Pharmacologic and Parenteral Therapies; **Cognitive Level:** Analysis; **Nursing Process:** Evaluation/Outcomes

8. **Answers: 1, 4**

Nonselective adrenergic agonist medication acts primarily on beta receptors with some alpha receptor interaction to improve coronary output and constrict blood vessels.

2 Although used to treat nasal congestion, improved coronary output and constriction of blood vessels are the primary foci of nonselective adrenergic agonist medication. **3** Although used to treat bronchospasms, improved coronary output and constriction of blood vessels are the primary foci of nonselective adrenergic agonist medication. **5** Although used to manage anaphylactic shock, improved coronary output and constriction of blood vessels are the primary foci of nonselective adrenergic agonist medication.

Client Need: Pharmacologic and Parenteral Therapies; **Cognitive Level:** Analysis; **Nursing Process:** Assessment/Analysis

9. **Answers: 1, 2**

Closed angle glaucoma, and hyperthyroidism are conditions that would be exacerbated by epinephrine's vasoconstricting actions and so would be contraindicated.

3 Hypotension is a contraindication for norepinephrine therapy. **4** Trachydysrhythmias are contraindications for norepinephrine therapy. **5** Lactation is a condition where the use of norepinephrine therapy is given serious consideration.

Client Need: Pharmacologic and Parenteral Therapies; **Cognitive Level:** Analysis; **Nursing Process:** Assessment/Analysis

10. **1 A serotonin/norepinephrine reuptake inhibitor would create a major drug interaction if taken in combination with pseudoephedrine.**

2 A tricyclic antidepressant would create a major drug interaction if taken in combination with ephedrine not pseudoephedrine. **3** A beta blocker would create a major drug interaction if taken in combination with ephedrine not pseudoephedrine. **4** Digoxin would create a major drug interaction if taken in combination with ephedrine not pseudoephedrine.

Client Need: Pharmacologic and Parenteral Therapies; **Cognitive Level:** Analysis; **Nursing Process:** Assessment/Analysis

11. **Answers: 1, 2, 3, 5**

Potential side effects to nonselective adrenergic agonist medication includes dizziness, anorexia, insomnia, and restlessness.

5 Diarrhea rather than constipation is a possible side effect to this medication.

Client Need: Pharmacologic and Parenteral Therapies; **Cognitive Level:** Application; **Integrated Process:** Teaching/Learning; **Nursing Process:** Assessment/Analysis

12. **1 The client's safety is dependent of their ability to recognize and promptly report any potential adverse effects of the medication therapy.**

    2 Although appropriate to include instructions about medication administration, doing so focuses on medication effectiveness more than client safety. **3** Although appropriate to include instructions about missed dosage, doing so focuses on medication effectiveness more than client safety. **4** Although appropriate to encourage the client to stop the use of tobacco products, this information is not directly associated with the medication therapy.

    Client Need: Pharmacologic and Parenteral Therapies; **Cognitive Level:** Application; **Integrated Process:** Teaching/Learning; **Nursing Process:** Planning/Implementation

13. **3 Sympathomimetics are vasopressors that induce arterial constriction, which increases venous return and cardiac output.**

    1 Diuretics promote excretion of fluid, which will exacerbate hypovolemia associated with hypovolemic shock. **2** Cardiac glycosides slow and strengthen the heartbeat; they do not increase the blood pressure and may decrease the blood pressure. **4** Alpha-adrenergic blockers decrease peripheral resistance, resulting in a decreased blood pressure.

    Client Need: Pharmacologic and Parenteral Therapies; **Cognitive Level:** Analysis; **Nursing Process:** Planning/Implementation

14. **3 The beta adrenergic blocking effect of atenolol decreases the heart's rate and contractility; it may result in orthostatic hypotension and decreased cerebral perfusion, causing dizziness.**

    1 Depleting acetylcholine is not an action of atenolol. **2** Stimulating histamine release is not an action of atenolol. **4** Decreasing adrenal release of epinephrine is not an action of atenolol.

    Client Need: Pharmacologic and Parenteral Therapies; **Cognitive Level:** Comprehension; **Nursing Process:** Assessment/Analysis

 Study Tip: To remember that beta adrenergic blockers decrease heart rate and contractility, think of blocking adrenaline. You know that adrenaline gives you the fight-or-flight boost of energy, so when it's blocked you become more relaxed and your heart rate decreases.

15. **1 Atenolol, a beta blocker, slows the rate of SA node discharge and AV node conduction, thus decreasing the heart rate; it prevents angina by decreasing the cardiac workload and myocardial oxygen consumption.**

    2 Atenolol does not alter the respiratory rate, but its side effects may include bronchospasm and wheezing. **3** Atenolol is not an antipyretic. **4** Atenolol does not directly affect gas exchange in the lungs.

    Client Need: Pharmacologic and Parenteral Therapies; **Cognitive Level:** Application; **Nursing Process:** Evaluation/Outcomes

16. **2 Beta blockers block stimulation of beta$_1$ (myocardial) adrenergic receptors, which decreases the heart rate and blood pressure. The client should be monitored for bradycardia, which can progress to heart failure or cardiac arrest.**

    1 Excessive growth of hair or presence of hair in unusual places does not occur with this medication; however, absence or loss of hair (alopecia) may occur. **3** A side effect of this medication is fatigue, not restlessness. **4** Propranolol may produce hypotension, not hypertension.

    Client Need: Pharmacologic and Parenteral Therapies; **Cognitive Level:** Application; **Nursing Process:** Evaluation/Outcomes

Study Tip: Think **BBB: b**eta **b**lockers can bring **b**radycardia.

17. **3 Monoamine oxidase inhibitors increase certain chemicals (catecholamines) in the brain that help manage the symptoms of depression.**

    1 A beta-blocker is not used to treat depression as it is not effective at increasing catecholamine metabolism. **2** An alpha block is not used to treat depression as it is not effective at increasing catecholamine metabolism. **4** A selective adrenergic agonist is not used to treat depression as it is not effective at increasing catecholamine metabolism.

    Client Need: Pharmacologic and Parenteral Therapies; **Cognitive Level:** Application; **Nursing Process:** Planning/Implementation

18. **1 Angina is a contraindication to receptor antagonist therapy with phentolamine.**

    2 Pneumonia is a contraindication to receptor antagonist therapy with phenoxybenzamine. **3** Kidney disease is a contraindication to receptor antagonist therapy with Phenoxybenzamine. **4** Cerebral arteriosclerosis is a contraindication to receptor antagonist therapy with Phenoxybenzamine.

    Client Need: Pharmacologic and Parenteral Therapies; **Cognitive Level:** Analysis; **Nursing Process:** Planning/Implementation

Cholinergic and Cholinergic-blocking Drugs 7

INTRODUCTION TO CHOLINERGIC AND CHOLINERGIC-BLOCKING DRUGS

Central Nervous System (CNS)
- Composed of the brain and spinal cord

Peripheral Nervous System (PNS)
- Composed of cranial nerves, spinal nerves
- Includes autonomic nervous system (ANS)

Autonomic Nervous System (see Chapter 6)
Acetylcholine
- Located at the ganglions and parasympathetic terminal nerve endings
- Innervates cholinergic receptors in organs, tissues, glands
- Causes skeletal muscle contraction in PNS and inhibits activation of cholinergic system in CNS
- Axons that release acetylcholine are called cholinergic
- Two types of cholinergic receptors that bind acetylcholine and transmit its signal
  - Muscarinic
    - Muscarinic receptors are found in smooth muscle of GI tract, genitourinary tract, glands, and heart
    - Stimulates smooth muscle and slows heart rate
  - Nicotinic
    - Secretes epinephrine and norepinephrine into blood
    - Affects skeletal muscles

Major Disorders of Parasympathetic Nervous System
- Myasthenia Gravis
  - Cause: reduced acetylcholine receptors, autoimmune response
  - Clinical findings: remission and exacerbation of symptoms: increased pulse, respirations, and blood pressure; respiratory distress with cyanosis; loss of cough and swallowing reflexes; increased respiratory secretions; diaphoresis; increased lacrimation; dysarthria; restlessness; bowel and bladder incontinence; extreme muscle weakness
  - Therapeutic interventions: corticosteroids, cholinesterase inhibitors, immunosuppressives, radiation/surgical removal of thymus gland
- Dementia
  - Cause: decreased acetylcholine, anatomic brain changes, infections, toxins, not a normal sign of aging
  - Clinical findings: forgetfulness, aphasia, apraxia, amnesia, ataxia, agnosia, flat affect, delusions, sundowning phenomena, slow and progressive mental deterioration
  - Therapeutic interventions: reduction of causative agent (toxins), high calorie/protein diet, medications

Cholinergic Drugs

- Affect the nervous system
- Cholinergic agonists (also called muscarinic agonists or parasympathomimetics)
  - Mimic the neurotransmitter acetylcholine
  - Nonselective and affect both muscarinic and nicotinic receptors
  - Stimulate bladder and GI tone, constrict pupils, increase neuromuscular transmission
  - Decrease heart rate and blood pressure; increase salivary, GI, bronchial secretions
- Two types
  - Direct acting: act on muscarinic receptors to activate a tissue response
  - Indirect acting: inhibit action of cholinesterase (acetylcholinesterase) and allows acetylcholine to accumulate at receptor sites
  - Cholinergic muscle stimulants are used to treat myasthenia gravis; other cholinergics are used to reduce urinary retention, reverse effects of muscle relaxants used in surgery, and treat glaucoma (Fig. 7.1, A)
- Cholinergic antagonists (also called muscarinic antagonists, parasympatholytics, or anticholinergics)
  - Inhibit acetylcholine by occupying acetylcholine receptors
  - Block parasympathetic nerves allowing domination of sympathetic nervous system
  - Decrease in GI motility, salivation, dilation of pupils, bladder contraction, and increase in pulse rate
  - Can act as antidote to toxicity of cholinesterase inhibitors
  - Used to decrease secretions in certain disorders (ulcers, urethritis, Chronic Obstructive Pulmonary Disease [COPD]) and surgical procedures; also used to treat insomnia and dizziness
- Cholinesterases (also called cholinesterase inhibitors, acetylcholinesterase inhibitors) (Fig. 7.1, B)
  - Break down acetylcholine into choline and acetic acid
  - Bind with cholinesterase, allowing acetylcholine to activate muscarinic and nicotinic cholinergic receptors
  - Increase skeletal muscle contraction, GI motility, bradycardia, miosis, bronchial constriction, micturition
  - Two types

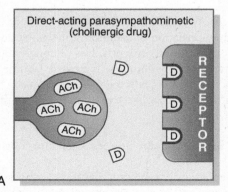
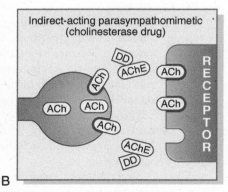

FIG. 7.1 **A,** Direct-acting parasympathomimetic (cholinergic agonist). Cholinergic agonists resemble acetylcholine and act directly on the receptor. **B,** Indirect-acting parasympathomimetic (cholinesterase inhibitor). (From McCuistion, L., Vuljoin-DiMaggio, K., Winton, M.B., Yeager, J.J. [2018]. *Pharmacology: A patient-centered nursing process approach* [9th ed.]. St. Louis: Elsevier.)

- Reversible inhibitors: bind cholinesterase for several minutes to hours
  - Used to treat myasthenia gravis, dementia, glaucoma
- Irreversible inhibitors: bind cholinesterase permanently
  - Used to treat glaucoma

CHOLINERGIC AGONISTS

- Used to treat urinary retention (bethanecol), glaucoma (carbachol, pilocarpine), dry mouth (cevimeline)
- Available in PO, IM, ophthalmic preparations

Mode of Action

- Increases actylcholine at muscarinic receptors

Contraindications, Precautions and Drug Interactions of Cholinergic Agonists*

Drug	Contraindications/Precautions	Drug Interaction
bethanecol	*Contraindications:* Hypersensitivity, severe bradycardia, asthma, severe hypotension, hyperthyroidism, peptic ulcer, parkinsonism, seizure disorders, CAD, COPD *Precautions:* Breastfeeding, children <8 yr, hypertension *Pregnancy:* Only given after risks to the fetus are considered; animal studies have shown adverse reactions; no human studies available	Ganglionic blockers, cholinergic agonists, anticholinesterase agents
carbachol	*Contraindications:* Hypersensitivity, acute iritis, acute inflammatory disease of anterior chamber *Precautions:* Breastfeeding, children, retinal detachment; cataracts; uveitis; hyperthyroidism; urinary tract obstruction *Pregnancy:* Only given after risks to the fetus are considered; animal studies have shown adverse reactions; no human studies available	Atropine, bethanecol
cevimeline	*Contraindications:* Hypersensitivity, acute iritis *Precautions:* Breastfeeding, children, asthma, COPD, glaucoma *Pregnancy:* Only given after risks to the fetus are considered; animal studies have shown adverse reactions; no human studies available	Beta blockers
pilocarpine	*Contraindications:* Hypersensitivity, acute iritis *Precautions:* Breastfeeding, children, asthma, COPD, glaucoma *Pregnancy:* Only given after risks to the fetus are considered; animal studies have shown adverse reactions; no human studies available	Beta blockers

*Pregnancy categories have been revised. See http://www.fda.gov/Drugs/DevelopmentApprovalProcess/DevelopmentResources/Labeling/ucm093307.htm for more information.

Adverse/Side Effects

- Dizziness
- Headache
- Malaise
- Hypotension
- Bradycardia
- Diaphoresis
- Increased salivation
- Rash
- Urticaria
- Flushing

Nursing Care

- Assess urinary patterns
- Monitor vital signs
- Monitor I&O

- Teach patient to take medication 1 hour before or 2 hours after meals
- Teach patient to change positions slowly
- Teach patient to avoid driving and hazardous activities

CHOLINERGIC ANTAGONISTS

- Used to decrease secretions (scopolamine, methscopolamine, glycopyrrolate), used to treat bronchospam, COPD (ipratropium)
- Examples: scopolamine, methscopolamine, glycopyrrolate, ipratropium
- Available in PO, IM, IV, subcutaneous, transdermal, intranasal, inhalation preparations

Mode of Action

- Blocks activity of the muscarinic acetylcholine receptor

Contraindications, Precautions and Drug Interactions of Cholinergic Antagonists*

Drug	Contraindications/Precautions	Drug Interaction
scopolamine	*Contraindications:* Hypersensitivity, closed-angle glaucoma, myasthenia gravis, GI/GU obstruction *Precautions:* Enlarged prostate, hyperthyroid, hypertension *Pregnancy:* No adverse effects in animals; no human studies available	Belladonna, barbiturates
methscopolamine	*Contraindications:* Hypersensitivity, closed-angle glaucoma *Precautions:* Enlarged prostate, hyperthyroid, hypertension *Pregnancy:* No adverse effects in animals; no human studies available	Potassium, pramlintide
glycopyrrolate	*Contraindications:* Hypersensitivity to glycopyrrolate, closed-angle glaucoma, myasthenia gravis *Precautions:* Enlarged prostate, hyperthyroid, hypertension, spastic paralysis *Pregnancy:* No adverse effects in animals; no human studies available	Antidepressants, ipratropium, potassium, CNS depressants
ipratropium	*Contraindications:* Hypersensitivity, atropine, bromide, soybean/peanut products *Precautions:* Breastfeeding, children <12 yr, angioedema, heart failure, bladder obstruction, closed-angle glaucoma, urinary retention *Pregnancy:* No adverse effects in animals; no human studies available	Other bronchodilators, phenothiazines, antihistamines, disopyramide

*Pregnancy categories have been revised. See http://www.fda.gov/Drugs/DevelopmentApprovalProcess/DevelopmentResources/Labeling/ucm093307.htm for more information.

Adverse/Side Effects

- Anxiety
- Nervousness
- Headache
- Palpitation
- Dry eyes
- Dry mouth
- Constipation
- Blurred vision
- Nasal congestion
- Rash

Nursing Care

- Monitor patient's respiratory status
- Monitor I&O
- Administer hard candy, gum, frequent drinks for dry mouth
- Shake liquids before administering

- Use a spacer when administering aerosols
- Teach patient correct method of inhalation
- Teach patient to avoid alcohol, driving, and other hazardous activities

ACETYLCHOLINESTERASE INHIBITORS

Treatment of Myasthenia Gravis

- Examples: edrophonium, neostigmine, pyridostigmine, ambednonium
- Available in PO, IM, IV preparations

Mode of Action

- Acetylcholinesterase inhibitors bind to cholinesterase resulting in increased acetylcholine in the synapses, causing increased parasympathetic activity (vasodilatation; constriction of pupils; increased sweat, saliva, and tear secretion; decreased heart rate; mucus secretion in the respiratory tract; constriction of bronchioles)

Contraindications, Precautions, and Drug Interactions of Acetylcholinesterase Inhibitors (Myasthenia Gravis)*

Drug	Contraindications/Precautions	Drug Interaction
edrophonium	*Contraindications:* Hypersensitivity, GI/GU obstruction *Precautions:* Asthma, cardiac arrythmia *Pregnancy:* Only given after risks to the fetus are considered; animal studies have shown adverse reactions; no human studies available	Sulfites
neostigmine	*Contraindications:* Hypersensitivity, GI/GU obstruction, bradycardia, heart blockage *Precautions:* Urinary tract infection (UTI) *Pregnancy:* Only given after risks to the fetus are considered; animal studies have shown adverse reactions; no human studies available	Anesthetics, procainamide, beta blockers, succinylcholine, quinolones
pyridostigmine	*Contraindications:* Hypersensitivity, bradycardia, hypotension, GI obstruction, adrenal insufficiency *Precautions:* Seizure disorders, asthma, hyperthyroidism, dysthythmias, poor GI motility *Pregnancy:* Only given after risks to the fetus are considered; animal studies have shown adverse reactions; no human studies available	Quinolones, succinylcholine, atropine, aminoglycosides, anesthetics, corticosteroids, antidysrhythmics
ambenonium	*Contraindications:* Hypersensitivity, GI/GU obstruction, bradycardia *Precautions:* COPD, coronary occlusion, hyperthyroidism, Parkinson's, peptic ulcer disease, cardiac arrhthymias *Pregnancy:* Only given after risks to the fetus are considered; animal studies have shown adverse reactions; no human studies available	Atropine, belladonna, mecamylamine

*Pregnancy categories have been revised. See http://www.fda.gov/Drugs/DevelopmentApprovalProcess/DevelopmentResources/Labeling/ucm093307.htm for more information.

Adverse/Side Effects

- Nausea
- Vomiting
- Abdominal cramps
- Diarrhea
- Hypersalivation
- Hypotension
- Bradycardia
- Miosis
- Muscle cramps
- Seizures
- Acute toxicity
- Dizziness
- Headache
- Sweating
- Blurred vision
- Urinary frequency/incontinence

Nursing Care
- Administer on time exactly as prescribed
  - Have atropine sulfate available for treatment of overdose
  - Administer with food (reduces GI irritation)
  - Instruct patient to take medication before meals
- Encourage patient diet rich in nutrient-dense foods (e.g., fruits, vegetables, whole grains, and legumes)
- Teach patient to report respiratory distress immediately

APPLICATION AND REVIEW

1. A client with myasthenia gravis has been receiving neostigmine and asks about its action. What information about its action should the nurse consider when formulating a response?
   1. Stimulates the cerebral cortex
   2. Blocks the action of cholinesterase
   3. Replaces deficient neurotransmitters
   4. Accelerates transmission along neural sheaths

2. A client is prescribed a cholinergic medication affecting the parasympathetic nervous system. What physical processes are stimulated by this system? **Select all that apply.**
   1. Digestion
   2. Heart rate
   3. Urination
   4. Defecation
   5. Fight-or-Flight

3. What effect should the nurse expect to see in a client who was administered a cholinergic agonist?
   1. Dilated pupils
   2. Urinary retention
   3. Decrease in heart rate
   4. Hypoactive bowel sounds

4. A client has been prescribed a cholinergic antagonist medication. What side effect of this medication class should the nurse discuss with the client?
   1. Anxiety
   2. Insomnia
   3. Dry mouth
   4. A faster pulse rate

5. A client has been prescribed a cholinesterase inhibitor to serve as an irreversible inhibitor. Which disorder has the client most likely been diagnosed with?
   1. Glaucoma
   2. Dementia
   3. Myasthenia gravis (MG)
   4. Chronic Obstructive Pulmonary Disease (COPD)

6. What is the mode of action for the cholinergic agonist classification of medications?
   1. Increases acetylcholine in the brain
   2. Increases acetylcholine in the synapses
   3. Increases acetylcholine at muscarinic receptors
   4. Blocks activity of the muscarinic acetylcholine receptor

7. What classification of medications can act as an antidote for toxicity caused by cholinesterase inhibitor therapy?
   1. Cholinesterases
   2. Cholinergic agonists
   3. Cholinergic antagonists
   4. Acetylcholinesterase inhibitors

8. A client is prescribed edrophonium, an acetylcholinesterase inhibitor, for a newly diagnosed myasthenia gravis (MG). Which assessment data poses a contraindication for this medication?
   1. Photosensitivity
   2. Urinary retention
   3. Dysrhythmia
   4. Asthma

9. Which intervention is required for a client prescribed an acetylcholinesterase inhibitor?
   1. Instructing to take medication without food
   2. Providing laxative for anticipated constipation
   3. Educating client that wheezing is an expected side effect
   4. Having atropine sulfate available for treatment of overdose
10. Which medication classification is likely to produce a drug interaction with the acetylcholinesterase inhibitor, donepezil?
    1. NSAIDs
    2. Beta blockers
    3. Corticosteroids
    4. Tricyclic antidepressants

See Answers on pages 128-129.

Treatment of Mild to Moderate Dementia

- Examples: rivastigmine, donepezil, galantamine
- Available in PO preparations

Mode of Action

- Increases acetylcholine in the brain

Contraindications, Precautions and Drug Interactions of Acetylcholinesterase Inhibitors (Dementia)*

Drug	Contraindications/Precautions	Drug Interaction
rivastigmine	**Contraindications:** Hypersenstivity to rivastigmine/carbamates **Precautions:** Asthma, breastfeeding, children, cardiac/hepatic/renal/ respiratory disease, GI bleeding, increased intracranial pressure, jaundice, peptic ulcer, seizure disorder, surgery, urinary obstruction **Pregnancy:** No adverse effects in animals; no human studies available	Anticholinergics, cholinergic agonists, other cholinesterase inhibitors, nicotine, NSAIDs, phenothiazines, sedating H1 blockers, tricyclics
donepezil	**Contraindications:** Hypersensitivity, hypersensitivity to piperidine derivatives **Precautions:** Breastfeeding, children, Parkinson's, GI bleeding, hepatic disease, GI/GU obstruction, asthma, COPD **Pregnancy:** Only given after risks to the fetus are considered; animal studies have shown adverse reactions; no human studies available	Succinylcholine, cholinergic agonists, NSAIDs, phenobarbital, rifampin
galantamine	**Contraindications:** Hypersensitivity, GI bleeding, jaundice, renal failure, children **Precautions:** Breastfeeding, geriatric patients, respiratory/renal/ hepatic/cardiac disease, seizure disorder, peptic ulcer, asthma, bradycardia, GU obstruction **Pregnancy:** No adverse effects in animals; no human studies available	Cholinomimetics, NSAIDs, anticholinergics

*Pregnancy categories have been revised. See http://www.fda.gov/Drugs/DevelopmentApprovalProcess/DevelopmentResources/Labeling/ucm093307.htm for more information.

Adverse/Side Effects

- AV block
- Dizziness
- Cardiac arrest
- MI
- Insomnia
- Headache
- Fatigue
- Syncope
- Atrial fibrillation
- Hypo/hypertension
- Nausea
- Vomiting
- GI bleeding/obstruction
- Pancreatitis
- Urinary frequency
- Rash
- Arthralgia
- QT prolongation

Nursing Care

- Monitor vital signs
- Monitor mental status
- Monitor I&O
- Monitor renal/hepatic function
- Monitor GI effects
- Monitor for anorexia and weight loss
- Assist patient with ambulation
- Teach patient not to increase or abruptly decrease dose
- Teach patient to notify prescriber of any adverse effects
- Teach patient that medication is not a cure but relieves symptoms

ANSWER KEY: REVIEW QUESTIONS

1. **2 Neostigmine, an anticholinesterase, inhibits the breakdown of ACh, thus prolonging neurotransmission.**
   1 Neostigmine's action is at the myoneural junction, not the cerebral cortex. **3** Neostigmine prevents neurotransmitter breakdown but is not a neurotransmitter. **4** Neostigmine's action is at the myoneural junction, not the sheath.
   Client Need: Pharmacologic and Parenteral Therapies; **Cognitive Level:** Application; **Integrated Process:** Teaching/Learning; **Nursing Process:** Planning/Implementation

> **Study Tip:** Say this sentence aloud, sounding the *n*'s out with extra emphasis: **N**eostigmi**n**e (Prostigmi**n**) prolo**n**gs **n**eurotransmissio**n**.

2. **Answers: 1, 3, 4**
   The parasympathetic nervous system stimulates digestion, urination, and defecation.
   2 The sympathetic nervous system stimulates the heart to increase its rate. **5** The sympathetic nervous system controls the fight or flight response.
   Client Need: Pharmacologic and Parenteral Therapies; **Cognitive Level:** Analysis; **Nursing Process:** Assessment/Analysis

3. **3 Cholinergic agonists decrease heart rate and blood pressure.**
   1 Cholinergic agonists constrict pupils. **2** Cholinergic antagonists decrease bladder contraction resulting in decreased urinary retention. **4** Cholinergic agonists stimulate GI tone resulting in hyperactive bowel sounds.
   Client Need: Pharmacologic and Parenteral Therapies; **Cognitive Level:** Analysis; **Nursing Process:** Assessment/Analysis

4. **3 Cholinergic antagonists decrease salivation causing dry mouth.**
   1 Cholinergic antagonists are not associated with causing anxiety. **2** Cholinergic antagonists are sometimes prescribed for insomnia. **4** Cholinergic antagonists stimulate pulse rate.
   Client Need: Pharmacologic and Parenteral Therapies; **Cognitive Level:** Analysis; **Integrated Process:** Teaching/Learning; **Nursing Process:** Planning/Implementation

5. **1 There are two types of cholinergic antagonists; irreversible inhibitors bind cholinesterase permanently and are used to treat glaucoma.**
   2 Reversible inhibitors bind cholinesterase for several minutes to hours and are used to treat dementia. **3** Reversible inhibitors bind cholinesterase for several minutes to hours and are used to treat MG. **4** Cholinergic antagonists are used to decrease secretions in certain disorders like COPD.
   Client Need: Pharmacologic and Parenteral Therapies; **Cognitive Level:** Analysis; **Nursing Process:** Planning/Implementation

6. **3 Cholinergic agonists increase acetylcholine at muscarinic receptors.**

   1 Acetylcholinesterase inhibitors bind to cholinesterase resulting in increased acetylcholine in the brain. 2 Acetylcholinesterase inhibitors bind to cholinesterase resulting in increased acetylcholine in the synapses. 4 Cholinergic antagonists block activity of the muscarinic acetylcholine receptor.

   Client Need: Pharmacologic and Parenteral Therapies; **Cognitive Level:** Analysis; **Nursing Process:** Assessment/Analysis

   > **Study Tip:** Look at the bolded *a's* and *c's* in this sentence: **C**holinergic **A**gonists block **A**cetyl**C**holine at mus**CA**rinic receptors. Visualize the highlighted *a's* and *c's* in this sentence as you say it aloud to reinforce the message.

7. **3 Cholinergic antagonists can be prescribed to treat cholinesterase inhibitor induced toxicity.**

   1 Be aware that the term cholinesterases refers to cholinesterase inhibitors and so would not manage toxicity. 2 The action of a cholinergic agonist would not serve to manage the toxicity resulting from cholinesterase inhibitor therapy. 4 Be aware that the term acetylcholinesterase inhibitors refers to cholinesterase inhibitors and so would not manage toxicity.

   Client Need: Pharmacologic and Parenteral Therapies; **Cognitive Level:** Analysis; **Nursing Process:** Assessment/Analysis

8. **2 Genitourinary obstruction resulting in urinary retention is a contraindication for this medication.**

   1 Photosensitivity is not a recognized contraindication for this medication. 3 Dysrhythmias are considered precautions associated with this medication. The risks must be weighed against the benefits before a prescription is written. 4 Asthma is considered a precaution associated with this medication. The risks must be weighed against the benefits before a prescription is written.

   Client Need: Pharmacologic and Parenteral Therapies; **Cognitive Level:** Analysis; **Nursing Process:** Assessment/Analysis

9. **4 Considering mode of action, atropine sulfate is the treatment for acetylcholinesterase inhibitor overdose**

   1 An acetylcholinesterase inhibitor should be administer with food to reduce GI irritation. 2 An acetylcholinesterase inhibitor is likely to cause diarrhea rather than constipation. 4 Wheezing is not considered an expected side effect and the client should be taught to report respiratory distress immediately.

   Client Need: Pharmacologic and Parenteral Therapies; **Cognitive Level:** Analysis; **Nursing Process:** Implementation/Planning

10. **2 Beta blockers are known to produce drug interactions when administered with donepezil.**

   1 NSAIDs are not recognized as producing drug interactions when administered with donepezil. 3 Corticosteroids are not known to produce drug interactions when administered with donepezil. 4 Tricyclic antidepressants are not known to produce drug interactions when administered with donepezil.

   Client Need: Pharmacologic and Parenteral Therapies; **Cognitive Level:** Analysis; **Integrated Process:** Teaching/Learning; **Nursing Process:** Assessment/Analysis

8 Antihypertensive Drugs and Diuretic

OVERVIEW OF HYPERTENSION (FIG. 8.1)

- Etiology is complex; begins insidiously; changes in arteriolar bed cause increased resistance; increased blood volume may result from hormonal or renal dysfunction; arteriolar thickening causes increased peripheral vascular resistance; abnormal renin release constricts arterioles
- 90% to 95% have an unidentifiable cause (essential or primary hypertension); multiple factors such as the renin-angiotensin-aldosterone mechanism, sympathetic nervous system activity, and insulin resistance may be involved
- 5% to 10% have identifiable causes (secondary hypertension); pathophysiology is related to condition causing the rise in pressure; conditions include renovascular disease; primary hyperaldosteronism; Cushing's syndrome; diabetes mellitus; neurologic disorders; dysfunction of thyroid, pituitary, or parathyroid glands; coarctation of the aorta; and pregnancy
- Risk factors
  - Stress
  - Abdominal obesity
  - Diet: high sodium, low calcium, low magnesium, and low potassium
  - Substance abuse (e.g., cigarettes, alcohol, cocaine)
  - Family history
  - Increasing age
  - Gender
  - Sedentary lifestyle
  - Hyperlipidemia: increased LDL and cholesterol levels, decreased HDL level
  - African American heritage
  - Type 2 diabetes
  - Renal disorders
    - Often asymptomatic; diagnosis requires three assessments of elevated BP on separate occasions
  - Classification of BP by the Joint National Committee on Prevention, Detection, Evaluation, and Treatment of High Blood Pressure (JNC)
    - Normal: systolic less than 120 mm Hg and diastolic less than 80 mm Hg
    - Prehypertension: systolic 120 to 139 mm Hg or diastolic 80 to 89 mm Hg
    - Stage 1 hypertension: systolic 140 to 159 mm Hg or diastolic 90 to 99 mm Hg
    - Stage 2 hypertension: systolic 160 mm Hg or more, or diastolic 100 mm Hg or more
- Hypertension increases risk for coronary artery disease, heart failure, myocardial infarction, brain attacks (CVAs), retinopathy, and nephropathy
- Clinical findings
  - Subjective: headache (occipital area); light-headedness; tinnitus; easy fatigue; visual disturbances; palpitations
  - Objective: BP more than 140/90 mm Hg obtained on three separate occasions; retinal changes; renal pathology (e.g., azotemia); epistaxis; cardiac hypertrophy
- Therapeutic interventions
  - Lifestyle modifications
  - Weight control or reduction to attain a body mass index of 18.5 to 24.9 kg/m^2

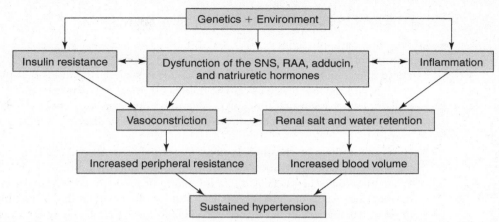

FIG. 8.1 Pathophysiology of Hypertension. (From Huether, S.E., McCance, K.L., Brashers, V.L., Rote, N.S. [2012]. *Understanding pathophysiology* [5th ed.]. St. Louis: Mosby.)

- Dietary Approaches to Stop Hypertension (DASH) eating plan: increased fruits, vegetables, and low-fat dairy products that are rich in calcium and potassium
- Sodium restriction (less than 2.4 g daily)
- Aerobic exercise at least 30 minutes on most days
- Alcohol moderation (no more than one drink daily for women, two for men)
- Assessment/Analysis
  - Vital signs in both upright and recumbent positions; use appropriate cuff (width should be 40% of the arm's circumference); avoid errors of parallax when reading sphygmomanometer
  - Baseline weight
  - Presence of risk factors and clinical evidence of target organ damage
- Planning/Implementation
  - Monitor levels of electrolytes, blood urea nitrogen (BUN), creatinine, lipid profile, and urine for protein
  - Encourage weight reduction if indicated; weigh daily to monitor fluid balance when there is threat of heart failure
  - Teach to monitor own BP; a BP of 180/120 mm Hg or higher represents a hypertensive emergency; advise to change position slowly and avoid hot showers to prevent orthostatic hypotension when taking antihypertensives
  - Support expression of emotions; encourage relaxation techniques
  - Reinforce that hypertension is not cured, but controlled
  - Educate client and family regarding drugs, follow-up care, activity restrictions, smoking cessation, limiting alcohol intake, and diet; note that many salt substitutes contain potassium chloride rather than sodium chloride and may be permitted by health care provider if there is no renal impairment; caution about use of nonsteroidal antiinflammatory drugs (NSAIDs), which can cause hypertension
- Evaluation/Outcomes
  - Maintains BP at an acceptable level
  - Adheres to therapeutic regimen
  - Verbalizes need for stress reduction

OVERVIEW OF HEART FAILURE

- Etiology and pathophysiology
  - Inability of heart to meet oxygen demands of the body
  - Pump failure may be caused by cardiac abnormalities or conditions that place increased demands on the heart such as cardiac muscle disorders, valvular defects (e.g., mitral valve prolapse with regurgitation, aortic stenosis), hypertension, coronary atherosclerosis, hyperthyroidism, obesity, chronic obstructive pulmonary disease (COPD), and circulatory overload
  - Heart failure may be classified as diastolic (impaired ventricular filling) or systolic (impaired ventricular contraction); determined by ejection fraction
  - When one side of heart "fails," there is buildup of pressure in the vascular system feeding into that side; signs of right ventricular failure are first evident in the systemic circulation; those of left ventricular failure are first evident in the pulmonary system, causing pulmonary edema; eventually affects both pulmonary and systemic circulation
  - Decreased cardiac output activates the renin-angiotensin-aldosterone mechanism and sympathetic nervous system, leading to vasoconstriction and retention of sodium and water thus increasing cardiac workload (Fig. 8.2)

Clinical Findings

- Left ventricular heart failure
  - Subjective: dyspnea from fluid within lungs; orthopnea; fatigue; restlessness; paroxysmal nocturnal dyspnea
  - Objective: decreased oxygen saturation; crackles; peripheral cyanosis; Cheyne-Stokes respirations; frothy, blood-tinged sputum; dry, nonproductive cough; decreased ejection fraction; dyspnea; decreased urine output; S3/S4 summation gallop
- Right ventricular failure
  - Subjective: abdominal pain; fatigue; bloating; nausea
  - Objective: jugular vein distention (JVD); dependent, pitting edema that often subsides at night when legs are elevated; ankle edema is frequently the first sign of HF; ascites from increased hydrostatic pressure within portal system; hepatomegaly; anorexia; respiratory distress (e.g., use of accessory muscles of respiration); increased central venous pressure (CVP); diminished urinary output

Diagnostic Tests

- B-type natriuretic peptide (BNP) rises (normal value is <100 pg/mL); produced by myocardium in response to increased ventricular end-diastolic pressure; functions to promote diuresis and vasodilation, which reduces cardiac workload

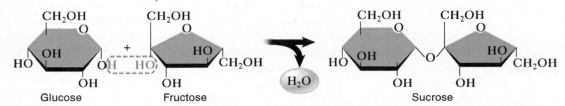

FIG. 8.2 The Renin-Angiotensin-Aldosterone System. (From Patton, K.T., Thibodeau, G.A. [2016]. *Anatomy and physiology* [8th ed.]. St. Louis: Elsevier.)

- Echocardiogram to assess ventricular function/hypertrophy; assesses ejection fraction
- Hemodynamic monitoring for cardiogenic shock
- Electrolytes, hematocrit, hemoglobin, BUN, creatinine, complete blood count, thyroid-stimulating hormone, and ECGs are done to identify underlying causes

Therapeutic Interventions

- Rest in high-Fowler or orthopneic position to reduce cardiac workload
- Morphine to reduce anxiety and dyspnea
- Oxygen therapy; endotracheal intubation and a ventilator for acute ventricular failure
- Decrease cardiac workload with diuretics, vasodilators, angiotensin-converting enzyme inhibitors (ACEIs), angiotensin II receptor blockers (ARBs), beta blockers, phosphodiesterase inhibitors
- Increase pump performance with digitalis or dobutamine (Dobutrex)
- Potassium supplements to prevent digitalis toxicity and hypokalemia
- Hemodynamic monitoring through a multilumen pulmonary artery catheter
- Sodium-restricted diet to limit fluid retention and promote fluid excretion
- Paracentesis if ascites exists and is causing respiratory distress
- Cardiac resynchronization therapy: use of right and left ventricular pacemaker leads to synchronize contractions and improve cardiac output

Assessment/Analysis

- Baseline vital signs, breath sounds, oxygen saturation (Sao$_2$)
- Daily weight, extent of pitting edema, circumference of edematous extremities, abdominal girth, JVD
- Hemodynamic status (e.g., CVP, PCWP)
- Electrolyte levels (e.g., sodium, chloride, potassium)
- I&O

Planning/Implementation

- Maintain in high-Fowler or orthopneic position; administer supplemental oxygen
- Elevate extremities except when in acute distress
- Monitor vital signs, breath sounds, JVD, Sao$_2$
- Change position slowly and frequently
- Monitor I&O, daily weight, electrolytes
- Restrict fluids as ordered
- Provide small, frequent, low-sodium meals
- Monitor invasive lines
- Administer medications as prescribed: cardiac glycosides, antihypertensives, diuretics, and phosphodiesterase inhibitors (see Related Pharmacology)
- Help to establish balanced schedule of rest and activity; lifestyle modifications (e.g., weight control, smoking cessation)
- Teach importance of continued health care provider supervision

Evaluation/Outcomes

- Maintains adequate tissue perfusion
- Reduces peripheral edema/ascites
- Adheres to pharmacologic and dietary regimen

Antihypertensive Drugs

- Promote dilation of peripheral blood vessels, thus decreasing BP, peripheral vascular resistance, and afterload
- Reduce cardiac contractility
- Antihypertensive drug classes include ACEIs, ARBs, $alpha_1$ blockers, alpha-beta blockers, central $alpha_2$ agonists, vasodilators
  - ACEIs stop conversion of angiotensin I to II, blocking vasoconstriction and fluid retention from aldosterone secretion
  - ARBs block angiotensin II from binding to specific vascular smooth muscle and adrenal gland receptor sites; stop vasoconstriction and fluid retention; similar antihypertensive effect of ACEIs but less likely to cause chronic cough
  - $Alpha_1$ blockers inhibit effects of norepinephrine by blocking receptors that control vasomotor tone; cause vasodilation
  - Alpha-beta blockers combine effects of $alpha_1$ and beta blockers, leading to vasodilation, decreased contractility, and decreased heart rate
  - Central $alpha_2$ agonists decrease sympathetic activity from CNS
  - Vasodilators relax smooth muscles of blood vessels, resulting in decreased peripheral vascular resistance
- Antihypertensives may be combined with diuretics to potentiate their effects

Diuretic Drugs

- Interfere with sodium reabsorption in kidney
- Increase urine output, which reduces hypervolemia; decrease preload and afterload
- Diuretic drug classes include thiazides, thiazide-like diuretics, loop diuretics, potassium-sparing diuretics, osmotic diuretics, carbonic anhydrase inhibitors
- Thiazides interfere with sodium ion transport at loop of Henle and inhibit carbonic anhydrase activity at distal tubule sites
- Potassium-sparers interfere with aldosterone-induced reabsorption of sodium ions at distal nephron sites to increase sodium chloride excretion and decrease potassium ion loss
- Loop diuretics interfere with active transport of sodium ions in loop of Henle and inhibit sodium chloride and water reabsorption at proximal tubule sites
- Osmotic diuretics cause water to be retained within the proximal tubule and descending limb of loop of Henle
- Carbonic anhydrase inhibitors inhibit carbonic anhydrase, thus reducing renal bicarbonate resorption in the proximal tubule

ANTIHYPERTENSIVE DRUGS

ACE Inhibitors

- Used to treat hypertension
- Examples include captopril, enalapril, benazepril, lisinopril, quinapril, fosinopril
- Available in PO, IV, transdermal preparations

Mode of Action

- Prevent conversion of angiotensin I to angiotensin II

Contraindications, Precautions, and Drug Interactions of ACE Inhibitors*

Drug	Contraindications/Precautions	Drug Interaction
captopril	**Contraindications:** Hypersensitivity, breastfeeding, children, heart block, potassium-sparing diuretics, angioedema **Precautions:** Pregnancy first trimester, African descent, bilateral renal artery stenosis, blood dyscrasias, CHF, collagen vascular disease, diabetes mellitus, dialysis patients, hyponatremia, hypovolemia, hyperkalemia, leukemia, SLE, thyroid/renal/hepatic disease **Pregnancy:** **First trimester:** Only given after risks to the fetus are considered; animal studies have shown adverse reactions; no human studies available **Second/Third trimester:** Definite fetal risks, may be given in spite of risks if needed in life-threatening conditions	Acute alcohol ingestion, antacids, antihypertensives, digoxin, insulin, lithium, MAOIs, nitrates, NSAIDs, oral antidiabetics, phenothiazines, potassium-sparing diuretics, potassium supplements, salicylates, sympathomimetics
enalapril	**Contraindications:** Hypersensitivity, history of angioedema **Precautions:** Breastfeeding, bilateral renal artery/aortic stenosis, dehydration, hepatic failure, hyperkalemia, renal diseae **Pregnancy:** Definite fetal risks, may be given in spite of risks if needed in life-threatening conditions	Allopurinol, antihypertensives, diuretics, phenothiazines, nitrates, acute alcohol ingestion, general anesthesia, salt substitutes, potassium-sparing diurectics, potassium supplements, cyclosporine, NSAIDs, lithium, digoxin, antacids, rifampin
benazepril	**Contraindications:** Hypersensitivity to ACE inhibitors, breastfeeding, children, angioedema **Precautions:** Geriatric patients, dialysis patients, renal/hepatic disease, blood dyscrasias, hypovolemia, CHF, asthma, bilateral renal artery stenosis **Pregnancy:** Definite fetal risks, may be given in spite of risks if needed in life-threatening conditions	Acute alcohol ingestion, antihypertensives, diuretics, nitrates, phenothiazines, potassium-sparing diuretics, potassium supplements, azathioprine, digoxin, lithim, NSAIDs
lisinopril	**Contraindications:** Hypersensitivity, angioedema **Precautions:** Breastfeeding, pregnancy 1st trimester, renal disease, CHF, renal artery stenosis, aortic stenosis **Pregnancy:** Definite fetal risks, may be given in spite of risks if needed in life-threatening conditions	Acute alcohol ingestion, allopurinol, aspirin, NSAIDs, indomethacin, potassium salt substitutes, potassium-sparing diuretics, potassium supplements, cyclosporine, lithium, antihypertensives, diuretics, probenecid, phenothiazines, nitrates
quinapril	**Contraindications:** Hypersensitivity to ACE inhibitors, children, angioedema **Precautions:** Breastfeeding, geriatric patients, renal/hepatic disease, dialysis patients, bilateral renal artery stenosis, aortic stenosis, hypovolemia, blood dyscrasias, cough, hyperkalemia, African descent **Pregnancy:** Definite fetal risks, may be given in spite of risks if needed in life-threatening conditions	Vasodilators, hydralazine, prazosin, potassium-sparing diuretics, sympathomimetics, potassium supplements, ACE/angiotensin II receptor agonists, aliskiren, diuretics, antihypertensives, ganglionic blockers, adrenergic blockers, phenothiazines, nitrates, acute alcohol ingestion, lithium, tetracycline, quinolones, quinapril, NSAIDs
fosinapril	**Contraindications:** Hypersensitivity to ACE inhibitors, children, angioedema **Precautions:** Geriatric patients, renal/hepatic disease, blood dyscrasias, hypovolemia, CHF, COPD, asthma, angioedema, renal artery stenosis, hyperkalemia, aortic stenosis, febrile illness, autoimmune disorders, collagen vascular disease **Pregnancy:** Definite fetal risks, may be given in spite of risks if needed in life-threatening conditions	Acute alcohol ingestion, antacids, potassium-sparing diuretics, potassium supplements, antihypertensives, diuretics, nitrates, adrenergic blockers, ganglionic blockers, vasodilators, hydralazine, prazosin, digoxin, NSAIDs, lithium, sympathomimetics, salicylates

*Pregnancy categories have been revised. See http://www.fda.gov/Drugs/DevelopmentApprovalProcess/DevelopmentResources/Labeling/ucm093307.htm for more information.

Adverse/Side Effects

- Fever
- Chills
- Hypotension
- Postural hypotension
- Tachycardia
- Angina
- Dysrhythmias
- Angioedema
- Bronchospasm
- Dyspnea
- Cough
- Loss of taste
- Dysuria
- Nocturia
- Proteinuria
- Polyuria
- Oliguria
- Urinary frequency
- Hepatotoxicity
- Nephrotic syndrome
- Acute reversible renal failure
- Neutropenia
- Agranulocytosis
- Pancytopenia
- Thrombocytopenia
- Anemia
- Hyperkalemia
- Toxic epidermal necrolysis
- Stevens-Johnson syndrome

Nursing Care

- Administer 1 hour before or 2 hours after meals
- If using patch, remove old patch first before applying new one
- Weigh patient daily
- Monitor for blood dyscrasias
- Monitor for hypo/hypertension
- Monitor for allergic reaction
- Monitor for congested heart failure (CHF)
- Monitor for infection
- Teach patient not to discontinue drug abruptly
- Teach patient not to miss or double doses
- Teach patient not to use OTC products without prescriber's consent
- Teach patient to change positions slowly
- Teach patient to report signs and symptoms of infection
- Teach patient how to self-monitor BP
- Teach patient to avoid sun exposure
- Teach patient to avoid high-potassium foods, if indicated
- Teach patient to maintain sodium restriction, calorie reduction, exercise program, stress management

APPLICATION AND REVIEW

1. A client is being considered for ACE inhibitor therapy to manage their diagnosis of hypertension. Which medical diagnosis should the nurse recognize as a contraindication for this medication therapy? **Select all that apply.**
   1. Leukemia
   2. Angioedema
   3. Diabetes mellitus
   4. Congestive heart failure
2. A client being treated for hypertension reports having a persistent hacking cough. What class of antihypertensive should the nurse identify as a possible cause of this response when reviewing a list of this client's medications?
   1. ACE inhibitors
   2. Thiazide diuretics
   3. Calcium channel blockers
   4. Angiotensin receptor blockers

3. A client has been prescribed ACE inhibitor therapy to manage their diagnosis of hypertension. What information should the nurse provide when discussing medication-related safety needs with the client? **Select all that apply.**
   1. Need to regularly self-monitor blood pressure
   2. Need to move from sitting to standing positions slowly
   3. Need to identify and report signs and symptoms of infection
   4. Need to double dosing medication to deal with a missed dose
   5. Need to avoid sun exposure with appropriate hat and clothing

4. The nurse managing care for a client prescribed ACE inhibitor therapy should include which specific monitoring as part of the client's plan of care? **Select all that apply.**
   1. Reports of urinary retention
   2. Signs and symptoms of infection
   3. Adherence to dietary recommendations
   4. Reports of dizziness when standing up
   5. Signs and symptoms of congested heart failure (CHF)

See Answers on pages 153-155.

Angiotensin II Receptor Blockers (ARBs)

- Used to treat hypertension
- Examples include candesartan, irbesartan, losartan, valsartan
- Available in PO, IV preparations

Mode of Action

- Blocks angiotensin II from binding to angiotensin II receptor

Contraindications, Precautions, and Drug Interactions of ARBs*

Drug	Contraindications/Precautions	Drug Interaction
candesartan	**Contraindications:** Hypersensitivity **Precautions:** Pregnancy first trimester, breastfeeding, children, geriatric patients, renal/hepatic disease, renal artery stenosis, hypersensitivity to ACE inhibitors, hypotension, volume depletion, electrolyte abnormalities **Pregnancy:** **First trimester:** Only given after risks to the fetus are considered; animal studies have shown adverse reactions; no human studies available **Second/Third trimester:** Definite fetal risks, may be given in spite of risks if needed in life-threatening conditions	Potassium-sparing diuretics, ACE inhibitors, beta blockers, calcium channel blockers, alpha blockers, MAOIs, NSAIDs, salicylates
irbesartan	**Contraindications:** Hypersensitivity **Precautions:** Pregnancy first trimester, breastfeeding, children, geriatric patients, renal/hepatic disease, renal artery stenosis, hypersensitivity to ACE inhibitors, angioedema, African descent **Pregnancy:** **First trimester:** Only given after risks to the fetus are considered; animal studies have shown adverse reactions; no human studies available **Second/Third trimester:** Definite fetal risks, may be given in spite of risks if needed in life-threatening conditions	Potassium-sparing diuretics, ACE inhibitors, potassium salt substitutes, CYP2C9 inhibitors, NSAIDs

Continued

Contraindications, Precautions, and Drug Interactions of ARBs—cont'd

Drug	Contraindications/Precautions	Drug Interaction
losartan	*Contraindications:* Hypersensitivity *Precautions:* Pregnancy first trimester, breastfeeding, children, geriatric patients, renal/hepatic disease, renal artery stenosis, hypersensitivity to ACE inhibitors, hypotension, angioedema, African descent *Pregnancy:* **First trimester:** Only given after risks to the fetus are considered; animal studies have shown adverse reactions; no human studies available **Second/Third trimester:** Definite fetal risks, may be given in spite of risks if needed in life-threatening conditions	Potassium-sparing diuretics, potassium supplements, ACE inhibitors, NSAIDs, lithium, fluconazole, phenobarbital, rifamycin, salicylates
Valsartan	*Contraindications:* Hypersensitivity, bilateral renal artery stenosis, severe hepatic disease *Precautions:* Breastfeeding, children, geriatric patients, renal/hepatic disease, hypertrophic cardiomyopathy aortic/mitral valve stenosis, hypersensitivity to ACE inhibitors, CAD, CHF, African descent, angioedema, hyperkalemia, hypovolemia *Pregnancy:* Definite fetal risks, may be given in spite of risks if needed in life-threatening conditions	Potassium-sparing diuretics, potassium supplements, ACE inhibitors, NSAIDs, salicylates, lithium, antidiabetics, cyclosporine, rifampin, ritonavir, gemfibrozil, telithromycin

*Pregnancy categories have been revised. See http://www.fda.gov/Drugs/DevelopmentApprovalProcess/DevelopmentResources/Labeling/ucm093307.htm for more information.

Adverse/Side Effects

- Headache
- Dizziness
- Fatigue
- Syncope
- Angioedema
- Hypotension
- Angina
- Palpitations
- MI
- Cerebrovascular accident
- Dysrhythmias
- Cough
- Upper respiratory infection
- Pharyngitis
- Sinusitis
- Rhinitis
- Nausea
- Vomiting
- Diarrhea
- Abdominal pain
- Thrombocytopenia
- Renal failure
- Arthralgia

Nursing Care

- Weigh patient daily
- Monitor for hypo/hypertension
- Monitor for allergic reaction
- Monitor for CHF
- Monitor for infection
- Monitor I&O
- Teach patient not to discontinue drug abruptly, even if feeling better
- Teach patient not to miss or double doses
- Teach patient not to use OTC products without prescriber's consent
- Teach patient to change positions slowly
- Teach patient that drug may cause dizziness, fainting, light-headedness and to implement safety precautions accordingly
- Teach patient to report signs and symptoms of infection
- Teach patient to avoid sun exposure, wear sunscreen, protective clothing, sunglasses
- Teach patient how to self-monitor BP

- Teach patient events that can adversely affect BP (vomiting, diarrhea, excessive perspiration, dehydration)
- Teach patient to maintain sodium restriction, calorie reduction, exercise program, stress management

APPLICATION AND REVIEW

5. What should the nurse assess to determine whether a client is experiencing the therapeutic effect of valsartan?
   1. Lipid profile
   2. Apical pulse
   3. Urinary output
   4. Blood pressure

See Answers on pages 153–155.

Alpha₁ Blockers

- Used to treat hypertension
- Examples include doxazosin, prazosin, terazosin
- Available in PO preparations

Mode of Action

- Lowers peripheral resistance by dilating peripheral blood vessels

Contraindications, Precautions, and Drug Interactions of Alpha₁ Blockers*

Drug	Contraindications/Precautions	Drug Interaction
Doxazosin	**Contraindications:** Hypersensitivity to quinazolines **Precautions:** Breastfeeding, children, geriatric patients, hepatic disease **Pregnancy:** Only given after risks to the fetus are considered; animal studies have shown adverse reactions; no human studies available	Alcohol, antihypertensives, clonidine, nitrates, PDE-5 inhibitors
prazosin	**Contraindications:** Hypersensitivity **Precautions:** Breastfeeding, children, geriatric patients, orthostatic hypotension, ocular surgery, prostate cancer **Pregnancy:** Only given after risks to the fetus are considered; animal studies have shown adverse reactions; no human studies available	Alcohol, beta blockers, nitroglycerin, diuretics, antihypertensives, MAOIs, phosphodiesterase inhibitors
Terazosin	**Contraindications:** Hypersensitivity **Precautions:** Breastfeeding, children, prostate cancer, syncope **Pregnancy:** Only given after risks to the fetus are considered; animal studies have shown adverse reactions; no human studies available	Beta blockers, antihypertensives, alcohol, nitroglycerin, verapamil, PDE5 inhibitors, NSAIDs, salicylates, estrogens

*Pregnancy categories have been revised. See http://www.fda.gov/Drugs/DevelopmentApprovalProcess/DevelopmentResources/Labeling/ucm093307.htm for more information.

Adverse/Side Effects

- Headache
- Dizziness
- Fatigue
- Weakness
- Drowsiness
- Anxiety
- Depression
- Syncope
- Vertigo
- Asthenia
- Dysrhythmia
- Angina
- Tachycardia
- Palpitations
- Edema
- Orthostatic hypotension
- Dry mouth
- Red sclera
- Nausea
- Vomiting
- Diarrhea
- Constipation
- Pancreatitis
- Hepatitis
- Incontinence
- Polyuria
- Priapism
- Impotence

Nursing Care

- Weigh patient daily
- Monitor for hypo/hypertension
- Monitor for CHF
- Monitor for BPH
- Monitor I&O
- Teach patient that fainting may occur
- Teach patient to avoid driving and other hazardous activities
- Teach patient to change positions slowly
- Teach patient not to abruptly discontinue drug
- Teach patient to avoid OTC products, alcohol unless prescriber approves

Alpha-Beta Blockers

- Used to treat hypertension
- Examples include labetalol, carvedilol
- Available in PO, IV preparations

Mode of Action

- Utilizes alpha- and beta-blocking effects to lower blood pressure

Contraindications, Precautions, and Drug Interactions of Alpha-Beta Blockers*

Drug	Contraindications/Precautions	Drug Interaction
labetalol	**Contraindications:** Hypersensitivity to beta blockers, bronchial asthma, cardiogenic shock, CHF, heart block, sinus bradycardia **Precautions:** Breastfeeding, geriatric patients, COPD, diabetes mellitus, hepatic/renal/thyroid disease, major surgery, nonallergic bronchospasm, peripheral vascular disease, well-compensated heart failure **Pregnancy:** Only given after risks to the fetus are considered; animal studies have shown adverse reactions; no human studies available	Class I antidysrhythmics, MAOIs, tricyclics, hydantoins, general anesthetics, diuretics, verapamil, antihypertensives, alcohol, nitrates, nitroglycerin, cimetidine, beta blockers, xanthines, bronchodialtors, lidocaine, theophylline, sympathomimetics, antidiabetics, NSAIDs, salicylates
carvedilol	**Contraindications:** Hypersensitivity, asthma, cardiogenic shock, heart block, severe bradycardia, heart failure, pulmonary edema, severe hepatic disease, sick sinus symptoms **Precautions:** Breastfeeding, children, geriatric patients, diabetes mellitus, renal disease, hepatic injury, major surgery, peripheral vascular disease, cardiac failure, anesthesia, thyrotoxicosis, emphysema, chronic bronchitis **Pregnancy:** Only given after risks to the fetus are considered; animal studies have shown adverse reactions; no human studies available	Calcium channel blockers, MAOIs, reserpine, levodopa, antidiabetic agents, digoxin, cyclosporine, CYP2D6 inhibitors, cimetidine, antihypertensives, nitrates, acute alcohol ingestion, clonidine, thyroid medications, rifampin, NSAIDs

*Pregnancy categories have been revised. See http://www.fda.gov/Drugs/DevelopmentApprovalProcess/DevelopmentResources/Labeling/ucm093307.htm for more information.

Adverse/Side Effects

- Headache
- Dizziness
- Drowsiness
- Fatigue
- Lethargy
- Anxiety
- Depression
- Nightmares
- Bronchospasm

- Dyspnea
- Wheezing
- Pulmonary edema
- CHF
- Angina
- AV block
- Ventricular dysrhythmias
- Bradycardia

- Visual changes
- Nausea
- Vomiting
- Diarrhea
- Hepatotoxicity
- Agranulocytosis
- Thrombocytopenia
- Purpura

- Impotence
- Dysuria
- Ejaculatory failure
- Rash
- Alopecia
- Urticaria
- Exfoliative dermatitis

Nursing Care

- Weigh patient daily
- Monitor for hypo/hypertension
- Monitor renal/hepatic function
- Monitor for CHF
- Monitor I&O
- Teach patient to report bradycardia, dizziness, confusion, depression, fever
- Teach patient to report signs and symptoms of heart failure
- Teach patient to avoid driving and other hazardous activities
- Teach patient to change positions slowly
- Teach patient not to abruptly discontinue drug, even if feeling better
- Teach patient to avoid OTC products unless prescriber approves
- Teach patient how to self-monitor pulse
- Teach diabetic patients to monitor blood sugar closely
- Teach patient to avoid smoking, alcohol
- Teach patient to maintain sodium restriction, calorie reduction, exercise program, stress management

Central Alpha$_2$ Agonists

- Used to treat hypertension
- Examples include clonidine, methyldopa
- Available in PO, IV, transdermal, epidural preparations

Mode of Action

- Decreases sympathetic activity from CNS

Contraindications, Precautions, and Drug Interactions of Central Alpha$_2$ Agonists*

Drug	Contraindications/Precautions	Drug Interaction
Clonidine	**Contraindications:** Hypersensitivity, anticoagulants, bleeding disorders (epidural preparation) **Precautions:** Breastfeeding, children <12 yr (transdermal preparation), geriatric patients, noncompliant patients, diabetes mellitus, COPD, recent MI, chronic renal failure, depression, asthma, thyroid disease, phenochromocytoma, Raynaud's disease **Pregnancy:** Only given after risks to the fetus are considered; animal studies have shown adverse reactions; no human studies available	Diuretics, antihypertensive nitrates, verapamil, diltiazem, beta blockers, MAOIs, tricyclics, antipsychotics, opiates, sedatives, hypnotics, alcohol, anesthetics, levodopa, amphetamines, appetite suppressants, prazosin

Continued

Contraindications, Precautions, and Drug Interactions of Central Alpha$_2$ Agonists—cont'd

Drug	Contraindications/Precautions	Drug Interaction
methyldopa	*Contraindications:* Hypersensitivity, active hepatic disease, MAOI therapy *Precautions:* Geriatric patients, autoimmune disease, cardiac disease, depression, dialysis, hemolytic anemia, Parkinson's disease, pheochromocytoma, sulfite hypersensitivity *Pregnancy:* No adverse effects in animals; no human studies available	MAOIs, lithium, sympathomimetic amines, levodopa, diuretic, antihypertensives, haloperidol, alcohol, antihistamines, antidepressants, analgesics, sedatives, hypnotics, iron, tolbutamide, barbiturates, tricyclics, NSAIDs, amphetamines, beta blockers, phenothiazines

*Pregnancy categories have been revised. See http://www.fda.gov/Drugs/DevelopmentApprovalProcess/DevelopmentResources/Labeling/ucm093307.htm for more information.

Adverse/Side Effects
- Headache
- Dizziness
- Drowsiness
- Fatigue
- Sedation
- Malaise
- Drug fever
- Anxiety
- Depression
- Delirium
- Mental changes
- Withdrawal symptoms
- CHF
- ECG abnormalities
- Orthostatic hypotension
- Palpitations
- Sinus tachycardia
- Myocarditis
- Hepatic dysfunction
- Pancreatitis
- Hyperglycemia
- Nausea
- Vomiting
- Constipation
- Dry mouth
- Dysuria
- Nocturia
- Gynecomastia
- Impotence
- Leukopenia
- Thrombocytopenia
- Hemolytic anemia
- Granulocytopenia
- Arthralgia
- Myalgia
- Rash
- Alopecia
- Pruritus
- Hives
- Edema
- Toxic epidermal necrolysis

Nursing Care
- Weigh patient daily
- Monitor for hypo/hypertension
- Monitor cardiac conduction
- Monitor blood studies
- Monitor renal/hepatic function
- Monitor for CHF
- Monitor I&O
- Monitor for allergic reaction
- Teach patient to avoid driving and other hazardous activities
- Teach patient to change positions slowly
- Teach patient to report signs and symptoms of infection to prescriber
- Teach patient not to abruptly discontinue drug, even if feeling better
- Teach patient to avoid OTC products unless prescriber approves
- Teach patient to avoid smoking, alcohol
- Teach patient to maintain sodium restriction, calorie reduction, exercise program, stress management

Vasodilators

- Used to treat hypertension
- Examples include hydralazine, minoxidil, nitroprusside
- Available in PO, IV preparations

Mode of Action

- Vasodilates vascular smooth muscle

Contraindications, Precautions, and Drug Interactions of Vasodilators*

Drug	Contraindications/Precautions	Drug Interaction
Hydralazine	**Contraindications:** Hypersensitivity to hydralazines, CAD, mitral valvular rheumatic heart disease **Precautions:** Breastfeeding, geriatric patients, advanced renal disease, CVA, dissecting aortic aneurysm, hepatic disease, SLE **Pregnancy:** Only given after risks to the fetus are considered; animal studies have shown adverse reactions; no human studies available	MAOIs, sympathomimetics, alcohol, antihypertensives, thiazide diuretics, beta blockers, estrogens NSAIDs
Minoxidil	**Contraindications:** Hypersensitivity, dissecting aortic aneurysm, pheochromocytoma **Precautions:** Breastfeeding, children, geriatric patients, CVD, renal disease **Pregnancy:** Only given after risks to the fetus are considered; animal studies have shown adverse reactions; no human studies available	Antihypertensives, MAOIs, estrogens, NSAIDs, salicylates
nitroprusside	**Contraindications:** Hypersensitivity, acute CHF, AV shunt, Leber's disease, toxic amblyopia **Precautions:** Breastfeeding, children, geriatric patients, anemia, electrolyte imbalances, hepatic/renal disease, hypothyroidism, hypovolemia, **Pregnancy:** Only given after risks to the fetus are considered; animal studies have shown adverse reactions; no human studies available	Circulatory depressants, enflurane, ganglionic blockers, halothane, volatile liquid anesthetics

*Pregnancy categories have been revised. See http://www.fda.gov/Drugs/DevelopmentApprovalProcess/DevelopmentResources/Labeling/ucm093307.htm for more information.

Adverse/Side Effects

- Headache
- Dizziness
- Depression
- Anxiety
- Fever
- Chills
- Dyspnea
- Pulmonary edema
- Shock
- CHF
- Pericardial effusion
- Palpitations
- Reflex tachycardia
- Angina
- Rebound hypertension
- Nausea
- Vomiting
- Diarrhea
- Constipation
- Paralytic ileus
- Hepatotoxicity
- Urinary retention
- Hematuria
- Glomerulonephritis
- Leukopenia
- Thrombocytopenia
- Anemia
- Agranulocytosis
- Cyanide/thiocyanate toxicity
- Arthralgia
- Muscle cramps
- Rash
- Pruritus
- Urticaria
- Edema
- Stevens-Johnson syndrome

Nursing Care
- Administer with food
- Weigh patient daily
- Monitor for hypo/hypertension
- Monitor cardiac blood studies
- Monitor renal/hepatic function
- Monitor for CHF
- Monitor I&O
- Monitor electrolyte status
- Monitor for mental status changes
- Monitor for edema, fluid overload
- Teach patient to protect nitroprusside from light
- Teach patient that nitroprusside may have a brown discoloration
- Teach patient to avoid driving and other hazardous activities
- Teach patient to change positions slowly
- Teach patient not to abruptly discontinue drug, even if feeling better
- Teach patient to report signs and symptoms of edema, fluid overload
- Teach patient body hair will increase during therapy and decrease after therapy
- Teach patient to avoid OTC products unless prescriber approves
- Teach patient to avoid smoking, alcohol
- Teach patient to maintain sodium restriction, calorie reduction, exercise program, stress management

APPLICATION AND REVIEW

6. What client response indicates to the nurse that a vasodilator medication is effective?
    1. Pulse rate decreases from 110 to 75
    2. Absence of adventitious breath sounds
    3. Increase in the daily amount of urine produced
    4. Blood pressure changes from 154/90 to 126/72
7. What information from a client's history would contraindicate a prescription for alpha-beta blocker therapy with labetalol? **Select all that apply.**
    1. Female
    2. 76 years of age
    3. Being treated for bronchial asthma
    4. History of congestive heart failure (CHF)
    5. History of peripheral vascular disease (PVD)

See Answers on pages 153-155.

DIURETIC DRUGS

Thiazide Diuretics
- Used to rid body of excess fluid and electrolytes
- Examples include chlorothiazide, hydrochlorothiazide
- Available in PO preparations

Mode of Action
- Acts on distal tubule and loop of Henle to excrete water and electrolytes
- Lowers blood pressure by reducing total body sodium and secondarily inducing vascular relaxation

Contraindications, Precautions, and Drug Interactions of Thiazide Diuretics*

Drug	Contraindications/Precautions	Drug Interaction
chlorothiazide	***Contraindications:*** Hypersensitivity to thiazides/ sulfonamides, anuria, preeclampsia, renal decompensation ***Precautions:*** Breastfeeding, COPD, diabetes mellitus, gout, hepatic/renal disease, hyperlipidemia, hypokalemia, hypomagnesemia, LE, sympathectomy ***Pregnancy:*** No adverse effects in animals; no human studies available	Amphotericin B, corticosteroids, piperacillin, ticarcillin, diazoxide, lithium, cardiac glycosides, nondepolarizing skeletal muscle relaxants, NSAIDs, loop diuretics, antidiabetics, cholestyramine, colestipol
hydrochlorothiazide	***Contraindications:*** Hypersensitivity to thiazides/ sulfonamides, anuria, preeclampsia, renal decompensation ***Precautions:*** Breastfeeding, COPD, diabetes mellitus, gout, hepatic/renal disease, hyperlipidemia, hypokalemia, hypomagnesemia, LE ***Pregnancy:*** No adverse effects in animals; no human studies available	Amphotericin B, corticosteroids, piperacillin, ticarcillin, diazoxide, lithium, cardiac glycosides, nondepolarizing skeletal muscle relaxants, NSAIDs, loop diuretics, antidiabetics, cholestyramine, colestipol

*Pregnancy categories have been revised. See http://www.fda.gov/Drugs/DevelopmentApprovalProcess/DevelopmentResources/Labeling/ucm093307.htm for more information.

Adverse/Side Effects

- Headache
- Dizziness
- Depression
- Fever
- Hyperuricemia
- Orthostatic hypotension
- Palpitations
- Blurred vision
- Hypokalemia
- Hypercalcemia
- Hyponatremia
- Hypochloremia
- Hypomagnesemia
- Nausea
- Vomiting
- Diarrhea
- Constipation
- Pancreatitis
- Hepatitis
- Jaundice
- Urinary frequency
- Uremia
- Glucosuria
- Hyperglycemia
- Renal failure
- Erectile dysfunction
- Leukopenia
- Thrombocytopenia
- Anemia
- Agranulocytosis
- Neutropenia
- Rash
- Urticaria
- Alopecia
- Stevens-Johnson syndrome

Nursing Care

- Administer with food or milk
- Administer early in the day at the same time each day
- Weigh patient daily
- Monitor I&O
- Monitor electrolyte status
- Monitor for hypo/hypertension
- Monitor renal/hepatic function
- Monitor for mental status changes
- Monitor for skin changes, rashes
- Teach patient to change positions slowly
- Teach patient to notify prescriber of muscle weakness/cramps, nausea, dizziness
- Teach patient to use sunscreen, protective clothing, sunglasses
- Teach diabetic patient to monitor blood glucose levels
- Teach patient to avoid OTC products, alcohol unless prescriber approves

- Teach patient to monitor weight daily and report to prescriber
- Teach patient dietary requirements (sodium, potassium restrictions)
- Teach patient self-blood pressure monitoring
- Teach patient to maintain calorie reduction, exercise program, stress management

Thiazide-Like Diuretics

- Used to rid body of excess fluid and electrolytes
- Examples include metolazone, indapamide
- Available in PO preparations

Mode of Action

- Acts on distal tubule to excrete water and electrolytes

Contraindications, Precautions, and Drug Interactions of Thiazide-Like Diuretics*

Drug	Contraindications/Precautions	Drug Interaction
metolazone	*Contraindications:* Hypersensitivity to thiazides/sulfonamides, anuria, coma, hepatic encephalopathy *Precautions:* Breastfeeding, geriatric patients, COPD, diabetes mellitus, electrolyte imbalance, gout, hepatic/renal disease, hypokalemia, hypotension, hypersensitivity to sulfonamides, LE, thiazides *Pregnancy:* No adverse effects in animals; no human studies available	Antidiabetics, mezlocillin, piperacillin, amphotericin B, glucocorticoids, digoxin, stimulant laxatives, alcohol (large amounts), nitrates, antihypertensives, opioids, barbiturates, lithium, loop diuretics, NSAIDs, salicylates
indapamide	*Contraindications:* Hypersensitivity to thiazides/sulfonamides, anuria, hepatic coma *Precautions:* Breastfeeding, ascites, dehydration, diabetes mellitus, dysrhythmias, gout, hepatic/renal disease, hypokalemia *Pregnancy:* Only given after risks to the fetus are considered; animal studies have shown adverse reactions; no human studies available	Lithium, digoxin, diazoxide, steroids, toxicity of muscle relaxants, corticosteroids, loop diuretics, thiazide diuretics, amphotericin B, antidiabetics, anticoagulants, antigout agents, cholestyramine, colestipol, indomethacin, NSAIDs

*Pregnancy categories have been revised. See http://www.fda.gov/Drugs/DevelopmentApprovalProcess/DevelopmentResources/Labeling/ucm093307.htm for more information.

Adverse/Side Effects

- Headache
- Dizziness
- Fatigue
- Weakness
- Anxiety
- Depression
- Orthostatic hypotension
- Palpitations
- Volume depletion
- Blurred vision
- Hypokalemia
- Hyponatremia
- Hypercalcemia
- Nausea
- Vomiting
- Diarrhea
- Constipation
- Anorexia
- Pancreatitis
- Hepatitis
- Jaundice
- Urinary frequency
- Uremia
- Glucosuria
- Hyperglycemia
- Renal failure
- Erectile dysfunction
- Leukopenia
- Thrombocytopenia
- Aplastic anemia
- Hemolytic anemia
- Agranulocytosis
- Neutropenia
- Rash
- Urticaria
- Alopecia
- Toxic epidermal necrolysis
- Stevens-Johnson syndrome
- Muscle cramps
- Arthralgia

Nursing Care

- Administer with food or milk
- Administer early in the day at the same time each day
- Weigh patient daily
- Monitor I&O
- Monitor electrolyte status
- Monitor for CHF
- Monitor for hypo/hypertension
- Monitor renal/hepatic function
- Monitor for infection
- Monitor for mental status changes
- Monitor for skin changes, rashes
- Teach patient to change positions slowly
- Teach patient to notify prescriber of muscle weakness/cramps, nausea, dizziness
- Teach patient to use sunscreen, protective clothing, sunglasses
- Teach diabetic patient to monitor blood glucose levels
- Teach patient not to abruptly discontinue drug, even if feeling better
- Teach patient to avoid OTC products, alcohol unless prescriber approves
- Teach patient to monitor weight daily and report to prescriber
- Teach patient dietary requirements (sodium, potassium)
- Teach patient to report signs and symptoms of infection to prescriber
- Teach patient self-blood pressure monitoring
- Teach patient to maintain calorie reduction, exercise program, stress management

Loop Diuretics

- Used to rid body of excess fluid and electrolytes
- Examples include furosemide, bumetanide, torsemide
- Available in PO, IM, IV preparations

Mode of Action

- Inhibits sodium and water reabsorption at proximal tubule sites and ascending loop of Henle

Contraindications, Precautions, and Drug Interactions of Loop Diuretics*

Drug	Contraindications/Precautions	Drug Interaction
furosemide	**Contraindications:** Anuria **Precautions:** Breastfeeding, infants, ascites, cirrhosis, diabetes mellitus, dehydration, electrolyte imbalance, gout, severe renal disease, hypovolemia, hypersensitivity to sulfonamides/thiazides **Pregnancy:** Only given after risks to the fetus are considered; animal studies have shown adverse reactions; no human studies available	Antihypertensives, nitrates, aminoglycosides, cisplatin, vancomycin, anticoagulants, salicylates, lithium, nondepolarizing skeletal muscle relaxants, digoxin, probenecid
bumetanide	**Contraindications:** Hypersensitivity to thiazides/sulfonamides, anuria, hepatic coma **Precautions:** Breastfeeding, neonates, ascites, blood dyscrasias, hepatic cirrhosis, hyperuricemia, ototoxicity, hypokalemia, hyperglycemia, oliguria, hypomagnesemia, hypovolemia **Pregnancy:** Only given after risks to the fetus are considered; animal studies have shown adverse reactions; no human studies available	Aminoglycosides, cisplatin, potassium-wasting products, lithium, digoxin, metolazone, indomethacin, NSAIDs, probenecid, antidiabetics

Continued

Contraindications, Precautions, and Drug Interactions of Loop Diuretics—cont'd

Drug	Contraindications/Precautions	Drug Interaction
torsemide	*Contraindications:* Hypersensitivity to sulfonamides, anuria, infants *Precautions:* Breastfeeding, dehydration, diabetes mellitus, dysrhythmias, electrolyte depletion, renal disease, hypovolemia, syncope *Pregnancy:* No adverse effects in animals; no human studies available	Lithium, nondepolarizing skeletal muscle relaxants, digoxin, antihypertensives, nitrates, aminoglycosides, cisplatin, vancomycin, anticoagulants, indomethacin, carbamazepine, phenobarbital, phenytoin, rifampin, NSAIDs

*Pregnancy categories have been revised. See http://www.fda.gov/Drugs/DevelopmentApprovalProcess/DevelopmentResources/Labeling/ucm093307.htm for more information.

Adverse/Side Effects

- Headache
- Fatigue
- Weakness
- Orthostatic hypotension
- Circulatory collapse
- Blurred vision
- Loss of hearing
- Hypokalemia
- Hyponatremia
- Hypocalcemia
- Hypochloremic alkalosis
- Hypomagnesemia
- Hyperuricemia
- Metabolic alkalosis
- Nausea
- Vomiting
- Dry mouth
- Anorexia
- Pancreatitis
- Polyuria
- Renal failure
- Glucosuria
- Hyperglycemia
- Leukopenia
- Thrombocytopenia
- Anemia
- Agranulocytosis
- Neutropenia
- Rash
- Pruritus
- Urticaria
- Photosensitivity
- Toxic epidermal necrolysis
- Stevens-Johnson syndrome
- Muscle cramps
- Arthralgia

Nursing Care

- Administer with food or milk
- Administer early in the day at the same time each day
- Weigh patient daily
- Monitor I&O
- Monitor electrolyte status
- Monitor for CHF
- Monitor for hypo/hypertension
- Monitor renal/hepatic function
- Monitor for mental status changes
- Monitor for vision/hearing changes
- Monitor for skin changes, rashes
- Teach patient to change positions slowly
- Teach patient to notify prescriber of muscle weakness/cramps, nausea, dizziness
- Teach patient to use sunscreen, protective clothing, sunglasses
- Teach diabetic patient to monitor blood glucose levels
- Teach patient not to abruptly discontinue drug, even if feeling better
- Teach patient to avoid OTC products, alcohol unless prescriber approves
- Teach patient to monitor weight daily and report to prescriber
- Teach patient dietary requirements (sodium, potassium)
- Teach patient self-blood pressure monitoring
- Teach patient to maintain calorie reduction, exercise program, stress management

8. A nurse identifies signs of electrolyte depletion in a client with heart failure who is receiving bumetanide and digoxin. What does the nurse determine is the cause of the depletion?

   1. Diuretic therapy
   2. Sodium restriction
   3. Continuous dyspnea
   4. Inadequate oral intake

9. A client is admitted to the intensive care unit with acute pulmonary edema. Which rapidly acting intravenous diuretic should the nurse anticipate will be prescribed?

   1. Furosemide
   2. Chlorothiazide
   3. Spironolactone
   4. Acetazolamide

See Answers on pages 153-155.

Potassium-Sparing Diuretics

- Used to rid body of excess fluid and electrolytes
- Examples include spironolactone, triamterene, amiloride
- Available in PO preparations

Mode of Action

- Inhibits sodium, potassium ion exchange in distal tubule to increase sodium excretion and decrease potassium loss

Contraindications, Precautions, and Drug Interactions of Loop Diuretics*

Drug	Contraindications/Precautions	Drug Interaction
spironolactone	**Contraindications:** Hypersensitivity, anuria, hyperkalemia, severe renal disease **Precautions:** Breastfeeding, dehydration, electrolyte imbalances, gynecomastia, hepatic disease, metabolic acidosis, renal impairment **Pregnancy:** Only given after risks to the fetus are considered; animal studies have shown adverse reactions; no human studies available	Antihypertensives, digoxin, lithium, cholestyramine, potassium-sparing diuretics, potassium products, ACE inhibitors, sodium substitutes, anticoagulants, NSAIDs, salicylates
triamterene	**Contraindications:** Hypersensitivity to triamterene/thiazides, anuria **Precautions:** Breastfeeding, diabetes, gout, glaucoma, hyperkalemia, renal/hepatic disease, SLE **Pregnancy:** Only given after risks to the fetus are considered; animal studies have shown adverse reactions; no human studies available	Lithium, amphotericin B, methenamine, allopurinol, colchicine, probenecid, prednisone, potassium-sparing diuretics, potassium products,
Amiloride	**Contraindications:** Hypersensitivity, anuria, diabetic neuropathy, renal failure **Precautions:** Breastfeeding, children, geriatric patients, dehydration, diabetes, hyponatremia, impaired renal function, respiratory acidosis **Pregnancy:** No adverse effects in animals; no human studies available	Potassium-sparing diuretics, potassium products, ACE inhibitors, sodium substitutes, cyclosporine, tacrolimus, lithium, antihypertensives, NSAIDs

*Pregnancy categories have been revised. See http://www.fda.gov/Drugs/DevelopmentApprovalProcess/DevelopmentResources/Labeling/ucm093307.htm for more information.

Adverse/Side Effects

- Headache
- Drowsiness
- Confusion
- Lethargy
- Ataxia
- Parathesias
- Encephalopathy
- Hyperkalemia
- Hyponatremia
- Hypochloremic metabolic acidosis
- Nausea
- Vomiting
- Diarrhea
- Anorexia
- Abdominal cramps
- GI bleeding
- Gastritis
- Hepatocellular toxicity
- Agranulocytosis
- Aplastic anemia
- Neutropenia
- Impotence
- Gynecomastia
- Irregular menses
- Amenorrhea
- Postmenopausal bleeding
- Hirsutism
- Breast pain
- Deepening voice
- Rash
- Pruritus
- Urticaria

Nursing Care

- Administer with food or milk to decrease GI upset
- Administer early in the day at the same time each day
- Weigh patient daily
- Monitor I&O
- Monitor electrolyte status
- Monitor for hypo/hypertension
- Monitor for dysrhythmias
- Monitor renal/hepatic function
- Monitor for mental status changes
- Teach patient to change positions slowly
- Teach patient to notify prescriber of muscle weakness/cramps, nausea, dizziness
- Teach patient not to abruptly discontinue drug, even if feeling better
- Teach patient to avoid hazardous activities until reaction is known
- Teach patient to monitor weight daily and report to prescriber
- Teach patient to monitor diet potassium
- Teach patient to avoid salt substitutes
- Teach patient self-blood pressure monitoring
- Teach patient to maintain calorie reduction, exercise program, stress management

Osmotic Diuretics

- Used to decrease edema
- Examples include mannitol
- Available in IV preparations

Mode of Action

- Increases osmotic pressure of glomerular filtrate, which inhibits reabsorption of water and sodium

Contraindications, Precautions, and Drug Interactions of Osmotic Diuretics*

Drug	Contraindications/Precautions	Drug Interaction
Mannitol	**Contraindications:** Hypersensitivity, acute MI, aneurysm, anuria, active intracranial bleeding, edema, severe dehydration, severe pulmonary congestion, stroke **Precautions:** Breastfeeding, geriatric patients, CHF, dehydration, electrolyte imbalances, severe renal disease **Pregnancy:** Only given after risks to the fetus are considered; animal studies have shown adverse reactions; no human studies available	Lithium, salicylates, barbiturates, imipramine, bromides, arsenic trioxide, cardiac glycosides, levomethadyl

*Pregnancy categories have been revised. See http://www.fda.gov/Drugs/DevelopmentApprovalProcess/DevelopmentResources/Labeling/ucm093307.htm for more information.

Adverse/Side Effects

- Headache
- Drowsiness
- Confusion
- Seizures
- Fever
- Chills
- Rebound increased ICP
- Pulmonary congestion
- Cough
- Dyspnea
- Edema
- Tachycardia
- CHF
- Circulatory overload
- PVCs
- Thrombophlebitis
- Hypo/hypertension
- Nausea
- Vomiting
- Diarrhea
- Dry mouth
- Blurred vision
- Hearing loss
- Decreased intraocular pressure
- Electrolyte imbalances
- Fluid imbalances
- Acidosis
- Dehydration
- Hypo/hyperkalemia
- Diuresis
- Urinary retention
- Thirst

Nursing Care

- Weigh patient daily
- Monitor I&O
- Monitor electrolyte status
- Monitor for hypo/hypertension
- Monitor renal/hepatic function
- Monitor neurologic/mental status
- Teach patient to change positions slowly
- Teach patient to notify prescriber of muscle weakness/cramps, nausea, dizziness
- Teach patient not to abruptly discontinue drug, even if feeling better
- Teach patient to monitor weight daily and report to prescriber

Carbonic Anhydrase Inhibitors

- Used to decrease edema
- Examples include acetazolamide, methazolamide
- Available in PO, IV preparations

Mode of Action

- Inhibits carbonic anhydrase activity in proximal renal tubules to decrease reabsorption of water/electrolytes

Contraindications, Precautions, and Drug Interactions of Carbonic Anhydrase Inhibitors*

Drug	Contraindications/Precautions	Drug Interaction
acetazolamide	**Contraindications:** Hypersensitivity to sulfonamides, acidemia, Addison's disease, adrenocortical insufficiency, anuria, electrolyte imbalances, hyperchloremic acidosis, metabolic acidosis, severe hepatic/renal disease **Precautions:** Breastfeeding, COPD, emphysema, hypercalciuria, pulmonary obstruction, respiratory acidosis **Pregnancy:** Only given after risks to the fetus are considered; animal studies have shown adverse reactions; no human studies available	Amphetamines, beta blockers, carbamazepine, cyclosporine, ethotoin, lithium, salicylates, primidone, flecainide, memantine, phenytoin, procainamide, quinidine, anticholinergics, methenamine, mexiletine, folic acid antagonists, topiramate, corticosteroids, amphotericin B, corticotropin, ACTH, arsenic trioxide, cardiac glycosides, levomethadyl
methazolamide	**Contraindications:** Hypersensitivity to sulfonamides, acidemia, Addison's disease, adrenocortical insufficiency, anuria, electrolyte imbalances, hyperchloremic acidosis, metabolic acidosis, severe hepatic/renal disease **Precautions:** Breastfeeding, COPD, emphysema **Pregnancy:** Only given after risks to the fetus are considered; animal studies have shown adverse reactions; no human studies available	Amphetamines, beta blockers, carbamazepine, cyclosporine, ethotoin, lithium, salicylates, primidone, flecainide, memantine, phenytoin, procainamide, quinidine, anticholinergics, methenamine, mexiletine, folic acid antagonists, topiramate, corticosteroids, amphotericin B, corticotropin, ACTH, arsenic trioxide, cardiac glycosides, levomethadyl

*Pregnancy categories have been revised. See http://www.fda.gov/Drugs/DevelopmentApprovalProcess/DevelopmentResources/Labeling/ucm093307.htm for more information.

Adverse/Side Effects

- Headache
- Dizziness
- Drowsiness
- Confusion
- Seizures
- Anxiety
- Depression
- Fatigue
- Paresthesia
- Myopia
- Tinnitus
- Hypo/hyperglycemia
- Nausea
- Vomiting
- Diarrhea
- Anorexia
- Melena
- Weight loss
- Hepatic insufficiency
- Hepatic necrosis
- Jaundice
- GI bleeding
- Taste alterations
- Urinary frequency
- Polyuria
- Uremia
- Glucosuria
- Hematuria
- Dysuria
- Crystalluria
- Renal calculi
- Aplastic anemia
- Hemolytic anemia
- Leukopenia
- Thrombocytopenia
- Purpura
- Pancytopenia
- Hypokalemia
- Hyperchloremic acidosis
- Hyponatremia
- Metabolic acidosis
- Hyperuricemia
- Hypercalcemia
- Rash
- Pruritus
- Urticaria
- Photosensitivity
- Flushing
- Stevens-Johnson syndrome
- Toxic epidermal necrolysis

Nursing Care

- Weigh patient daily
- Monitor I&O
- Monitor electrolyte status
- Monitor for hypo/hypertension
- Monitor renal/hepatic function

- Monitor neurologic/mental status
- Teach patient not to skip, double doses
- Teach patient to change positions slowly
- Teach diabetic patient to monitor blood glucose
- Teach patient not to abruptly discontinue drug, even if feeling better
- Teach patient to monitor weight daily and report to prescriber
- Teach patient to report to prescriber signs and symptoms of Stevens-Johnson syndrome and toxic epidermal necrolysis
- Teach patient to avoid hazardous activities if drowsiness occurs
- Teach patient to avoid prolonged sun exposure

APPLICATION AND REVIEW

10. What information concerning possible side effects should the nurse provide a client being prescribed a loop diuretic? **Select all that apply.**
    1. Need to report suicidal ideations
    2. Dizziness when changing positions
    3. Importance of reporting any skin rash
    4. Protect eyes and exposed skin from sun exposure
    5. Notify primary health provider of any vision changes

See Answers on pages 153-155.

ANSWER KEY: REVIEW QUESTIONS

1. **2 An ACE inhibitor is prescribed to convert angiotensin I to angiotensin II in an effort to manage hypertension. Angioedema is considered a contraindication for ACE therapy. Research has determined that the risks caused by ACE therapy to clients diagnosed with angioedema far exceed the potential benefits.**
   1 Leukemia is recognized as a precautionary condition when considering ACE therapy with captopril. The decision to prescribe the medication is determined after weighing the potential benefits versus the potential risks. 3 Diabetes mellitus is recognized as a precautionary condition when considering ACE therapy with captopril. The decision to prescribe the medication is determined after weighing the potential benefits versus the potential risks. 4 Congestive heart failure is recognized as a precautionary condition when considering ACE therapy with captopril. The decision to prescribe the medication is determined after weighing the potential benefits versus the potential risks.
   Client Need: Pharmacologic and Parenteral Therapies; **Cognitive Level:** Analysis; **Nursing Process:** Assessment/Analysis

2. **1 ACE (angiotensin-converting enzyme) increases the sensitivity of the cough reflex, leading to the common adverse effect sometimes referred to as an ACE cough.**
   2, 3, 4 A cough is not a side effect of angiotensin-converting enzymes.
   Client Need: Pharmacologic and Parenteral Therapies; **Cognitive Level:** Application; **Nursing Process:** Evaluation/Outcomes

 Study Tip: Don't cough up any aces! ACE inhibitors inCrease the Cough reflex.

3. **Answers: 1, 2, 3, 5**
   Safety issues associated with the administration of an ACE inhibitor include adverse reactions like orthostatic hypotension, increased risk for infections, and an increased sensitivity to sunlight. Regular monitoring of blood pressure is necessary to be alert for unsafe changes that may occur.

4 Clients should be instructed to avoid missing medication doses but that double dosing is not to be implemented as a "catch up" technique.

Client Need: Pharmacologic and Parenteral Therapies; **Cognitive Level:** Analysis; **Integrated Process:** Teaching/Learning; **Nursing Process:** Assessment/Analysis

4. **Answers: 2, 3, 4, 5**

ACE inhibitor therapy may include adverse reactions like orthostatic hypotension, increased risk for infections, and an increased risk of CHF. Regular monitoring of adherence to dietary recommends to limit sodium and calories is appropriate and contribute to the goal of managing the client's blood pressure.

1 ACE inhibitors are likely to cause signs and symptoms associated with urinary frequency and oliguria than actually urinary retention.

Client Need: Pharmacologic and Parenteral Therapies; **Cognitive Level:** Analysis; **Nursing Process:** Planning/Implementation

5. **4 Angiotensin II receptor blockers (ARBs) lower the blood pressure; they block the receptor sites in smooth muscles and adrenal glands so vasoconstriction is prevented.**

1, 2, 3 ARBs do not directly affect lipid profile, apical pulse, or blood pressure.

Client Need: Pharmacologic and Parenteral Therapies; **Cognitive Level:** Application; **Nursing Process:** Evaluation/Outcomes

6. **4 Vasodilation will lower the blood pressure.**

1 The pulse rate is not decreased and may increase. **2** Breath sounds are not directly affected by vasodilation, although vasodilator medications can decrease preload and afterload, which could indirectly affect breath sounds in heart failure. **3** The urine output is not affected immediately, although control of blood pressure can help preserve renal function over time.

Client Need: Pharmacologic and Parenteral Therapies; **Cognitive Level:** Application; **Nursing Process:** Evaluation/Outcomes

7. **Answers: 3, 4**

Contraindications for labetalol therapy include bronchial asthma and CHF.

1 Being female is neither a contraindication nor a precautionary condition for the alpha-beta blocker labetalol. **2** Advanced age is recognized as a precautionary condition when considering alpha-beta blocker therapy with labetalol. The decision to prescribe the medication is determined after weighing the potential benefits versus the potential risks. **5** A history of PVDs is recognized as a precautionary condition when considering alpha-beta blocker therapy with labetalol. The decision to prescribe the medication is determined after weighing the potential benefits versus the potential risks.

Client Need: Pharmacologic and Parenteral Therapies; **Cognitive Level:** Analysis; **Nursing Process:** Assessment/Analysis

8. **1 Diuretic therapy that affects the loop of Henle generally involves the use of drugs (e.g., bumetanide [Bumex]) that directly or indirectly increase urinary sodium, chloride, and potassium excretion.**

2 Sodium restriction does not necessarily accompany administration of bumetanide. **3** Dyspnea does not directly result in a depletion of electrolytes. **4** Unless otherwise ordered, oral intake is unaffected.

Client Need: Pharmacologic and Parenteral Therapies; **Cognitive Level:** Analysis; **Nursing Process:** Evaluation/Outcomes

9. **1 Furosemide acts on the loop of Henle by increasing the excretion of chloride and sodium.**

2 Although used in the treatment of edema and hypertension, chlorothiazide is not as potent as furosemide. **3** Spironolactone is a potassium-sparing diuretic; it is less potent than thiazide diuretics. **4** Acetazolamide is used in the treatment of glaucoma to lower intraocular pressure.

Client Need: Pharmacologic and Parenteral Therapies: **Cognitive Level:** Analysis; **Nursing Process:** Planning/Implementation

10. **Answers: 2, 3, 4, 5**

    Client education related to the prescription of a loop diuretic should include information regarding both the reporting and management of orthostatic hypotension, photosensitivity, rashes, and visual changes.

    1 Although depression and suicidal ideations are serious and need immediate professional attention, neither is generally associated with loop diuretic therapy.

    Client Need: Pharmacologic and Parenteral Therapies; **Cognitive Level:** Analysis; **Integrated Process:** Teaching/Learning; **Nursing Process:** Planning/Implementation

9 Antianginal Drugs

INTRODUCTION TO CORONARY ARTERY DISEASES (CAD)

Etiology and Pathophysiology

- Coronary atherosclerosis: deposition of fatty plaques along inner wall of coronary arteries leads to inflammation; macrophages infiltrate endothelium, causing further damage and development of atheromas (fibrous caps over fatty deposits); narrowing and possible obstruction occur; also affects peripheral and cerebral vessels
- Angina pectoris (also known as stable angina): episodic pain experienced when the blood oxygen level cannot meet metabolic demands of muscles. In addition to atherosclerosis, this temporary ischemia may be precipitated by coronary artery spasms, strenuous exercise, heavy meals, hyperthyroidism, exposure to cold, and emotional stress; classified as stable, unstable (preinfarction), refractory, variant (Prinzmetal)
  - Unstable angina: unexpected chest pain while resting or sleeping
  - Refractory angina: does not respond to medication and is debilitating
  - Variant (Prinzmetal) angina: angina at rest that occurs in cycles
- Myocardial infarction (MI): acute necrosis of heart muscle caused by interruption of oxygen supply to the area (ischemia), resulting in altered function and reduced cardiac output (Fig. 9.1)
- Risk factors
  - Family history
  - Increasing age, particularly women
  - Gender: men; women, especially after menopause (estrogen seems to provide some protection)
  - Race; risk appears higher in African Americans
  - Cigarette smoking contributes to vasoconstriction, platelet activation, arterial smooth muscle cell proliferation, and reduced oxygen availability
  - Hypertension; widened QRS complex (bundle branch block)
  - Hyperlipidemia: increased total cholesterol; increased LDL (high: 130–150 mg/dL; very high: 160 mg/dL or more); increased ratio of total cholesterol or LDL to HDL; low HDL (less than 40 mg/dL); HDL greater than 60 mg/dL seems to help protect against coronary artery disease (CAD); increased triglycerides (high: 200–499 mg/dL; very high: 500 mg/dL or more)
  - Obesity (particularly abdominal obesity)
  - Sedentary lifestyle (contributes to obesity and reduced HDL)
  - Type 2 diabetes
  - Stress; an innate, competitive, aggressive type A personality seems less important than amount of stress and client's psychologic response
  - Metabolic syndrome: cluster of signs including hyperlipidemia, low HDL level, abdominal obesity, increased BP, insulin resistance, increased levels of C-reactive protein, and increased fibrinogen level

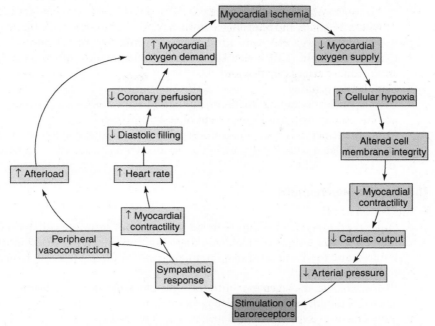

FIG. 9.1 Effects of prolonged myocardial ischemia. (From Monahan, F.D., Sands, J., Neighbors, M., Marek, J., Green-Nigro, C. [2007]. *Phipps' medical-surgical nursing: Health and illness* perspectives [8th ed.]. St. Louis: Mosby.)

Clinical Findings

- Subjective
  - Retrosternal chest pain that may radiate to arms, jaw, neck, shoulder, or back; pain described as "pressure," "crushing," or "viselike"; palpitations, apprehension, feeling of dread/impending doom, dyspnea, nausea, vomiting; pain of angina can be associated with activity and generally subsides with rest; asymptomatic with silent ischemia
  - Atypical symptoms of angina in women include exertion-related discomfort above waist; burning or tenderness to touch in back, shoulders, arm, jaw, abdomen; overwhelming fatigue; indigestion; feeling of unease
  - Aytypical symptoms of angina in clients with diabetes mellitus include blunted perception of ischemic chest pain; prolongation of the angina perceptual threshold during exercise
- Objective
  - ECG changes may reveal ischemia (inverted T wave, elevated ST segment) or evidence of MI (presence of Q wave); a Holter monitor may be used to detect changes associated with activities of daily living (ADLs)
  - Elevated levels of serum enzymes and isoenzymes with MI
    - Cardiac troponin T (cTnT) levels increase within 3 to 6 hours and remain elevated for 14 to 21 days; accurate for assessing myocardial damage
    - Cardiac troponin I (cTnI) levels rise 7 to 14 hours after an MI and remain elevated for 5 to 7 days; specific for myocardial damage
    - Creatinine kinase (CK) levels elevate 3 to 6 hours after infarction, peaking at 24 hours, and returning to normal within 72 hours

- MB isoenzyme of creatine kinase (CK-MB) levels elevate 4 to 6 hours after pain, peaking within 24 hours, and returning to normal within 72 hours; specific for myocardial damage
  - Myoglobin levels elevate in 1 to 3 hours; returning to normal within 12 hours
- C-reactive protein (CRP): elevation suggests inflammation of the vascular endothelium and coronary artery calcification
- Doppler flow studies
- Cardiac nuclear scanning (thallium, multigated acquisition scan [MUGA]) or echocardiographic studies help determine extent of vessels involved
- Sympathetic nervous system responses: pallor, tachycardia, diaphoresis, vomiting
- Signs associated with MI: dysrhythmia, elevated temperature, elevated sedimentation rate, and increased WBCs

Therapeutic Interventions

- Prevention of MI
  - Supervised exercise program to avoid ischemia but promote collateral circulation and increase HDL; weight control; smoking cessation; dietary restriction of sodium, cholesterol, and total and saturated fat; management of hypertension, hyperlipidemia, and diabetes
  - Pharmacologic management: nitrates, beta-blocking agents, calcium channel blocking agents, antilipidemics, antiplatelet agents, ACEIs
  - Supplemental oxygen during anginal attack as needed
  - Percutaneous coronary interventions (PCIs) such as percutaneous transluminal coronary angioplasty (PTCA), coronary artery stent placement, and atherectomy to revascularize myocardium
  - Coronary artery bypass graft (CABG) if medical regimen not successful
- Management of acute MI
  - Improvement of perfusion
    - Administration of aspirin immediately
    - Beta blockers or angiotensin II receptor blockers for left ventricular systolic dysfunction (LVSD)
    - Thrombolytic therapy within 30 minutes of arrival; anticoagulants
    - IV nitroglycerin
    - ACEIs
    - Antidysrhythmics to maintain cardiac function
    - PCI within 90 minutes of arrival at emergency department
    - Intraaortic balloon pump that inflates during diastole and deflates during systole to decrease cardiac workload by decreasing afterload and increasing myocardial perfusion for cardiogenic shock
    - Aspirin, beta blocker, and possible antilipidemic prescribed at discharge
  - Promotion of comfort and rest
    - Analgesics (e.g., IV morphine) to reduce pain, anxiety, and cardiac workload by decreasing preload and afterload
    - Oxygen to improve tissue oxygenation
    - Maintenance of bed or chair rest to decrease oxygen tissue demands
    - Diet therapy: 2 g sodium diet or clear liquids, depending on presence of nausea
  - Continuous monitoring
    - Pulse oximetry
    - Cardiac monitoring: rate, evidence of ischemia, and dysrhythmias

- ▪ Vital signs
- ▪ Hemodynamic monitoring with pulmonary artery catheter
- • Assessment for complications of MI
  - ▪ Dysrhythmias
  - ▪ Cardiogenic shock
  - ▪ Pulmonary edema caused by acute heart failure
  - ▪ Thromboembolism
  - ▪ Extension of MI
  - ▪ Pericardial effusion and cardiac tamponade

APPLICATION AND REVIEW

1. A client is admitted with chest pain unrelieved by nitroglycerin, an elevated temperature, decreased blood pressure, and diaphoresis. A myocardial infarction is diagnosed. Which should the nurse consider as a valid reason for one of this client's physiologic responses?
   1. Parasympathetic reflexes from the infarcted myocardium cause diaphoresis.
   2. Inflammation in the myocardium causes a rise in the systemic body temperature.
   3. Catecholamines released at the site of the infarction cause intermittent localized pain.
   4. Constriction of central and peripheral blood vessels causes a decrease in blood pressure.

2. What information should the nurse include when teaching a client with heart disease about cholesterol?
   1. Can be found in both plant and animal sources
   2. Causes an increase in serum high-density lipoprotein
   3. Should be eliminated because it causes the disease process
   4. Decreases when unsaturated fats are substituted for saturated fats

3. A nurse is providing dietary instruction to a client with cardiovascular disease. Which dietary selection by the client indicates the need for further instruction?
   1. Whole milk with oatmeal
   2. Garden salad with olive oil
   3. Tuna fish with a small apple
   4. Soluble fiber cereal with skim milk

4. A nurse asks a client with ischemic heart disease to identify the foods that are **most** important to restrict. The nurse determines that the client understands the dietary instructions when the client identifies the following foods. **Select all that apply.**
   1. Olive oil
   2. Chicken broth
   3. Enriched whole milk
   4. Red meats, such as beef
   5. Vegetables and whole grains
   6. Liver and other glandular organ meats

5. What should the nurse identify as the **primary** cause of the pain experienced by a client with a coronary occlusion?
   1. Arterial spasm
   2. Heart muscle ischemia
   3. Blocking of the coronary veins
   4. Irritation of nerve endings in the cardiac plexus

6. For which common complication of myocardial infarction should the nurse monitor clients in the coronary care unit?
   1. Dysrhythmia
   2. Hypokalemia
   3. Anaphylactic shock
   4. Cardiac enlargement

7. A client with a bundle branch block is on a cardiac monitor. What ECG change should the nurse identify on the client's cardiac monitor?
   1. Sagging ST segments
   2. Absence of P wave configurations
   3. Inverted T waves following each QRS complex
   4. Widening of QRS complexes to a minimum of 0.12 second

8. A nurse is providing discharge instructions to a client who experienced an anterior septal myocardial infarction. What statement by the client indicates to the nurse that there is a need for further teaching?
   1. "I want to stay as pain-free as possible."
   2. "I am not good at remembering to take medications."
   3. "I should not have any problems in reducing my salt intake."
   4. "I wrote down my medication information for future reference."

9. A client is admitted with the diagnosis of possible myocardial infarction, and a series of diagnostic tests is ordered. Which blood level should the nurse expect will increase **first** if this client has had a myocardial infarction?
   1. ALT
   2. AST
   3. Total LDH
   4. Troponin T

10. A nurse is leading a discussion in a senior citizen center about the risk factors for developing coronary heart disease (CHD) for women versus men. What should the nurse respond when asked to identify the **most** significant risk factor?
    1. Obesity
    2. Diabetes
    3. Elevated CRP levels
    4. High levels of HDL-C

11. A client enters the emergency department, reporting shortness of breath and epigastric distress. What should be the triage nurse's **first** intervention?
    1. Assess vital signs.
    2. Insert a saline lock.
    3. Place client on oxygen.
    4. Draw blood for troponins.

See Answers on pages 169-172.

ANTIANGINAL AGENTS

Nitrates
- Used to relieve angina
- Categories are short-acting and long-acting
- Examples: isosorbide dinitrate, isosorbide moninitrate, nitroglycerin
- Available in sublingual (most common), aerosol spray, intravenous, oral, topical, transdermal, and translingual preparations

Mode of Action
- Causes vascular and coronary vasodilation

Contraindications, Precautions, and Drug Interactions of Nitrates*

Drug	Contraindications/Precautions	Drug Interaction
Short-Acting		
nitroglycerin	*Contraindications:* Anemia, cardiomyopathy, increased intracranial pressure, shock *Precautions:* Acute myocardial infarction, breastfeeding, head trauma, hypotension, hypovolemia, pregnancy, renal or hepatic disease *Pregnancy:* Only given after risks to the fetus are considered	Alcohol, antihypertensives, aspirin, benzodiazepines, beta blockers, calcium channel blockers, heparin, sildenafil, tadalofil, vasodilators, verdanafil
Long-Acting		
isosorbide dinitrate	*Contraindications:* Closed-angle glaucoma, hypersensitivity to isosorbide mononitrate or nitrates, severe anemia *Precautions:* Acute myocardial infarction, breastfeeding, cerebral hemorrhage, children, chronic heart failure, gastrointestinal disease, geriatrics, hypotension, increased intracranial pressure, orthostatic myocardial infarction, pregnancy, severe renal/hepatic disease, syncope *Pregnancy:* Only given after risks to the fetus are considered	Alcohol, rosiglitazone, sildenafil, tadalofil, vardenafil
isosorbide mononitrate	*Contraindications:* Closed-angle glaucoma, hypersensitivity to isosorbide mononitrate or nitrates, severe anemia *Precautions:* Acute myocardial infarction, breastfeeding, cerebral hemorrhage, children, chronic heart failure, gastrointestinal disease, geriatrics, hypotension, increased intracranial pressure, orthostatic myocardial infarction, pregnancy, severe renal/hepatic disease, syncope *Pregnancy:* No human studies available, but no adverse effects in animals; only given after risks to the fetus are considered	Alcohol, rosiglitazone, sildenafil, tadalofil, vardenafil

*Pregnancy categories have been revised. See http://www.fda.gov/Drugs/DevelopmentApprovalProcess/DevelopmentResources/Labeling/ucm093307.htm for more information.

Adverse/Side Effects
- Circulatory collapse (life threatening)
- Diaphoresis
- Dizziness
- Flushing
- Headache
- Nausea and vomiting
- Orthostatic hypotension
- Pallor
- Rash
- Syncope
- Tachycardia
- Tolerance
- Weakness

Nursing Care
- Monitor orthostatic blood pressure, pulse
- Assess pain, check for tolerance over extended periods
- Monitor for headache, light-headedness, decreased blood pressure; may indicate a need for a lower dosage

- Isosorbide dinitrate/isosorbide mononitrate: monitor for methemoglobinemia (rare): assess for cyanosis, coma, seizures, shock; more common at high doses, may occur with normal doses.
- Teach to avoid alcohol and to never use erectile dysfunction products (may cause severe hypotension, death)
- Teach that product may cause headache; tolerance usually develops; use nonopioid analgesic
- Teach that stinging may occur when first placing sublingual tab against mucous membranes
- Teach avoiding hazardous activities if dizziness occurs
- Teach changing positions slowly to prevent fainting

APPLICATION AND REVIEW

12. What instructions about the use of nitroglycerin should the nurse provide to a client with angina?
    1. "Identify when pain occurs, and place two tablets under the tongue."
    2. "Place one tablet under the tongue, and swallow another when pain is intense."
    3. "Before physical activity place one tablet under the tongue, and repeat the dose in 5 minutes if pain occurs."
    4. "Place one tablet under the tongue when pain occurs, and use an additional tablet after the attack to prevent recurrence."
13. A nurse is providing discharge instructions for a client with angina who has a prescription for sublingual nitroglycerin tablets. The nurse should teach the client that the nitroglycerin sublingual tablets have lost their potency when:
    1. sublingual tingling is experienced.
    2. the tablets are more than 3 months old.
    3. the pain is unrelieved, but facial flushing is increased.
    4. onset of relief is delayed, but the duration of relief is unchanged.
14. What instructions should a nurse give a client for whom nitroglycerin tablets are prescribed?
    1. Limit the number of tablets to four per day.
    2. Discontinue the medication if a headache develops.
    3. Ensure that the medication is stored in a dark container.
    4. Increase the number of tablets if dizziness is experienced.

See Answers on pages 169-172.

Beta Blockers

- Used as antianginal, antidysrhythmic, and antihypertensive drugs
- Categories: selective and nonselective
- Examples: atenolol (beta$_1$), emtoprolol (beta$_1$), nadolol (beta$_1$ and beta$_2$), propranolol (beta$_1$ and beta$_2$)
- Available in oral and IV preparations

Mode of Action

- Decrease the effects of the sympathetic nervous system by blocking the action of the catecholamines, epinephrine and norepinephrine, thereby decreasing the heart rate and blood pressure.

Contraindications, Precautions, and Drug Interactions of Beta-Blockers*

Drug	Contraindications/Precautions	Drug Interaction
Selective		
atenolol (beta₁)	**Contraindications:** Cardiac failure, cardiogenic shock, hypersensitivity to β-blockers, heart block (second and third degree), sinus bradycardia, pregnancy **Precautions:** Asthma, breastfeeding, diabetes mellitus, major surgery, renal disease, thyroid disease, congestive heart failure, chronic obstructive pulmonary disease, asthma, well-compensated heart failure, dialysis, myasthenia gravis, Raynaud's disease, pulmonary edema **Pregnancy:** Evidence of fetal risk, but benefits out-weigh risks	Amphetamines, anticholinergics, antihypertensives, antidiabetic agents, digoxin, diltiazem, dopamine, ephedrine, hydralazine, insulin, methyldopa, prazosin, pseudoephedrine, reserpine, sympathomemetics, theophylline, verapamil,
metoprolol (beta₁)	**Contraindications:** Cardiogenic shock, heart block (second and third degree), hypersensitivity to β-blockers, pheochromocytoma, sick sinus syndrome, sinus bradycardia **Precautions:** Breastfeeding, bronchial asthma, cerebrovascular accident, children, chronic obstructive pulmonary disease, congestive heart failure, coronary artery disease, depression, diabetes mellitus, geriatric, major surgery, nonallergic bronchospasm, pregnancy, thyroid/renal/hepatic disease, vasospastic angina **Pregnancy:** Only given after risks to the fetus are considered	Antidiabetics (oral), amphetamines, barbiturates, calcium channel blockers, cimetidine, epinephrine, histamine Hx antagonists, hydralazine, insulin, MAOIs (do not use together), methyldopa prazosin, reserpine, NSAIDs, salicylates, xanthines.
Nonselective		
nadolol (beta₁ and beta₂)	**Contraindications:** Asthma, cardiac failure, cardiogenic shock, heart block (second and third degree), hypersensitivity to nadolol, sinus bradycardia, chronic obstructive pulmonary disease, congestive heart failure **Precautions:** Breastfeeding, diabetes mellitus, hyperthyroidism, myasthenia gravis, major surgery, nonallergic bronchospasm, peripheral vascular disease, pregnancy, renal disease **Pregnancy:** Only given after risks to the fetus are considered	Antihypertensives, clonidine, epinephrine, ergots, digoxin, MAOIs, NSAIDs, phenothiazines, thyroid
propranolol (beta₁ and beta₂)	**Contraindications:** Asthma, atrioventricular heart block, bronchospasm, bronchospastic disease, hydrochloride, hypersensitivity to propranolol cardiogenic shock, sinus bradycardia **Precautions:** Breastfeeding, cardiac failure, children, chronic obstructive pulmonary disease, diabetes mellitus, hyperthyroidism, hypotension, myasthenia gravis, peripheral vascular disease, pregnancy, renal/hepatic disease, Raynaud's disease, sick sinus syndrome, smoking, thyrotoxicosis, vasospastic angina, Wolff-Parkinson-White syndrome **Pregnancy:** Only given after risks to the fetus are considered	Barbiturates, calcium channel blockers, cimetidine, disopyramide, haloperidol, propafenone, phenothiazines, smoking

MAOI, monoamine oxidase inhibitor; *NSAIDs,* nonsteroidal antiinflammatory drugs.
*Pregnancy categories have been revised. See http://www.fda.gov/Drugs/DevelopmentApprovalProcess/DevelopmentResources/Labeling/ucm093307.htm for more information.

Adverse/Side Effects

- Agitation
- Agranulocytosis
- Blurred vision
- Bradycardia
- Bronchospasm
- Congestive heart failure
- Depression
- Dizziness/drowsiness/fatigue
- Dysrhythmias

- Heart failure
- Hypotension
- Insomnia
- Impotence
- Laryngospasm
- Mental changes
- Peripheral edema
- Pulmonary edema
- Stevens-Johnson syndrome
- Thrombocytopenia
- Toxic epidermal necrolysis

Nursing Care

- Monitor vital signs (especially blood pressure and heart rate) closely in the early stages of beta-blocker therapy
- Check baselines in renal and liver function tests
- Monitor for edema in lower extremities daily; monitor I&O, daily weight; check for jugular vein distention, crackles bilaterally, dyspnea (CHF)
- Monitor for headache, lightheadedness, decreased blood pressure, which may indicate a need for a lower dosage
- Teach patient to taper dose for 1 to 2 weeks when discontinuing medication; take at same time each day
- Teach patient not to use over the counter products containing α-adrenergic stimulants
- Teach patient to limit alcohol, smoking, and sodium intake as required
- Teach patient how to monitor pulse and blood pressure at home; advise when to notify healthcare provider
- Teach patient to comply with weight control, diet, and exercise requirements
- Advise patient to obtain emergency identification identifying products, allergies, conditions being treated
- Teach patient to change position slowly; avoid hazardous activities if dizziness occurs
- Teach patient to report symptoms of congestive heart failure
- Teach patient to take product as prescribed, not to double doses, skip doses; take any missed doses as remembered if at least 6 hr until next dose
- Teach patient that product may mask symptoms of hypoglycemia in diabetic patients
- Teach patient to use contraception while taking this product and avoid breastfeeding

APPLICATION AND REVIEW

15. Which client's health problem motivates the nurse to question a prescription for a beta blocker?
    1. Heart failure
    2. Hypertension
    3. Sinus tachycardia
    4. Coronary artery disease

16. A nurse provides instruction when the beta blocker atenolol (Tenormin) is prescribed for a client with moderate hypertension. What action identified by the client indicates to the nurse that the client needs further teaching?
    1. Move slowly when changing positions.
    2. Take the medication before going to bed.
    3. Expect to feel drowsy when taking this drug.
    4. Count the pulse before taking the medication.

17. Atenolol 150 mg by mouth is prescribed for a client with angina. Each tablet contains 50 mg. How many tablets should the nurse administer? **Record your answer using a whole number.**

    Answer: _____ tablets

18. Metoprolol is prescribed for a client. The nurse should question the prescription if the client has which diagnosis?
   1. Hypertension
   2. Angina pectoris
   3. Sinus bradycardia
   4. Myocardial infarction

See Answers on pages 169-172.

Calcium Channel Blockers (Dihydropyridines)

- Used to treat stable and variant angina pectoris, certain dysrhythmias, and hypertension
- Examples: amlodipine, felodipine, isradipine, nicardipine, nifedipine, nisoldipine
- Available in oral and IV preparations

Mode of Action

- Controls variant (vasospastic) angina by relaxing coronary arteries and controls classic (stable) angina by decreasing oxygen demand
- Reduces systemic vascular resistance and arterial pressure

Contraindications, Precautions, and Drug Interactions of Calcium Channel Blockers*

Drug	Contraindications/Precautions	Drug Interaction
amlodipine	*Contraindications:* Hypersensitivity to amlodipine, hypersensitivity to dihydropyridine, severe aortic stenosis, severe obstructive coronary artery disease *Precautions:* Breastfeeding, children, congestive heart failure, gastroesophageal reflux disease, geriatric, hepatic injury, hypotension, pregnancy *Pregnancy:* Only given after risks to the fetus are considered	Alcohol, antihypertensives, beta blockers, diltiazem, fentanyl, lithium, nitrates, NSAIDs, quinidine
felodipine	*Contraindications:* Hypersensitivity to this felodipine or dihydropyridines, hypotension <90 mm Hg systolic, sick sinus syndrome, second- or third-degree heart block *Precautions:* Breastfeeding, children, congestive heart failure, coronary artery disease, geriatric, hepatic injury, pregnancy, renal disease *Pregnancy:* Only given after risks to the fetus are considered	Alcohol, beta-adrenergic blockers, carbamazepine, cimetidine, clarithromycin, conivaptan, cyclosporine, dalfopristin, delavirdine, digoxin, diltiazem, disopyramide, erythromycin, itraconazole, ketoconazole, miconazole, nitrates, NSAIDs, phenytoin, propranolol, quinidine, quinupristin, zileuton
isradipine	*Contraindications:* Hypersensitivity to isradipine, hypersensitivity to other dihydropyridines *Precautions:* Pregnancy, breastfeeding, children, congestive heart failure, hypertension *Pregnancy:* Only given after risks to the fetus are considered	Dolasetron, fentanyl, isoniazid, itraconazole, pyrazinamide, rifabutin, rifampin, tizanidine
nicardipine	*Contraindications:* Advanced aortic stenosis, dihydropyridine, sick sinus syndrome, second- or third-degree heart block, hypersensitivity to nicardipine hydrochloride *Precautions:* Pregnancy, breastfeeding, children, geriatric, congestive heart failure, hypotension, hepatic injury, renal disease *Pregnancy:* Only given after risks to the fetus are considered	Alcohol, antihypertensives, carbamazepine, cimetidine, cyclosporine, digoxin, neuromuscular blocking agents, nitrates, NSAIDs, prazosin, propranolol, quinidine, rifampin

Continued

Contraindications, Precautions, and Drug Interactions of Calcium Channel Blockers—cont'd

Drug	Contraindications/Precautions	Drug Interaction
nifedipine	**Contraindications:** Cardiogenic shock, hypersensitivity to this nifedipine or dihydropyridine **Precautions:** Acute MI, aortic stenosis, breastfeeding, children, hypotension, hypotension <90 mm Hg systolic, GERD, heart failure, hepatic injury, pregnancy sick sinus syndrome, second- or third-degree heart block, renal disease **Pregnancy:** Only given after risks to the fetus are considered	Antihypertensives, beta-adrenergic blockers, carbamazepine, cimetidine, cyclosporine, digoxin, NSAIDs phenytoin, prazosin, quinidine, ranitidine, smoking, strong CYP3A4 inducers
nisoldipine	**Contraindications:** Aortic stenosis, hypersensitivity to this nisoldipine or dihydropyridines, sick sinus syndrome, second- or third-degree heart block **Precautions:** Acute myocardial infarction, breastfeeding, cardiogenic shock children, congestive heart failure, coronary artery disease, geriatric, hepatic injury, hypotension <90 mm Hg systolic, pregnancy, renal disease, unstable angina **Pregnancy:** Only given after risks to the fetus are considered	Antifungals, antihypertensives, beta-adrenergic blockers, cimetidine, CYP3A4 inducers, digoxin, hydantoins, ranitidine

NSAIDs, nonsteroidal antiinflammatory drugs.
*Pregnancy categories have been revised. See http://www.fda.gov/Drugs/DevelopmentApprovalProcess/DevelopmentResources/Labeling/ucm093307.htm for more information.

Adverse/Side Effects

- Angina
- Bradycardia
- Changes in liver and kidney function
- Congestive heart failure
- Dizziness
- Dysrhythmias
- Fatigue
- Flushing
- Headache
- Hypotension
- Myocardial infarction
- Palpitations
- Peripheral edema
- Pulmonary edema
- Reflex tachycardia
- Syncope

Nursing Care

- Assess angina pain, fluid volume status
- Assess for extravasation
- Monitor ALT, AST, bilirubin daily; if these are elevated, hepatotoxicity is suspected
- Monitor cardiac status, congestive heart failure, GI obstruction
- Monitor for serious skin disorders (discontinue in case of sudden rash, fever, cutaneous lesions)
- Monitor platelets
- Monitor renal/hepatic function tests, serum potassium
- Monitor vital signs
- Teach patient capsules may appear in stool
- Teach patient not to discontinue abruptly; taper instead
- Teach patient to change positions slowly and avoid hazardous activities when dizzy
- Teach patient to comply with instructions on diet (limit alcohol, caffeine, avoid grapefruit juice), exercise, stress reduction, and take medication as directed
- Teach patient to implement oral hygiene to prevent gingival hyperplasia; increase fluid intake to prevent constipation

Calcium Channel Blockers (Non-dihydropyridines)

- Used to treat atrial fibrillation, dysrhythmias, hypertension
- Examples: verapamil, diltiazem
- Available in oral and IV preparations

Mode of Action

- Decreases heart rate and contractility
- Increases the refractory period of the AV node, which decreases ventricular response

Contraindications, Precautions, and Drug Interactions of Calcium Channel Blockers (Non-dihydropyridines)*

Drug	Contraindications/Precautions	Drug Interaction
verapamil	*Contraindications:* Cardiogenic shock, hypotension <90 mm Hg systolic, Lown-Ganong-Levine syndrome, sick sinus syndrome, second- or third-degree heart block, severe congestive heart failure, Wolff-Parkinson-White syndrome *Precautions:* Breastfeeding, children, concomitant beta-blocker therapy, congestive heart failure, geriatric, hepatic injury, hypotension, pregnancy, renal disease *Pregnancy:* Only given after risks to the fetus are considered	Antihypertensive, beta-adrenergic blockers, carbamazepine, cimetidine, clarithromycin, cyclosporine, digoxin, erythromycin, fentanyl, lithium, nitrates, nondepolarizing muscle relaxants, NSAIDs, prazosin, quinidine, theophylline
diltiazem	*Contraindications:* Acute myocardial infarction, cardiogenic shock, hypotension <90 mm Hg systolic, pulmonary congestion, sick sinus syndrome, second- or third-degree heart block *Precautions:* Aortic stenosis, bradycardia, breastfeeding, children, congestive heart failure, geriatric, GERD, hepatic disease, hiatal hernia, pregnancy ventricular dysfunction *Pregnancy:* Only given after risks to the fetus are considered	Anesthetics, beta-adrenergic blockers, benzodiazepines, carbamazepine, cimetidine, cyclosporine, digoxin, HMC-CoA reductase inhibitors, lithium, lovastatin, methylprednisolone, theophylline

Adverse/Side Effects

- Acute renal failure
- Anxiety
- Asthenia
- AV block
- Bleeding
- Bradycardia
- Bruising
- Confusion
- CHF
- Constipation
- Depression
- Diarrhea
- Dizziness
- Drowsiness
- Dyspnea
- Dysrhythmias
- Edema
- Fatigue
- Flushing
- Gastric upset
- Gingival hyperplasia
- Gynecomastia
- Headache
- Heart block
- Hypotension
- Increased LFTs
- Impotence
- Insomnia
- Lightheadedness
- Nausea
- Nocturia
- Palpitations
- Parathesia
- Petechiae
- Pharangytis
- Photosensitivity
- Polyuria
- Rash
- Rhinitis
- Tremor
- Vomiting
- Weakness

Nursing Care

- Assess cardiac and respiratory status
- Monitor I&O
- Monitor daily weights

- Monitor for edema
- Monitor renal/hepatic studies
- Teach patient to increase fluids, fiber to decrease constipation
- Teach patient how to monitor blood pressure and pulse before taking medication
- Teach patient to keep record of vital signs
- Teach patient to avoid hazardous activities until dizziness dissipates
- Teach patient to avoid alcohol and caffeine
- Teach patient to consult physician before taking OTC and grapefruit products
- Teach patient to change positions slowly
- Teach patient to report adverse effects
- Teach patient not to discontinue medication abruptly
- Teach patient to comply with diet, exercise, stress reduction, and product therapy

APPLICATION AND REVIEW

19. What should the nurse include in a teaching plan for a client taking calcium channel blockers such as nifedipine? **Select all that apply.**
    1. Reduce calcium intake.
    2. Change positions slowly.
    3. Report peripheral edema.
    4. Expect temporary hair loss.
    5. Avoid drinking grapefruit juice.
20. What should the nurse include in a teaching plan to help reduce the side effects associated with diltiazem?
    1. Lie down after meals.
    2. Change positions slowly.
    3. Avoid dairy products in diet.
    4. Take the drug with an antacid.

See Answers on pages 169-172.

Piperazineacetamides

- Used as an antianginal, antiischemic for chronic chest pain
- Example: ranolazine
- Available in oral preparations

Mode of Action

- Unknown, may act by inhibiting portal fatty-acid oxidation, improves blood flow

Contraindications, Precautions, and Drug Interactions of Piperazineacetamides*

Drug	Contraindications/Precautions	Drug Interaction
ranolazine	**Contraindications:** Hepatic cirrhosis, hepatic disease (Child-Pugh class A, B, C), hypersensitivity, hypokalemia, preexisting QT prolongation, renal failure, torsades de pointes, ventricular dysrhythmia, ventricular tachycardia **Precautions:** Breastfeeding, children, females at risk for torsades de pointes, geriatric, hypotension, pregnancy, renal disease. **Pregnancy:** Only given after risks to the fetus are considered	Antiretroviral protease inhibitors, arsenic trioxide, beta-agonists, chloroquine, clarithromycin, class IA/III anti-dysrhythmics, CYP3A4 inhibitors, CYP3A4 substrates, digoxin, diltiazem, dofetilide, droperidol, erythromycin, haloperidol, ketoconazole, levomethadyllocal anesthetics, macrolide antibiotics, macrolides, methadone, paroxetine, pentamidine, pimozide, protease inhibitors, quetiapine, quinidine, risperidone, simvastatin, some phenothiazines, sotalol, thioridazine, tricyclics, troleandomycinverapamil, ziprasidone

*Pregnancy categories have been revised. See http://www.fda.gov/Drugs/DevelopmentApprovalProcess/DevelopmentResources/Labeling/ucm093307.htm for more information.

Adverse/Side Effects

- Dizziness
- Dyspnea
- Headache
- Orthostatic hypotension
- Palpitations
- Peripheral edema
- QT prolongation

Nursing Care

- Assess cardiac status, angina, QT prolongation
- Teach patient to comply with medical regimen
- Teach patient not to chew or crush medication, and avoid grapefruit juice; may be taken without regard to meals
- Teach patient to avoid hazardous activities until dizziness no longer occurs
- Teach patient to avoid over the counter drugs and drugs prolonging QTc, unless directed by prescriber
- Teach patient to notify all health care providers of use of ranolazine
- Teach patient to notify prescriber of palpitations, dizziness, fainting, edema, dyspnea

ANSWER KEY: REVIEW QUESTIONS

1. **2 Temperature may increase within the first 24 hours as a result of the inflammatory response to tissue destruction and persist as long as a week.**

   1 Diaphoresis is caused by activation of the sympathetic, not parasympathetic, nervous system and may indicate cardiogenic shock. **3** Pain is persistent and constant, not intermittent; it is caused by oxygen deprivation and the release of lactic acid. **4** The blood pressure increases initially but then drops because there is a decrease in cardiac output.

   Client Need: Physiologic Adaptation; **Cognitive Level:** Comprehension; **Nursing Process:** Assessment/Analysis

2. **4 Cholesterol is a sterol found in tissue; it is attributed in part to diets high in saturated fats.**

   1 Only animal foods furnish dietary cholesterol. **2** Exercise, not cholesterol, increases HDL levels and helps decrease the risk of heart disease. **3** Cholesterol is also produced by the body and is needed for the synthesis of bile salts, adrenocortical and steroid sex hormones, and provitamin D.

   Client Need: Health Promotion and Maintenance; **Cognitive Level:** Comprehension; **Integrated Process:** Teaching/Learning; **Nursing Process:** Planning/Implementation

3. **1 Although oatmeal is a soluble fiber, whole milk is high in saturated fat and should be avoided.**

   2 Olive oil contains unsaturated fat. **3** Most fish have a low fat content; fruit does not contain fat. **4** Soluble fiber helps to lower cholesterol; skim milk does not contain fat.

   Client Need: Basic Care and Comfort; **Cognitive Level:** Analysis; **Integrated Process:** Teaching/Learning; **Nursing Process:** Evaluation/Outcomes

4. **Answers: 2, 3, 4, 6**

   2 Chicken broth is high in sodium and should be avoided to prevent fluid retention and an elevated blood pressure. **3** Enriched whole milk is high in saturated fats and contributes to hyperlipidemia; skim milk is the healthier choice. **4** Red meats, such as beef, are high in saturated fats and should be avoided. **6** Liver and other glandular organ meats are high in cholesterol and should be avoided.

   1 Olive oil is an unsaturated fat, which is a healthy choice. **5** Vegetables and whole grains are low in fat and have soluble fiber, which may reduce the risk for heart disease.

   Client Need: Basic Care and Comfort; **Cognitive Level:** Analysis; Integrated Process: Teaching/Learning; **Nursing Process:** Evaluation/Outcomes

5. **2 Ischemia causes tissue injury and the release of chemicals, such as bradykinin, that stimulate sensory nerves and produce pain.**

   1 Arterial spasm, resulting in tissue hypoxia and pain, is associated with angina pectoris. **3** Arteries, not veins, are involved in the pathology of a myocardial infarction. **4** Tissue injury and pain occur in the myocardium.

   Client Need: Physiologic Adaptation; **Cognitive Level:** Comprehension; **Nursing Process:** Assessment/Analysis

6. **1 Myocardial infarction (MI) may cause increased irritability of tissue or interruption of normal transmission of impulses. Dysrhythmias occur in about 90% of clients after an MI.**

   2 Hypokalemia may result when clients are taking cardiac glycosides and diuretics; this is a complication associated with therapy, not a pathologic entity related to the MI itself. **3** Anaphylactic shock is caused by an allergic reaction, not by an MI. **4** Cardiac enlargement is a slow process, so it will not be evident in the coronary care unit.

   Client Need: Physiologic Adaptation; **Cognitive Level:** Analysis; **Nursing Process:** Assessment/Analysis

7. **4 Bundle branch block interferes with the conduction of impulses from the AV node to the ventricle supplied by the affected bundle. Conduction through the ventricles is delayed, as evidenced by a widened QRS complex.**

   1, 3 Changes in the T waves and/or sagging ST segments usually occur as a result of cardiac damage. **2** P waves, produced when the SA node fires to begin a cycle, are present in bundle branch block.

   Client Need: Physiologic Adaptation; **Cognitive Level:** Analysis; **Nursing Process:** Assessment/Analysis

8. **2 Not adhering to the treatment regimen may interfere with effective resolution of the MI, and further intervention is necessary.**

   1, 3, 4 The statements "I want to stay as pain-free as possible," "I should not have any problems in reducing my salt intake," and "I wrote down my medication information for future reference," are appropriate responses related to teaching concerning self-care after an MI.

   Client Need: Health Promotion and Maintenance; **Cognitive Level:** Analysis; **Integrated Process:** Teaching/Learning; **Nursing Process:** Evaluation/Outcomes

9. **4 Troponin T (cTnT) has an extraordinarily high specificity for myocardial cell injury. Cardiac troponins elevate sooner and remain elevated longer than many of the other enzymes that reflect myocardial injury.**

   1 ALT (alanine aminotransferase) is found predominantly in the liver; it is found in lesser quantities in the kidneys, heart, and skeletal muscles; it is used primarily to diagnose and monitor liver, not heart, disease. **2** AST (serum aspartate aminotransferase), also known as SGOT (serum glutamic-oxaloacetic transaminase), is elevated 8 hours after a myocardial infarction. **3** Total LDH (lactate dehydrogenase) levels elevate 24 to 48 hours after a myocardial infarction.

   Client Need: Reduction of Risk Potential; **Cognitive Level:** Analysis; **Nursing Process:** Assessment/Analysis

   > **Test-Taking Tip:** Key words or phrases in the stem of the question such as *first, primary, early,* or *best* are important. For this question, other choices may also elevate (such as AST and LDH), but they are not the FIRST ones to elevate.

10. **2 Diabetes is twice as high a predictor of coronary heart disease in women than in men. Diabetes cancels the cardiac protection that estrogen provides premenopausal women.**

    1 Obesity is common to both women and men. **3** An elevated C-reactive protein level, a marker of the inflammatory process, is heart-specific in predicting the likelihood of future coronary events in both women and men. **4** Low, not high, levels of HDL-C, a lipid factor, (less than 35 mg/dL) have a greater bearing on predicting CHD in women than in men.

    Client Need: Health Promotion and Maintenance; **Cognitive Level:** Knowledge; **Integrated Process:** Teaching/Learning; **Nursing Process:** Planning/Implementation

11. **1 Assessment is the first step of the nursing process, and vital signs provide vital information about the client's cardiopulmonary status.**

    2, 4 Although inserting a saline lock and drawing blood for troponins may be done, they are not the priority. **3** Although placing a client on oxygen may be done, it is not the priority. Administration of oxygen may alter the client's baseline vital sign results.

    Client Need: Physiologic Adaptation; **Cognitive Level:** Analysis; **Nursing Process:** Assessment

12. **3** Anginal pain, which can be anticipated during certain activities, may be prevented by dilating the coronary arteries immediately before engaging in the activity.

1 One tablet is generally administered at a time; doubling the dosage may produce severe hypotension and headache. **2** The sublingual form of nitroglycerin is absorbed directly through the mucous membranes and should not be swallowed. **4** When the pain is relieved, rest will generally prevent its recurrence by reducing oxygen consumption of the myocardium.

Client Need: Pharmacologic and Parenteral Therapies; **Cognitive Level:** Application; **Integrated Process:** Teaching/Learning; **Nursing Process:** Planning/Implementation

13. **2** Nitroglycerin tablets are affected by light, heat, and moisture. Loss of potency can occur after 3 months, reducing the drug's effectiveness in relieving pain. A new supply should be obtained routinely.

1 Sublingual tingling indicates the tablets have retained their potency. **3, 4** Unrelieved pain/increased facial flushing and delayed onset of relief with the same duration of relief do not necessarily indicate loss of potency.

Client Need: Pharmacologic and Parenteral Therapies; **Cognitive Level:** Application; **Integrated Process:** Teaching/Learning; **Nursing Process:** Planning/Implementation

14. **3** Nitroglycerin is sensitive to light and moisture, so it must be stored in a dark, airtight container.

1 Nitroglycerin usually is taken prn. If more than three tablets are necessary in a 15-minute period, emergency medical attention should be received. **2** Headache may be an expected side effect, and the medication should not be discontinued. **4** Dizziness indicates the dosage may need to be decreased by the health care provider.

Client Need: Pharmacologic and Parenteral Therapies; **Cognitive Level:** Application; **Integrated Process:** Teaching/Learning; **Nursing Process:** Planning/Implementation

15. **1** Beta blockers reduce cardiac output, so they are contraindicated for clients with uncontrolled heart failure.

2 Beta blockers are used to treat hypertension because they cause vasodilation and decrease cardiac contractility. **3** Beta blockers lower heart rate. **4** Beta blockers are used to treat coronary artery disease because they decrease myocardial oxygen demand by reducing peripheral resistance and cardiac contractility.

Client Need: Management of Care; **Cognitive Level:** Analysis; **Integrated Process:** Communication/Documentation; **Nursing Process:** Planning/Implementation

16. **2** Beta blockers (BBs) should not be taken at night because the blood pressure usually decreases when sleeping. This medication blocks beta-adrenergic receptors in the heart, which ultimately lowers the blood pressure. Therefore the drug should be taken early in the morning to maximize its therapeutic effect.

1 Orthostatic hypotension is a side effect of BBs, and the client should change positions slowly to prevent dizziness and falls. **3** Drowsiness is a side effect of BBs, and the client should be taught precautions to prevent injury. **4** The pulse rate should be taken before administration because ventricular dysrhythmias and heart block may occur with BBs.

Client Need: Pharmacologic and Parenteral Therapies; **Cognitive Level:** Application; **Integrated Process:** Teaching/Learning; **Nursing Process:** Evaluation/Outcomes

17. **Answer: 3 tablets.**

Use the "Desire over Have" formula of ratio and proportion to solve the problem.

$$\frac{\text{Desire}}{\text{Have}} \frac{150 \text{ mg}}{50 \text{ mg}} = \frac{\text{x tablets}}{1 \text{ tablet}}$$

$$50x = 150$$

$$x = 3 \text{ tablets}$$

Client Need: Pharmacologic and Parenteral Therapies; **Cognitive Level:** Application; **Nursing Process:** Planning/Implementation

18. **3** Metoprolol is a beta blocker; it decreases the heart rate and thus is contraindicated with bradycardia.

1 Metoprolol is an antihypertensive agent. **2, 4** By reducing cardiac output, metoprolol reduces myocardial oxygen consumption, which helps prevent ischemia and anginal pain.

Client Need: Management of Care; **Cognitive Level:** Analysis; **Integrated Process:** Communication/Documentation; **Nursing Process:** Planning/Implementation

19. **Answers: 2, 3, 5**

2 Changing positions slowly helps reduce orthostatic hypotension. **3** Peripheral edema may occur as a result of heart failure and must be reported. **5** Grapefruit juice affects the metabolism of calcium channel blockers and should be avoided.

1 Reducing calcium intake is unnecessary because calcium levels are not affected. **4** Hair loss does not occur.

Client Need: Pharmacologic and Parenteral Therapies; **Cognitive Level:** Analysis; **Integrated Process:** Teaching/Learning; **Nursing Process:** Planning/Implementation

20. **2 Changing positions slowly will help prevent the side effect of orthostatic hypotension.**

1 Diltiazem can relax the esophagus and lead to acid reflux; lying down after meals may intensify this effect. **3, 4** It is not necessary to avoid dairy products or take the drug with an antacid.

Client Need: Pharmacologic and Parenteral Therapies; **Cognitive Level:** Application; **Integrated Process:** Teaching/Learning; **Nursing Process:** Planning/Implementation

---

Study Tip: To recall that orthostatic hypotension occurs when changing positions suddenly, remember that to *test for* orthostatic hypotension, you check the patient's blood pressure with him/her lying down, sitting, and standing. It is the change in position that causes the change in blood pressure.

Antihyperlipidemic and Antidysrhythmic Drugs

INTRODUCTION TO ANTIHYPERLIPIDEMIC AND ANTIDYSRHYTHMIC DRUGS

Overview of Hyperlipidemia

- Lipids: cholesterol, triglycerides, phospholipids
- The old way of treating hyperlipidemia was to recommend target cholesterol levels for the four categories of lipoproteins
  - High density lipoprotein (HDL)
    - "Good" lipoprotein
    - Removes cholesterol from bloodstream and delivers it to liver for excretion in the bile
  - Low density lipoprotein (LDL)
    - "Bad" lipoprotein
    - Elevated levels put patient at risk for atherosclerosis and heart disease
  - Very low density lipoprotein (VLDL)
    - Carries mostly triglycerides
  - Chylomicrons
    - Transport fatty acids and cholesterol to the liver
    - Composed mostly of triglycerides
- Hyperlipidemia: excess of one or more lipids in the blood; increased total cholesterol; increased ratio of LDL to HDL
- Today's guidelines define four groups of patients for primary and secondary prevention of hyperlipidemia
  - For each group, there is a recommended intensity level for statin therapy
  - Statin therapy is now considered the first-line treatment for lowering cholesterol levels
  - Other cholesterol-lowering agents (fibrates, bile acid sequestrants, and niacin) are reserved for patients who are statin intolerant or for when statins fail to reach the desired outcome
- Patient groupings for hyperlipidemia prevention with statins include
  - Atherosclerotic cardiovascular disease
    - Target reduction of LDL: greater than or equal to 50%
    - Recommended statin therapy: high intensity
  - LDL cholesterol greater than or equal to 190 mg/dL
    - Target reduction of LDL: greater than or equal to 50%
    - Recommended statin therapy: high intensity
  - Age 40–75, diabetes, LDL cholesterol 70–189 mg/dL
    - Target reduction by 30%–49%
    - Recommended statin therapy: moderate intensity
  - No atherosclerotic cardiovascular disease or diabetes, 10-year risk for cardiovascular disease greater than or equal to 7.5%, LDL cholesterol 70–189 mg/dL
    - Target reduction by 30%–50%
    - Recommended statin therapy: moderate to high intensity
- Increased cholesterol, triglycerides, LDLs put patient at risk for CAD
- Causes: diet high in saturated fat and cholesterol; disorders such as diabetes mellitus, kidney disease, hypothyroidism

- Clinical findings: increased homocysteine levels; increased high-sensitivity C-reactive protein (hsCRP) levels
- Treatment: try nonpharmacologic methods before medications
  - Low fat diet: total fat intake 25%–35% of caloric intake; calories from saturated fat should be less than 7%
  - Replacing trans fats with polyunsaturated fats is most important way to improve blood lipid profiles
  - Exercise
    - When exercise is combined with a low-saturated-fat diet, LDL cholesterol levels can decrease by 7%–15% and triglycerides by 4%–18%. HDL cholesterol levels can increase 5%–18%
  - Smoking cessation
  - Decreased alcohol consumption

Antihyperlipidemic Drugs

- Drugs that lower blood lipid levels are called antihyperlipidemics, antilipidemics, antilipemics, hypolipidemics
- Improve lipid profile by reducing cholesterol or triglyceride synthesis and/or increasing high-density lipoprotein (HDL) level
- Used to attain recommended goals for low-density lipoprotein (LDL) levels established by the National Cholesterol Education Program's (NCEP) Adult Treatment Panel
  - Patients with coronary heart disease: less than 100 mg/dL with optional lower goal of less than 70 mg/dL
  - Patients with two or more risk factors: less than 130 mg/dL with optional lower goal of less than 100 mg/dL
  - Patients with zero to one risk factor: less than 160 mg/dL
- Antilipemic drugs are classified as bile acid sequestrants, 3-hydroxy-3-methylglutaryl coenzyme A (HMG-CoA) reductase inhibitors, fibric acid derivatives, nicotinic acids, cholesterol absorption inhibitors, miscellaneous agents
- HMG-CoA reductase inhibitors are also known as statins
- Statins decrease serum cholesterol, LDL, VLDL, triglycerides; elevate HDLs
- Bile acid sequestrants may be combined with statins to increase lipid-lowering effects
- Statins may be combined with other drugs to decrease blood pressure, blood clotting
- Antihyperlipidemic therapy is lifelong; stopping these drugs will result in increased cholesterol, LDL levels
- Abruptly stopping statins can result in death from acute myocardial infarction (AMI)

Overview of Dysrhythmia

- Normal cardiac rhythm: conduction from SA node through atria causes atrial contraction and gives rise to the P wave; conduction from AV node down bundle of His and bundle branches to Purkinje's fibers, which extend to lateral walls of the ventricles, causes ventricular contraction, which gives rise to the QRS wave; ventricular repolarization is associated with the T wave; late ventricular repolarization is associated with the U wave
- Normal sinus rhythm (NSR): ventricular and atrial rate of 60 to 100 beats/min; regular rhythm; a P wave (representing atrial depolarization) precedes each QRS complex (representing ventricular depolarization); PR interval (representing conduction of an impulse from the SA node through the AV node) is 0.12 to 0.20 seconds; T wave after each QRS complex (representing repolarization of the ventricles)

- Sinus bradycardia: same as NSR, but rate less than 60; atropine may be administered if symptomatic
- Sinus tachycardia: same as NSR, but with rate greater than 100; beta blockers, calcium channel blockers may be administered and catheter ablation may be performed if severe
- Premature atrial complexes or beats
  - An ectopic focus fires an impulse before the next sinus impulse is due; a pause follows the premature atrial complex; may cause palpitations; atrial irritability often caused by stress, fatigue, caffeine, nicotine, alcohol
- Treatment includes elimination of causative agent, antidysrhythmics
- Atrial fibrillation and flutter
  - Results from rapid firing of atrial ectopic foci; not all impulses conducted to ventricles
    - Fibrillation: atrial rate of 300 to 600/min; ECG shows no P waves, rather irregular forms; pulse deficit is common; danger from blood pooling in quivering atria leads to emboli formation (Fig. 10.1).
    - Flutter: atrial rate of 250 to 400/min, P waves on ECG have saw-tooth appearance
  - Administer prescribed medications: antidysrhythmics; anticoagulant until rhythm is controlled to reduce risk of brain attack (cerebral vascular accident [CVA]) caused by atrial thrombi; prepare for cardioversion; catheter ablation if dysrhythmia is prolonged
    - Monitor vital signs, oxygen saturation, and potassium levels
- First-degree atrioventricular (AV) block: conduction of impulse from atria is slowed; PR interval on ECG is consistent, but greater than 0.20 seconds
- Second-degree AV block type I (Wenckebach): repeating pattern in which conduction of atrial impulse is progressively prolonged until it is completely blocked; ECG shows increasingly long PR interval until a QRS complex does not follow a P wave
- Second-degree AV block type II: conduction of atrial impulses is intermittently blocked every second, third, fourth beat, etc.; P waves may precede each QRS complex
- Third-degree atrioventricular block (complete heart block)
  - No electric communication between atria and ventricles and each beat independently; does not provide long-term adequate circulation; syncope, heart failure, or cardiac arrest may ensue
  - Document dysrhythmia and notify health care provider; administer medications per protocol; prepare for pacemaker insertion (see Implantable Cardiac Devices under Related Procedures)
- Premature ventricular complexes or beats
  - Originate in ventricles and occur before next expected sinus beat; can be life-threatening when they occur close to a T wave because cardiac repolarization is disrupted and ventricular fibrillation may ensue
  - Administer medications per protocol; document dysrhythmia and notify health care provider; institute antidysrhythmics as prescribed; monitor vital signs, oxygen saturation, and potassium levels

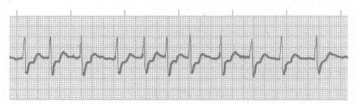

FIG. 10.1   Atrial fibrillation. (From Monahan, F.D., Sands, J., Neighbors, M., Marek, J., Green-Nigro, C. [2007]. *Phipps' medical-surgical nursing: Health and illness perspectives* [8th ed.]. St. Louis: Mosby.)

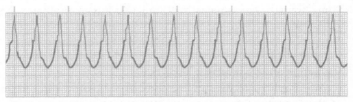

FIG. 10.2   Ventricular tachycardia. (From Monahan, F.D., Sands, J., Neighbors, M., Marek, J., Green-Nigro, C. [2007]. *Phipps' medical-surgical nursing: Health and illness perspectives* [8th ed.]. St. Louis: Mosby.)

- Ventricular tachycardia (Fig. 10.2)
  - Series of three or more bizarre premature ventricular complexes that occur in a regular rhythm; results in decreased cardiac output and may rapidly convert to ventricular fibrillation
  - Administer medications per protocol (e.g., amiodarone [Cordarone]); perform cardioversion if medications fail; be prepared to perform defibrillation and cardiopulmonary resuscitation; document dysrhythmia and notify health care provider; prepare for possible implantable cardioverter defibrillator (ICD) insertion; monitor vital signs, provide oxygen
- Ventricular fibrillation
  - Repetitive rapid stimulation from ectopic ventricular foci to which ventricles are unable to respond; ventricular contraction is replaced by uncoordinated twitching; circulation ceases and death ensues without treatment; death may be prevented by cardiopulmonary resuscitation (CPR) and defibrillation
  - Defibrillate immediately; inject medications per protocol; institute CPR; document dysrhythmia and notify health care provider; monitor oxygen saturation, and potassium levels
- Cardiac standstill (asystole)
  - No cardiac activity (flat line on ECG tracing); terminates in death unless intervention is immediate
  - Institute CPR; document dysrhythmia and notify health care provider; cardiac stimulants may be given via IV or intracardiac route; pacemaker insertion may be indicated (see Implantable Cardiac Devices under Related Procedures)

Antidysrhythmic Drugs

- Treat abnormal variations in cardiac rate and rhythm; also prevent dysrhythmias
- Class IA antidysrhythmics suppress ectopic foci by increasing refractory period and slowing depolarization; Class IA antidysrhytmic drugs are also known as sodium channel blockers
- Class IB antidysrhythmics suppress ventricular dysrhythmias by decreasing automaticity and increasing ventricular electrical stimulation threshold
- Class IC antidysrhythmics slow conduction and increase ventricular refractoriness
- Class II antidysrhythmics decrease heart rate, contractility, and automaticity by blocking beta-adrenergic receptor sites from catecholamines; decrease myocardial workload and oxygen requirements; indicated for tachydysrhythmias, hypertension, angina
- Class III antidysrhythmics prolong repolarization
- Class IV antidysrhythmics block calcium influx into muscle cells during depolarization; control atrial dysrhythmias by decreasing cardiac automaticity and impulse conduction; reduce peripheral vascular resistance in treatment of hypertension

Bile Acid Sequestrants

- Used to lower high blood levels of lipids
- Examples include cholestyramine, colesevelam, colestipol
- Available in PO preparations

Mode of Action

- Combine with bile acids in the intestine to decrease blood cholesterol levels

Contraindications, Precautions, and Drug Interactions of Bile Acid Sequestrants*

Drug	Contraindications/Precautions	Drug Interaction
cholestyramine	**Contraindications:** Hypersensitivity; hyperlipidemia III, IV, V; complete biliary obstruction **Precautions:** Breastfeeding, children, renal disease, PKU, coagulopathy **Pregnancy:** Only given after risks to the fetus are considered; animal studies have shown adverse reactions; no human studies available	Warfarin, thiazides, vitamins A/D/E/K, glipizide, corticosteroids, cardiac glycosides, propranolol, thyroid hormones, iron, penicillin G, tertracyclines, acetaminophen, amiodarone, vancomycin, clofibrate, gemfibrozil
colesevelam	**Contraindications:** Hypersensitivity, biliary obstruction, biliary cirrhosis, hypertriglycerides, bowel disease/obstruction, pancreatitis, dysphagia, fat-soluble vitamin deficiency **Precautions:** Breastfeeding, children **Pregnancy:** No adverse effects in animals; no human studies available	Oral contraceptives, warfarin, glyburide, fluoroquinolones, diltiazem, phenytoin, thiazides, tetracyclines, iron, corticosteroids, gemfibrozil, mycophenolate, propranolol, digoxin, penicillin G, thyroid hormones, fat-soluble vitamins
colestipol	**Contraindications:** Hypersensitivity, bowel disease/obstruction, fat-soluble vitamin deficiency **Precautions:** Breastfeeding, children, renal diseasea **Pregnancy:** No adverse effects in animals; no human studies available	Fat-soluble vitamins, digoxin, corticosteroids, propranolol, tetracycline, furosemide, gemfibrozil, penicillin G, hydrochlorothiazide

*Pregnancy categories have been revised. See http://www.fda.gov/Drugs/DevelopmentApprovalProcess/DevelopmentResources/Labeling/ucm093307.htm for more information.

Adverse/Side Effects

- Headache
- Dizziness
- Anxiety
- Vertigo
- Drowsiness
- Tinnitus
- Nausea
- Vomiting
- Constipation
- Abdominal pain
- Hemorrhoids
- Fecal impaction
- Flatulence
- Steatorrhea
- Peptic ulcer
- Bleeding
- GI obstruction
- Increased prothombin time
- Hyperchloremic acidosis
- Hypertrigylcerides
- Hypoglycemia
- Joint/muscle pain
- Rash

Nursing Care

- Administer with food
- Mix powder forms of medication with 120 to 180 mL liquid
- Monitor blood lipid levels
- Monitor for signs of vitamin A/D/E/K deficiency
- Monitor for bleeding
- Monitor electrolyte balance
- Ensure PKU patients avoid products with phenylalanine
- Manage constipation with stool softeners
- Teach patient to report signs and symptoms of bleeding
- Teach patient to avoid tobacco products, alcohol, high fat foods
- Encourage patients to exercise

APPLICATION AND REVIEW

1. Which instructions should the nurse include in the teaching plan for a client with hyperlipidemia who is being discharged with a prescription for cholestyramine (Questran)?
   1. "Increase your intake of fiber and fluid."
   2. "Take the medication before you go to bed."
   3. "Check your pulse before taking the medication."
   4. "Contact your health care provider if your skin or sclera turn yellow."

2. Which class of antidysrhythmics increase the heart's refractory period thus slowing depolarization?
   1. Class 1A
   2. Class 1B
   3. Class 1C
   4. Class III

3. Which action is the Class IV antidysrhythmics capable of producing? **Select all that apply.**
   1. Blocks calcium influx into muscle cells
   2. Reduces peripheral vascular resistance
   3. Decreases blood cholesterol levels
   4. Decreases cardiac automaticity
   5. Controls atrial dysrhythmias

4. Which instructions should the nurse provide to a client prescribed a bile acid sequestrant to lower blood cholesterol levels? **Select all that apply.**
   1. Avoid alcohol
   2. Avoid tobacco products
   3. Take the medication with food
   4. Diarrhea is a common side effect
   5. Be aware that bleeding may be difficult to control

5. Which client statement demonstrates an understanding of the safe compliance when on Class II antidysrhythmic therapy? **Select all that apply.**
   1. "I take my medication on an empty stomach."
   2. "I know what the signs of cardiac distress are."
   3. "I can take over-the-counter medication for a cold."
   4. "I understand that alcohol in any amount is bad for me."
   5. "I should always have enough medication available when I travel."

See Answers on pages 196-197.

HMG-CoA Reductase Inhibitors

- Used to lower high blood levels of lipids
- Examples include atorvastatin, fluvastatin, lovastatin, pitavastatin, pravastatin, rosuvastatin, simvastatin
- Available in PO preparations

Mode of Action

- Inhibits MHG-CoA reductase enzyme in the liver, thus interfering with cholesterol synthesis

Contraindications, Precautions, and Drug Interactions of HMG-CoA Reductase Inhibitors*

Drug	Contraindications/Precautions	Drug Interaction
atorvastatin	*Contraindications:* Hypersensitivity, breastfeeding, pregnancy hepatic disease *Precautions:* Alcoholism, severe infections, hepatic/metabolic disease, trauma, electrolyte imbalance *Pregnancy:* Absolute fetal abnormalities; not to be used at any time during pregnancy	Cyclosporine, erythromycin, azole antifungals, niacin, gemfibrozil, clofibrate, digoxin, oral contraceptives, CYP3A4 inhibitors, warfarin, colestipol

Contraindications, Precautions, and Drug Interactions of HMG-CoA Reductase Inhibitors—cont'd

Drug	Contraindications/Precautions	Drug Interaction
fluvastatin	**Contraindications:** Hypersensitivity, breastfeeding, pregnancy, hepatic disease **Precautions:** Alcoholism, severe infections, hypotension, metabolic disease, uncontrolled seizures, trauma, electrolyte imbalance, myopathy, rhabdomyolysis **Pregnancy:** Absolute fetal abnormalities; not to be used at any time during pregnancy	Warfarin, digoxin, phenytoin, cyclosporine, protease inhibitors, niacin, colchicine, erythromycin, fibric acid derivatives, fluconazole, ketoconazole, itraconazole, alcohol, cimetidine, ranitidine, rifampin, omeprazole, cholestyramine, colestipol
lovastatin	**Contraindications:** Hypersensitivity, breastfeeding, pregnancy, hepatic disease **Precautions:** Children, hepatic disease, severe infection, alcoholism, hypotension, uncontrolled seizures, metabolic disease, trauma, electrolyte imbalance, visual disorders **Pregnancy:** Absolute fetal abnormalities; not to be used at any time during pregnancy	Warfarin, diltiazem, bosentan, bile acid sequestrants, exonatide, azole antifungals, verapamil, erythromycin, cyclosporine, clofibrate, clarithromycin, cyclosporine, protease inhibitors, telithromycin, gemfibrozil, niacin, danazol, quinupristin-dalfopristin
pitavastatin	**Contraindications:** Hypersensitivity, breastfeeding, pregnancy, hepatic disease, cholestasis **Precautions:** Females, hepatic/renal disease, severe infection, alcoholism, hypotension, seizures, metabolic disease, endocrine disease, trauma, surgery, organ transplant, electrolyte imbalance **Pregnancy:** Absolute fetal abnormalities; not to be used at any time during pregnancy	Erythromycin, cyclosporine, azole antifungals, niacin, gemfibrozil, clofibrate
pravastatin	**Contraindications:** Hypersensitivity, breastfeeding, pregnancy, hepatic disease **Precautions:** Hepatic/renal disease, severe infection, alcoholism, metabolic disease, trauma, electrolyte imbalance **Pregnancy:** Absolute fetal abnormalities; not to be used at any time during pregnancy	Erythromycin, cyclosporine, niacin, gemfibrozil, clofibrate, clarithromycin, itraconazole, protease inhibitors
rosuvastatin	**Contraindications:** Hypersensitivity, breastfeeding, pregnancy, hepatic disease **Precautions:** Children, geriatric patients, Asian patients, hepatic/renal disease, severe infection, alcoholism, metabolic disease, trauma, electrolyte imbalance, hypotension, hypothyroidism **Pregnancy:** Absolute fetal abnormalities; not to be used at any time during pregnancy	Alcohol, warfarin, cyclosporine, clofibrate, gemfibrozil, azole antifungals, fibric acid derivatives, antiretroviral protease inhibitors
simvastatin	**Contraindications:** Hypersensitivity, breastfeeding, pregnancy, hepatic disease **Precautions:** Hepatic disease, severe infection, alcoholism, metabolic disease, trauma, electrolyte imbalance, Chinese patients **Pregnancy:** Absolute fetal abnormalities; not to be used at any time during pregnancy	Gemfibrozil, digoxin, warfarin, CYP3A4 inhibitors, niacin, erythromycin, clarithromycin, clofibrate, ketoconazole, itraconazole, macrolide antibiotics, protease inhibitors, danazol, delavirdine, verapamil, nefazodone, diltiazem, azole antifungals, amiodarone, telithromycin, voriconazole, ATP1B1 inhibitors

*Pregnancy categories have been revised. See http://www.fda.gov/Drugs/DevelopmentApprovalProcess/DevelopmentResources/Labeling/ucm093307.htm for more information.

Adverse/Side Effects

- Headache
- Dizziness
- Confusion
- Insomnia
- Asthenia
- Vision changes
- Pharyngitis
- Sinusitis
- Nausea
- Constipation
- Diarrhea
- Abdominal cramps
- Heartburn
- Dyspepsia
- Flatulence
- Pancreatitis
- Hepatic dysfunction
- Thrombocytopenia
- Leukopenia
- Hemolytic anemia
- Impotence
- Gynecomastia (child)
- Rhabdomyolysis
- Arthralgia
- Myalgia
- Myositis
- Rash
- Pruritus
- Alopecia
- Photosensitivity

Nursing Care

- Administer before meals and in the evening or at bedtime
- Monitor blood lipid levels
- Monitor renal/hepatic function
- Monitor for muscle pain, tenderness
- Manage constipation with stool softeners
- Teach patient to avoid drugs if pregnant or breastfeeding
- Teach patient to wear sunscreen, protective clothing, and sunglasses while outdoors
- Teach patient to avoid tobacco products, alcohol, high fat foods
- Encourage patient to exercise

Fibric Acid Derivatives

- Used to reduce high triglyceride and mildly lower LDL levels; slightly improve HDL
- Examples include fenofibrate, gemfibrozil
- Available in PO preparations

Mode of Action

- Decrease synthesis of cholesterol, lipoproteins, triglycerides in the liver and then speeds up removal of triglycerides in the blood

Contraindications, Precautions, and Drug Interactions of Fibric Acid Inhibitors*

Drug	Contraindications/Precautions	Drug Interaction
fenofibrate	**Contraindications:** Hypersensitivity, breastfeeding, renal/hepatic disease, gallbladder disease, biliary cirrhosis **Precautions:** Geriatric patients, renal/hepatic disease, diabetes mellitus, peptic ulcer, pancreatitis **Pregnancy:** Only given after risks to the fetus are considered; animal studies have shown adverse reactions; no human studies available	Cyclosporine, colchicine, HMG-CoA reductase inhibitors, oral anticoagulants, antidiabetics, bile acid sequestrants
gemfibrozil	**Contraindications:** Hypersensitivity, breastfeeding, renal/hepatic disease, gallbladder disease, biliary cirrhosis **Precautions:** Breastfeeding, renal disease, cholelithiasis **Pregnancy:** Only given after risks to the fetus are considered; animal studies have shown adverse reactions; no human studies available	Repaglinide, simvastatin, sulfonylureas, warfarin, HMG-CoA reductase inhibitors, bile acid sequestrants

*Pregnancy categories have been revised. See http://www.fda.gov/Drugs/DevelopmentApprovalProcess/DevelopmentResources/Labeling/ucm093307.htm for more information.

Adverse/Side Effects

- Dizziness
- Drowsiness
- Insomnia
- Fatigue
- Weakness
- Depression
- Vertigo
- Paresthesia
- Bronchitis
- Cough
- Taste changes
- Pharyngitis
- Angioedema
- Angina
- Hypo/hypertension
- Flulike syndrome
- Infection
- Nausea
- Vomiting
- Dyspepsia
- Flatulence
- Gastritis
- Increased liver enzymes
- Hepatomegaly
- Pancreatitis
- Cholelithiasis
- Dysuria
- Urinary frequency
- Thrombolysis
- Pulmonary embolism
- Anemia
- Leukopenia
- Polyphagia
- Weight gain
- Myalgia
- Arthralgia
- Myopathy
- Rhabdomyolysis
- Exfoliative dermatitis
- Rash
- Urticaria
- Pruritus
- Photosensitivity

Nursing Care

- Administer medication at prescribed times
- Administer fenofibrate with meals
- Administer gemfibrozil 30 minutes before breakfast and dinner
- Monitor blood lipid levels
- Monitor renal/hepatic function
- Monitor for muscle pain/tenderness
- Teach patient to report GU signs and symptoms: decreased libido, impotence, dysuria, proteinuria, oliguria, hematuria
- Teach patient not to skip or double dose
- Teach patient to avoid tobacco products, alcohol, high fat foods
- Encourage patient to exercise
- Teach patient to report signs and symptoms of flu
- Teach patient to avoid driving and other hazardous activities

Nicotinic Acids

- Used to lower triglyceride levels
- Example includes niacin
- Available in PO preparations

Mode of Action

- Reduces production of triglycerides and VLDL in the liver

Contraindications, Precautions, and Drug Interactions of Nicotinic Acids*

Drug	Contraindications/Precautions	Drug Interaction
niacin	*Contraindications:* Hypersensitivity, breastfeeding, renal/hepatic disease, severe hypotension, hemorrhage *Precautions:* Children, hepatic disease, CAD, angina, gout, peptic ulcer, pancreatitis, glaucoma, diabetes mellitus, hemophilia, alcoholism, myasthenia gravis *Pregnancy:* Only given after risks to the fetus are considered; animal studies have shown adverse reactions; no human studies available	Colestipol, cholestyramine, alcohol

*Pregnancy categories have been revised. See http://www.fda.gov/Drugs/DevelopmentApprovalProcess/DevelopmentResources/Labeling/ucm093307.htm for more information.

Adverse/Side Effects

- Dizziness
- Headache
- Flushing
- GI upset
- Postural hypotension
- Diarrhea
- Pruritus

Nursing Care

- Administer with meals to prevent GI distress
- Administer with aspirin to decrease flushing
- Do not administer with alcohol, hot beverages, hot/spicy foods
- Do not crush or chew tablets
- Monitor hepatic/renal function
- Monitor blood lipid levels
- Teach patient that warmth and flushing is normal effect of drug
- Teach patient that a hot shower and/or exercise can exacerbate flushing
- Teach patient to change positions slowly
- Teach patient to avoid tobacco products, alcohol, high fat foods
- Encourage patient to exercise

Cholesterol Absorption Inhibitors

- Used to lower cholesterol levels
- Example includes ezetimibe
- Available in PO preparations

Mode of Action

- Reduces absorption of cholesterol by the small intestine

Contraindications, Precautions, and Drug Interactions of Cholesterol Absorption Inhibitors*

Drug	Contraindications/Precautions	Drug Interaction
ezetimibe	*Contraindications:* Hypersensitivity, severe hepatic disease *Precautions:* Breastfeeding, children, hepatic disease *Pregnancy:* Only given after risks to the fetus are considered; animal studies have shown adverse reactions; no human studies available	HMG-CoA reductase inhibitors, fibric acid derivatives, cyclosporine, antacids, bile acid sequestrants

*Pregnancy categories have been revised. See http://www.fda.gov/Drugs/DevelopmentApprovalProcess/DevelopmentResources/Labeling/ucm093307.htm for more information.

Adverse/Side Effects
- Angioedema
- Angina
- Pharyngitis
- Nasopharyngitis
- Sinusitis
- Cough
- Upper respiratory infection
- Diarrhea
- Abdominal pain
- Myalgias
- Arthralgias
- Back pain
- Rhabdomyolysis

Nursing Care
- Monitor blood lipid levels
- Monitor for muscle pain/tenderness
- Teach patient to avoid tobacco products, alcohol, high fat foods
- Encourage patient to exercise

Miscellaneous Antihyperlipidemic Agents
- Used to lower cholesterol and triglyceride levels
- Examples include icosapent, mipomersen, alirocumab, evolocumab
- Available in PO, SUBCUT preparations

Mode of Action
- Inhibit cholesterol and triglyceride synthesis in the liver

Contraindications, Precautions, and Drug Interactions of Miscellaneous Antihyperlipidemic Agents*

Drug	Contraindications/Precautions	Drug Interaction
icosapent	*Contraindications:* Hypersensitivity *Precautions:* Breastfeeding, children, hepatic disease, bleeding, thrombolytic/anticoagulation therapy, fish/shellfish hypersensitivity *Pregnancy:* Only given after risks to the fetus are considered; animal studies have shown adverse reactions; no human studies available	Anticoagulants, thrombolytics, platelet inhibitors
mipomersen	*Contraindications:* Hypersensitivity, hepatic disease *Precautions:* Breastfeeding, geriatric patients, proteinuria, renal disease, dialysis, alcohol ingestion, low density lipoprotein apheresis *Pregnancy:* No adverse effects in animals; no human studies available	Acetaminophen, methotrexate, tamoxifen, tetracycline
alirocumab	*Contraindications:* Hypersensitivity *Precautions:* Breastfeeding, pregnancy *Pregnancy:* No adverse effects in animals; no human studies available	No known drug interactions
evolocumab	*Contraindications:* Hypersensitivity *Precautions:* Breastfeeding, pregnancy, latex sensitivity *Pregnancy:* No adverse effects in animals; no human studies available	No known drug interactions

*Pregnancy categories have been revised. See http://www.fda.gov/Drugs/DevelopmentApprovalProcess/DevelopmentResources/Labeling/ucm093307.htm for more information.

Adverse/Side Effects

- Headache
- Fever
- Confusion
- Memory impairment
- Fatigue
- Pharyngitis
- Sinusitis
- Cough

- Palpitations
- Hypertension
- Angioedema
- Ecchymosis
- Epistaxis
- Vomiting
- Diarrhea
- Abdominal pain

- Edema
- Infection
- Antibody formation
- Proteinuria
- Glomerulonephritis
- Arthralgia
- Myalgia
- Pruritus

Nursing Care

- Do not crush, break, open, dissolve capsules
- Monitor renal/hepatic function
- Monitor blood lipid levels
- Monitor for bleeding
- Monitor for infection
- Teach patient to avoid tobacco products, alcohol, high fat foods
- Encourage patient to exercise

APPLICATION AND REVIEW

6. Which classification of medications focus on affective function of the small intestines?
   1. Nicotinic acids
   2. Fibric acid inhibitors
   3. HMG-CoA reductase inhibitors
   4. Cholesterol absorption inhibitors
7. Which client diagnosis is considered a contraindication for the common HMG-CoA reductase inhibitors?
   1. Alcoholism
   2. Hepatic disease
   3. Uncontrolled seizures
   4. Severe systemic infection
8. Which client statement demonstrates an understanding of the safe administration of an antihyperlipidemic agent?
   1. "I shouldn't crush or dissolve this medication."
   2. "I need to limit my intake of potassium rich foods."
   3. "The medication should be taken each day at bedtime."
   4. "I need to limit my alcohol intake to a couple beers a week."

See Answers on pages 196-197.

Class IA Antidysrhythmic Agents

- Used to treat atrial and ventricular dysrhythmias
- Examples include disopyramide phosphate, procainamide, quinidine sulfate, quinidine gluconate
- Available in PO, IM, IV preparations

Mode of Action

- Block the sodium channels in the cardiac cell membrane during an action potential
- ECG changes: widens QRS complex, prolongs QT interval

Contraindications, Precautions, and Drug Interactions of Class IA Antidysrhythmic Agents*

Drug	Contraindications/Precautions	Drug Interaction
disopyramide phosphate	*Contraindications:* Hypersensitivity, CHF, torsades de pointes, severe heart block, cardiogenic shock, QT prolongation *Precautions:* Breastfeeding, children, hypotension, glaucoma, myasthenia gravis *Pregnancy:* Only given after risks to the fetus are considered; animal studies have shown adverse reactions; no human studies available	Phenytoin, quinidine, CYP3A4 inhibitors, clarithromycin, erythromycin
procainamide	*Contraindications:* Hypersensitivity, severe heart block, torsades de pointes *Precautions:* Breastfeeding, children, renal/hepatic disease, respiratory depression, CHF, digoxin toxicity, dysrhythmia due to digoxin toxicity, cytopenia, myasthenia gravis *Pregnancy:* Only given after risks to the fetus are considered; animal studies have shown adverse reactions; no human studies available	Neuromuscular blockers, cimetidine, quinidine, beta blockers, trimethoprim, ranitidine
quinidine sulfate	*Contraindications:* Hypersensitivity, AV block, digoxin toxicity, myasthenia gravis, blood dyscrasias, idiosyncratic response *Precautions:* Breastfeeding, children, geriatric patients, renal/hepatic disease, CHF, respiratory depression, bradycardia, hypotension, syncope, electrolyte imbalance *Pregnancy:* Only given after risks to the fetus are considered; animal studies have shown adverse reactions; no human studies available	Anticholinergic blockers, phenothiazines, reserpine, other antidysrhythmics, neuromuscular blockers, digoxin, warfarin, propranolol, tricyclics, macrolides, quinolones, procainamide, antipsychotics, cimetidine, sodium bicarbonate, carbonic anhydrase inhibitors, antacids, hydroxide suspensions, amiodarone, verapamil, nifedipine, protease inhibitors, barbiturates, phenytoin, rifampin, sucralfate, cholinergics
quinidine gluconate	*Contraindications:* Hypersensitivity, AV block, digoxin toxicity, myasthenia gravis, blood dyscrasias, idiosyncratic response *Precautions:* Breastfeeding, children, geriatric patients, renal/hepatic disease, CHF, respiratory depression, bradycardia, hypotension, syncope, electrolyte imbalance *Pregnancy:* Only given after risks to the fetus are considered; animal studies have shown adverse reactions; no human studies available	Anticholinergic blockers, phenothiazines, reserpine, other antidysrhythmics, neuromuscular blockers, digoxin, warfarin, propranolol, tricyclics, macrolides, quinolones, procainamide, antipsychotics, cimetidine, sodium bicarbonate, carbonic anhydrase inhibitors, antacids, hydroxide suspensions, amiodarone, verapamil, nifedipine, protease inhibitors, barbiturates, phenytoin, rifampin, sucralfate, cholinergics

*Pregnancy categories have been revised. See http://www.fda.gov/Drugs/DevelopmentApprovalProcess/DevelopmentResources/Labeling/ucm093307.htm for more information.

Adverse/Side Effects

- Headache
- Dizziness
- Confusion
- Psychosis
- Depression
- Restlessness
- Irritability
- Weakness
- Flushing
- Respiratory depression
- Hypotension
- Heart block
- Cardiac arrest
- Cardiovascular collapse
- Ventricular tachycardia
- Torsades de pointes
- Angioedema
- Nausea
- Vomiting
- Diarrhea
- Anorexia

- Bitter taste
- Impotence
- Hepatomegaly
- Hepatoxicity
- SLE syndrome
- Thrombocytopenia
- Neutropenia

- Hemolytic anemia
- Agranulocytosis
- Rash
- Edema
- Urticaria
- Pruritus

Nursing Care

- Do not crush or chew extended release tablets
- Administer IV preparation to treat acute dysrhythmias
- Monitor for cardiac dysrhythmias
- Monitor for cardiac/respiratory distress
- Monitor cardiac blood levels
- Monitor for CNS changes
- Monitor heart rhythm
- Monitor for infection/SLE signs and symptoms
- Monitor hepatic function
- Monitor I&O
- Monitor electrolyte status
- Teach patient not to discontinue medication abruptly
- Teach patient that waxy substance may appear in stools
- Teach patient how to monitor pulse
- Teach patient not to drive or engage in other hazardous activities
- Teach patient to wear sunglasses to decrease photosensitivity
- Teach patient to avoid grapefruit products

Class IB Antidysrhythmic Agents

- Used to treat ventricular dysrhythmias
- Examples include lidocaine, phenytoin, mexiletine
- Available in PO, IM, IV preparations

Mode of Action

- Increases electrical stimulation threshold of ventricle
- ECG changes: accelerates repolarization

Contraindications, Precautions, and Drug Interactions of Class IB Antidysrhythmic Agents*

Drug	Contraindications/Precautions	Drug Interaction
lidocaine	**Contraindications:** Hypersensitivity, hypersensitivity to amides, severe heart block, supraventricular dysrhythmias, Wolff-Parkinson-White syndrome, Adams-Stokes syndrome **Precautions:** Breastfeeding, children, geriatric patients, renal/hepatic disease, CHF, respiratory depression, myasthenia gravis, malignant hyperthermia **Pregnancy:** No adverse effects in animals; no human studies available	Amiodarone, phenytoin, procainamide, propranolol, MAOIs, antihypertensives, tubocurarine, neuromuscular blockers, cimetidine, beta blockers, protease inhibitors, ritonavir, voriconazole, ciprofloxacin, barbiturates, cyclosporine

Contraindications, Precautions, and Drug Interactions of Class IB Antidysrhythmic Agents—cont'd

Drug	Contraindications/Precautions	Drug Interaction
phenytoin	*Contraindications:* Hypersensitivity, Adams-Stokes syndrome, SA and AV block, bradycardia, psychiatric conditions *Precautions:* Geriatric patients, renal/hepatic disease, hepatic failure, petit mal seizures, allergies, hypotension, myocardial insufficiency, acute intermittent porphyria, Asian patients positive for HLA-B1502 *Pregnancy:* Definite fetal risks, may be given in spite of risks if needed in life-threatening conditions	Delavirdine, benzodiazepines, cimetidine, tricyclics, salicylates, valproate, cycloserine, diazepam, chloramphenicol, disulfiram, alcohol, amiodarone, sulfonamides, fluoxetine, gabapentin, H2 agonists, azole antifungals, estrogens, succinamides, phenothiazines, methylphenidate, felbamate, trazadone, alcohol, antacids, barbiturates, carbamazepine, rifampin, calcium, folic acid
mexiletine	*Contraindications:* Hypersensitivity, cardiogenic shock, AV block *Precautions:* Geriatric patients, renal/hepatic disease, heart failure, allergies, seizure disorder *Pregnancy:* Only given after risks to the fetus are considered; animal studies have shown adverse reactions; no human studies available	Cimetidine, fluvoxamine, propafenone, rifampin, phenobarbital

*Pregnancy categories have been revised. See http://www.fda.gov/Drugs/DevelopmentApprovalProcess/DevelopmentResources/Labeling/ucm093307.htm for more information.

Adverse/Side Effects

- Headache
- Dizziness
- Confusion
- Drowsiness
- Euphoria
- Vision changes
- Shivering
- Seizures
- Suicidal tendencies
- Tremor
- Hypotension
- Bradycardia
- Heart block
- CV collapse

- CV arrest
- Ventricular fibrillation
- Dyspnea
- Respiratory depression
- Tinnitus
- Nausea
- Vomiting
- Anorexia
- Methemoglobinemia
- Hepatitis
- Nephritis
- Diabetes insipidus
- Agranulocytosis
- Leukopenia

- Aplastic anemia
- Thrombocytopenia
- Megablastic anemia
- Rash
- Urticaria
- Edema
- Pruritus
- Petechiae
- Lupus erythematosus
- Stevens-Johnson syndrome
- Toxic epidermal necrolysis
- Purple glove syndrome
- DRESS
- Anaphylaxis

Nursing Care

- Use IV form to treat acute dysrhythmia
- Administer IM injection in deltoid
- Do not crush sustained-release tablets
- Monitor for cardiac dysrhythmias
- Monitor for cardiac/respiratory distress
- Monitor cardiac blood levels
- Monitor for CNS changes
- Monitor heart rhythm
- Monitor hepatic function

- Monitor I&O
- Monitor electrolyte status
- Monitor for malignant hyperthermia
- Monitor for skin changes/disorders
- Monitor for seizures
- Monitor for blood dyscrasias
- Teach patient to monitor blood glucose, if diabetic
- Teach patient to report signs and symptoms of toxicity
- Teach patient proper use of autoinjector
- Teach patient that urine may turn pink (phenytoin)
- Teach patient not to abruptly discontinue product
- Teach patient not to drive or engage in hazardous activities
- Teach patient to use nonhormonal contraception

Class IC Antidysrhythmic Agents

- Used to treat severe ventricular dysrhythmias
- Examples include flecainide, propafenone
- Available in PO preparations

Mode of Action

- Slows conduction in all parts of the heart
- ECG changes: delays ventricular repolarization

Contraindications, Precautions, and Drug Interactions of Class IC Antidysrhythmic Agents*

Drug	Contraindications/Precautions	Drug Interaction
flecainide	***Contraindications:*** Hypersensitivity, cardiogenic shock, AV bundle branch block ***Precautions:*** Breastfeeding, children, geriatric patients, renal/hepatic disease, CHF, QT prolongation, MI, bundle branch block, atrial fibrillation, sick sinus syndrome, torsades de pointes, respiratory depression, myasthenia gravis, electrolyte abnormalities ***Pregnancy:*** Only given after risks to the fetus are considered; animal studies have shown adverse reactions; no human studies available	Class IA/III antidysrhythmics, phenothiazines, beta agonists, local anesthetics, tricyclics, haloperidol, chloroquine, droperidol, pentamidine, CYP3A4 inhibitors, arsenic trioxide, levomethadyl, CYP3A4 substrates, propranolol, beta blockers, disopyramide, verapamil, amiodarone, cimetidine, ritonavir, digoxin, urinary alkalinizing agents, urinary acidifying agents
propafenone	***Contraindications:*** Hypersensitivity, cardiogenic shock, AV bundle branch block, right bundle branch block, bradycardia, uncontrolled CHF, sick sinus syndrome, hypotension, bronchospastic disorders, Brugada syndrome, electrolyte imbalance ***Precautions:*** Breastfeeding, children, geriatric patients, renal/hepatic disease, CHF, COPD, bronchospasm, myasthenia gravis, hypo/hyperkalemia, hematologic disorders ***Pregnancy:*** Only given after risks to the fetus are considered; animal studies have shown adverse reactions; no human studies available	CYP1A2, CYP2D6, CYP3A4 inhibitors, other IA/IC antidysrhythmics, arsenic trioxide, warfarin, chloroquine, clarithromycin, droperidol, erythromycin, haloperidol, levomethadyl, methadone, pentamidine, chlorpromazine, mesoridazine, thioridazine, local anesthetics, digoxin, propranolol, metoprolol, cyclosporine, rifampin, cimetidine, quinidine

*Pregnancy categories have been revised. See http://www.fda.gov/Drugs/DevelopmentApprovalProcess/DevelopmentResources/Labeling/ucm093307.htm for more information.

Adverse/Side Effects

- Headache
- Dizziness
- Confusion
- Psychosis
- Restlessness
- Irritability
- Parathesias
- Somnolence
- Depression
- Anxiety
- Malaise
- Fatigue
- Asthenia
- Tremors
- Ataxia
- Flushing
- Seizures
- Dyspnea
- Respiratory depression
- Hypotension
- Bradycardia
- Angina
- PVCs
- Heart block
- CV collapse
- CV arrest
- Dysrhythmias
- CHF
- Fatal ventricular tachycardia
- Palpitations
- QT prolongation
- Torsades de pointes
- Supraventricular dysrhythmia
- Ventricular dysrhythmia
- Asystole
- Tinnitus
- Blurred vision
- Hearing loss
- Dry eyes
- Nausea
- Vomiting
- Diarrhea
- Constipation
- Abdominal pain
- Anorexia
- Flatulence
- Change in taste
- Decreased libido
- Impotence
- Polyuria
- Urinary retention
- Leukopenia
- Thrombocytopenia
- Agranulocytosis
- Granulocytopenia
- Rash
- Urticaria
- Edema

Nursing Care

- Administer with food to minimize adverse reactions
- Do not crush sustained-release tablets
- Monitor for cardiac dysrhythmias
- Monitor for cardiac/respiratory distress
- Monitor heart rhythm
- Monitor cardiac blood levels
- Monitor for CNS changes
- Monitor hepatic function
- Monitor I&O
- Monitor electrolyte status
- Monitor digoxin levels, if applicable
- Notify prescriber if PR interval or QRS complex increases by more than 25%
- Teach patient not to drive or engage in hazardous activities
- Teach patient to change positions slowly
- Teach patient to take as prescribed; do not skip or double doses
- Teach patient not to abruptly discontinue drug
- Teach patient to avoid grapefruit products
- Teach patient to report signs and symptoms of infection

Class II Antiarrhythmic Agents

- Used to treat superventricular tachycardia, sinus tachycardia, arterial fibrillation/flutter
- Examples include esmolol, propranolol, metoprolol, atenolol, timolol, nadolol, sotalol
- Available in PO, IV preparations

Mode of Action
- Blocks beta-adrenergic receptor sites in the heart
- ECG changes

Contraindications, Precautions, and Drug Interactions of Class II Antidysrhythmic Agents*

Drug	Contraindications/Precautions	Drug Interaction
esmolol	**Contraindications:** Hypersensitivity, cardiogenic shock, heart block, CHF, cardiac failure, severe bradycardia **Precautions:** Breastfeeding, geriatric patients, renal/cardiac disease, hypotension, atrial fibrillation, peripheral vascular disease, bronchospasm, asthma, COPD, hypoglycemia, diabetes, thyrotoxicosis, hyperthyroidism, myasthenia gravis, pheochromocytoma, abrupt discontinuation **Pregnancy:** Only given after risks to the fetus are considered; animal studies have shown adverse reactions; no human studies available	MAOIs, sotalol, antidiabetics, clonidine, dilitiazem, verapamil, general anesthetics, digoxin, ephedrine, epinephrine, amphetamine, norepinephrine, phenylephrine, pseudoephedrine, thyroid hormones, salicylates, calcium channel blockers
propranolol	**Contraindications:** Hypersensitivity, cardiogenic shock, AV heart block, sinus bradycardia, bronchospastic disease, bronchospasm, asthma **Precautions:** Breastfeeding, children, renal/cardiac disease, hypotension, cardiac failure, sick sinus syndrome, peripheral vascular disease, vasospastic angina, COPD, diabetes mellitus, hyperthyroidism, myasthenia gravis, Raynaud's disease, Wolff-Parkinson-White syndrome, smoking, thyrotoxicosis **Pregnancy:** Only given after risks to the fetus are considered; animal studies have shown adverse reactions; no human studies available	Phenothiazines, propafenone, calcium channel blockers, neuromuscular blockers, disopyramide, cimetidine, quinidine, haloperidol, prazosin, barbiturates, smoking, calcium channel blockers
metoprolol	**Contraindications:** Hypersensitivity, hypersensitivity to beta blockers, cardiogenic shock, heart block, sinus bradycardia, sick sinus syndrome, pheochromocytoma **Precautions:** Breastfeeding, children, geriatric patients, renal/hepatic/thyroid disease, CAD, CVA, vasospastic angina, COPD, bronchospasm, bronchial asthma, depression **Pregnancy:** Only given after risks to the fetus are considered; animal studies have shown adverse reactions; no human studies available	MAOIs, insulin, oral antidiabetics, cimetidine, reserpine, hydralazine, methyldopa, prazosin, amphetamines, epinephrine, calcium channel blockers, H2 agonists, cimetidine, benzodiazepines, barbiturates, salicylates, NSAIDs, xanthines, calcium channel blockers
atenolol	**Contraindications:** Hypersensitivity, hypersensitivity to beta blockers, cardiogenic shock, heart block, sinus bradycardia, cardiac failure **Precautions:** Breastfeeding, renal/thyroid disease, CHF, COPD, pulmonary edema, asthma, diabetes mellitus, dialysis, myasthenia gravis, Raynaud's disease **Pregnancy:** Definite fetal risks, may be given in spite of risks if needed in life-threatening conditions	MAOIs, sympathomimetics, reserpine, hydralazine, methyldopa, prazosin, anticholinergics, digoxin, diltiazem, verapamil, antihypertensives, cardiac glycosides, insulins, oral antidiabetics, amphetamines, ephedrine, pseudoephedrine, theophylline, dopamine, calcium channel blockers
timolol	**Contraindications:** Hypersensitivity, hypersensitivity to beta blockers, cardiogenic shock, heart block, sinus bradycardia, cardiac failure, CHF, COPD, asthma **Precautions:** Breastfeeding, renal/hepatic/thyroid disease, well-compensated heart failure, peripheral vascular disease, COPD, nonallergic bronchospasm, diabetes mellitus, major surgery **Pregnancy:** Only given after risks to the fetus are considered; animal studies have shown adverse reactions; no human studies available	Beta blockers, calcium channel blockers, NSAIDs, salicylates, sympathomimetics, thyroid, hydralazine, methyldopa, prazosin, anticholinergics, alcohol, reserpine, nitrates, insulin, sulfonylureas, theophyllines, calcium channel blockers

Contraindications, Precautions, and Drug Interactions of Class II Antidysrhythmic Agents—cont'd

Drug	Contraindications/Precautions	Drug Interaction
nadalol	*Contraindications:* Hypersensitivity, cardiac failure, cardiogenic shock, heart block, sinus bradycardia, CHF, COPD, bronchospastic disease *Precautions:* Breastfeeding, renal disease, peripheral vascular disease, nonallergic bronchospasm, diabetes mellitus, major surgery, hyperthyroidism, myasthenia gravis *Pregnancy:* Only given after risks to the fetus are considered; animal studies have shown adverse reactions; no human studies available	MAOIs, ergots, digoxin, clonidine, epinephrine, phenothiazines, antihypertensives, NSAIDs, thyroid hormones, calcium channel blockers
sotalol	*Contraindications:* Hypersensitivity, hypersensitivity to beta blockers, cardiogenic shock, heart block, sinus bradycardia, CHF, bronchial asthma *Precautions:* Breastfeeding, renal/thyroid disease, CAD, COPD, peripheral vascular disease, well-compensated heart failure, bradycardia, nonallergic bronchospasm, diabetes mellitus, major surgery, electrolyte disturbances *Pregnancy:* No adverse effects in animals; no human studies available	Class IA/III antidysrhythmics, phenothiazines, beta agonists, tricyclics, haloperidol, local anesthetics, chloroquine, droperidol, pentamidine, CYP3A4 inhibitors, insulin, lidocaine, nitroglycerin, diuretics, antihypertensives, sympathomimetics, theophylline, beta 2 agonists, sulfonylureas, calcium channel blockers

*Pregnancy categories have been revised. See http://www.fda.gov/Drugs/DevelopmentApprovalProcess/DevelopmentResources/Labeling/ucm093307.htm for more information.

Adverse/Side Effects

- Headache
- Dizziness
- Confusion
- Light-headedness
- Paresthesias
- Somnolence
- Insomnia
- Fatigue
- Depression
- Anxiety
- Mental changes
- Hallucinations
- Nightmares
- Seizures
- Fever
- Flushing
- Bronchospasm
- Laryngospasm
- Dyspnea
- Cough
- Wheeziness
- Nasal stuffiness
- Pulmonary edema
- Hypotension
- Bradycardia
- Angina
- Peripheral ischemia
- Heart block
- CHF
- Dysrhythmias
- Conduction disturbances
- Palpitations
- Nausea
- Vomiting
- Constipation
- Gastric pain
- Anorexia
- Heartburn
- Bloating
- Flatulence
- Hyper/hypoglycemia
- Urinary retention
- Dysuria
- Impotence
- Agranulocytosis
- Thrombocytopenia
- Purpura
- Edema
- Rash
- Pruritus
- Alopecia
- Stevens-Johnson syndrome
- Toxic epidermal necrolysis

Nursing Care

- Administer IV preparations for acute dysrhythmias
- Administer medication with food
- Assess apical pulse before administering medication
- Assess blood pressure before administering medication

- Monitor I&O
- Monitor heart rhythm
- Monitor daily weight
- Monitor blood glucose, if diabetic
- Monitor for lung changes
- Monitor for dysrhythmias
- Monitor renal/hepatic function
- Monitor for cardiac/respiratory distress
- Monitor for CNS changes
- Teach patient to report signs and symptoms of cardiac/respiratory distress
- Teach patient not to discontinue medication abruptly
- Teach patient to avoid alcohol
- Teach patient to avoid OTC products
- Teach patient to avoid driving and other hazardous activities
- Teach patient to change positions slowly
- Teach patient how to correctly monitor pulse and blood pressure
- Teach patient to comply with diet and exercise program

Class III Antiarrhythmic Agents

- Used to treat ventricular arrhythmias
- Examples include amiodarone, dofetilide, ibutilide
- Available in PO, IV preparations

Mode of Action

- Delays repolarization and prolongs duration of action potential
- ECG changes: widens QRS, prolongs PR and QT intervals

Contraindications, Precautions, and Drug Interactions of Class III Antidysrhythmic Agents*

Drug	Contraindications/Precautions	Drug Interaction
amiodarone	**Contraindications:** Hypersensitivity, sensitivity to iodine/benzyl alcohol, breastfeeding, neonates, infants, cardiogenic shock, severe sinus node dysfunction, AV block, bradycardia **Precautions:** Children, CHF, torsades de pointes, respiratory disease, goiter, Hashimoto's thyroiditis **Pregnancy:** Definite fetal risks, may be given in spite of risks if needed in life threatening conditions	Azoles, fluoroquinolones, macrolides, protease inhibitors, HMG-CoA reductase inhibitors, beta blockers, calcium channel blockers, dabigatran, warfarin, cyclosporine, dextromethorphan, digoxin, disopyramide, flecainide, methotrexate, phenytoin, procainamide, quinidine, theophylline, class I antidysrhythmics
dofetilide	**Contraindications:** Hypersensitivity, children, digoxin toxicity, aortic stenosis, severe renal disease/failure, pulmonary hypertension, QT prolongation, torsades de pointes **Precautions:** Breastfeeding, AV block, bradycardia, electrolyte imbalance, dysrhythmia **Pregnancy:** Definite fetal risks, may be given in spite of risks if needed in life threatening conditions	Cimetidine, ketoconazole, verapamil, prochlorperazine, trimethoprim-sulfamethoxazole, megestrol, hydrochlorothiazide, class IA/III antidysrhythmics, arsenic trioxide, chloroquine, clarithromycin, droperidol, erythromycin, halofantrine, haloperidol, methadone, pentamidine, phenothiazines, ziprasidone, ciprofloxacin, potassium depleting diuretics, antiretroviral protease inhibitors, amloride, metformin, entecavir, lamivudine, memantine, triamterene, procainamide, trospium

Contraindications, Precautions, and Drug Interactions of Class III Antidysrhythmic Agents—cont'd

Drug	Contraindications/Precautions	Drug Interaction
ibutilide	**Contraindications:** Hypersensitivity **Precautions:** Breastfeeding, children, geriatric patients, renal/hepatic disease, CHF, AV block, sinus node dysfunction, bradycardia, electrolyte imbalance **Pregnancy:** Only given after risks to the fetus are considered; animal studies have shown adverse reactions; no human studies available	Phenothiazines, tricyclics, tetracyclines, antidepressants, H1-receptor agonists, antihistamines, digoxin, class IA/III antidysrhythmics

*Pregnancy categories have been revised. See http://www.fda.gov/Drugs/DevelopmentApprovalProcess/DevelopmentResources/Labeling/ucm093307.htm for more information.

Adverse/Side Effects

- Headache
- Dizziness
- Insomnia
- Malaise
- Fatigue
- Tremors
- Peripheral neuropathy
- Parathesias
- Flushing
- Abnormal taste/smell
- Stroke
- Angioedema
- Hypotension
- Bradycardia
- Sinus arrest
- CHF
- Dysrhythmias
- SA node dysfunction
- AV block
- QT prolongation
- Torsades de pointes
- Ventricular dysrhythmias
- Pulmonary fibrosis/toxicity
- ARDS
- Pulmonary inflammation
- Vision changes
- Dry eyes
- Hypo/hyperthyroidism
- Nausea
- Vomiting
- Diarrhea
- Constipation
- Abdominal pain
- Anorexia
- Hepatotoxicity
- Pancreatitis
- Erectile dysfunction
- Epididymitis
- Rash
- Urticaria
- Alopecia
- Toxic epidermal necrolysis
- Blue-gray skin discoloration

Nursing Care

- Monitor for cardiac/respiratory arrest
- Monitor heart rhythm
- Monitor chest x-ray results
- Monitor pulmonary function test results
- Monitor eye exam results
- Monitor electrolytes
- Monitor I&O
- Monitor renal/hepatic function
- Monitor for CNS changes
- Monitor for thyroid changes
- Teach patient to take drug as directed
- Teach patient to avoid grapefruit products
- Teach patient not to abruptly discontinue drug
- Teach patient to change positions slowly
- Teach patient to avoid sun exposure, to wear sunscreen/protective clothing/sunglasses
- Teach patient that skin discoloration is reversible

9. A client who had a myocardial infarction is in the coronary care unit on a cardiac monitor. The nurse observes ventricular irritability on the screen. What medication should the nurse prepare to administer?
   1. Digoxin
   2. Furosemide
   3. Amiodarone
   4. Norepinephrine
10. For what client response must the nurse monitor to determine the effectiveness of amiodarone?
    1. Results of fasting lipid profile
    2. Presence of cardiac dysrhythmias
    3. Degree of blood pressure control
    4. Incidence of ischemic chest pain

See Answers on pages 196-197.

Class IV Antiarrhythmic Agents

- Used to treat supraventricular dysrhythmias
- Examples include diltiazem, nifedipine, verapamil, felodipine
- Available in PO, IV preparations

Mode of Action

- Inhibits calcium influx into cardiac muscle cells during depolarization
- ECG changes: reduce SA nodal automaticity; delay AV nodal conduction; prolong PR interval

Contraindications, Precautions, and Drug Interactions of Class IV Antidysrhythmic Agents*

Drug	Contraindications/Precautions	Drug Interaction
dilitiazem	**Contraindications:** Hypersensitivity, AV heart block, hypotension, acute MI, cardiogenic shock, pulmonary congestion, sick sinus syndrome **Precautions:** Breastfeeding, children, geriatric patients, hepatic disease, ventricular dysfunction, CHF, aortic stenosis, bradycardia, GERD, hiatal hernia **Pregnancy:** Only given after risks to the fetus are considered; animal studies have shown adverse reactions; no human studies available	Theophylline, beta blockers, digoxin, lithium, carbamazepine, cyclosporine, HMG-CoA reductase inhibitors, anesthetics, methylprednisone, lovastatin, benzodiazepines, cimetidine
nifedipine	**Contraindications:** Hypersensitivity, hypersensitivity to dihydropyridine, cardiogenic shock **Precautions:** Breastfeeding, children, renal disease, hepatic injury, acute MI, aortic stenosis, heart failure, hypotension, sick sinus syndrome, heart block, GERD **Pregnancy:** Only given after risks to the fetus are considered; animal studies have shown adverse reactions; no human studies available	CYP3A4 inducers, digoxin, phenytoin, cyclosporine, prazosin, carbamazepine, cimetidine, ranitidine, beta blockers, antihypertensives, quinidine, smoking
verapamil	**Contraindications:** Hypersensitivity, cardiogenic shock, severe CHF, sick sinus syndrome, heart block, hypotension, Lown-Ganong-Levine syndrome, Wolff-Parkinson-White syndrome **Precautions:** Breastfeeding, children, geriatric patients, renal disease, hepatic injury, CHF, hypotension, beta blocker therapy **Pregnancy:** Only given after risks to the fetus are considered; animal studies have shown adverse reactions; no human studies available	Beta blockers, cimetidine, clarithromycin, erythromycin, prazosin, quinidine, fentanyl, nitrates, antihypertensives, digoxin, theophylline, cyclosporine, carbamazepine, nondepolarizing muscle relaxants, lithium, NSAIDs

Contraindications, Precautions, and Drug Interactions of Class IV Antidysrhythmic Agents—cont'd

Drug	Contraindications/Precautions	Drug Interaction
felodipine	*Contraindications:* Hypersensitivity, hypersensitivity to dihydropyridines, sick sinus syndrome, heart block, hypotension *Precautions:* Breastfeeding, children, geriatric patients, renal/hepatic disease, CHF, coronary artery disease *Pregnancy:* Only given after risks to the fetus are considered; animal studies have shown adverse reactions; no human studies available	Beta blockers, digoxin, phenytoin, disopyramide, nitrates, alcohol, quinidine, zileuton, miconazole, diltiazem, delavirdine, conivaptan, quinupristin-dalfopristin, cimetidine, cyclosporine, clarithromycin, antiretroviral protease inhibitors, MAOIs, antihypertensives, propranolol, ketoconazole, itraconazole, erythromycin

*Pregnancy categories have been revised. See http://www.fda.gov/Drugs/DevelopmentApprovalProcess/DevelopmentResources/Labeling/ucm093307.htm for more information.

Adverse/Side Effects
- Headache
- Dizziness
- Fatigue
- Drowsiness
- Insomnia
- Weakness
- Depression
- Tremor
- Paresthesia
- Flushing
- Vision changes
- Dysrhythmia
- CHF
- Edema
- Dyspnea
- Pharyngitis
- Rhinitis
- Bradycardia
- Heart block
- Hypotension
- Palpitations
- Nausea
- Vomiting
- Diarrhea
- Constipation
- Gastric upset
- Acute renal failure
- Nocturia
- Polyuria
- Rash
- Pruritus
- Photosensitivity
- Stevens-Johnson syndrome
- Toxic epidermal necrolysis
- Exfoliative dermatitis

Nursing Care
- Monitor for cardiac/respiratory arrest
- Monitor heart rhythm
- Monitor electrolytes
- Monitor I&O
- Monitor renal/hepatic function
- Monitor for CNS changes
- Monitor for skin changes/disorders
- Teach patient to avoid grapefruit products
- Teach patient to avoid caffeine and alcohol
- Teach patient to report signs and symptoms of gingival hyperplasia
- Teach patient not to abruptly discontinue drug
- Teach patient to change positions slowly
- Teach patient to avoid driving and other hazardous activities
- Teach patient how to correctly take pulse and BP

ANSWER KEY: REVIEW QUESTIONS

1. **1 Fiber and fluids help prevent the most common adverse effect of constipation and its complication—fecal impaction.**

    2 Cholestyramine should be taken with meals. **3** The pulse is not affected. **4** Cholestyramine binds bile in the intestine; therefore, it reduces the incidence of jaundice.

    Client Need: Pharmacologic and Parenteral Therapies; **Cognitive Level:** Application; **Integrated Process:** Teaching/Learning; **Nursing Process:** Planning/Implementation

2. **1 Class IA antidysrhythmics suppress ectopic foci by increasing refractory period and slowing depolarization.**

    2 Class IB antidysrhythmics suppress ventricular dysrhythmias by decreasing automaticity and increasing ventricular electrical stimulation threshold. **3** Class IC antidysrhythmics slow conduction and increase ventricular refractoriness. **4** Class III antidysrhythmics prolong repolarization.

    Client Need: Pharmacologic and Parenteral Therapies; **Cognitive Level:** Analysis; **Nursing Process:** Assessment/Analysis

3. **Answers: 1, 2, 4, 5**

    Class IV antidysrhythmics block calcium influx into muscle cells during depolarization; control atrial dysrhythmias by decreasing cardiac automaticity and impulse conduction; reduce peripheral vascular resistance in treatment of hypertension.

    3 Bile acid sequestrants not antidysrhythmics decrease blood cholesterol levels.

    Client Need: Pharmacologic and Parenteral Therapies; **Cognitive Level:** Analysis; **Nursing Process:** Assessment/Analysis

4. **Answers: 1, 2, 3, 5**

    Client education regarding a bile acid sequestrant should include avoiding alcohol and tobacco products, taking the medication with food, and being cautious as bleeding may occur.

    4 Constipation, not diarrhea, may occur and can be managed with stool softeners.

    Client Need: Pharmacologic and Parenteral Therapies; **Cognitive Level:** Analysis; **Integrated Process:** Teaching/Learning; **Nursing Process:** Planning/implementation

5. **Answers: 2, 4, 5**

    Safe compliance associated with Class II antidysrhythmic therapy includes; knowing and reporting the signs/symptoms of cardiac and respiratory distress; avoiding all alcohol; and the medication should never be discontinued abruptly.

    1 Class II antidysrhythmic agents should be taken with food. **3** A client prescribed a Class II antidysrhythmic should not self-medicate with over-the-counter medications.

    Client Need: Pharmacologic and Parenteral Therapies; **Cognitive Level:** Analysis; **Integrated Process:** Teaching/Learning; **Nursing Process:** Evaluation/Outcomes

6. **4 Cholesterol absorption inhibitors inhibit absorption of cholesterol by the small intestine.**

    1 Nicotinic acids reduce production of triglycerides; this process does not occur in the small intestines. **2** Fibric acid inhibitors decrease synthesis of cholesterol, lipoproteins, triglycerides; this process does not occur in the small intestines **3** HMG-CoA reductase inhibitors interfere with cholesterol synthesis; this process does not occur in the small intestines.

    Client Need: Pharmacologic and Parenteral Therapies; **Cognitive Level:** Analysis; **Nursing Process:** Assessment/Analysis

7. **2 Hepatic disease is a contraindication for the common HMG-CoA reductase inhibitors.**

    1 Alcoholism is a precautionary diagnosis that would require consideration before many of HMG-CoA reductase inhibitors could be prescribed. **3** Uncontrolled seizures are a precautionary diagnosis that would require consideration before many of HMG-CoA reductase inhibitors could be prescribed. **4** Severe systemic infection is a precautionary diagnosis that would require consideration before many of HMG-CoA reductase inhibitors could be prescribed.

    Client Need: Pharmacologic and Parenteral Therapies; **Cognitive Level:** Analysis; **Nursing Process:** Assessment/Analysis

8. **1 Safe administration of antihyperlipidemic medication includes not crushing, breaking, opening, or dissolving the capsule.**

   2 High fat foods, not potassium rich foods, need to be limited to facilitate the effectiveness of the antihyperlipidemic medication. **3** Antihyperlipidemic medications need not be taken at bedtime. **4** Alcohol should be avoided when on an antihyperlipidemic medication.

   Client Need: Pharmacologic and Parenteral Therapies; **Cognitive Level:** Analysis; **Integrated Process:** Teaching/Learning; **Nursing Process:** Evaluation/Outcomes

9. **3 Amiodarone decreases the irritability of the ventricles by prolonging the duration of the action potential and refractory period. It is used in the treatment of ventricular dysrhythmias.**

   1 Digoxin slows and strengthens ventricular contractions; it will not rapidly correct ectopic beats. **2** Furosemide, a diuretic, does not affect ectopic foci. **4** Norepinephrine is a sympathomimetic and is not the drug of choice for ventricular irritability.

   Client Need: Pharmacologic and Parenteral Therapies; **Cognitive Level:** Analysis; **Nursing Process:** Planning/Implementation

---

Study Tip: Use associations already in your brain (and your sense of humor!) and repurpose them to remember which drugs have which effects. For instance: Have you ever had an irritable friend that you helped calm, perhaps by using a *Ven*n diagram? Did you know the word *ami* in French means friend? That's how you can remember that *Ami*odarone decreases the irritability of the *ven*tricles.

---

10. **2 Amiodarone is a class III antidysrhythmic used to treat ventricular and supraventricular tachycardia, and conversion of atrial fibrillation.**

    1 Results of fasting lipid profile is expected with antilipidemics. **3** Degree of blood pressure control is expected with antihypertensives. **4** Incidence of ischemic chest pain is expected with antianginal agents such as nitrates.

    Client Need: Pharmacologic and Parenteral Therapies; **Cognitive Level:** Application; **Nursing Process:** Evaluation

11 Drugs Affecting the Blood

OVERVIEW OF THE BLOOD

- Blood
  - Volume: males: 5 to 6 L; females: 4.5 to 5.5 L
  - Viscosity: about 5.5 times as viscous as pure water; reflected by hematocrit (percentage of blood volume made up of red blood cells [RBCs])
  - Males: 45% to 52%
  - Females: 37% to 48%
  - Hematopoiesis
    - Location: red marrow of vertebrae, sternum, ribs, iliac crests, clavicles, scapulae, and skull
    - Pluripotential stem cell differentiates into myeloid and lymphoid stem cells
    - Myeloid stem cells further differentiate into erythrocytes, platelets, neutrophils, monocytes, eosinophils, basophils, and mast cells
    - Lymphoid stem cells further differentiate into B and T lymphocytes
- Blood components
  - Plasma
  - Water: 3 L in average adult; 90% of plasma
  - Ions
  - Albumin (major plasma protein)
    - Acts as a buffer
    - Maintains plasma colloid osmotic pressure
    - Glucose: prime oxidative metabolite
    - Serum: plasma with fewer or no coagulating proteins
    - Erythrocytes (RBCs)
    - Shape: pliable biconcave disk that maximizes surface area proportional to volume for ease of diffusion of gases
    - Number: males: 4.5 to 6.2 $\times$ 106/mm^3; females: 4.0 to 5.5 $\times$ 106/mm^3
    - Formation (erythropoiesis): liver and kidneys secrete proteins that help form erythropoietin, which stimulates erythrocyte production by red bone marrow
    - Principal component is hemoglobin; functions to bind oxygen through iron in heme and carbon dioxide through globulin portion; can carry both simultaneously
    - Erythrocytes live for about 120 days; old or deteriorated ones are removed by reticuloendothelial cells of liver, spleen, and bone marrow; heme is converted to bilirubin, which is excreted from liver as part of bile
  - Leukocytes white blood cells [WBCs]
    - Granulocytes (polymorphonuclear): neutrophils, eosinophils, and basophils
    - Agranulocytes (mononuclear): monocytes that become macrophages in tissue spaces and lymphocytes
    - Phagocytosis of bacteria by neutrophils and macrophages; phagocytosis of antigen-antibody complexes by eosinophils
    - Antibody synthesis: B lymphocytes become plasma cells, which produce most circulatory antibodies

- Destruction of transplanted tissues and cancer cells by T lymphocytes, which form in lymphoid tissue and mature in the thymus
- Leukocytes live for a few hours or days; some T lymphocytes live for many years and provide long-term immunity
- Platelets (thrombocytes)
  - Number: 150,000 to 450,000/mm^3
  - Function in blood coagulation (agglutination, adhesiveness, aggregation)
  - Adhere to each other and to damaged areas of circulatory system to limit or
  - prevent blood loss
  - Release chemicals that constrict damaged blood vessels
- Blood groups
  - Four blood types: A, B, AB, and O; type indicates antigens on or in the RBC membrane (e.g., type A blood has A antigens; type O blood has no antigens)
  - Blood can be either Rh-positive or Rh-negative; usually blood does not contain anti-Rh antibodies. However, Rh-negative blood will contain anti-Rh antibodies if the individual has been transfused with Rh-positive blood or has carried an Rh-positive fetus without treatment; Rh-positive blood never contains anti-Rh antibodies; people with Rh-positive blood can receive blood from an Rh-negative donor; people with Rh-negative blood cannot receive blood from an Rh-positive donor.
  - Plasma: usually contains no antibodies against antigens present on its own RBCs, but does contain antibodies against other A or B antigens not present on its RBCs
  - The potential danger in transfusing blood is that the donor's blood may be agglutinated (clumped) by the recipient's antibodies.
  - Hemostasis: process to arrest blood loss using vasoconstriction
  - Aggregation of platelets: adhere to damaged blood vessel walls, forming plugs
  - Blood coagulation (clotting): blood becomes gel as soluble fibrinogen is converted to insoluble fibrin
  - Extrinsic clotting mechanism: trigger is blood contacting damaged tissue
  - Intrinsic clotting mechanism: trigger is release of chemicals (platelet factors such as thromboplastin) from platelets aggregated at site of injury
  - Liver cells synthesize prothrombin, fibrinogen, and other clotting factors; adequate amounts of vitamin K must be present in blood for liver to produce prothrombin; calcium acts as a catalyst to convert prothrombin to thrombin
  - Prothrombin is converted to thrombin, which converts fibrinogen to fibrin; fibrin is an insoluble protein formed from soluble protein fibrinogen in the presence of thrombin; fibrin appears as a tangled mass of threads in which blood cells become enmeshed.
  - When new endothelial cells form, the fibrin clot is destroyed by plasmin, which is formed from plasminogen.
- Blood vessels
  - Arteries
    - Carry blood away from heart (all arteries except pulmonary artery carry oxygenated blood)
    - Branch into smaller and smaller vessels called arterioles, which branch into microscopic capillaries
    - Structure: lining (tunica intima) of endothelium; middle coat (tunica media) of smooth muscle, elastic, and fibrous tissues, which permits constriction and dilation; outer coat (tunica adventitia or externa) of fibrous tissue; this firmness allows arteries to remain open instead of collapsing when cut

- Peripheral pulses can be felt wherever an artery lies near the surface of the skin and over a firm background such as bone; sites: radial—at wrist; carotid—along anterior edge of sternocleidomastoid muscle, at level of lower margin of thyroid cartilage; brachial—at bend of the elbow, along inner margin of biceps muscle; femoral—in groin; popliteal—behind knee; posterior tibial—behind medial malleolus; dorsalis pedis—on anterior surface of foot, just below bend of the ankle; volume or amplitude of pulse may be absent, thready, diminished, have an acceptable volume, or bounding
    - Pulse deficit: difference between apical and radial pulses
    - Blood pressure: systolic—pressure within arteries when heart is contracting; diastolic—pressure within arteries when heart is at rest between contractions; pulse pressure—difference between systolic and diastolic pressures
- Veins
    - Carry blood toward heart (all veins except pulmonary veins carry deoxygenated blood)
    - Branch into venules, which collect blood from capillaries; veins in cranial cavity formed by dura mater are called sinuses
    - Structure: same three coats as arteries, but thinner and fewer elastic and muscle fibers, allowing veins to collapse when cut; semilunar valves present in most veins more than 2 mm in diameter prevent backward flow of blood
- Capillaries
    - Carry blood from arterioles and unite to form small veins or venules, which in turn unite to form veins
    - Exchange of substances between blood and interstitial fluid occurs in capillaries
    - Structure: only lining coat present (intima); wall only one cell thick to allow for diffusion of gases and small molecules

COMMON DISORDERS OF THE BLOOD

Venous Disorders

- Etiology and pathophysiology
    - Thrombus: a clot composed of platelets, fibrin, clotting factors, and cellular debris attached to interior wall of an artery or vein
    - Embolus: a clot or solid particle carried by bloodstream; may interfere with tissue perfusion in an artery or vein
    - Interfere with transportation of blood back to the heart from the capillary beds; pathophysiologic changes may include impaired smooth muscle around vessels, lack of muscular contraction, damage to intima, incompetent valves; risk factors include immobility, venous stasis, vessel trauma, oral contraceptive use, pregnancy, obesity, orthopedic surgery, and pelvic surgery
        - Thrombophlebitis: inflammation of a vein
        - Deep vein thrombosis (DVT): thrombophlebitis associated with clot formation
        - Venous thromboembolism (VTE): DVT associated with pulmonary embolism
- Clinical findings
    - Thrombophlebitis or DVT
        - Subjective: may be asymptomatic until embolus is released and occludes organ; calf pain on dorsiflexion of ankle (Homan's sign) is not a reliable indicator; this sign should not be elicited because dorsiflexion may dislodge the thrombus
        - Objective: edema of one leg; redness and warmth of area along the vein; Doppler studies/flow studies of lower extremities indicate obstruction or decreased flow from the area, suggesting thrombus formation; positive D-dimer assay, which indicates products of

fibrin degradation in the blood (normal value is ,250 mcg/L). The normal range of D-dimer assay may be higher in elderly patients.

- Therapeutic intervention
  - Thrombophlebitis
    - Prophylactic interventions: antiembolism stockings and exercises to promote venous return
    - Moist heat to promote vasodilation
    - Elevation of extremity to reduce edema
    - Anticoagulants to prevent recurrence
    - Vasodilators to prevent vascular spasm
    - Thrombolytic therapy to dissolve clot
    - Transvenous filter or thrombectomy
- Assessment/Analysis
  - Risk factors and subjective data
  - Affected extremity for pulses, color, temperature, and circumference; a Doppler scan facilitates attainment of peripheral pulses
  - Mobility of involved extremity
- Planning/Implementation
  - Observe for signs of vascular impairment (e.g., pallor, cyanosis, coolness of involved extremities, and amplitude and symmetry of peripheral pulses)
  - Instruct to avoid cigarette smoking (nicotine constricts vessels, massaging legs), maintaining one position for long periods, and wearing tight clothing that can affect peripheral vessels; reduce weight when indicated; control diabetes, hypertension, and lipid levels; maintain adequate hydration; perform ankle exercises so muscle contractions prevent venous stasis
  - Venous insufficiency: elevate legs to limit edema; apply antiembolism stockings before arising; apply sequential compression device for clients on prescribed bed rest; if thrombophlebitis is suspected, maintain bed rest and notify health care provider
  - Observe for clinical manifestations of thrombophlebitis and pulmonary embolism (e.g., sudden chest pain, cyanosis, hemoptysis, shock); maintain client on bed rest and notify health care provider if thrombophlebitis or pulmonary embolism is suspected
  - Provide specific care if undergoing vascular surgery: monitor for hemorrhage; notify health care provider if bleeding is suspected; assess neurovascular status of extremity; keep extremity elevated in immediate postoperative period; allow out of bed as ordered
  - Administer prescribed medications

Anemias

- Etiology and pathophysiology
- Anemia is a symptom and not a disease; the underlying cause of the anemia must be identified.
  - Anemia: reduction in concentration of erythrocytes (RBCs) or hemoglobin
    - Iron deficiency anemia: most common causes are GI bleeding, menstruation, malignancy; other causes include inadequate dietary intake, malabsorption, and increased demand (e.g., pregnancy)
    - Megaloblastic anemia
      - Folate deficiency: insufficient amount of folic acid absorbed or ingested to synthesize DNA, RNA, and proteins; associated with alcoholism, malabsorption, pregnancy, lactation
    - Pernicious anemia: lack of intrinsic factor in the stomach prevents absorption of vitamin B_{12}, reducing the formation of adequate numbers of erythrocytes
    - Aplastic (hypoplastic) anemia: bone marrow is depressed or destroyed by a chemical or drug, leading to leukopenia, thrombocytopenia, decreased erythrocytes, and decreased leukocytes (agranulocytosis)

- Hemolytic anemia: excessive or premature destruction of RBCs; causes include sickle cell anemia, thalassemia, glucose-6-phosphate dehydrogenase (G-6-PD) deficiency, antibody reactions, infection, and toxins
- Sickle cell anemia: inheritance of autosomal recessive gene mutation that produces defective hemoglobin molecule (hemoglobin S)
  - Polycythemia vera: sustained increase in number of erythrocytes, leukocytes, and platelets, with an increased blood viscosity
  - Idiopathic thrombocytopenic purpura: appears to result from production of an antiplatelet antibody that coats surface of platelets and facilitates their destruction by phagocytic leukocytes
- Clinical findings
  - Subjective: fatigue, headache, paresthesias, dyspnea; sore mouth with pernicious anemia; bleeding gums, epistaxis with thrombocytopenic purpura, and neuro changes (altered sensation/paresthesias) with pernicious anemia
  - Objective
    - Ankle edema
    - Dry, pale mucous membranes
    - Pallor except with polycythemia vera and hemolytic anemia
    - Iron deficiency anemia: decreased levels of hemoglobin, erythrocytes, ferritin; increased iron-binding capacity; megaloblastic condition of blood
    - Pernicious anemia: beefy red tongue, lack of intrinsic factor, positive Romberg's test (loss of balance with eyes closed)
    - Aplastic anemia: fever; bleeding from mucous membranes; decreased levels of leukocytes, erythrocytes, and platelets
    - Hemolytic anemia: increased reticulocytes and unconjugated bilirubin levels; jaundice
    - Sickle cell anemia: chronic fatigue, unexplained dyspnea, pain, frequent infections; sickled cells on stained blood smear
    - Polycythemia vera: increased hemoglobin level, purple-red complexion
    - Thrombocytopenic purpura: low platelet count, ecchymotic areas, hemorrhagic petechiae
- Therapeutic interventions
  - Improvement of diet: include ascorbic acid, which enhances iron uptake
  - Supplements: iron, vitamin B_{12}, folic acid
  - Blood transfusions (except for polycythemia vera)
  - Oxygen as needed
  - Epoetin to stimulate bone marrow function
  - Aplastic anemia: bone marrow transplant (BMT); peripheral blood stem cell transplant (PBSCT); immunosuppressive therapy
  - Hemolytic anemia: splenectomy if indicated
  - Sickle cell anemia: analgesics and warm compresses to relieve pain
  Polycythemia vera: routine phlebotomy; low-iron diet; hydroxyurea to suppress bone marrow
- Assessment/Analysis
  - History of dietary habits, symptoms, and causative agents
  - Status of skin, mucous membranes, and sclera
  - Baseline vital signs
- Planning/Implementation
  - Teach dietary modifications and medication administration; emphasize foods high in iron (e.g., spinach, raisins, liver)
  - Help to balance rest and activity
  - Explain need for prevention of hemorrhage related to thrombocytopenia

- Provide postoperative care if splenectomy is performed; encourage deep breathing and coughing; assess for abdominal distention that may reflect hemorrhage
  - Polycythemia vera: explain need for repeated phlebotomies and interventions to prevent DVTs

Disseminated Intravascular Coagulation (DIC)

- Etiology and pathophysiology
  - Response to overstimulation of clotting and anticlotting processes as a result of injury or disease; massive amounts of microthrombi affect microcirculation
  - Complicated by hemorrhage at various sites as a result of fibrinolytic response
  - Multiple system failure may occur (e.g., circulatory, respiratory, GI, renal, neurologic) from bleeding or thrombosis
- Clinical findings
  - Subjective: restlessness, anxiety
  - Objective
    - Low fibrinogen level; prolonged prothrombin and partial thromboplastin times; reduced platelets; positive D-dimer assay
    - Hemorrhage, both subcutaneous and internal; petechiae; signs of organ failure
- Therapeutic interventions
  - Relieve underlying cause
  - Heparin to prevent formation of thrombi
  - Transfusion of blood products
  - Antifibrinolytic therapy to prevent bleeding if necessary
  - Assessment/Analysis
    - History of causative factors (e.g., septicemia, obstetric emergencies, and septic shock)
    - Bleeding; abnormal coagulation profile
- Planning/Implementation
  - Observe for bleeding; replace fluids as ordered
  - Minimize skin punctures; prevent injury
  - Monitor for renal, cerebral, and respiratory complications
  - Provide emotional support

Hemophilia

- Etiology and pathophysiology
  - Hereditary: X-linked genetic disease; mostly affects males
  - Two types
  - Hemophilia A: most common; caused by deficiency/nonfunctioning of clotting factor VIII
  - Hemophilia B: least common; caused by deficiency/nonfunctioning of clotting factor IX
  - Lack of clotting factor prevents fibrin clot from forming at bleeding site
- Clinical findings
  - Subjective: pain in joints, muscles
  - Objective
  - Delayed bleeding
  - Spontaneous bleeding
  - Hematuria
  - Hematemesis
  - Red or tarry stools
  - Hematomas on torso, extremities
  - Prolonged PTT (hemophilia A)
  - Factor IX assay deficiency (hemophilia B)
- Therapeutic interventions
  - Antihemophilic factors
  - Fresh frozen plasma
  - Analgesics
  - Clothing with padded patches (children)
  - Assessment/Analysis
  - Bleeding; abnormal coagulation profile

- Planning/Implementation
  - Observe for bleeding; replace fluids as ordered
  - Minimize skin punctures; prevent injury
  - Provide emotional support

Overview of Anticoagulants

- Anticoagulants
  - Prevent fibrin formation by interfering with production of various clotting factors in the coagulation process
  - Prevent platelet aggregation and clot extension
  - Used for prevention and treatment of thrombus and embolus
  - Parenteral preparations may be given with oral medications until oral medications reach therapeutic
  - Monitor blood work when client is receiving warfarin (Coumadin)
    - International normalized ratio (INR): therapeutic value should be 2.0 to 3.5; change in drug regimen requires more frequent INRs because many drugs have interactive effects
  - Monitor blood work when client is receiving heparin derivatives
    - Prothrombin time (PT); therapeutic value should be 1.5 to 2 times the normal value
    - Activated partial thromboplastin time (aPTT); therapeutic value should be 1.5 to 2 times normal value when given as a continuous IV drip
  - Monitor blood work if surgery cannot be delayed when client is receiving dabigatran to evaluate bleeding risk
    - Ecarin clotting time (ECT)
    - Activated thromboplastin time (aPTT)
    - Thrombin time (TT)
  - Administer subcutaneous heparin in the abdomen; do not aspirate or massage the area
  - Have appropriate antidote available: vitamin K for warfarin; protamine sulfate for heparin
  - Avoid intramuscular injections and salicylates with the concomitant administration of anticoagulants to prevent bleeding

Overview of Blood Transfusion

- Purpose: restores blood volume after hemorrhage; maintains hemoglobin levels in clients with severe anemia; replaces specific blood components
- Sources of blood for transfusion
  - Homologous: random collection of blood by volunteer donors
- Autologous: donation of a client's own blood before hospitalization; possible when donor's hemoglobin remains higher than 11 g/dL; donations can be saved for 5 weeks
- Directed donation: donation of blood by a donor for a specific client
- Blood salvage: client's blood is suctioned from a closed body cavity (e.g., operative site, trauma site, joint) into a cell-saver machine, processed, and transfused back into the client; must be used within 6 hours of collection; contains high levels of potassium
- Blood components and use
  - Whole blood: volume replacement for blood loss
- Packed RBCs: increase RBC mass
- Platelets: increase platelets to prevent bleeding related to thrombocytopenia
- Fresh frozen plasma: contains plasma, antibodies, clotting factors
- Cryoprecipitate: contains factor VIII, fibrinogen, and factor XIII to treat hemophilia
- Albumin: volume expander to treat hypoproteinemia
- Plasma protein factor: to treat some types of hemophilia
- IV gamma globulin: contains immunoglobulin G (IgG) antibodies to treat immunodeficiency

- Nursing care
  - Obtain and document informed consent
- Check that blood or blood components are typed and cross-matched for compatibility; follow agency policy; two nurses should verify blood type, Rh factor, client identification, blood numbers, and expiration date
- Blood must be administered within 30 minutes of arrival on unit
- Obtain baseline vital signs before administration and monitor every 5 minutes for 15 minutes and then every 15 minutes during the transfusion
- Initiate an IV with normal saline infusing through a large-bore catheter and a blood administration set containing a filter; solutions containing glucose should not be used
- Maintain standard precautions when handling blood and IV equipment; assure client that risk for acquired immunodeficiency syndrome (AIDS) is minimal because blood is screened
- Invert blood container gently to suspend RBCs within the plasma
- Administer at appropriate rate
  - Platelets, plasma, and cryoprecipitate may be infused rapidly; assess for signs of circulatory overload
    - Blood transfusions should be completed within 4 hours because potential for bacterial contamination increases over time
    - Administer slowly for first 15 minutes to detect transfusion reaction
    - Use IV controller to provide safe infusion rate; ensure that IV controller is appropriate for blood administration
- Monitor for signs of hemolytic reaction: usually occurs within first 10 to 15 minutes; shivering, headache, flank pain, increased pulse and respiratory rates, hemoglobinuria, oliguria, progressive signs of shock and renal failure
- Monitor for signs of febrile reaction: usually occurs within 30 minutes; chills, fever, muscle stiffness
- Monitor for allergic reaction: hives, wheezing, flushing, pruritus, joint pain
- If reaction occurs: stop infusion immediately; replace IV tubing containing blood; maintain patency of IV tubing with normal saline; monitor vital signs and I&O frequently; send blood to the laboratory; send urine specimen to laboratory if a hemolytic reaction is suspected; evaluate hemoglobin and hematocrit laboratory results; monitor urine output; notify health care provider

APPLICATION AND REVIEW

1. A client who is pale and moaning is diagnosed with esophageal varices and is admitted to the hospital. The health care provider orders a blood transfusion. What nursing actions should be taken?
   1. Take the vital signs, verify the blood product with another nurse against the client's ID bracelet, and monitor the vital signs according to agency policy.
   2. Because the vital signs were recorded during admission, hang the blood and monitor the client's vital signs every 15 minutes until the transfusion is absorbed.
   3. Record the vital signs in accordance with facility policy and check the blood product against the client's ID bracelet in the presence of the nursing supervisor.
   4. Take the vital signs after hanging the blood because the client is pale and moaning and is in critical condition; return in 15 minutes to monitor the vital signs.
2. The spouse of a client with an intracranial hemorrhage asks the nurse, "Why aren't they administering an anticoagulant?" How should the nurse respond?
   1. "It is contraindicated because bleeding will increase."
   2. "If necessary it will be started to enhance circulation."
   3. "If necessary it will be started to prevent pulmonary thrombosis."
   4. "It is inadvisable because it masks the effects of the hemorrhage."

See Answers on pages 219-221.

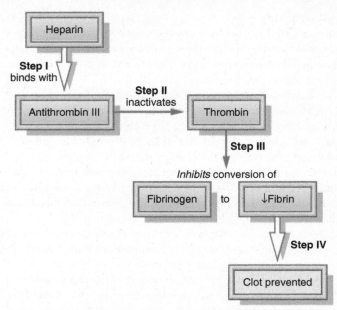

FIG. 11.1 Action of the parenteral anticoagulant heparin. (From Kee, J.L., Hayes, E.R., McCuistion, L.E. [2015]. *Pharmacology: A patient-centered nursing process approach* [8th ed.]. St. Louis: Saunders.)

DRUGS USED TO TREAT BLOOD DISORDERS

Anticoagulants

- Used to prevent and treat thrombosis
- Examples include heparin, enoxaparin, dalteparin, fondaparinux, dabigatran, warfarin (Fig. 11.1)
- Available in PO, IV, SUBCUT preparations

Mode of Action

- Inhibits production of vitamin K in the liver that interferes with the blood clotting mechanism by blocking thrombin

Contraindications, Precautions, and Drug Interactions of Anticoagulants*

Drug	Contraindications/Precautions	Drug Interaction
heparin	*Contraindications:* Hypersensitivity to heparin/corn/porcine protein, bleeding *Precautions:* Children, geriatric patients, benzyl alcohol products in neonates/infants/pregnancy/lactation, alcoholism, blood dyscrasias, diabetes, hyperlipidemia, renal disease, hemophilia, leukemia with bleeding, heparin-induced thrombocytopenia (HIT), peptic ulcer disease, severe renal/hepatic disease, severe thrombocytopenic purpura, severe hypertension, acute nephritis, subacute bacterial endocarditis *Pregnancy:* Only given after risks to the fetus are considered; animal studies have shown adverse reactions; no human studies available	Dextran, oral anticoagulants, NSAIDs, salicylates, platelet inhibitors, cephalosporins, penicillins, SSRIs, SNRIs, ticlopidine, dipyridamole, antineoplastics, valproic acid, quinidine, clopidogrel, antihistamines, digoxin, cardiac glycosides, nicotine, nitroglycerin, tetracyclines

Contraindications, Precautions, and Drug Interactions of Anticoagulants—cont'd

Drug	Contraindications/Precautions	Drug Interaction
enoxaparin	**Contraindications:** Hypersensitivity to enoxaparin/heparin/pork, active major bleeding, hemophilia, heparin-induced thrombocytopenia, leukemia with bleeding, thrombocytopenic purpura **Precautions:** Breastfeeding, children, geriatric patients, acute nephritis, hypersensitivity to benzyl alcohol, indwelling catheter, low weight males/females, severe hypertension, severe renal/hepatic disease, recent burn, spinal surgery, subacute bacterial endocarditis **Pregnancy:** No adverse effects in animals, no human studies available	Anticoagulants, antiplatelets, NSAIDs, RU-486, salicylates, thrombolytics
dalteparin	**Contraindications:** Hypersensitivity to dalteparin/heparin/pork, active major bleeding, hemophilia, heparin-induced thrombocytopenia, leukemia with bleeding, thrombocytopenic purpura, cerebral vascular hemorrhage, hemorrhagic stroke, cerebral aneurysm, non-Q wave MI, regional anesthesia for unstable angina **Precautions:** Breastfeeding, children, geriatric patients, recent childbirth, blood dyscrasias, renal/hepatic disease, bacterial endocarditis, uncontrolled hypertension, nephritis, peptic ulcer disease, severe cardiac disease, HIT, pericarditis, recent lumbar puncture, pericardial effusion, vasculitis, other bleeding **Pregnancy:** No adverse effects in animals, no human studies available	Oral anticoagulants, platelet inhibitors, salicylates, NSAIDs, thrombolytics, cephalosporins
fondaparinux	**Contraindications:** Hypersensitivity, active major bleeding, hemophilia, leukemia with bleeding, thrombocytopenic purpura, peptic ulcer disease, hemorrhagic stroke, surgery, low weight, severe renal disease, bacterial endocarditis **Precautions:** Breastfeeding, children, geriatric patients, alcoholism, blood dyscrasias, severe hepatic disease, heparin-induced thrombocytopenia, uncontrolled severe hypertension, acute nephritis, moderate renal disease **Pregnancy:** No adverse effects in animals, no human studies available	NSAIDs, salicylates, abciximab, valproic acid, quinidine, eptifibatide, tirofiban, clopidogrel, dipyridamole
dabigatran	**Contraindications:** Hypersensitivity, active major bleeding, hemophilia, leukemia with bleeding, thrombocytopenic purpura, peptic ulcer disease, hemorrhagic stroke, surgery, low weight, severe renal disease, bacterial endocarditis **Precautions:** Breastfeeding, children, geriatric patients, labor, obstetric delivery, anticoagulant therapy, renal disease, surgery **Pregnancy:** Only given after risks to the fetus are considered; animal studies have shown adverse reactions; no human studies available	Anticoagulants, amiodarone, clopidogrel, ketoconazole, quinidine, thrombolytics, verapamil, rifampin, tipranavir, carbamazepine
warfarin	**Contraindications:** Breastfeeding, hypersensitivity, hemophilia, leukemia with bleeding, thrombocytopenic purpura, peptic ulcer disease, stroke, surgery, severe hepatic disease, malignant hypertension, acute nephritis, subacute bacterial endocarditis, eclampsia, preeclampsia, aneurysm, spinal puncture **Precautions:** Geriatric patients, Asian patients, CHF, indwelling catheter, severe hypertension, trauma, active infection, vasculitis, severe diabetes, polycythemia vera, protein C/S deficiency **Pregnancy:** Absolute fetal abnormalities; not to be used at any time during pregnancy	Phenytoin, oral sulfonylureas, allopurinol, amiodarone, chloramphenicol, cimetidine, clofibrate, COX-2 selective inhibitors, disulfiram, erythromycin, furosemide, glucagon, heparin, HMG-CoA reductase inhibitors, NSAIDs, penicillins, quinidine, salicylates, sulfonamides, SSRIs, steroids, thrombolytics, tricyclics

*Pregnancy categories have been revised. See http://www.fda.gov/Drugs/DevelopmentApprovalProcess/DevelopmentResources/Labeling/ucm093307.htm for more information.

Adverse Effects/Side Effects

- Fever
- Confusion
- Anaphylaxis
- Edema
- Peripheral edema
- Intracranial bleeding
- Nausea
- Hematuria

- HIT
- Hematoma
- Hemorrhage
- Hypochromic anemia
- Heparin-induced thrombocytopenia
- Thrombocytopenia
- Agranulocytosis

- Leukopenia
- Eosinophilia
- Major bleeding
- Hepatitis
- Osteoporosis
- Hyperkalemia
- Exfoliative dermatitis
- Purple toe syndrome

Nursing Care

- Administer at same time each day to maintain blood levels
- Monitor blood studies
- Monitor renal/hepatic studies
- Monitor blood clotting studies
- Monitor for bleeding
- Monitor for signs and symptoms of infection, sensitivity
- Monitor for injection site reactions
- Teach patient to avoid bleeding (use soft-bristled tooth brush and electric razor)
- Teach patient to report any signs of bleeding to prescriber
- Teach patient not to abruptly discontinue medication
- Teach patient to avoid OTC products containing aspirin, NSAIDs
- Teach patient importance of diet and to include foods rich in vitamin K

APPLICATION AND REVIEW

3. An older adult with cerebral arteriosclerosis is admitted with atrial fibrillation and is started on a continuous heparin infusion. What clinical finding enables the nurse to conclude that the anticoagulant therapy is effective?
   1. A reduction of confusion
   2. An aPTT twice the usual value
   3. An absence of ecchymotic areas
   4. A decreased viscosity of the blood
4. A client is receiving warfarin. Which test result should the nurse use to determine whether the daily dose of this anticoagulant is therapeutic?
   1. INR
   2. aPTT
   3. Bleeding time
   4. Sedimentation rate

See Answers on pages 219-221.

Thrombolytics

- Used to promote thrombolysis
- Examples include alteplase, streptokinase tenecteplase
- Available in IV preparations

Mode of Action

- Lyses thrombi, fibrinogen, and other plasma proteins

Contraindications, Precautions, and Drug Interactions of Thrombolytics*

Drug	Contraindications/Precautions	Drug Interaction
alteplase	**Contraindications:** Active internal bleeding, aneurysm, brain tumor, history of CVA, uncontrolled hypertension, intracranial/intraspinal surgery/trauma, low platelets, INR >1.7, PR >15 secs **Precautions:** Breastfeeding, children, geriatric patients, acute pericarditis, arrhythmias, CVA, diabetic retinopathy, GI/GU bleeding, hepatic disease, hypertension, mitral stenosis, recent surgery **Pregnancy:** Only given after risks to the fetus are considered; animal studies have shown adverse reactions; no human studies available	Anticoagulants, NSAIDs, salicylates, dipyridamole, ACE inhibitors, abciximab, eptifibatide, clopidogrel, tirofiban, valproic acid, ticlopidine, plicamycin, nitroglycerin
streptokinase	**Contraindications:** Hypersensitivity, active internal bleeding, aneurysm, history of CVA, severe hypertension, intracranial/intraspinal surgery/trauma, severe renal/hepatic disease, cerebrovascular disease **Precautions:** Breastfeeding, children, geriatric patients, GI bleeding, mitral stenosis, bacterial endocarditis, any other bleeding disorder **Pregnancy:** Only given after risks to the fetus are considered; animal studies have shown adverse reactions; no human studies available	Salicylates, NSAIDs, anticoagulants, antiplatelets
tenecteplase	**Contraindications:** Hypersensitivity, active internal bleeding, aneurysm, history of CVA, severe hypertension, intracranial/intraspinal surgery/trauma, severe renal/hepatic disease **Precautions:** Breastfeeding, children, geriatric patients, dysrhythmias, hypertension, hypocoagulation, bacterial endocarditis, rheumatic valvular disease, cerebral embolism/thrombosis/hemorrhage **Pregnancy:** Only given after risks to the fetus are considered; animal studies have shown adverse reactions; no human studies available	Salicylates, NSAIDs, SSRIs, SNRIs, cefotetan, cefoperazone, anticoagulants, antithrombolytics, dipyridamole, clopidogrel, ticlopidine

*Pregnancy categories have been revised. See http://www.fda.gov/Drugs/DevelopmentApprovalProcess/DevelopmentResources/Labeling/ucm093307.htm for more information.

Adverse Effects/Side Effects

- Fever
- Anaphylaxis
- Angioedema
- Bleeding
- Pulmonary embolism
- Cardiogenic shock
- Cardiac arrest
- Heart failure
- Pericarditis
- Bradycardia
- Sinus bradycardia
- Ventricular tachycardia
- Hypotension
- Ischemic stroke
- Thrombosis
- Rash
- Urticaria
- Purple toe syndrome

Nursing Care

- Avoid invasive procedures, injections, rectal temperatures
- Use reconstituted IV solution within 8 hours
- Monitor vital signs every 4 hours
- Monitor for dysrhythmias/cardiac changes
- Monitor for bleeding
- Monitor for allergic reaction
- Monitor blood studies
- Monitor hepatic/renal function
- Monitor for cardiac/respiratory distress
- Monitor for purple toe syndrome
- Monitor for mental status changes

- Teach patient to report bleeding to prescriber
- Teach patient to report signs and symptoms of infection to prescriber
- Teach patient to avoid bleeding (use soft-bristled tooth brush and electric razor)
- Teach patient to report sudden, severe headache to prescriber

Antiplatelets

- Used to prevent arterial thromboembolism
- Examples include salicylic acid, clopidogrel, dipyridamole, ticlopidine
- Available in PO, IV, rectal preparations

Mode of Action
- Decreases platelet aggregation

Contraindications, Precautions, and Drug Interactions of Antiplatelets*

Drug	Contraindications/Precautions	Drug Interaction
salicylic acid	*Contraindications:* Hypersensitivity to salicylates, pregnancy third trimester, breastfeeding, children <12 years, children with flu symptoms, acute bronchospasm, agranulocytosis, bleeding disorders, GI bleeding, peptic ulcer, increased intracranial pressure, intracranial bleeding, nasal polyps, urticaria, vitamin K deficiency *Precautions:* Pregnancy first trimester, acetaminophen/ NSAIDs hypersensitivity, acid/base imbalance, alcoholism, anemia, ascites, asthma, dehydration, G6PD deficiency, gastritis, gout, heart failure, hepatic/renal disease *Pregnancy:* *First trimester:* Only given after risks to the fetus are considered; animal studies have shown adverse reactions; no human studies available *Third trimester:* Definite fetal risks, may be given in spite of risks if needed in life-threatening conditions	Alcohol, antiinflammatories, corticosteroids, NSAIDs, plicamycin, cefamandole, thrombolytics, ticlopidine, clopidogrel, tirofiban, eptifibatide, anticoagulants, thrombolytic agents, insulin, methotrexate, penicillins, phenytoin, valproic acid, sulfonamide, oral hypoglycemics, nizatidine, urinary acidifiers, ammonium chloride, nitroglycerin, antacids, ACE inhibitors, probenecid, spironolactone, sulfinpyrazone, sulfonyl amides, beta blockers, loop diuretics
clopidogrel	*Contraindications:* Hypersensitivity, active bleeding *Precautions:* Breastfeeding, children, Asian/Black/Caucasian patients, agranulocytosis, increased bleeding risk, neutropenia, previous hepatic disease, renal disease *Pregnancy:* No adverse effects in animals, no human studies available	Anticoagulants, aspirin, abciximab, eptifibatide, NSAIDs, tirofiban, thrombolytics, ticlopidine, rifampin, SSRIs, treprostinil, proton pump inhibitors
dipyridamole	*Contraindications:* Hypersensitivity *Precautions:* Breastfeeding, asthma, hepatic disease, hypotension, labor, unstable angina *Pregnancy:* No adverse effects in animals, no human studies available	Theophylline, anticoagulants, NSAIDs, digoxin, salicylates, cefotetan, sulfinpyrazone, valproic acid, thrombolytics
ticlopidine	*Contraindications:* Hypersensitivity, active bleeding, coagulopathy, severe hepatic disease *Precautions:* Breastfeeding, children, geriatric patients, past hepatic disease, increased bleeding risk, peptic ulcer disease, renal disease, surgery *Pregnancy:* No adverse effects in animals, no human studies available	

*Pregnancy categories have been revised. See http://www.fda.gov/Drugs/DevelopmentApprovalProcess/DevelopmentResources/Labeling/ucm093307.htm for more information.

Adverse Effects/Side Effects

- Headache
- Confusion
- Dizziness
- Drowsiness
- Flushing
- Seizures
- Coma
- Intracranial hemorrhage
- Anaphylaxis
- Laryngeal edema
- Angioedema
- Wheezing
- Bronchospasm
- Dysrhythmias
- Pulmonary edema
- Tinnitus
- Hearing loss
- Hypoglycemia
- Nausea
- Vomiting
- Diarrhea
- GI bleeding
- GI ulcer
- Hepatitis
- Jaundice
- Hepatic failure
- Pancreatitis
- Glomerulonephritis
- Thrombocytopenia
- Thrombocytopenic purpura
- Agranulocytosis
- Leukopenia
- Neutropenia
- Hemolytic anemia
- Aplastic anemia
- Rash
- Urticaria
- Bruising
- Toxic epidermal necrolysis
- Stevens-Johnson syndrome
- Reye's syndrome (children)

Nursing Care

- Administer with full glass of water
- Administer with food
- Do not administer to children/teens with flu-like symptoms
- Monitor for pain
- Monitor for fever
- Monitor renal/hepatic studies
- Monitor blood studies
- Monitor for allergic reaction
- Monitor for ototoxicity
- Monitor for MI, stroke
- Teach patient not to exceed recommended dosage
- Teach patient to avoid OTC products that contain aspirin/salicylates
- Teach patient to avoid alcohol
- Teach patient to change positions slowly
- Teach patients with allergies, nasal polyps, asthma to monitor for allergic reaction
- Teach patient to report unusual bruising, bleeding to prescriber
- Teach patient to report signs and symptoms of infection to prescriber
- Teach patient that medication may need to be discontinued before surgery

Antianemics

- Used to treat anemia
- Examples include epoetin alfa, darbepoetin alfa, methoxy polyethylene glycol-epoetin beta, ferrous gluconate, ferrous sulfate, cyanocobalamin (vitamin B_{12}), folic acid (vitamin B_9)
- Available in PO, IM, IV, SUBCUT preparations

Mode of Action
- Epoetins/vitamins B_9, B_{12}: increases red blood cell production
- Iron supplements: replace iron stores needed for red blood cell development

Contraindications, Precautions, and Drug Interactions of Antianemics*

Drug	Contraindications/Precautions	Drug Interaction
epoetin alfa	*Contraindications:* Hypersensitivity to human albumin/mammalian-cell-derived products, uncontrolled hypertension, pure red cell aplasia *Precautions:* Breastfeeding, children <1 mo, CV disease, hemodialysis, history of CABG, hypertension, porphyria, latex allergy, seizure disorder *Pregnancy:* Only given after risks to the fetus are considered; animal studies have shown adverse reactions; no human studies available	Increased heparin during hemodialysis
darbepoetin alfa	*Contraindications:* Hypersensitivity to human albumin/mammalian-cell-derived products, uncontrolled hypertension, pure red cell aplasia *Precautions:* Breastfeeding, bleeding, CHF, folic acid/iron/vitamin B_{12} deficiency *Pregnancy:* Only given after risks to the fetus are considered; animal studies have shown adverse reactions; no human studies available	Alcohol
methoxy polyethylene glycol-epoetin beta	*Contraindications:* Hypersensitivity, severe renal disease *Precautions:* Breastfeeding, hypertension, MI, stroke, CHF, CABG, thrombosis *Pregnancy:* Only given after risks to the fetus are considered; animal studies have shown adverse reactions; no human studies available	No known drug interactions
ferrous gluconate/ferrous sulfate	*Contraindications:* Hypersensitivity, hemosiderosis/hemochromatosis, sideroblastic anemia, thalassemia *Precautions:* Hemolytic anemia, cirrhosis, peptic ulcer disease, ulcerative colitis, sulfite sensitivity *Pregnancy:* No adverse effects in animals; no human studies available	Ascorbic acid, chloramphenicol, penicillamine, levodopa, methyldopa, tetracycline, fluoroquinolones, l-thyroxine, H_2 antagonists, proton pump inhibitors, antacids, cholestyramine, vitamin E
cyanocobalamin (vitamin B_{12})	*Contraindications:* Hypersensitivity to cyanocobalamin/cobalt/benzyl alcohol, optic nerve atrophy *Precautions:* Breastfeeding, children, folic acid deficiency anemia, iron deficiency anemia, infection, renal/hepatic disease *Pregnancy:* No risk demonstrated to the fetus in any trimester	Aminoglycosides, anticonvulsants, colchicine, chloramphenicol, aminosalicylic acid, potassium preparations, prednisone, cimetidine
folic acid (vitamin B_9)	*Contraindications:* Hypersensitivity, breastfeeding *Precautions:* Vitamin B_{12} deficiency anemia, uncorrected pernicious anemia, anemias other than megaloblastic/macrocytic anemia *Pregnancy:* No risk demonstrated to the fetus in any trimester	Estrogen, hydantoins, carbamazepine, glucocorticosteroids, methotrexate, sulfonamides, sulfasalazine, trimethoprim, phenytoin, fosphenytoin

*Pregnancy categories have been revised. See http://www.fda.gov/Drugs/DevelopmentApprovalProcess/DevelopmentResources/Labeling/ucm093307.htm for more information.

Adverse Effects/Side Effects

- Headache
- Dizziness
- Fatigue
- Diaphoresis
- Coldness
- Flushing
- Seizures
- Anaphylaxis
- Bronchospasm
- Optic nerve atrophy
- Pulmonary edema
- Cough
- CHF
- Edema
- DVT
- Hypertension

- Hypertensive encephalopathy
- Nausea
- Vomiting
- Diarrhea
- Constipation
- Epigastric pain
- Black/red tarry stools
- Iron deficiency
- Thromboembolism
- Peripheral vascular thrombosis
- Hypokalemia
- Arthralgia
- Myalgia
- Bone pain
- Rash
- Pruritus

Nursing Care

- Do not shake vial for IV, SUBCUT preparations
- Do not administer iron supplements with dairy products, eggs, caffeine
- Monitor GI function
- Monitor for cardiac/respiratory distress
- Monitor renal/hepatic function
- Monitor blood studies
- Monitor for hypertension
- Monitor for CNS changes
- Monitor for allergic, toxicity reaction
- Assess thrill/bruit of shunts in dialysis patients
- Teach patient to avoid driving and other hazardous activities
- Teach patient to avoid alcohol and tobacco
- Teach patient that iron supplements may cause constipation and turn stools black
- Teach patient that iron supplements may stain teeth
- Teach patient to follow high-iron, high folic-acid diet
- Teach patient that urine will turn bright yellow with folic acid use

APPLICATION AND REVIEW

5. What specifically should the nurse monitor when a client is receiving a platelet aggregation inhibitor such as clopidogrel (Plavix)?
   1. Nausea
   2. Epistaxis
   3. Chest pain
   4. Elevated temperature
6. A nurse is evaluating the results of treatment with erythropoietin (Epogen). Which client response is considered significant?
   1. Elevation in liver panel
   2. Increase in WBC counts
   3. Elevation in hematocrit level
   4. Decrease in Kaposi sarcoma lesions

7. A client with upper gastrointestinal (GI) bleeding develops mild anemia. What should the nurse expect to be prescribed for this client?
   1. Epogen
   2. Dextran
   3. Iron salts
   4. Vitamin B_{12}

8. Cyanocobalamin (vitamin B_{12}) 0.2 mg IM is prescribed for a client with pernicious anemia. A vial of the drug labeled "1 mL = 100 mcg" is available. How many milliliters should the nurse administer? **Record your answer using a whole number.**

9. A nurse determines that teaching regarding vitamin B_{12} injections to treat pernicious anemia is understood when a client states, "I must take the drug:
   1. when feeling fatigued."
   2. until my symptoms subside."
   3. monthly, for the rest of my life."
   4. during exacerbations of anemia."

See Answers on pages 219-221.

Miscellaneous Antianemics

- Used to treat sickle cell anemia, aplastic anemia
- Examples include hydroxyurea, cyclosporine, cyclophosphamide, filgrastim, sargramostim, lymphocyte immune globulin
- Available in PO, IV, SUBCUT preparations

Mode of Action

- Various modes of action to improve red blood cell production, reduce red blood cell destruction

Contraindications, Precautions, and Drug Interactions of Miscellaneous Antianemics*

Drug	Contraindications/Precautions	Drug Interaction
hydroxyurea	**Contraindications:** Hypersensitivity, breastfeeding, leukopenia, thrombocytopenia, severe anemia **Precautions:** Geriatric patients, anemia, bone marrow suppression, dental disease, HIV, hyperkalemia, hyperphosphatemia, hyperuricemia, hypocalcemia, infection, infertility, IM injection, tumor lysis syndrome, vaccinations **Pregnancy:** Definite fetal risks, may be given in spite of risks if needed in life-threatening conditions	Antineoplastics, radiation, didanosine, stavudine, anticoagulants, salicylates, NSAIDs, thrombolytics, platelet inhibitors, probenecid, sulfinpyrazone, live virus vaccines
cyclosporine	**Contraindications:** Hypersensitivity, breastfeeding **Precautions:** Geriatric patients, severe hepatic disease **Pregnancy:** Only given after risks to the fetus are considered; animal studies have shown adverse reactions; no human studies available	Allopurinol, amiodarone, amphotericin B, androgens, azole antifungals, beta blockers, bromocriptine, calcium channel blockers, carvedilol, cimetidine, colchicine, corticosteroids, fluoroquinolones, foscarnet, imipenem-cilastatin, macrolides, metoclopramide, oral contraceptives, NSAIDs, melphalan, SSRIs, digoxin, etoposide, methotrexate, potassium-sparing diuretics, HMG-CoA reductase inhibitors, aliskiren, sirolimus, tacrolimus, anticonvulsants, nafcillin, orlistat, phenobarbital, rifamycins, phenytoin, sulfamethoxazole, trimethoprim, terbinafine, ticlopidine, live virus vaccines

Contraindications, Precautions, and Drug Interactions of Miscellaneous Antianemics—cont'd

Drug	Contraindications/Precautions	Drug Interaction
cyclophosphamide	**Contraindications:** Hypersensitivity, bladder neck obstruction, prostatic hypertrophy **Precautions:** Breastfeeding, children, geriatric patients, anemia, cardiac disease, dysrhythmias, dialysis, dental disease, heart failure, hematuria, infection, leukopenia, tumor lysis syndrome, QT prolongation, severely depressed bone marrow function, vaccinations **Pregnancy:** Definite fetal risks, may be given in spite of risks if needed in life-threatening conditions	Barbiturates, warfarin, succinylcholine, thiazides, allopurinol, insulin, digoxin, chloramphenicol, corticosteroids, live virus vaccine
filgrastim	**Contraindications:** Hypersensitivity to *E. coli* proteins **Precautions:** Breastfeeding, children, chemotherapy, myeloid malignancies, radiation, sepsis, respiratory disease, sickle cell disease **Pregnancy:** Only given after risks to the fetus are considered; animal studies have shown adverse reactions; no human studies available	Antineoplastics, lithium
sargramostim	**Contraindications:** Hypersensitivity to GM-CSF/benzyl alcohol/yeast products, neonates **Precautions:** Breastfeeding, children, cardiac/hepatic/pulmonary/renal disease, leukocytosis, mannitol hypersensitivity, pericardial effusions, peripheral edema **Pregnancy:** Only given after risks to the fetus are considered; animal studies have shown adverse reactions; no human studies available	Corticosteroids, lithium
lymphocyte immune globulin	**Contraindications:** Hypersensitivity to lymphocyte immune globulin/equine protein/leporine protein **Precautions:** Breastfeeding, children, hepatic/renal disease, leukopenia, thrombocytopenia **Pregnancy:** Only given after risks to the fetus are considered; animal studies have shown adverse reactions; no human studies available	No known drug interactions

*Pregnancy categories have been revised. See http://www.fda.gov/Drugs/DevelopmentApprovalProcess/DevelopmentResources/Labeling/ucm093307.htm for more information.

Adverse Effects/Side Effects

- Headache
- Dizziness
- Confusion
- Hallucinations
- Tremors
- Encephalopathy
- Fever
- Chills
- Malaise
- Anaphylaxis
- Seizures
- Pulmonary fibrosis
- Diffuse pulmonary infiltrates
- Interstitial pneumonia
- ARDs
- Angina
- Ischemia
- Cardiotoxicity
- Myocardial fibrosis
- CHF
- Pericarditis
- Nausea
- Vomiting
- Diarrhea
- Constipation
- Anorexia
- Stomatitis
- Hepatotoxicity
- Pancreatitis
- Renal failure
- Renal tubular fibrosis
- Hemolytic uremic syndrome
- Hemorrhagic cystitis

- Nephrotoxicity
- Albuminuria
- Hematuria
- Proteinuria
- Leukopenia
- Anemia

- Thrombocytopenia
- Pancytopenia
- Myelosuppression
- Megaloblastic erythropoiesis
- Tumor lysis syndrome
- Secondary cancers

- Rash
- Urticaria
- Pruritus
- Facial erythema
- Dry skin

Nursing Care

- Administer antiemetic 30 to 60 minutes before drug
- Administer with food or milk to prevent GI upset
- Administer at same time every day
- Do not break, crush, chew tablets
- Monitor for bone marrow suppression
- Monitor renal/hepatic function
- Monitor I&O
- Monitor for infection
- Monitor for bleeding
- Monitor for cardiac/respiratory distress
- Monitor for allergic reaction, anaphylaxis
- Monitor for CNS changes
- Teach patient to brush teeth with soft-bristled toothbrush and use electric razor
- Teach patient to report signs and symptoms of infection
- Teach patient to report signs and symptoms of anemia
- Teach patient to report signs and symptoms of CNS changes
- Teach patient to report bleeding
- Teach patient to avoid aspirin, ibuprofen products
- Teach patient not to skip, double doses

Thrombopoietin Receptor Agonists

- Used to treat idiopathic thrombocytopenic purpura
- Examples include romiplostim
- Available in SUBCUT preparations

Mode of Action

- Aids bone marrow in platelet production

Contraindications, Precautions, and Drug Interactions of Thrombopoietin Receptor Agonists*

Drug	Contraindications/Precautions	Drug Interaction
romiplostim	**Contraindications:** Hypersensitivity to romiplostim/ mannitol **Precautions:** Breastfeeding, children, bleeding, bone marrow suppression, malignancies **Pregnancy:** Only given after risks to the fetus are considered; animal studies have shown adverse reactions; no human studies available	Anticoagulants, NSAIDs, platelet inhibitors, thrombolytics, salicylates

*Pregnancy categories have been revised. See http://www.fda.gov/Drugs/DevelopmentApprovalProcess/DevelopmentResources/Labeling/ucm093307.htm for more information.

Adverse Effects/Side Effects

- Headache
- Fatigue
- Insomnia
- Dizziness
- Diarrhea

- Abdominal pain
- Dyspepsia
- Thromboembolism
- Thrombosis
- Bleeding

- Myelofibrosis
- Erythromelalgia
- Myalgia
- Antibody formation
- Secondary malignancy

Nursing Care

- Monitor blood studies
- Monitor for infection
- Monitor for bleeding
- Teach patient to report signs and symptoms of infection
- Teach patient to report bleeding
- Teach patient to avoid activities that may cause bleeding
- Teach patient to report missed dose to prescriber (increased risk of bleeding)
- Teach patient that regular laboratory tests will be performed

Antifibrinolytics/Hemostatics

- Used to treat excessive bleeding, DIC
- Examples include tranexamic acid, aprotinin, ethamsylate
- Available in PO, IV preparations

Mode of Action

- Promotes platelet adhesion to maintain clots

Contraindications, Precautions, and Drug Interactions of Antifibrinolytics/Hemostatics*

Drug	Contraindications/Precautions	Drug Interaction
tranexamic acid	*Contraindications:* Hypersensitivity to tranexamic acid, bleeding *Precautions:* Renal disease *Pregnancy:* No adverse effects in animals; no human studies available	Estrogen, progestin, anticoagulants, hormonal contraceptives
aprotinin	*Contraindications:* Hypersensitivity to aprotinin, previous exposure to aprotinin in past 12 months, bleeding *Precautions:* Renal/hepatic disease *Pregnancy:* No adverse effects in animals; no human studies available	Fibrinolytic agents, captopril, heparin
ethamsylate	*Contraindications:* Hypersensitivity to aprotinin, previous exposure to aprotinin in past 12 months, bleeding *Precautions:* Renal/hepatic disease *Pregnancy:* No adverse effects in animals; no human studies available	Fibrinolytic agents

*Pregnancy categories have been revised. See http://www.fda.gov/Drugs/DevelopmentApprovalProcess/DevelopmentResources/Labeling/ucm093307.htm for more information.

Adverse Effects/Side Effects

- Headache
- Fatigue
- Anaphylaxis
- Angioedema
- Changes in color vision
- Pulmonary embolism

- Hypotension
- Vomiting
- Diarrhea
- Abdominal pain
- DVT
- Anemia

- Arthralgia
- Myalgia
- Rash
- Pruritus
- Urticaria

Nursing Care
- Ensure emergency life-saving equipment/medications are on hand
- Monitor renal/hepatic function
- Monitor I&O
- Monitor for infection
- Monitor for bleeding
- Monitor for cardiac/respiratory distress
- Monitor for allergic reaction, anaphylaxis
- Teach patient to report signs and symptoms of infection
- Teach patient to report signs and symptoms of anemia
- Teach patient to report bleeding

Antihemophiliacs
- Used to prevent and treat bleeding in hemophilia A and B
- Examples include desmopressin, clotting factor VII, clotting factor IX
- Available in PO, IV, SUBCUT, intranasal preparations

Mode of Action
- Increases platelet aggregation

Contraindications, Precautions, and Drug Interactions of Antihemophiliacs*

Drug	Contraindications/Precautions	Drug Interaction
desmopressin	**Contraindications:** Hypersensitivity, hyponatremia, nephrogenic diabetes insipidus, severe renal disease **Precautions:** Breastfeeding, male infertility, CAD, cystic fibrosis, hypertension, electrolyte imbalance, thrombus **Pregnancy:** No adverse effects in animals; no human studies available	Carbamazepine, chlorpropamide, clofibrate, lamotrigine, SSRIs, pressor products, alcohol, lithium, heparin, demeclocycline
clotting factor VII	**Contraindications:** Hypersensitivity, hyponatremia, nephrogenic diabetes insipidus, severe renal disease **Precautions:** Breastfeeding, male infertility, CAD, cystic fibrosis, hypertension, electrolyte imbalance, thrombus **Pregnancy:** Only given after risks to the fetus are considered; animal studies have shown adverse reactions; no human studies available	Antifibrinolytics
clotting factor IX	**Contraindications:** Hypersensitivity, hyponatremia, nephrogenic diabetes insipidus, severe renal disease **Precautions:** Breastfeeding, male infertility, CAD, cystic fibrosis, hypertension, electrolyte imbalance, thrombus **Pregnancy:** Only given after risks to the fetus are considered; animal studies have shown adverse reactions; no human studies available	Antifibrinolytics

*Pregnancy categories have been revised. See http://www.fda.gov/Drugs/DevelopmentApprovalProcess/DevelopmentResources/Labeling/ucm093307.htm for more information.

Adverse Effects/Side Effects
- Headache
- Lethargy
- Drowsiness
- Fever
- Confusion
- Flushing
- Seizures
- Anaphylaxis
- Hypo/hypertension
- Paresthesias
- Palpitation
- Tachycardia
- Nasal congestion
- Rhinitis
- Nausea

- Vomiting
- Abdominal cramps
- Heartburn

- Hyponatremia
- Oliguria
- Bleeding

- Arthralgia
- Rash
- Urticaria

Nursing Care

- Weigh patient daily
- Monitor bleeding times
- Monitor for I&O
- Monitor for edema, water intoxication
- Monitor for allergic reaction, anaphylaxis

- Monitor vitals when administering IV, SUBCUT
- Teach patient to avoid OTC products
- Teach patient to wear emergency ID specifying therapy
- Teach patient not to skip, double doses

APPLICATION AND REVIEW

10. A client has been prescribed medication to increase platelet aggregation. Which medical diagnosis should the nurse recognize as a contraindication for this medication therapy? **Select all that apply.**
    1. Hypertension
    2. Hyponatremia
    3. Cystic fibrosis
    4. Diabetes insipidus
    5. Severe renal disease

See Answers on pages 219-221.

ANSWER KEY: REVIEW QUESTIONS

1. **1 Baseline vital signs should be obtained immediately before administering the blood product for future comparison purposes. Two licensed nurses should confirm the verifying data between the client and the blood product. The nurse should remain with and monitor the client's vital signs during the first 15 minutes of administration of the blood product and then follow the institution's protocol to monitor for a transfusion reaction or fluid overload.**

   2 Vital signs must be taken immediately before the blood product infusion is begun for accurate future comparisons. 3 It is not necessary for the licensed nurse verifying the data between the client and the blood product to be a supervisor. 4 Blood should not be hung without following the appropriate protocol for ensuring accuracy of the blood product for the client; the nurse should remain with and monitor the client's vital signs during the first 15 minutes of administration of the blood product to monitor for a transfusion reaction or fluid overload.

   Client Need: Pharmacologic and Parenteral Therapies; Cognitive Level: Analysis; Integrated Process: Communication/Documentation; Nursing Process: Planning/Implementation

2. **1 An anticoagulant should not be administered to a client who is bleeding because it will interfere with clotting and will increase hemorrhage.** 2 "If necessary it will be started to enhance circulation" is unsafe; it will not be used in this situation. 3 "If necessary it will be stated to prevent pulmonary thrombosis" is unsafe; it will not be used in this situation. 4 An anticoagulant is contraindicated because, if given, it will increase, not mask, the effects of the hemorrhage.

   Clinical Area: Medical-Surgical Nursing; Client Needs: Pharmacologic and Parenteral Therapies; Cognitive Level: Application; Nursing Process: Planning/Implementation

3. **2 Desired anticoagulant effect is achieved when the activated partial thromboplastin time is 1.5 to 2 times normal.**

   1 Although anticoagulants help prevent thrombi that could block cerebral circulation, they do not increase cerebral perfusion, and so will not affect existing confusion. 3 Although absence of bleeding suggests

that the drug has not reached toxic levels, it does not indicate its effectiveness. **4** Continuous heparin infusion does not affect the viscosity of blood.
Client Need: Pharmacologic and Parenteral Therapies; **Cognitive Level:** Application; **Nursing Process:** Evaluation/ Outcomes

4. **1 Warfarin (Coumadin) initially is prescribed day by day, based on international normalized ratio (INR) blood test results. This test provides a standard system to interpret prothrombin times.**
   2 aPTT (accelerated partial thromboplastin time) is used to evaluate the effects of heparin, which acts on the intrinsic pathway. **3** Bleeding time is the time required for blood to cease flowing from a small wound; it is not used for warfarin dosage calculation. **4** Sedimentation rate is a test used to determine the presence of inflammation or infection; it does not indicate clotting ability.
   Client Need: Reduction of Risk Potential; **Cognitive Level:** Analysis; **Nursing Process:** Evaluation/Outcomes

5. **2 The high vascularity of the nose, combined with its susceptibility to trauma (e.g., sneezing, nose blowing), makes it a frequent site of hemorrhage.**
   1, 3, 4 Nausea, chest pain, and elevated temperature are not associated with anticoagulant therapy.
   Client Need: Pharmacologic and Parenteral Therapies; **Cognitive Level:** Application; **Nursing Process:** Evaluation/ Outcomes

6. **3 Erythropoietin (Epogen) stimulates red blood cell production, thereby elevating hematocrit levels.**
   1 An increased liver panel may signify liver disease; it is not affected by erythropoietin. **2** WBC counts are not affected by erythropoietin. **4** Kaposi sarcoma lesions signify progression of HIV and are not affected by erythropoietin.
   Clinical Area: Medical-Surgical Nursing; **Client Needs:** Pharmacologic and Parenteral Therapies; **Cognitive Level:** Analysis; **Nursing Process:** Evaluation/Outcomes

> **Study Tip:** Remember medical terminology word parts! Erythr/o means "red" (red blood cell); think "erythema". And -poietin means "that which stimulates". So erythropoietin literally means "that which stimulates red blood cells"— which make the hematocrit increase.

7. **3 Iron is needed in the formation of hemoglobin.**
   1 The client's anemia is caused by GI bleeding, not impaired RBC production. **2** Dextran is a plasma volume expander; it does not affect erythrocyte production. **4** Vitamin B_{12} is a water-soluble vitamin that must be used as a supplement when an individual has pernicious anemia.
   Client Need: Pharmacologic and Parenteral Therapies; **Cognitive Level:** Analysis; **Nursing Process:** Planning/ Implementation

8. **Answer: 2**
   First, convert milligrams to micrograms by moving the decimal point three places to the right (0.2 mg = 200 mcg). Use ratio and proportion to solve the problem.

$$\frac{\text{Desired}}{\text{Have}} \quad \frac{200\,\text{mc}}{100\,\text{mcg}} = \frac{x\,\text{mL}}{1\,\text{mL}}$$

$$100\,x = 200$$
$$x = 200 \div 100$$
$$x = 2\,\text{mL}$$

   Clinical Area: Medical-Surgical Nursing; **Client Needs:** Pharmacologic and Parenteral Therapies; **Cognitive Level:** Application; **Nursing Process:** Planning/Implementation

9. **3 Because the intrinsic factor does not return to gastric secretions even with therapy, B_{12} injections will be required for the remainder of the client's life.**
   1, 2, 4 B_{12} injections must be taken on a regular basis for the rest of the client's life.

Clinical Area: Medical-Surgical Nursing; **Client Needs:** Pharmacologic and Parenteral Therapies; **Cognitive Level:** Application; **Nursing Process:** Evaluation/Outcomes

> **Study Tip:** Use this silly mnemonic to recall that B_{12} injections are needed on a lifelong basis: **Be** happy you can get **B_{12}** injections, **Be**cause it will help you **Be** well for the rest of your life—which could **Be 12** years or longer!

10. **Answers: 2, 4, 5**

Antihemophiliac therapy is prescribed to increase platelet aggregation. Diabetes insipidus, hyponatremia and severe renal disease are considered contraindications for the antihemophiliac therapy. Research has determined that the risks caused by antihemophiliac therapy to clients diagnosed with these conditions far exceed the potential benefits.

1 Hypertension is recognized as a precautionary condition when considering antihemophiliac therapy. The decision to prescribe the medication is determined after weighing the potential benefits versus the potential risks. **3** Cystic fibrosis is recognized as a precautionary condition when considering antihemophiliac therapy. The decision to prescribe the medication is determined after weighing the potential benefits versus the potential risks.

Client Need: Pharmacologic and Parenteral Therapies; **Cognitive Level:** Analysis; **Nursing Process:** Assessment/Analysis

12 Antidiabetic Drugs

INTRODUCTION TO DIABETES MELLITUS

Etiology and Pathophysiology

- Hyperglycemia occurs with insufficient secretion of insulin, peripheral cells become insulin-resistant, and/or hepatic glucose production is increased
- Body attempts to excrete excess glucose via kidneys; osmotic force is created because of excess glucose in urine, resulting in polyuria
- If body is unable to use carbohydrates for cellular function, fat is oxidized as an energy source; oxidation of fats produces ketone bodies
- Risk factors
  - Type 1: genetic predisposition; environmental factors (e.g., toxins, viruses); age younger than 30 years
  - Type 2: family history, obesity, usually age 45 years or older, history of gestational diabetes, increasing incidence in childhood and adolescence
- Classification
  - Type 1: formerly known as insulin-dependent diabetes mellitus (IDDM); destruction of beta cells leads to inability to produce insulin; requires exogenous insulin
  - Type 2: formerly known as non–insulin-dependent diabetes mellitus (NIDDM); has gradual onset and pancreas produces some insulin so that ketoacidosis is unlikely; may be controlled with adherence to diet and exercise program that promotes maintenance of desirable weight; accounts for 90% of diabetes
  - Gestational: detected during 24 to 28 weeks' gestation; glucose levels generally are normal 6 weeks postpartum; more likely to develop type 2 diabetes 5 to 10 years after birth of fetus; neonate exhibits macrosomia, hypoglycemia, hypocalcemia, and hyperbilirubinemia
  - Diabetes mellitus associated with other conditions or syndromes (formerly known as secondary diabetes): associated with glucocorticoid medication and conditions such as Cushing syndrome and pancreatic disease
  - Impaired glucose tolerance: high glucose levels but not sufficiently high to be diagnostic for diabetes; prediabetes—fasting serum glucose level of 100 to 125 mg/dL
- Acute increases in serum glucose levels: diabetic ketoacidosis (DKA) and hyperglycemic hyperosmolar nonketotic syndrome (HHNS) constitute medical emergencies
  - Causes: insufficient insulin, major stresses (e.g., infection, surgery, trauma, pregnancy, emotional turmoil, nausea and vomiting); drugs (steroids); glucose load
  - Pathophysiology
    - DKA is associated with type 1; inadequate insulin to support basal needs; proteins and fats are used for energy; ketones are excreted via urine and breathing; dehydration and electrolyte imbalances occur; serum glucose level 300 to 600 mg/dL; acidosis with pH<7.35
    - HHNS is associated with type 2; hyperglycemia increases intravascular osmotic pressure, leading to polyuria and cellular dehydration; serum glucose level 500 to 900 mg/dL
- Acute decrease in serum glucose level: hypoglycemia
  - Causes: excess insulin or oral antidiabetic medications; too little food or too much exercise when receiving antidiabetic medications

- Pathophysiology: excessive insulin lowers serum glucose level as glucose is carried into cells; decreased food intake in relation to prescribed antidiabetic medications results in hypoglycemia; excessive exercise uses glucose for metabolism, decreasing serum glucose level
- Long-term complications: all types subject to same complications; microangiopathy (e.g., retinopathy, nephropathy), macroangiopathy (e.g., peripheral vascular diseases, arteriosclerosis, coronary heart disease, cerebral vascular disease), neuropathy, skin problems (e.g., cellulitis, fungal infections, boils), periodontal disease (Fig. 12.1)

Clinical Findings

- Subjective: polydipsia; polyphagia; fatigue; blurred vision (retinopathy; osmotic changes); peripheral neuropathy
- Objective
  - Polyuria; weight loss; glycosuria; peripheral vascular changes; ulcers; delayed wound healing; infection; gangrene

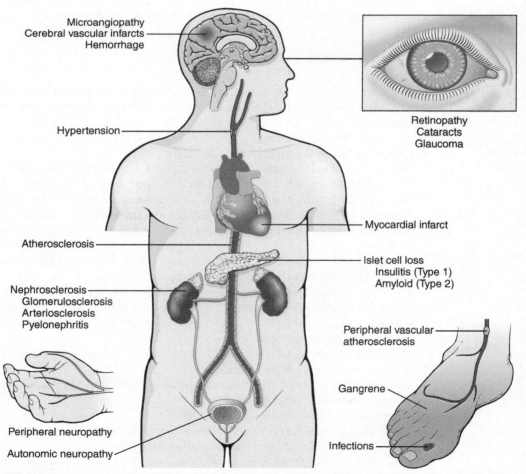

FIG. 12.1   Long-term complications of diabetes mellitus. (From Kumar, V., Abbas, A. K., Aster, J. C. [2015]. *Robbins and Cotran pathologic basis of disease* [9th ed.]. Philadelphia: Saunders.)

- Hyperglycemia: detected by casual plasma glucose measurement of 200 mg/dL or higher, fasting plasma glucose level of 126 mg/dL or higher, and 2-hour postload glucose level of 200 mg/dL or higher; monitored by hemoglobin A$_{1c}$ (Hb A$_{1c}$, glycosylated hemoglobin) measurement, which reflects average glucose level over preceding 2 to 3 months and should not exceed 7%
- DKA and HHNS
  - Hyperglycemia, glycosuria, polyuria
  - Dehydration (e.g., flushed, hot, dry skin; decreased skin turgor [tenting]); hyperosmolar blood; hypotension; tachycardia; thirst; headache; confusion; drowsiness
  - Metabolic acidosis (DKA only): Kussmaul respirations as body attempts to blow off carbon dioxide; ketonuria, sweet breath odor, anorexia, nausea, vomiting, decreased serum pH, decreased PCO_2, decreased HCO_3
- Hypoglycemia
  - Insulin shock or reaction because of excessive insulin, deficient glucose, or excessive exercise
  - Clinical findings result from sympathetic nervous system (SNS) stimulation or reduced cerebral glucose supply
  - CNS effects (e.g., mental confusion, blurred vision, diplopia, slurred speech, fatigue, seizures)
  - SNS (adrenergic) effects (e.g., nervousness, weakness, pallor, diaphoresis, tremor, tachycardia, hunger)

Therapeutic Interventions

- Lifestyle changes
  - Weight control: obesity leads to insulin resistance that can be reversed by weight loss
  - Regular exercise: increases insulin sensitivity; brisk walking, swimming, and bicycling are recommended
  - Diet: current recommendations
    - Caloric control to maintain ideal body weight
    - 50% to 60% of caloric intake from carbohydrates with emphasis on complex carbohydrates, high-fiber foods rich in water-soluble fiber (e.g., oat bran, peas, all forms of beans, pectin-rich fruits and vegetables); avoidance of foods with high glycemic index (glycemic index refers to effect of particular foods on blood glucose level)
    - Protein: consistent with the U.S. Dietary Guidelines, usually 60 to 85 g; 12% to 20% of daily calories
    - Fat intake not to exceed 30% of daily calories (70 to 90 g/day); replace saturated fats with monounsaturated and polyunsaturated fats
    - Dietary ratio: carbohydrate to protein to fat ratio usually about 5:1:2
    - Distribute food evenly throughout the day in three or four meals, with snacks added between meals and at bedtime as needed in accordance with total food allowance and therapy (insulin or oral hypoglycemics)
    - Consistent, regulated food intake is basic to disease control with consistent exercise, medication, and glucose monitoring
    - Basic tools for planning diet: food composition tables showing nutrient content and glycemic index of commonly used foods
  - Self-monitoring of blood glucose (SMBG) level
    - Blood glucose monitoring: finger stick—a drop of blood from the fingertip is put on a special reagent strip, which is read by glucose monitor
    - Interstitial glucose monitoring: continuous interstitial testing (via biosensor inserted subcutaneously) or intermittent transdermal testing (via interstitial fluid drawn through skin and tested with electrochemical sensor)

- Alternate site testing: forearm, upper arm, abdomen, thigh, base of thumb; rests fingertips; alternate sites have less capillary blood flow than fingertips and may not reflect glucose levels that rapidly rise and fall; rotate site within one area consistently unless otherwise instructed because results at various areas differ
  - Use fingertip if hypoglycemia is expected or if client is experiencing rapid change in glucose level
  - Rub forearm vigorously until warm before testing
  - Use monitor designed for alternate site testing
  - Avoid use in arm on side of mastectomy; results may be lower; reduces risk of infection and lymphedema
- Insulin administration
  - Adjusted after considering physical and emotional stresses; a specific type of insulin and schedule are prescribed; aggressive insulin therapy regimens are gold standard of care
  - Insulin pump
    - External battery-operated device delivers insulin through needle inserted into subcutaneous tissue
    - Small (basal) doses of regular insulin programmed into computer and delivered every few minutes; bolus doses (extra preset amounts) delivered before meals
    - Improves glucose control for clients with wide variations in insulin need as result of irregular schedules, pregnancy, or growth requirements
    - Prescribed amount of insulin for 24 hours plus priming is drawn into syringe
    - Administration set is primed and needle inserted aseptically, usually into subcutaneous tissue of abdomen
  - Jet injectors: deliver medication through skin under pressure
- Oral antidiabetics for certain clients with type 2 diabetes who cannot be managed with lifestyle changes alone; must have some functioning beta cells in islets of Langerhans
- Other therapies: pancreatic islet cell grafts, pancreas transplants, implantable insulin pumps that continually monitor blood glucose level and release insulin accordingly, cyclosporin therapy to prevent beta cell destruction in type 1 diabetes
- Management of DKA and HHNS
  - IV to provide fluid replacement and direct access to circulatory system, and indwelling urinary catheter to monitor urine output
  - Titration of IV regular insulin according to serum glucose levels
  - Replacement of lost electrolytes, particularly sodium and potassium, using blood studies to determine dosage; when insulin is administered, potassium reenters the cell, resulting in hypokalemia
  - Cardiac monitoring if circulatory collapse is imminent or dysrhythmias associated with electrolyte imbalance occur
  - Acidosis treated according to cause
  - Monitoring for hypoglycemia as result of treatment
- Management of hypoglycemia (insulin shock or reaction)
  - 15 g of carbohydrate (e.g., glucose gel, 3 glucose tablets, 4 to 6 ounces of juice or soda, hard candy, 1 cup milk, ½ banana, 6 saltine crackers, 1 tablespoon of sugar or honey)
  - Insertion of an intravenous line for circulatory access if hemodynamically unstable
  - Administration of 50% dextrose solution for profound hypoglycemia
  - If unconscious, glucagon injection to stimulate glycogenolysis
- Management of Somogyi effect
  - Insulin-induced hypoglycemia rebounds to hyperglycemia

- • Epinephrine and glucagon are released in response to hypoglycemia
- • Causes mobilization of liver's stored glucose, which induces hyperglycemia
- • Treated by gradually lowering insulin dosage while monitoring blood glucose level, particularly during night when hypoglycemia is most likely to occur
- • Management of Dawn phenomenon
  - • Early morning hyperglycemia attributed to increased secretion of GH
  - • Treated by delaying administration of PM insulin or increased dosage
- • Acetylcysteine therapy when contrast radiologic studies are performed to prevent contrast medium nephrotoxicity

APPLICATION AND REVIEW

1. What principle of teaching specific to an older adult should the nurse consider when providing instruction to such a client recently diagnosed with diabetes mellitus?
   1. Knowledge reduces general anxiety
   2. Capacity to learn decreases with age
   3. Continued reinforcement is advantageous
   4. Readiness of the learner precedes instruction

2. A nurse is caring for two clients newly diagnosed with diabetes. One client has type 1 diabetes and the other client has type 2 diabetes. The nurse determines that the main difference between newly diagnosed type 1 and type 2 diabetes is that in type 1 diabetes:
   1. onset of the disease is slow.
   2. excessive weight is a contributing factor.
   3. short-term complications may be present at the time of diagnosis.
   4. treatment involves diet, exercise, and oral medications.

3. A client tells the nurse during the admission history that an oral hypoglycemic agent is taken daily. For which condition does the nurse conclude that an oral hypoglycemic agent may be prescribed by the health care provider?
   1. Ketosis
   2. Obesity
   3. Type 1 diabetes
   4. Reduced insulin production

4. A nurse is caring for a client with a diagnosis of type 1 diabetes who has developed diabetic coma. Which element excessively accumulates in the blood to precipitate the signs and symptoms associated with this condition?
   1. Sodium bicarbonate, causing alkalosis
   2. Ketones as a result of rapid fat breakdown, causing acidosis
   3. Nitrogen from protein catabolism, causing ammonia intoxication
   4. Glucose from rapid carbohydrate metabolism, causing drowsiness

5. A client with untreated type 1 diabetes mellitus may lapse into a coma because of acidosis. An increase in which component in the blood is a direct cause of this type of acidosis?
   1. Ketones
   2. Glucose
   3. Lactic acid
   4. Glutamic acid

6. A client with diabetes asks the nurse whether the new forearm stick glucose monitor gives the same results as a fingerstick. What is the nurse's **best** response to this question?
   1. "There is no difference between readings."
   2. "These types of monitors are meant for children."
   3. "Readings are on a different scale for each monitor."
   4. "Faster readings can be obtained from a fingerstick."

7. A nurse is planning to teach facts about hyperglycemia to a client with the diagnosis of diabetes. What information should the nurse include in the discussion about what causes diabetic acidosis?
   1. Breakdown of fat stores for energy
   2. Ingestion of too many highly acidic foods
   3. Excessive secretion of endogenous insulin
   4. Increased amounts of cholesterol in the extracellular compartment

8. A nurse is caring for a client with diabetes who is scheduled for a radiographic study requiring contrast. Which should the nurse expect the health care provider to prescribe?
   1. Acetylcysteine before the test
   2. Renal-friendly contrast medium for the test
   3. Forced diuresis with mannitol after the test
   4. Hydration with dextrose and water throughout the test

9. A nurse is caring for a client with type 1 diabetes, and the health care provider prescribes one tube of glucose gel. What is the **primary** reason for the administration of glucose gel to this client?
   1. Diabetic acidosis
   2. Hyperinsulin secretion
   3. Insulin-induced hypoglycemia
   4. Idiosyncratic reactions to insulin

10. A nurse is caring for a client newly diagnosed with type 1 diabetes. When the health care provider tries to regulate this client's insulin regimen, the client experiences episodes of hypoglycemia and hyperglycemia, and 15 g of a simple sugar is prescribed. What is the reason this is administered when a client experiences hypoglycemia?
    1. Inhibits glycogenesis
    2. Stimulates release of insulin
    3. Increases blood glucose levels
    4. Provides more storage of glucose

11. A nurse working in the diabetes clinic is evaluating a client's success with managing the medical regimen. Which is the **best** indication that a client with type 1 diabetes is successfully managing the disease?
    1. Reduction in excess body weight
    2. Stabilization of the serum glucose
    3. Demonstrated knowledge of the disease
    4. Adherence to the prescription for insulin

12. A client with type 1 diabetes mellitus has a fingerstick glucose level of 258 mg/dL at bedtime. A prescription for sliding scale regular insulin exists. What should the nurse do?
    1. Call the health care provider.
    2. Encourage the intake of fluids.
    3. Administer the insulin as prescribed.
    4. Give the client a half cup of orange juice.

13. A client with diabetes is given instructions about foot care. The nurse determines that the instructions are understood when the client states, "I will:
    1. cut my toenails before bathing."
    2. soak my feet daily for 1 hour."
    3. examine my feet using a mirror at least once a week."
    4. break in my new shoes over the course of several weeks."

14. The nurse identifies that the dietary teaching provided for a client with diabetes is understood when the client states, "My diet:
    1. should be rigidly controlled to avoid emergencies."
    2. can be planned around a wide variety of commonly used foods."

3. is based on nutritional requirements that are the same for all people."

4. must not include eating any combination dishes and processed foods."

15. A client with diabetes states, "I cannot eat big meals; I prefer to snack throughout the day." What information should the nurse include in a response to this client's statement?

1. Regulated food intake is basic to control.

2. Salt and sugar restriction is the main concern.

3. Small, frequent meals are better for digestion.

4. Large meals can contribute to a weight problem.

16. A client with type 1 diabetes comes to the clinic because of concerns regarding erratic control of blood glucose with the prescribed insulin therapy. The client has been experiencing a sudden fall in the blood glucose level, followed by a sudden episode of hyperglycemia. Which complication of insulin therapy should the nurse conclude that the client is experiencing?

1. Somogyi effect
3. Diabetic ketoacidosis

2. Dawn phenomenon
4. Hyperosmolar nonketotic syndrome

17. A nurse is formulating a teaching plan for a client recently diagnosed with type 2 diabetes. What interventions should the nurse include that will decrease the risk of complications? **Select all that apply.**

1. Examining the feet daily
4. Powdering the feet after showering

2. Wearing well-fitting shoes
5. Visiting the health care provider weekly

3. Performing regular exercise
6. Testing bathwater with the toes before bathing

18. Which is an independent nursing action that should be included in the plan of care for a client after an episode of ketoacidosis?

1. Monitoring for signs of hypoglycemia as a result of treatment

2. Withholding glucose in any form until the situation is corrected

3. Giving fruit juices, broth, and milk as soon as the client is able to take fluids orally

4. Regulating insulin dosage according to the amount of ketones found in the client's urine

19. A client's problem with ineffective control of type 1 diabetes is identified when a sudden decrease in blood glucose level is followed by rebound hyperglycemia. What should the nurse do when this event occurs?

1. Give the client a glass of orange juice.

2. Seek an order to increase the insulin dose at bedtime.

3. Encourage the client to eat smaller, more frequent meals.

4. Collaborate with the health care provider to alter the insulin prescription.

See Answers on pages 237-242.

ANTIDIABETIC AGENTS

Insulin

- Used to improve glycemic control in patients with diabetes mellitus
- Categories are rapid acting, short acting, intermediate acting, and long acting
- Examples: insulin lispro, insulin aspart, insulin glulisine, insulin regular, insulin isophane NPH, insulin glargine, insulin detemir, insulin degludec
- Available in subcutaneous injection and IV preparations

Mode of Action

- Causes decreased blood glucose by transport of glucose into body cells and conversion of glucose into glycogen in the liver and muscle

Contraindications, Precautions, and Drug Interactions of Insulin*

Drug	Contraindications/Precautions	Drug Interaction
Rapid-Acting Insulins		
insulin lispro	**Contraindications:** Hypersensitivity to protamine **Precautions:** Pregnancy **Pregnancy:** No human studies available, but no adverse effects in animals	Alcohol, anabolic steroids, beta-adrenergic blockers, corticosteroids, diuretics, dobutamine, epinephrine, estrogen, fenfluramine, MAOIs, oral contraceptives, oral hypoglycemics, salicylates, thyroid hormones
insulin aspart	**Contraindications:** Creosol, hypersensitivity to protamine **Precautions:** Pregnancy **Pregnancy:** No human studies available, but no adverse effects in animals	Alcohol, anabolic steroids, beta-adrenergic blockers, corticosteroids, diuretics, dobutamine, epinephrine, estrogen, fenfluramine, MAOIs, oral contraceptives, oral hypoglycemics, salicylates, thyroid hormones
insulin glulisine	**Contraindications:** Hypersensitivity to protamine **Precautions:** Pregnancy **Pregnancy:** Only given after risks to the fetus are considered	Alcohol, anabolic steroids, beta-adrenergic blockers, corticosteroids, diuretics, dobutamine, epinephrine, estrogen, fenfluramine, MAOIs, oral contraceptives, oral hypoglycemics, salicylates, thyroid hormones
Short-Acting Insulins		
insulin regular	**Contraindications:** Hypersensitivity to protamine **Precautions:** Pregnancy **Pregnancy:** No human studies available, but no adverse effects in animals	Alcohol, anabolic steroids, beta-adrenergic blockers, corticosteroids, diuretics, dobutamine, epinephrine, estrogen, fenfluramine, MAOIs, oral contraceptives, oral hypoglycemics, salicylates, thyroid hormones
Intermediate-Acting Insulins		
insulin isophane NPH	**Contraindications:** Hypersensitivity to protamine **Precautions:** Pregnancy **Pregnancy:** Only given after risks to the fetus are considered	Alcohol, anabolic steroids, beta-adrenergic blockers, corticosteroids, diuretics, dobutamine, epinephrine, estrogen, fenfluramine, MAOIs, oral contraceptives, oral hypoglycemics, salicylates, thyroid hormones
Long-Acting Insulins		
insulin glargine	**Contraindications:** Hypersensitivity to protamine **Precautions:** Pregnancy **Pregnancy:** Only given after risks to the fetus are considered	Alcohol, anabolic steroids, beta-adrenergic blockers, corticosteroids, diuretics, dobutamine, epinephrine, estrogen, fenfluramine, MAOIs, oral contraceptives, oral hypoglycemics, salicylates, thyroid hormones
insulin detemir	**Contraindications:** Hypersensitivity to protamine **Precautions:** Pregnancy **Pregnancy:** No human studies available, but no adverse effects in animals	Alcohol, anabolic steroids, beta-adrenergic blockers, corticosteroids, diuretics, dobutamine, epinephrine, estrogen, fenfluramine, MAOIs, oral contraceptives, oral hypoglycemics, salicylates, thyroid hormones
insulin degludec	**Contraindications:** Hypersensitivity to insulin **Precautions:** Pregnancy **Pregnancy:** Only given after risks to the fetus are considered	Alcohol, anabolic steroids, beta-adrenergic blockers, corticosteroids, diuretics, dobutamine, epinephrine, estrogen, fenfluramine, gatifloxacin, MAOIs, oral contraceptives, oral hypoglycemics, salicylates, thyroid hormones

MAOI, monoamine oxidase inhibitor.

*Pregnancy categories have been revised. See http://www.fda.gov/Drugs/DevelopmentApprovalProcess/DevelopmentResources/Labeling/ucm093307.htm for more information.

Adverse Effects/Side Effects

- Blurred vision
- Dry mouth
- Flushing
- Hypoglycemia
- Lipodystrophy
- Lipohypertrophy
- Peripheral edema
- Rash
- Swelling
- Urticaria
- Warmth

Nursing Care

- Assess fasting blood glucose to identify treatment effectiveness
- Assess for hyperglycemia
- Teach patient blurred vision occurs, stabilizes 1 to 2 mo
- Teach patient to carry a glucagon kit/sugar in case of hypoglycemia
- Teach patient to carry diabetic emergency ID
- Teach patient to comply with medication, diet, exercise instructions
- Teach patient to perform blood glucose testing
- Teach patient to recognize hypoglycemia/hyperglycemia reactions; ketoacidosis symptoms

APPLICATION AND REVIEW

20. A health care provider prescribes 36 units of NPH insulin and 12 units of regular insulin. The nurse plans to administer these drugs in one syringe. Identify the steps in this procedure by listing the numbers by each picture next to the following step in **priority** order. (Start with the number of the picture that represents the first step and end with the number by the picture that represents the last step.)

    Step 1 _____ Step 2 _____ Step 3 _____ Step 4 _____

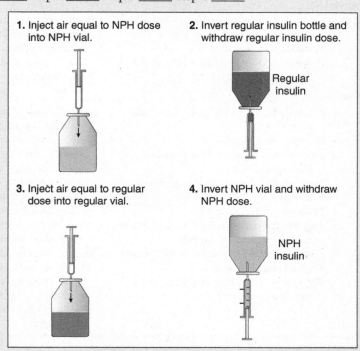

1. Inject air equal to NPH dose into NPH vial.

2. Invert regular insulin bottle and withdraw regular insulin dose.

Regular insulin

3. Inject air equal to regular dose into regular vial.

4. Invert NPH vial and withdraw NPH dose.

NPH insulin

(From Nugent, P.M., Green, J.S., Hellmer Saul, M.A., Pelikan, P.K. [2012]. *Mosby's comprehensive review of nursing for the NCLEX-RN examination* [20th ed.]. St. Louis: Mosby.)

21. A nurse is caring for several clients with type 1 diabetes, and they each have a prescription for a specific type of insulin. Which insulin does the nurse conclude has the fastest onset of action?
    1. Insulin lispro
    2. Insulin glargine
    3. NPH insulin
    4. Regular insulin

22. A nurse plans an evening snack of milk, crackers, and cheese for a client who is receiving NPH insulin. What does this snack provide?
    1. Encouragement to stay on the diet
    2. Added calories to promote weight gain
    3. Nourishment to counteract late insulin activity
    4. High-carbohydrate nourishment for immediate use

23. A client with diabetes is being taught to self-administer a subcutaneous injection of insulin. Identify the preferred site for the self-administration of this drug.
    1. A
    2. B
    3. C
    4. D

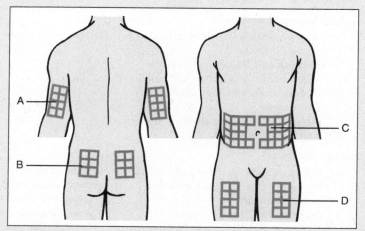

(From Nugent, P.M., Green, J.S., Hellmer Saul, M.A., Pelikan, P.K. [2012]. *Mosby's comprehensive review of nursing for the NCLEX-RN examination* [20th ed.]. St. Louis: Mosby.)

See Answers on pages 237-242.

Sulfonylureas

- Used to treat type 2 diabetes
- Categories are first-generation (short, intermediate and long acting) and second-generation
- Examples: tolbutamide, tolazamide, chlorpropamide, glipizide, glyburide, glimepiride
- Available in oral preparations

Mode of Action

- Causes pancreatic beta cells to secrete more insulin

Contraindications, Precautions, and Drug Interactions of Sulfonylureas*

Drug	Contraindications/Precautions	Drug Interaction
First-Generation Sulfonylureas: Short-Acting		
tolbutamide	**Contraindications:** Diabetic ketoacidosis, type 1 diabetes **Precautions:** Children, debilitated, G6PD deficiency, geriatric, malnourished, severe renal/hepatic disease, pregnancy **Pregnancy:** Only given after risks to the fetus are considered	Alcohol, gatifloxacin
First-Generation Sulfonylureas: Intermediate-Acting		
tolazamide	**Contraindications:** Diabetic ketoacidosis, type 1 diabetes **Precautions:** Breastfeeding, children, debilitated, G6PD deficiency, geriatric, malnourished, severe renal/hepatic disease, pregnancy **Pregnancy:** Only given after risks to the fetus are considered	Alcohol, gatifloxacin
First-Generation Sulfonylureas: Long-Acting		
chlorpropamide	**Contraindications:** Diabetic ketoacidosis, type 1 diabetes **Precautions:** Children, debilitated, G6PD deficiency, geriatric, malnourished, severe renal/hepatic disease, pregnancy **Pregnancy:** Only given after risks to the fetus are considered	Alcohol, gatifloxacin
Second-Generation Sulfonylureas		
glipizide	**Contraindications:** Hypersensitivity to sulfonylureas, diabetic ketoacidosis, type 1 diabetes **Precautions:** Cardiac disease, G6PD deficiency, geriatric, pregnancy, severe renal/hepatic disease **Pregnancy:** Only given after risks to the fetus are considered	Alcohol, androgens, anticoagulants, beta-blockers, charcoal, chloramphenicol, cholestyramine, cimetidine, clarithromycin, clofibrate, corticosteroids, diazoxide, digoxin, diuretics, fenfluramine, fibric acid derivatives, fluconazole, gemfibrozil, glycosides, guanethidine, H2-antagonists, hydantoins, insulin, isoniazid, magnesium salts, MAOIs, methyldopa, NSAIDs, phenylbutazone, probenecid, rifampin, salicylates, sulfinpyrazone, sulfonamides, tricyclics, urinary acidifiers, urinary alkalinizers, voriconazole

Contraindications, Precautions, and Drug Interactions of Sulfonylureas—cont'd

Drug	Contraindications/Precautions	Drug Interaction
Second-Generation Sulfonylureas		
glyburide	**Contraindications:** Hypersensitivity to sulfonylureas, diabetic ketoacidosis, renal failure, type 1 diabetes **Precautions:** Cardiac/thyroid disease, G6PD deficiency, geriatric, pregnancy, severe hypoglycemic reactions, severe renal/hepatic disease, sulfonamide/sulfonylurea hypersensitivity **Pregnancy:** Only given after risks to the fetus are considered	Alcohol, androgens, anticoagulants, antidepressants, beta-adrenergic blockers, beta-blockers, bosentan, charcoal, chloramphenicol, cholestyramine, clarithromycin, colesevelam, corticosteroids, cyclosporine, diazoxide, digoxin, diuretics, estrogens, fenfluramine, fluconazole, gemfibrozil, guanethidine, H2-antagonists, hydantoins, insulin, isoniazid, magnesium salts, MAOIs, methyldopa, NSAIDs, oral contraceptives, phenothiazines, phenylbutazone, probenecid, rifampin thyroid, salicylates, sulfinpyrazone, sulfonamides, urinary acidifiers, urinary alkalinizers, voriconazole
glimepiride	**Contraindications:** Hypersensitivity to sulfonylureas, diabetic ketoacidosis, type 1 diabetes **Precautions:** Cardiac disease, G6PD deficiency, geriatric, pregnancy, severe renal/hepatic disease **Pregnancy:** Only given after risks to the fetus are considered	Alcohol, androgens, anticoagulants, beta-blockers, charcoal, chloramphenicol, cholestyramine, cimetidine, clarithromycin, clofibrate, corticosteroids, diazoxide, digoxin, diuretics, fenfluramine, fibric acid derivatives, fluconazole, gemfibrozil, glycosides, guanethidine, H$_2$-antagonists, hydantoins, insulin, isoniazid, magnesium salts, MAOIs, methyldopa, NSAIDs, phenylbutazone, probenecid, rifampin, salicylates, sulfinpyrazone, sulfonamides, tricyclics, urinary acidifiers, urinary alkalinizers, voriconazole

MAOI, monoamine oxidase inhibitor; *NSAIDs,* nonsteroidal antiinflammatory drugs.
*Pregnancy categories have been revised. See http://www.fda.gov/Drugs/DevelopmentApprovalProcess/DevelopmentResources/Labeling/ucm093307.htm for more information.

Adverse Effects/Side Effects

- Blurred vision
- Dizziness
- Drowsiness
- Dysgeusia
- Fatigue
- Headache
- Hypoglycemia
- Gastrointestinal disturbances
- Paresthesia
- Pyrosis
- Tinnitus
- Vertigo
- Weakness
- Weight gain

Nursing Care

- Advise patient to carry emergency ID and carry a glucagon emergency kit for emergency purposes
- Assess for hypo/hyperglycemic reactions
- For blood dyscrasias: monitor CBC, check liver function tests, and renal studies during treatment
- Teach patient extended release tab may appear in stool
- Teach patient symptoms of hypo/hyperglycemia
- Teach patient to avoid alcohol; inform about disulfiram reaction

- Teach patient to avoid OTC medications unless approved by a prescriber
- Teach patient to check for symptoms of cholestatic jaundice
- Teach patient to eat all food included in diet plan to prevent hypoglycemia
- Teach patient to report bleeding, bruising, weight gain, edema, shortness of breath, weakness, sore throat
- Teach patient to take medication as prescribed, and not discontinue product abruptly
- Teach patient to take product in the morning to prevent hypoglycemic reactions at night
- Teach patient to use capillary blood glucose test

Other Antidiabetic Agents

- Used to improve blood sugar control in people with type 2 diabetes
- Categories are biguanides, thiazolidinediones, meglitinides, dipeptidyl peptidase 4 inhibitors, amylin analogs
- Examples: metformin, pioglitazone, repaglinide, nateglinide, sitagliptin, saxagliptin, linagliptin, alogliptin, pramlintide
- Available in oral and subcutaneous injection preparations

Mode of Action
- Affects the hepatic and GI production of glucose

Contraindications, Precautions, and Drug Interactions of Nonsulfonylureas*

Drug	Contraindications/Precautions	Drug Interaction
Biguanides		
metformin	*Contraindications:* Diabetic ketoacidosis, hypersensitivity, radiographic contrast administration *Precautions:* Alcoholism, cardiopulmonary insufficiency, children, concurrent infection, hepatic/renal dysfunction, lactation, pregnancy *Pregnancy:* No human studies available, but no adverse effects in animals	Beta-blockers, calcium channel blockers, cimetidine, contraceptives (oral), corticosteroids, digoxin, diuretics, dofetilide, estrogens, morphine, phenothiazines, phenytoin, procainamide, quinidine, radiologic contrast media, ranitidine, sympathomimetics, triamterene, vancomycin
Thiazolidinediones		
pioglitazone	*Contraindications:* Breastfeeding, class III and IV congestive heart failure, diabetic ketoacidosis, hypersensitivity to thiazolidinediones *Precautions:* Bladder cancer, edema, geriatric with cardiovascular disease, osteoporosis, pregnancy, polycystic ovary syndrome, pulmonary disease, secondary malignancy, thyroid/renal/hepatic disease. *Pregnancy:* Only given after risks to the fetus are considered	Atorvastatin, CYP2C8 inducers, fluconazole, itraconazole, ketoconazole, miconazole, oral contraceptives, voriconazole

Contraindications, Precautions, and Drug Interactions of Nonsulfonylureas—cont'd

Drug	Contraindications/Precautions	Drug Interaction
Meglitinides		
repaglinide	*Contraindications:* Diabetic ketoacidosis, hypersensitivity to meglitinides, type 1 diabetes *Precautions:* Breastfeeding, children, cardiac disease, geriatric, pregnancy, severe renal/hepatic disease, thyroid disease, severe hypoglycemic reactions *Pregnancy:* Only given after risks to the fetus are considered	Antifungals, barbiturates, beta-adrenergic blockers, calcium channel blockers, carbamazepine, chloramphenicol, corticosteroids, coumarins, CYP2C9 inhibitors, CYP3A4 inhibitors, CYP3A4 inducers, deferasirox, diuretics, erythromycin, estrogens, fenofibrate, gemfibrozil, isophane insulin (NPH), isoniazid, ketoconazole, levonorgestrel/ethinyl estradiol, macrolides, MAOIs, miconazole, NSAIDs, OATP1B1 inhibitors, oral contraceptives, rifampin, phenobarbital, phenothiazines, phenytoin, probenecid, salicylates, simvastatin, sulfonamides, sympathomimetics, thyroid preparations
nateglinide	*Contraindications:* Diabetic ketoacidosis, hypersensitivity to nateglinide, type 1 diabetes *Precautions:* Hepatic disease, hypoglycemia, infection *Pregnancy:* Only given after risks to the fetus are considered	Corticosteroids, CYP2C9 inhibitors, gatifloxacin, guanethidine, NSAIDs, monoamine oxidase inhibitors, nonselective beta-adrenergic-blocking agents, phenytoin salicylates, rifampin, somatropin, sympathomimetics, thiazides, thyroid products
Dipeptidyl Peptidase 4 Inhibitors		
sitagliptin phosphate	*Contraindications:* Angioedema, diabetic ketoacidosis (DKA) *Precautions:* Adrenal insufficiency, breastfeeding, burns, diabetic ketoacidosis, gastrointestinal obstruction, geriatric, hypercortisolism, hyperglycemia, hypersensitivity, hyperthyroidism, hypoglycemia, ileus, renal/hepatic disease, pancreatitis, pituitary insufficiency, pregnancy, thyroid disease, trauma, type 1 diabetes mellitus, surgery *Pregnancy:* No human studies available, but no adverse effects in animals	ACE inhibitors, androgens, aripiprazole, beta-blockers, cimetidine, clozapine, corticosteroids, digoxin, disopyramide, estrogens, fibric acid derivatives, fluoxetine, fosphenytoin, insulins, MAOIs, olanzapine, oral contraceptives, phenothiazines, phenytoin, progestins, protease inhibitors, quetiapine, risperidone, salicylates, sulfonylureas, sympathomimetics, thiazide diuretics, ziprasidone

Continued

Contraindications, Precautions, and Drug Interactions of Nonsulfonylureas—cont'd

Drug	Contraindications/Precautions	Drug Interaction
Dipeptidyl Peptidase 4 Inhibitors		
saxagliptin	**Contraindications:** Hypersensitivity, type 1 diabetes mellitus **Precautions:** Arthralgia, pancreatitis **Pregnancy:** No human studies available, but no adverse effects in animals	ACE inhibitors, alpha-lipoic agents, androgens, aprepitant, conivaptan, CYP3A4 inducers/inhibitors, dasatinib, fosaprepitant, fusidic acid, hyperglycemia-associated agents, hypoglycemia-associated agents, idelalisib, insulin, ivacaftor, luliconazole, lumacaftor, MAOIs, mifepristone, netupitant, palbociclib, pegvisomant, p-glycoprotein/ABCB1 inducers/inhibitors, quinolone antibiotics, ranolazine, salicylates, SSRIs, simeprevir, stiripentol, sulfonylureas, thiazide and thiazide-like diuretics
linagliptin	**Contraindications:** Hypersensitivity, angioedema **Precautions:** Diabetic ketoacidosis (DKA), geriatric, GI obstruction, renal/hepatic disease, pregnancy, thyroid disease, trauma, type 1 diabetes mellitus, surgery **Pregnancy:** No human studies available, but no adverse effects in animals	ACE inhibitors, androgens, aripiprazole, beta-blockers, cimetidine, clozapine, corticosteroids, digoxin, disopyramide, estrogens, fibric acid derivatives, fluoxetine, fosphenytoin, insulins, MAOIs, olanzapine, oral contraceptives, phenothiazines, phenytoin, progestins, protease inhibitors, quetiapine, risperidone, salicylates, sulfonylureas, sympathomimetics, thiazide diuretics, ziprasidone
alogliptin	**Contraindications:** Hypersensitivity **Precautions:** Adrenal insufficiency, breastfeeding, burns, children, diarrhea, fever, GI obstruction, hepatic disease, hypercortisolism, hyper/hypoglycemia, hyper/hypothyroidism, ileus, ketoacidosis, kidney disease, malnutrition, pancreatitis, pregnancy, surgery, trauma, type 1 diabetes, vomiting **Pregnancy:** No human studies available, but no adverse effects in animals	Bexarotene, gatifloxacin
Amylin Analog		
pramlintide	**Contraindications:** Hypersensitivity to pramlintide or cresol, gastroparesis **Precautions:** Breastfeeding, pregnancy **Pregnancy:** Only given after risks to the fetus are considered	ACE inhibitors, acetaminophen, alcohol, α-glucosidase inhibitors, antimuscarinics, dextrothyroxine, disopyramide, diphenoxylate, erythromycin, estrogens, insulin, loperamide, MAOIs, metoclopramide, niacin, octreotide, opiate agonist, oral contraceptives, phenothiazines, progestins, thiazide diuretics, triamterene, tricyclics

MAOI, monoamine oxidase inhibitor; *NSAIDs,* nonsteroidal antiinflammatory drugs.
*Pregnancy categories have been revised. See http://www.fda.gov/Drugs/DevelopmentApprovalProcess/DevelopmentResources/Labeling/ucm093307.htm for more information.

Adverse Effects/Side Effects

- Angina
- Anorexia
- Arthralgia
- Blurred vision
- Cough
- Dizziness
- Elevated liver enzymes
- Fatigue
- Fluid retention
- Fractures
- Gastrointestinal difficulties
- Headache
- Heart failure
- Hemolytic anemia
- Hypoglycemia
- Infection
- Lactic acidosis
- Leukopenia
- Myocardial infarction
- Palpitations
- Pulmonary and peripheral edema
- Systemic allergy
- Vitamin B_{12} deficiency
- Weight gain

Nursing Care

- Advise patient to avoid OTC medications, alcohol unless approved by the prescriber
- Advise patient to take product in morning to prevent hypoglycemic reactions at night
- Assess for hypoglycemic reactions/hyperglycemic reactions soon after meals
- Monitor CBC; check liver function tests and renal tests during treatment
- Monitor for lactic acidosis
- Teach patient symptoms of hypoglycemia/hyperglycemia
- Teach patient symptoms of lactic acidosis
- Teach patient to carry/wear emergency ID and glucagon emergency kit for emergencies
- Teach patient to self-monitor blood glucose
- Teach patient to take medication daily and not to abruptly discontinue
- Teach patient to take with meals, not to break, crush, chew extended release product, and that extended release tab may appear in stool

APPLICATION AND REVIEW

24. Metformin 2 g by mouth is prescribed for a client with type 2 diabetes. Each tablet contains 500 mg. How many tablets should the nurse administer? **Record your answer using a whole number.**
    Answer: _____ tablets
25. A client with type 2 diabetes develops gout, and allopurinol is prescribed. The client is also taking metformin and an over-the-counter nonsteroidal antiinflammatory drug (NSAID). When teaching about the administration of allopurinol, what should the nurse instruct the client to do?
    1. Decrease the daily dose of NSAIDs.
    2. Limit fluid intake to one quart a day.
    3. Take the medication on an empty stomach.
    4. Monitor blood glucose levels more frequently.

See Answers on pages 237-242.

ANSWER KEY: REVIEW QUESTIONS

1. **3 Neurologic aging causes forgetfulness and a slower response time; repetition increases learning.**
   1, 4 "Knowledge reduces general anxiety" and "Readiness of the learner precedes instruction" are principles applicable to all learning regardless of the client's age. **2** Learning occurs, but it may take longer.
   Client Need: Health Promotion and Maintenance; **Cognitive Level:** Application; **Integrated Process:** Teaching/Learning; **Nursing Process:** Planning/Implementation

2. **3 Clinical presentation of type 1 diabetes is characterized by acute onset. Short-term complications may be present (DKA, weight loss, etc.).**

   1 Clinical presentation of type 1 diabetes is rapid, not slow, as pancreatic beta cells are destroyed by an autoimmune process; in type 2 diabetes, the body is still producing some insulin, and therefore the onset of signs and symptoms is slow. **2** In type 1 diabetes, clients are generally lean or have an ideal weight; 80% to 90% of clients with type 2 diabetes are overweight. **4** type 1 diabetes requires diet control, exercise, and subcutaneous administration of insulin, not oral medications; oral medications are used for type 2 diabetes because some insulin is still being produced.
   Client Need: Physiologic Adaptation; **Cognitive Level:** Analysis; **Nursing Process:** Assessment/Analysis

3. **4 Oral hypoglycemics may be helpful when some functioning of the beta cells exists, as in type 2 diabetes.**

   1 Rapid-acting regular insulin is needed to reverse ketoacidosis. **2** Obesity does not offer enough information to determine the status of beta cell function. **3** Clients with type 1 diabetes have no functioning beta cells; the necessary treatment is insulin, not an oral hypoglycemic.
   Client Need: Pharmacologic and Parenteral Therapies; **Cognitive Level:** Application; **Nursing Process:** Assessment/Analysis

4. **2 Ketones are produced when fat is broken down for energy.**

   1 Although rarely used, sodium bicarbonate may be administered to correct the acid-base imbalance resulting from ketoacidosis; acidosis is caused by excess acid, not excess base bicarbonate. **3** Diabetes does not interfere with removal of nitrogenous wastes. **4** Carbohydrate metabolism is impaired in the client with diabetes.
   Client Need: Physiologic Adaptation; **Cognitive Level:** Comprehension; **Nursing Process:** Assessment/Analysis

5. **1 The ketones produced excessively in diabetes are a byproduct of the breakdown of body fats and proteins for energy; this occurs when insulin is not secreted or is unable to be utilized to transport glucose across the cell membrane into the cells. The major ketone, acetoacetic acid, is an alpha-ketoacid that lowers the blood pH, resulting in acidosis.**

   2 Glucose does not change the pH. **3** Lactic acid is produced as a result of muscle contraction; it is not unique to diabetes. **4** Glutamic acid is a product of protein metabolism.
   Client Need: Physiologic Adaptation; **Cognitive Level:** Comprehension; **Nursing Process:** Assessment/Analysis

6. **1 The forearm glucose monitor is calibrated to be consistent with results obtained from a fingerstick.**

   2 Individuals of all ages can use these glucose monitors. **3** A different scale is not used for each monitor; accompanying literature will indicate if the monitor reading reflects venous blood values even though capillary blood is used. **4** There is no difference in the time required to complete the test.
   Client Need: Reduction of Risk Potential; **Cognitive Level:** Application; **Integrated Process:** Teaching/Learning; **Nursing Process:** Planning/Implementation

7. **1 In the absence of insulin, which facilitates the transport of glucose into cells, the body breaks down proteins and fats to supply energy; ketones, a byproduct of fat metabolism, accumulate, causing metabolic acidosis (pH below 7.35).**

   2 The pH of food ingested has no effect on the development of acidosis. **3** Insufficient, not excessive, secretion of endogenous insulin causes metabolic acidosis. **4** Cholesterol level has no effect on the development of acidosis.
   Client Need: Physiologic Adaptation; **Cognitive Level:** Comprehension; **Integrated Process:** Teaching/Learning; **Nursing Process:** Planning/Implementation

8. **1 Acetylcysteine is an antioxidant that scavenges oxygen-free radicals, which are released when contrast medium causes cell death to renal tubular tissue; it also induces slight vasodilation.**

   2 Contrast that is renal friendly does not exist. **3** Mannitol is not necessary. Saline alone provides better protection of the kidneys from contrast-induced nephropathy. **4** Hydration with saline, not dextrose and water, affords some protection from kidney damage caused by contrast media; dextrose will increase the glucose level in an individual with diabetes and thus is contraindicated.

Client Need: Pharmacologic and Parenteral Therapies; **Cognitive Level:** Analysis; **Nursing Process:** Planning/Implementation

9. **3 Glucose gel delivers a measured amount of simple sugars to provide glucose to the blood for rapid action.**

   1 Acidosis occurs when there is an increased serum glucose level; therefore, glucose gel is not indicated. **2** Diabetes mellitus involves a decreased insulin production. **4** Glucose gel is not indicated in idiosyncratic reactions to insulin.

   Client Need: Pharmacologic and Parenteral Therapies; **Cognitive Level:** Application; **Nursing Process:** Planning/Implementation

10. **3 A simple sugar provides glucose to the blood for rapid action.**

    1 A simple sugar does not inhibit glycogenesis. **2** A simple sugar does not stimulate the release of insulin. **4** A simple sugar does not stimulate the storage of glucose.

    Client Need: Physiologic Adaptation; **Cognitive Level:** Comprehension; **Nursing Process:** Planning/Implementation

11. **2 A combination of diet, exercise, and medication is necessary to control the disease; the interaction of these therapies is reflected by the serum glucose level.**

    1 Weight loss may occur with inadequate insulin. **3** Acquisition of knowledge does not guarantee its application. **4** Insulin alone is not enough to control the disease.

    Client Need: Physiologic Adaptation; **Cognitive Level:** Analysis; **Nursing Process:** Evaluation/Outcomes

12. **3 A value of 258 mg/dL is above the expected range of 70 to 100 mg/dL; the nurse should administer the regular insulin as prescribed.**

    1 Calling the health care provider is unnecessary; a prescription for insulin exists and should be implemented. **2** Encouraging the intake of fluids is insufficient to lower a glucose level this high. **4** Giving the client a half cup of orange juice is contraindicated because it will increase the glucose level further; orange juice, a complex carbohydrate, and a protein should be given if the glucose level is too low.

    Client Need: Pharmacologic and Parenteral Therapies; **Cognitive Level:** Application; **Nursing Process:** Planning/Implementation

13. **4 A slower, longer period of time to break in new, stiff shoes will help prevent blisters and skin breakdown.**

    1 The toenails should be cut by a podiatrist; they usually are cut after a foot bath when the nails are softer. **2** Soaking feet for an hour will cause maceration of the skin and should be avoided. **3** Weekly is too long a period of time; the client should examine the feet daily for signs of trauma.

    Client Need: Reduction of Risk Potential; **Cognitive Level:** Application; **Integrated Process:** Teaching/Learning; **Nursing Process:** Evaluation/Outcomes

14. **2 Each client should be given an individually devised diet selecting commonly used foods from the American Diabetic Association diet; family members should be included in the diet teaching.**

    1 Rigid diets are difficult to follow; appropriate substitutions are permitted. **3** Nutritional requirements are different for each individual, depending on many factors, such as activity level, degree of compliance, and physical status. **4** These foods can be eaten when accounted for in the dietary regimen.

    Client Need: Basic Care and Comfort; **Cognitive Level:** Application; **Integrated Process:** Teaching/Learning; **Nursing Process:** Evaluation/Outcomes

15. **1 An understanding of the diet is imperative for adherence. A balance of carbohydrates, proteins, and fats usually apportioned over three main meals and two between-meal snacks needs to be tailored to the client's specific needs, with consideration of exercise and pharmacologic therapy.**

    2 A total dietary regimen proportioning carbohydrates, proteins, and fats must be followed, not just sugar restriction; salt is not restricted. **3** Small, frequent meals are better for digestion; however, digestion is not the basis for the client's problems. **4** Total caloric intake, rather than the size of meals, is the major factor in weight gain.

    Client Need: Basic Care and Comfort; **Cognitive Level:** Application; **Integrated Process:** Teaching/Learning; **Nursing Process:** Planning/Implementation

16. **1 The Somogyi effect is a response to hypoglycemia induced by too much insulin; the body responds to the hypoglycemia by counterregulatory hormones stimulating lipolysis, gluconeogenesis, and glycogenolysis, resulting in rebound hyperglycemia.**

2 The Dawn phenomenon is hyperglycemia that is present on awakening in the morning due to the release of counterregulatory hormones in the predawn hours; it is thought that growth hormone and/or cortisol are related to this phenomenon. **3** Diabetic ketoacidosis (diabetic coma) is a profound deficiency of insulin and is characterized by hyperglycemia, ketosis, acidosis, and dehydration. **4** Hyperosmolar nonketotic syndrome occurs in clients with type 2 diabetes. It is a condition in which the client produces enough insulin to prevent diabetic ketoacidosis but not enough to prevent severe hyperglycemia, osmotic diuresis, and extracellular fluid depletion.

Client Need: Pharmacologic and Parenteral Therapies; **Cognitive Level:** Analysis; **Nursing Process:** Evaluation/Outcomes

17. **Answers: 1, 2, 3**

1 Clients with diabetes often have peripheral neuropathies and are unaware of discomfort or pain in the feet; the feet should be examined every night for signs of trauma. **2** Well-fitting shoes prevent pressure and rubbing that can cause tissue damage and the development of ulcers. **3** Daily exercise increases the uptake of glucose by the muscles and improves insulin utilization.

4 Powdering the feet after showering may cause a pastelike residue between the toes that may macerate the skin and promote bacterial and fungal growth. **5** Visiting the health care provider weekly is generally unnecessary. **6** Clients with diabetes often have peripheral neuropathy and are unable to accurately evaluate the temperature of bathwater, which can result in burns if the water is too hot.

Client Need: Reduction of Risk Potential: **Cognitive Level:** Analysis; **Integrated Process:** Teaching/Learning; **Nursing Process:** Planning/Implementation

18. **1 During treatment for acidosis, hypoglycemia may develop; careful observation for this complication should be made by the nurse.**

2 Withholding all glucose may cause insulin coma. **3** Whole milk and fruit juices are high in carbohydrates, which are contraindicated immediately following ketoacidosis. **4** The regulation of insulin depends on the prescription for coverage; the prescription usually depends on the client's blood glucose level rather than ketones in the urine.

Client Need: Pharmacologic and Parenteral Therapies; **Cognitive Level:** Analysis; **Nursing Process:** Planning/Implementation

---

Test-Taking Tip: Start by reading each of the answer options carefully. Usually at least one of them will be clearly wrong. Eliminate this one from consideration. Now you have reduced the number of response choices by one and improved the odds. Continue to analyze the options. If you can eliminate one more choice in a four-option question, you have reduced the odds to 50/50. While you are eliminating the wrong choices, recall often occurs. One of the options may serve as a trigger that causes you to remember what a few seconds ago had seemed completely forgotten.

---

19. **4 The client is experiencing the Somogyi effect. It is a paradoxical situation in which sudden decreases in blood glucose are followed by rebound hyperglycemia. The body responds to the hypoglycemia by secreting glucagon, epinephrine, growth hormone, and cortisol to counteract the low blood sugar. This results in an excessive increase in the blood glucose level. It most often occurs in response to hypoglycemia when asleep. The health care provider may choose to decrease the insulin dose and then reassess the client.**

1 Giving the client a glass of orange juice will further increase the serum glucose level and is contraindicated. **2** Increasing the insulin dose at bedtime will further worsen the problem. **3** Encouraging the client to eat smaller, more frequent meals will not address the hypoglycemia and rebound hyperglycemia that occurs when sleeping. However, a bedtime snack may help minimize this event.

Client Need: Reduction of Risk Potential: **Cognitive Level:** Analysis; **Integrated Process:** Teaching/Learning; **Nursing Process:** Planning/Implementation

20. **Answers: 1, 3, 2, 4**

    1 Air should be injected into the NPH insulin vile first, which allows withdrawal of the NPH insulin at a later step in the procedure without having to instill air into the vial from a syringe that contains regular insulin. **3** Instilling air into the regular insulin vile increases the pressure in the vile, facilitating removal of the required dose. **2** Removing the desired dose of insulin while the needle is still in the vile reduces the risk of contamination by repeated punctures, and it maintains the sharpness of the needle. Having the syringe contain regular insulin first prevents the need to withdraw the regular insulin into a syringe that contains NPH insulin and inadvertently contaminating the regular insulin vial with the longer-acting NPH insulin; contaminating regular insulin with NPH insulin will reduce the speed at which the regular insulin functions, which in turn will delay treatment of a hyperglycemic event. **4** Finally, the required dose of NPH insulin can be removed from the NPH insulin vile.

    Client Need: Pharmacologic and Parenteral Therapies; **Cognitive Level:** Analysis; **Nursing Process:** Planning/Implementation

21. **1 Insulin lispro has an onset of 0.25 hours, a peak action of 0.5 to 1.5 hours, and a duration of 3 to 4 hours.**

    2 Insulin glargine has an onset of 1 to 1.5 hours, no peak action, and a duration of 20 to 24 hours. **3** NPH insulin has an onset of 1.5 hours, a peak action of 4 to 12 hours, and a duration of 18 to 24 hours. **4** Regular insulin has an onset of 0.5 hours, a peak action of 1 to 5 hours, and a duration of 6 to 10 hours.

    Client Need: Pharmacologic and Parenteral Therapies; **Cognitive Level:** Comprehension; **Nursing Process:** Planning/Implementation

---

 Study Tip: Insulin lis**pro** is a **pro** at quick onset!

---

22. **3 The protein in milk and cheese may be slowly converted to glucose (gluconeogenesis), providing the body with some glucose during sleep while the NPH insulin is still acting.**

    1 The purpose of an evening snack is to cover for insulin activity during sleep. **2** Adding calories to promote weight gain is not the purpose of an evening snack for a person taking insulin. **4** The foods chosen are rich in protein and will be utilized slowly.

    Client Need: Pharmacologic and Parenteral Therapies; **Cognitive Level:** Application; **Nursing Process:** Planning/Implementation

23. **3 The abdomen is the preferred site for an insulin injection because it is easily accessible and absorption is more even and rapid than when it is injected in the extremities.**

    1, 2, 4 The arms, thighs and buttocks are not the preferred sites for the administration of insulin.

    Client Need: Pharmacologic and Parenteral Therapies; **Cognitive Level:** Analysis; **Nursing Process:** Planning/Implementation

24. **Answer: 4 tablets.**

    First convert 2 g to its equivalent in mg by multiplying by 1000 (move the decimal 3 places to the right). Use the "Desired over Have" formula of ratio and proportion to solve this problem.

    $$\frac{\text{Desire}}{\text{Have}} \quad \frac{2000\,\text{mg}}{500\,\text{mg}} = \frac{x \text{ tablets}}{1 \text{ tablet}}$$

    $$500\,x = 2000$$

    $$x = 2000 \div 500$$

    $$x = 4 \text{ tablets}$$

    Client Need: Pharmacologic and Parenteral Therapies; **Cognitive Level:** Application; **Nursing Process:** Planning/Implementation

25. **4 Allopurinol can potentiate the effect of oral hypoglycemics, causing hypoglycemia; the blood glucose level should be monitored more frequently.**

    1 NSAIDs can be taken concurrently with allopurinol. **2** A daily fluid intake of 2500 to 3000 mL will limit the risk of developing renal calculi. **3** Allopurinol should be taken with milk or food to decrease GI irritation.

    Client Need: Pharmacologic and Parenteral Therapies; **Cognitive Level:** Application; **Integrated Process:** Teaching/Learning; **Nursing Process:** Planning/Implementation

Endocrine Drugs 13

REVIEW OF THE ENDOCRINE SYSTEM

Endocrine glands continuously secrete products called hormones, which are chemical messengers that deliver stimulatory or inhibitory signals to target cells as a result of a feedback mechanism; once secreted, hormones usually remain present in the body for 4 to 6 hours.

Structures of the Endocrine System (Fig. 13.1)

Pineal Gland
- Located in midbrain attached to third ventricle
- Pineal hormone (melatonin)
  - May regulate diurnal fluctuations of hypothalamic-hypophyseal hormones
  - Inhibits numerous endocrine functions, particularly gonadotropic hormones

Thymus Gland
- Located at root of neck and anterior thorax
- Thymic hormone (thymosin)
  - Regulates immunologic processes
  - T lymphocytes produced after birth migrate to lymph nodes and spleen to provide cell-mediated immunity
  - Synthesizes hormones that regulate rate of development of lymphoid cells, particularly T cells

Pituitary Gland
- Known as the "master gland" because it secretes hormones that stimulate other glands' responses, including secretion of their hormones
- Located in cranial cavity in sella turcica of sphenoid bone; near optic chiasm
- Two lobes: **A**nterior lobe (**a**denohypophysis) and posterior lobe (neurohypophysis)
- Pituitary hormones
  - Hormones secreted by anterior lobe
    - Growth hormone (GH)
      - Promotes protein anabolism
      - Promotes fat mobilization and catabolism
      - Slows carbohydrate metabolism
      - Promotes skeletal and muscle growth
    - Thyroid-stimulating hormone (TSH): stimulates synthesis and secretion of thyroid hormones
    - Adrenocorticotropic hormone (ACTH)
      - Stimulates growth of adrenal cortex
      - Stimulates secretion of glucocorticoids; slightly stimulates mineralocorticoid secretion
    - Follicle-stimulating hormone (FSH)
      - Stimulates primary Graafian follicle to grow and develop
      - Stimulates follicle cells to secrete estrogen
      - Stimulates development of seminiferous tubules and spermatogenesis

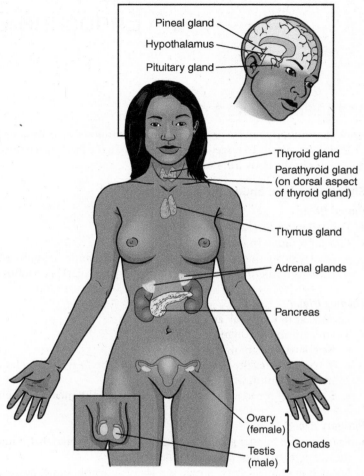

FIG. 13.1   Principal endocrine glands. (From McCance, K.L., Huether S.E., Brashers, V.L., Rote, N.S. [2002]. *Pathophysiology: The biological basis for disease in adults and children* [4th ed.]. St. Louis: Mosby.)

- Luteinizing hormone (LH)
  - Stimulates maturation of follicle and ovum; required for ovulation
  - Forms corpus luteum in ruptured follicle following ovulation; stimulates corpus luteum to secrete progesterone
  - In males, LH is called interstitial cell–stimulating hormone (ICSH); stimulates testes to secrete testosterone
- Prolactin (PRL)
  - Promotes breast development during pregnancy
  - Initiates milk production after delivery
  - Stimulates progesterone secretion by corpus luteum
  - Hormones secreted by posterior lobe
- Antidiuretic hormone (ADH, vasopressin)
  - Increases water reabsorption by distal and collecting tubules of kidneys
  - Stimulates vasoconstriction, raising blood pressure

- ▪ Oxytocin
  - ▪ Stimulates contractions by pregnant uterus
  - ▪ Stimulates milk ejection from alveoli of lactating breasts into ducts
- ▪ Melanocyte-stimulating hormone (MSH): stimulates synthesis and dispersion of melanin in skin, causing darkening

Thyroid Gland

- Overlies thyroid cartilage below larynx
- Thyroid hormones: accelerate cellular reactions in most body cells
  - Thyroxine (T_4): stimulates metabolic rate; essential for physical and mental development
  - Triiodothyronine (T_3): inhibits anterior pituitary secretion of thyroid-stimulating hormone
  - Calcitonin (thyrocalcitonin): decreases loss of calcium from bone; promotes hypocalcemia; *action opposite that of parathormone*

Parathyroid Gland

- Small glands (2 to 12) embedded in posterior part of thyroid
- Parathyroid hormone (parathormone)
  - Increases blood calcium concentration
    - ▪ Breakdown of bone with release of calcium into blood (requires active form of vitamin D)
    - ▪ Calcium absorption from intestine into blood
    - ▪ Kidney tubule reabsorption of calcium
  - Decreases blood phosphate concentration by slowing its reabsorption from kidneys, thereby decreasing calcium loss in urine

Testes and Ovaries

- See Chapter 14 on reproductive system medications

Adrenal Glands

- Two closely associated structures, adrenal medulla and adrenal cortex, positioned at each kidney's superior border
- Adrenal hormones
  - Adrenal medulla: produces two catecholamines, epinephrine and norepinephrine
    - ▪ Stimulate liver and skeletal muscle to break down glycogen to produce glucose
    - ▪ Increase oxygen use and carbon dioxide production
    - ▪ Increase blood concentration of free fatty acids through stimulation of lipolysis in adipose tissue
    - ▪ Cause constriction of most blood vessels of body, thus increasing total peripheral resistance and arterial pressure to shunt blood to vital organs
    - ▪ Increase heart rate and force of contraction, thus increasing cardiac output
    - ▪ Inhibit contractions of gastrointestinal and uterine smooth muscle
    - ▪ Epinephrine significantly dilates bronchial smooth muscle
  - Adrenal cortex: secretes adrenocortical agents: the mineralocorticoid aldosterone and the glucocorticoids cortisol and corticosterone
    - ▪ Aldosterone
      - (1) Markedly accelerates sodium and water reabsorption by kidney tubules
      - (2) Markedly accelerates potassium excretion by kidney tubules
      - (3) Secretion increases as sodium ions decrease or potassium ions increase

- Cortisol and corticosterone
  (1) Accelerate mobilization and catabolism of tissue protein and fats
  (2) Accelerate liver gluconeogenesis (hyperglycemic effect)
  (3) Decrease antibody formation (immunosuppressive, antiallergic effect)
  (4) Slow proliferation of fibroblasts characteristic of inflammation (antiinflammatory effect)
  (5) Decrease adrenocorticotropic hormone (ACTH) secretion
  (6) Mildly accelerate sodium and water reabsorption and potassium excretion by kidney tubules
  (7) Increase release of coagulation factors

Pancreas
- Retroperitoneal in abdominal cavity
- Pancreatic hormones: regulate glucose and protein homeostasis through action of insulin and glucagon (See Chapter 12)
  - Insulin: secreted by beta cells of islets of Langerhans in response to low level of blood glucose
    - Promotes cellular uptake of glucose
    - Stimulates intracellular macromolecular synthesis, such as glycogen synthesis (glyconeogenesis), fat synthesis (lipogenesis), and protein synthesis
    - Stimulates cellular uptake of sodium and potassium (latter is significant in treatment of diabetic coma with insulin)
  - Glucagon: secreted by alpha cells of islets of Langerhans
    - Induces liver glycogenolysis; antagonizes glycogen synthesis stimulated by insulin
    - Inhibits hepatic protein synthesis, which makes amino acids available for gluconeogenesis and increases urea production
    - Stimulates hepatic ketogenesis and release of glycerol and fatty acids from adipose tissue when cellular glucose level falls
  - Related Pharmacology: See Chapter 12

GROWTH HORMONE AGONIST

Hypopituitarism
- Deficiency of one or more anterior pituitary hormones
  - Decreased levels of GH, ACTH, TSH, FSH, and LH
- Total absence of pituitary hormones referred to as panhypopituitarism (Simmonds' disease)
- Occurs with destruction of anterior lobe of pituitary by trauma, tumor, or hemorrhage
- Clinical findings vary with target organs affected

Therapeutic Interventions
- Surgery if tumor is present
- Hormone replacement: Growth Hormone Agonist
  - Mode of Action: Stimulate tissue-building processes = stimulates growth, including protein synthesis, liver glycogenolysis, increasing glucose levels, lipid mobilization from fat stores, and retention of sodium, potassium, and phosphorus
    - Diabetogenic

Select Contraindications, Precautions, and Major Drug Interactions for Anterior Pituitary Hormone Replacement*

Drug	Contraindications/Precautions	Major Drug Interactions
growth hormone analogs	*Contraindications:* Hypersensitivity, neoplasia, closed epiphyses, acute critical illness (such as respiratory failure), intracranial lesions, scoliosis, Prader-Willi syndrome (especially if obese or with severe respiratory impairment) *Precautions:* Dosing depends on brand/trade name, so read brand and dosage carefully; newborns; geriatric; chronic illnesses including hypothyroidism, migraine headaches, epilepsy, respiratory diseases and asthma; chemotherapy *Pregnancy:* Varies with brand: No human studies available, but no adverse effects in animals; only given after risks to the fetus are considered	Androgens, anticonvulsants, corticosteroids, cyclosporine, estrogens, glucocorticoids, insulin, thyroid hormones

*Pregnancy categories have been revised. See http://www.fda.gov/Drugs/DevelopmentApprovalProcess/DevelopmentResources/Labeling/ucm093307.htm for more information.

Adverse Effects/Side Effects

- Development of neutralizing antibodies
- Flu-like syndrome
- Headache
- Hypercalcemia, hypercalciuria
- Hyperglycemia, ketosis
- Hypothyroidism
- Intracranial hypertension
- Joint pain, myalgia
- Pancreatitis
- Rash, urticaria
- Secondary malignancy
- Seizures

Nursing Care of Clients with Hypopituitarism

Assessment/Analysis

- Baseline vital signs
- Sexuality (e.g., loss of libido; painful intercourse; inability to maintain an erection)
- Past and present menstrual patterns
- Visual acuity
- Loss of secondary sexual characteristics
- Activity tolerance
- Monitor glucose levels

Planning/Implementation

- Monitor effects of hormone replacement therapy; adjust insulin therapy as needed
- Discuss importance of adhering to medical regimen on long-term basis
- Allow time to verbalize feelings regarding long-term nature of disease and effect on quality of life
- Provide adequate rest periods

Evaluation/Outcomes

- Adheres to medical regimen
- Expresses positive feelings of body image
- Establishes satisfying sexual functioning

GROWTH HORMONE ANTAGONISTS AND SOMATOSTATIN ANALOGS

Hyperpituitarism

- Excessive concentration of pituitary hormones (e.g., GH, ACTH, PRL) in the blood, glandular overactivity, an adenoma, or changes in the anterior lobe of the pituitary gland
- Classification of GH overproduction
  - Gigantism: generalized increase in size, especially in children; involves long bones
  - Acromegaly: occurs after epiphyseal closing, with subsequent enlargement of cartilage, bone, and soft tissues of body
- Cushing syndrome results from overproduction of ACTH (see following section)

Therapeutic interventions

- Surgical intervention: hypophysectomy
- Irradiation of pituitary gland
- Medications to relieve clinical findings of endocrine imbalances resulting from pituitary hyperfunction other than those of GH
- Medications' Mode of Action
  - Somatostatin analogs: lanreotide and octreotide; goal to normalize GH and IGF-1 levels
    - Octreotide: inhibits GH secretion
    - Lanreotide: acts similarly to somatostatin
  - GH receptor antagonists:
    - Pegvisomant: blocks GH receptor sites, which normalizes IGF-1 level
    - Bromocriptine (dopamine agonist): inhibits secretion of GH from pituitary adenomas

Select Contraindications, Precautions, and Major Drug Interactions for Pituitary Hormone Antagonists*

Drug	Contraindications/Precautions	Major Drug Interactions
Somatostatin Analogs (To Suppress Growth Hormone)		
lanreotide	***Contraindications:*** Hypersensitivity, breastfeeding ***Precautions:*** cardiac/liver/renal/thyroid/gallbladder disease, diabetes ***Pregnancy:*** Only given after risks to the fetus are considered	Antihypertensives, beta blockers, bromocriptine, cyclosporine
octreotide	***Contraindications:*** Hypersensitivity ***Precautions:*** Renal impairment; cardiac/liver/pancreatitis/thyroid/gallbladder disease, diabetes ***Pregnancy:*** No human studies available, but no adverse effects in animals	Bexarotene, ciprofloxacin, cyclosporine, thioridazine
GH Receptor Antagonist		
pegvisomant	***Contraindications:*** Hypersensitivity ***Precautions:*** Patients with tumors that secrete GH, diabetes, children, geriatrics, breastfeeding, liver disease ***Pregnancy:*** No human studies available, but no adverse effects in animals	Opioid analgesics, insulin

Select Contraindications, Precautions, and Major Drug Interactions for Pituitary Hormone Antagonists—cont'd

Drug	Contraindications/Precautions	Major Drug Interactions
Dopamine Agonist (To Suppress Prolactin) for Acromegaly, Pituitary Adenoma, Hyperprolactinemia		
bromocriptine	**Contraindications:** Hypersensitivity, hypersensitivity to ergot drugs, syncopal migraines, breastfeeding, diabetic ketoacidosis, **Precautions:** Hypotension/hypertension; psychosis; liver/kidney disease; stomach ulcer; pituitary tumor; discontinue if hypertension occurs during pregnancy; avoid abrupt discontinuation **Pregnancy:** No human studies available, but no adverse effects in animals; should be discontinued if hypertension occurs during pregnancy	Alcohol, antihypertensives, butyrophenones contraceptives, CYP3A4 inducers and inhibitors, dopamine agonists and antagonists, erythromycin, estrogens, MAOIs, neuroleptic agents, phenothiazines, progestins, salicylates, sulfonamides, sympathomimetics, thioxanthenes

*Pregnancy categories have been revised. See http://www.fda.gov/Drugs/DevelopmentApprovalProcess/DevelopmentResources/Labeling/ucm093307.htm for more information.

Adverse Effects/Side Effects
- Lanreotide: injection-site reactions, GI symptoms, bradycardia, hypo- or hyperglycemia; gallstone development
- Octreotide: arrhythmia, bradycardia, fatigue, hyperglycemia, malaise, headache, dyspnea, arthralgia, initially GI symptoms, gallbladder impairment, gallstone development months later, changing glucose levels, heart conduction abnormalities
- Pegvisomant: GI symptoms, injection-site reactions, flu-like symptoms, chest pain, hypertension, lipohypertrophy, and elevated hepatic transaminases
- Bromocriptine: hypertension, myocardial infarction, angina, stroke, seizure, somnolence, nausea, vomiting, fatigue, dizziness, headache, rash

Nursing Care of Clients with Hyperpituitarism
Assessment/Analysis
- Changes in energy level, sexual function, and menstrual patterns; signs of increased intracranial pressure
- Face, hands, and feet for thickening, enlargement; changes in the size of hat, gloves, rings, or shoes
- Dysphagia or voice changes
- Presence of hypogonadism as a result of hyperprolactinemia
- Reaction to changes in physical appearance and sexual function
- Monitor hepatic function if receiving pegvisomant
- Monitor IGF-1 serum levels within the age-adjusted normal range
- Monitor baseline and treatment levels of liver enzymes alanine aminotransferase (ALT) and aspartate aminotransferase (AST)

Planning/Implementation
- Help to accept altered body image that is irreversible
- Assist family to understand what client is experiencing

- Help to recognize that the need for medical supervision will be lifelong
- Help to understand the basis for the change in sexual functioning
- Encourage to express feelings
- Teach self-care after a hypophysectomy
  - Encourage to follow the established medical regimen, particularly hormone replacement
  - Limit stressful situations
  - Protect self from infection
- Provide care after intracranial surgery
  - Perform neurologic assessments; monitor for increased intracranial pressure
  - Monitor I&O and daily weight to identify complication of diabetes insipidus
  - Assess clear nasal drainage for glucose to determine presence of cerebrospinal fluid (CSF); CSF will test positive for glucose
  - Encourage deep breathing, but not coughing
  - Institute measures to prevent constipation because straining increases intracranial pressure
  - Maintain in no lower than semi-Fowler position

Evaluation/Outcomes
- Verbalizes an improved body image
- Reports satisfying sexual functioning
- Continues medical regimen and supervision

ANTIDIURETIC HORMONE REPLACEMENT

Diabetes Insipidus

- ADH promotes water reabsorption by distal renal tubules and causes vasoconstriction and increased muscle tone of bladder, GI tract, uterus, and blood vessels; ADH works *against* diuresis (fluid loss)

Types of Diabetes Insipidus
- *Deficient antidiuretic hormone* (ADH) by posterior pituitary gland, decreases reabsorption of water in nephron tubules; may be familial, idiopathic, or secondary to trauma, surgery, tumors, infections, or autoimmune disorders
- *Neurogenic diabetes insipidus:* renal tubular defect resulting in decreased water absorption; results in impaired renal concentrating ability; may be familial or result from renal disorders, primary aldosteronism, or excessive water intake (primary polydipsia)

Therapeutic interventions
- Treatment of underlying cause
- Hypophysectomy
- Antidiuretic hormone replacement
  - Administered orally, subcutaneously, intravenously, or intranasally
- Medication mode of action
  - Desmopressin and vasopressin: Promote reabsorption of water by acting on kidney
  - Antidiuretic effect: carbamazepine (unlabeled use; see Chapter 4) and others

Select Contraindications, Precautions, and Major Drug Interactions for Desmopressin and Vasopressin*

Drug	Contraindications/Precautions	Major Drug Interactions
desmopressin	*Contraindications:* Hypersensitivity, moderate to severe renal disease, hyponatremia *Precautions:* Heart disease, coronary artery disease, congestive heart failure, vascular diseases, kidney disease, cystic fibrosis, high or low blood pressure, electrolyte imbalances, breastfeeding, changes in nasal mucosa (for intranasal administration), children, geriatric, thrombus, male infertility *Pregnancy:* No human studies available, but no adverse effects in animals	Alcohol, carbamazepine, chlorpropamide, clofibrate, demeclocycline, heparin, lithium
vasopressin	*Contraindications:* Hypersensitivity, moderate to severe renal disease *Precautions:* Breastfeeding, seizure disorders, coronary artery disease, cardiac/renal/vascular disease, asthma, migraines; monitor serum cortisol levels; avoid injection into a blood vessel *Pregnancy:* Only given after risks to the fetus are considered	Alcohol, demeclocycline, fludrocortisones, haloperidol, heparin, lithium, norepinephrine, chlorpropamide, carbamazepine, tricyclics, urea

*Pregnancy categories have been revised. See http://www.fda.gov/Drugs/DevelopmentApprovalProcess/DevelopmentResources/Labeling/ucm093307.htm for more information.

Adverse Effects/Side Effects
- Increased blood pressure, facial flushing
- Headache, fever, vertigo, drowsiness, listlessness, tremor, sweating
- Hyponatremia (can lead to seizures)
- Nasal irritation, congestion, rhinitis, nosebleed (for intranasal administration)
- Nausea, diarrhea, heartburn/dyspepsia, mild abdominal cramps (GI irritation), vomiting
- Seizures
- Shock, hypovolemia (can lead to tachycardia and hypotension)
- Uterine cramping
- Vasopressin: angina pectoris, severe cardiovascular events: cardiac arrest, MI

Nursing Care of Clients with Diabetes Insipidus
Assessment/Analysis
- I&O, weight, urine, specific gravity, and urine and serum osmolality to establish baseline data
- Serum electrolyte levels
- Dryness of skin and mucous membranes
- Assess for side effects

Planning/Implementation
- Monitor fluid and electrolyte status (e.g., I&O, daily weight, skin turgor, electrolyte levels)
- Replace fluids as ordered

- Monitor response to ADH replacement
- Instruct client
  - Ensure long-term medical supervision
  - Obtain weight daily
  - Wear medical alert bracelet
  - Monitor for signs of polyuria; water retention and hyponatremia (overdosage of ADH medication may cause syndrome of inappropriate antidiuretic hormone [SIADH])
  - Avoid alcohol because it suppresses ADH secretion
  - Follow physician instruction on fluid intake; fluid intake needs to be *decreased* with pharmacologic therapy
  - Monitor urine specific gravity

Evaluation/Outcomes

- Maintains fluid balance
- States clinical findings if overmedication or undermedication with ADH replacement occurs

ANTIDIURETIC HORMONE ANTAGONIST

Syndrome of Inappropriate Antidiuretic Hormone Secretion (SIADH)

- Excessive ADH secretion leads to fluid retention and dilutional hyponatremia
- Caused by head trauma, tumors, or infection; malignant tumor cells may produce ADH

Therapeutic Interventions

- Fluid restriction; hypertonic parenteral fluids
- Treatment of symptoms (e.g., seizures, dysrhythmias)
- Medications = vasopressin receptor antagonists
  - Administered only in hospital environment
  - Used cautiously with clients with alcoholism and/or malnutrition
  - Mode of action: promotes renal excretion of water by blocking vasopressor receptors
    - Conivaptan: for treatment of symptomatic euvolemic hyponatremia from SIADH
    - Tolvaptan: for treatment of symptomatic hypervolemic or euvolemic hyponatremia from SIADH
    - Demeclocycline: tetracycline antibiotic used as off label treatment for SIADH

Select Contraindications, Precautions, and Major Drug Interactions for ADH Antagonists*

Drug	Contraindications/Precautions	Drug Interactions
Vasopressin Receptor Antagonists		
conivaptan (parenteral)	**Contraindications:** Hypersensitivity, corn allergy, concurrent CYP3A4 inhibitors, hypovolemia, urinary retention, severe renal impairment	All CYP3A4 substrates, digoxin
	Precautions: Alcoholism, breastfeeding, orthostatic/renal/hepatic disease, heart failure, alcoholism, malnutrition, HIV/AIDs; concurrent administration of anticholesterol medications or CYP3A4 substrates; administer only in large veins; rapid correction of serum sodium can cause neurologic deficits, so the rate of rise of serum sodium must not exceed 12 mEq/L/24 hr	
	Pregnancy: Only given after risks to the fetus are considered	

Select Contraindications, Precautions, and Major Drug Interactions for ADH Antagonists—cont'd

Drug	Contraindications/Precautions	Drug Interactions
Vasopressin Receptor Antagonists		
tolvaptan (oral)	**Contraindications:** Hypersensitivity, alcoholism, hepatic disease, malnutrition, hypovolemia, strong CYP3A4 inhibitors, diltiazem **Precautions:** Alcoholism, malnutrition, liver disease, dehydration, concurrent CYP3A4 moderate inhibitors and inducers; reduce dose if administered with P-gp inhibitors; rapid correction of serum sodium can cause neurologic deficits, so the rate of rise of serum sodium must not exceed 12 mEq/L/24 hr **Pregnancy:** Only given after risks to the fetus are considered	CYP3A4 inducers, digoxin
demeclocycline	**Contraindications:** Hypersensitivity to tetracyclines, breastfeeding **Precautions:** Benign intracranial hypertension **Pregnancy:** Positive evidence of human fetal risk; benefits may exceed risks in pregnant women	Acitretin, aluminum/calcium/magnesium antacids, anticoagulants, dicloxacillin, methoxyflurane, penicillin

*Pregnancy categories have been revised. See http://www.fda.gov/Drugs/DevelopmentApprovalProcess/DevelopmentResources/Labeling/ucm093307.htm for more information.

Adverse Effects/Side Effects
- Conivaptan: injection site reactions, including phlebitis, pain, edema, and pruritus; fever, headache, orthostatic hypotension, hypertension, atrial fibrillation, polyuria, electrolyte imbalances such as hypokalemia, constipation, diarrhea, vomiting
- Tolvaptan: polyuria; loss of fluids can produce thirst, dry mouth, constipation, hyperglycemia, dizziness, weakness

Nursing Care of Clients with Syndrome of Inappropriate Antidiuretic Hormone Secretion
Assessment/Analysis
- History of malignancy, infection, or increased intracranial pressure
- I&O, daily weight, vital signs
- Closely monitor serum and urine for sodium concentration and osmolality
- Neurologic evaluations

Planning/Implementation
- Monitor fluid and electrolyte status; weigh daily
- Monitor for altered level of consciousness
- Restrict fluid intake *unless taking conivaptan or tolvaptan;* administer hypertonic intravenous solutions (usually 3% sodium chloride) as ordered
- If taking conivaptan or tolvaptan, avoid fluid restriction
- Institute seizure precautions and protect from injury
- Provide supportive measures for related disorders
- Teach patients to avoid grapefruit juice if taking conivaptan or tolvaptan
- Teach patients that demeclocycline can discolor teeth

Evaluation/Outcomes
- Maintains fluid balance
- Remains seizure-free

OXYTOCIN

- A posterior pituitary hormone that stimulates contractions by pregnant uterus and stimulates milk ejection from alveoli of lactating breasts into ducts
- Synthetic versions, oxytocics, are used to induce or augment labor
  - Stimulate uterus to contract
  - Induce labor; infused slowly
  - Augment contractions that have already begun, increasing force, duration and frequency
  - Induce contraction of lacteal glands, which promotes let-down reflex for breastfeeding
  - Exert vasopressor and antidiuretic effects; control of postpartum hemorrhage
  - Enhance postpartum uterine contraction; infused rapidly
  - Available in IM, IV, oral, and nasal preparations

Mode of Action

- Oxytocin increases intracellular calcium in uterine myometrial tissue, enhancing contractility

Select Contraindications, Precautions, and Major Drug Interactions for Oxytocin*

Drug	Contraindications/Precautions	Major Drug Interactions
oxytocin	*Contraindications:* Hypersensitivity, proven cephalopelvic disproportion, fetal intolerance of labor, fetal malpresentation, umbilical cord prolapse, previous uterine surgery, anticipated nonvaginal delivery; intranasal spray is contraindicated in pregnancy; only for medical induction—not elective induction *Precautions:* Cervical/uterine surgery, uterine sepsis, primipara >35 yr, 1st/2nd stage of labor *Pregnancy:* Only given after risks to the fetus are considered	Cyclopropane anesthetics, vasopressors

*Pregnancy categories have been revised. See http://www.fda.gov/Drugs/DevelopmentApprovalProcess/DevelopmentResources/Labeling/ucm093307.htm for more information.

Adverse Effects/Side Effects

- Maternal
  - Hypertension (contracts smooth muscles of blood vessels)
  - Dysrhythmias; tachycardia (vasoconstriction)
  - Uterine hyperstimulation; hypertonic uterus; uterine rupture
  - Water intoxication (antidiuretic effect) may precipitate seizures and coma
  - Intracranial hemorrhage
- Fetal: caused by tetanic uterine contractions
  - Anoxia; asphyxia (vasoconstriction)
  - Dysrhythmias (premature ventricular complexes [PVCs], bradycardia)
  - Hyperbilirubinemia (hepatic dysfunction)
  - Fetal jaundice

Nursing Care Associated with Oxytocics

- Monitor vital signs every 30 to 60 minutes and with each dose increase
- Have oxygen and emergency resuscitative equipment available
- Maintain continuous fetal monitoring; assess uterine contractions and tone, and FHR every 15 minutes

- Use infusion-control device for IV administration; always given by secondary line (IV piggy back [IVPB])
- Discontinue infusion for prolonged uterine contractions, inadequate uterine resting tone, or nonreassuring fetal response to contractions

APPLICATION AND REVIEW

1. A nurse administers the drug desmopressin acetate (DDAVP) to a client with diabetes insipidus. What should the nurse monitor to evaluate the effectiveness of the drug?
   1. Arterial blood pH
   2. I&O
   3. Fasting serum glucose
   4. Pulse and respiratory rates
2. A client is admitted with a head injury. The nurse identifies that the client's urinary retention catheter is draining large amounts of clear, colorless urine. What does the nurse identify as the **most** likely cause?
   1. Increased serum glucose
   2. Deficient renal perfusion
   3. Inadequate ADH secretion
   4. Excess amounts of IV fluid
3. After a head injury a client develops a deficiency of antidiuretic hormone (ADH). What should the nurse consider about the response to secretion of ADH before assessing this client?
   1. Serum osmolarity increases
   2. Urine concentration decreases
   3. Glomerular filtration decreases
   4. Tubular reabsorption of water increases
4. After surgical clipping of a cerebral aneurysm, the client develops the syndrome of inappropriate secretion of antidiuretic hormone (ADH). For which manifestations of excessive levels of ADH should the nurse assess the client? **Select all that apply.**
   1. Polyuria
   2. Weight gain
   3. Hypotension
   4. Hyponatremia
   5. Decreased specific gravity
5. A client who has acromegaly and insulin-dependent diabetes undergoes a hypophysectomy. The nurse identifies that *further teaching about the hypophysectomy is necessary* when the client states, "I know I will:
   1. be sterile for the rest of my life."
   2. require larger doses of insulin than I did preoperatively."
   3. have to take cortisone or a similar drug for the rest of my life."
   4. have to take thyroxine or a similar medication for the rest of my life."

See Answers on pages 275-279.

THYROID HORMONES

Hypothyroidism

- Causes:
  - Deficient hormone synthesis
  - Congenital thyroid defects
  - Prenatal and postnatal iodine deficiency
  - Autoimmune diseases (e.g., Hashimoto disease, sarcoidosis)
- Classified according to time of life when it occurs
  - Cretinism: hypothyroidism found at birth
  - Lymphocytic thyroiditis: most often after 6 years of age and peaks during adolescence; generally self-limiting

- Hypothyroidism without myxedema: mild degree of thyroid failure in older children and adults; more common as one ages
  - Hypothyroidism with myxedema: severe degree of thyroid failure in older individuals
- Decreased levels of thyroid hormones (T_3 and T_4) slow basal metabolic rate (BMR); decreased BMR affects lipid metabolism, increases cholesterol and triglyceride levels, and affects RBC production, leading to anemia and folate deficiency
- Myxedema coma is most severe degree of hypothyroidism; exhibited by hypothermia, bradycardia, hypoventilation, progressive loss of consciousness; precipitated by severe physiologic stress; potentially fatal endocrine emergency

Therapeutic Interventions

- Thyroid hormones: levothyroxine (a synthetic preparation of thyroxine) is drug of choice; liothyronine; liotrix
  - Same mechanism as endogenous thyroid hormones
  - Regulate metabolic rate of body cells; aid in growth and development of bones and teeth; affect protein, fat, and carbohydrate metabolism
  - Replace thyroid hormone when there is a reduction in or absence of thyroid gland function
  - Available in oral and parenteral (IV) preparations
- Maintenance of vital functions
- Screening every 5 years after age 35 for thyroid hormone status

Select Contraindications, Precautions, and Major Drug Interactions for Thyroid Hormones*

Drug	Contraindications/Precautions	Major Drug Interactions
levothyroxine (synthetic thyroxine)	**Contraindications:** Hypersensitivity, hypersensitivity to beef, thyrotoxicosis, myocardial infarction, adrenal insufficiency, hyperthyroidism, obesity treatment **Precautions:** Cardiac arrhythmias, cardiac disease, hypertension, angina pectoris; diabetes mellitus; osteoporosis; hypopituitarism; dysphagia, breastfeeding, geriatric, ischemia, diabetes **Pregnancy:** No known adverse reactions	Sympathomimetics, aluminum and magnesium products, antacids, anticoagulants, antidiabetics, beta blockers, bile acid sequestrants, calcium and iron supplements, carbamazepine, cholestyramine, colestipol, corticosteroids, decongestants, digitalis products, epinephrine, estrogens, hepatic inducers, histamine receptor blockers, insulin, ketamines, phenytoin, rifampin sertraline, phenobarbital, proton pump inhibitors, simethicone, SSRIs, sucralfate, TCAs, vasopressors
liothyronine (synthetic T_3)	**Contraindications:** Hypersensitivity, adrenal insufficiency, MI, thyrotoxicosis, untreated hypertension, obesity treatment **Precautions:** Angina pectoris, breastfeeding, cardiac disease, diabetes, geriatric, hypertension, ischemia, adrenal or pituitary disease **Pregnancy:** No known adverse reactions	Oral anticoagulants, aluminum and magnesium products, antacids, calcium and iron supplements, cholestyramine, colestipol, decongestants, digitalis, estrogens, insulin, ketamine, oral hypoglycemic, oral contraceptives, sympathomimetics, TCAs, vasopressors
liotrix (mix of levothyroxine and liothyronine)	**Contraindications:** Hypersensitivity, adrenal insufficiency, MI, thyrotoxicosis, obesity treatment **Precautions:** Angina pectoris, breastfeeding, cardiac disease, congestive heart failure, geriatric, hypertension, ischemia, diabetes mellitus, adrenal or pituitary disease **Pregnancy:** No known adverse reactions	Amphetamines, antacids, carbamazepine, catecholamines, cholestyramine, colestipol, decongestants, estrogens, insulin, oral anticoagulants, oral hypoglycemics, oral contraceptives, phenytoin, rifampin, sympathomimetics, TCAs, vasopressors

*Pregnancy categories have been revised. See http://www.fda.gov/Drugs/DevelopmentApprovalProcess/DevelopmentResources/Labeling/ucm093307.htm for more information.

Adverse Effects/Side Effects

- Angina
- Anxiety
- Cardiac dysrhythmia, cardiac arrest
- Dysrhythmias
- Hyperactivity
- Hypertension
- Insomnia
- Osteoporosis
- Palpitations, tachycardia
- Thyroid storm
- Tremors

Nursing Care of Clients with Hypothyroidism

Assessment/Analysis

- History that may have contributed to condition
- Activity tolerance, bowel elimination, sleeping patterns, sexual function, and intolerance to cold
- Skin and hair for characteristic changes
- Weight and vital signs to establish baseline
- Clinical findings of anemia, atherosclerosis, or arthritis
- Assess for clinical findings of hypothyroidism
- Assess for potentiation of anticoagulant effect of thyroid hormone medication

Planning/Implementation

- Have patience with lethargic client
- Explain that activity tolerance and mental functioning will improve with therapy; explain importance of continued hormone replacement throughout life
- Review clinical findings of hypothyroidism and hyperthyroidism to help client identify clinical findings of undermedication or overmedication
- Note that levothyroxine dosages are in micrograms (mcg), not milligrams (mg)
- Offer emotional support; therapy is usually lifelong
- Instruct client
  - Report occurrence of side effects immediately
  - Take medication as scheduled at same time daily; do not stop abruptly
    - Teach patient to take thyroid hormones on an empty stomach at least 60 minutes before breakfast
  - Take pulse rate; notify health care provider if greater than 100 beats/min
  - Carry medical alert card
  - Continue routine medical supervision
  - Avoid OTC drugs unless approved by health care provider; have medical supervision when taking opioid analgesics and tranquilizers
  - Modify outdoor activities in cold weather; wear adequate clothing because of sensitivity to cold environments
  - Use moisturizers for dry skin
  - Restrict calories, cholesterol, and fat in diet to prevent weight gain
  - Avoid constipation (e.g., increase fluid intake and fiber in diet)
- Teach to seek medical supervision regularly and when clinical findings of illness develop; teach client and family clinical findings of complications
  - Angina pectoris: chest pain, indigestion
  - Cardiac failure: dyspnea, palpitations
  - Myxedema coma: weakness, syncope, slow pulse rate, subnormal temperature, slow respirations, lethargy

Evaluation/Outcomes

- Completes activities of daily living (ADLs) without fatigue
- Adheres to dietary, exercise, and medication regimen
- Establishes regular pattern of bowel elimination

ANTITHYROID AGENTS

Hyperthyroidism (Graves' Disease, Thyrotoxicosis)

- Excessive concentration of thyroid hormones (T_3 and T_4) in blood as result of thyroid disease or increased levels of TSH; leads to hypermetabolic state
- Autoimmune process of impaired regulation; mediated by immunoglobulin G (IgG) antibody that activates TSH receptors on surface of thyroid cells; associated with other autoimmune disorders
- Gland may enlarge (goiter) as a result of decreased iodine intake; there may or may not be an increase in secretion of thyroid hormones
- Hypothyroidism may result from therapy (e.g., radioactive iodine, thyroidectomy); treated with levothyroxine (Synthroid)

Therapeutic interventions

- Three main options: radioactive ablation, surgical excision, or antithyroid medications
- Radioactive iodine: ^{131}I (atomic cocktail); destroys thyroid gland cells, thereby decreasing production of thyroid hormone
- Surgical intervention: subtotal or total thyroidectomy; orbital decompression to reduce abnormal protrusion of the eyeball (exophthalmos); various procedures to correct vision or protect eye
- Medications to relieve clinical findings related to increased metabolic rate: adrenergic blocking agents (See Chapter 6)
- Graves' ophthalmopathy: prednisone to reduce inflammation behind the eye
- Well-balanced, high-calorie diet with vitamin and mineral supplements
- Antithyroid medications: Mode of action
  - Methimazole: interferes with synthesis and release of thyroid hormone by decreasing iodine use, but does not destroy existing thyroid hormone
  - Propylthiouracil (PTU): suppresses synthesis of thyroid hormones and inhibits conversion of T_4 to T_3
  - Iodine (potassium iodide); reduces vascularity of thyroid gland: suppresses thyroid release; inhibits oxidation of iodides to prevent their combination with tyrosine in formation of thyroxine; also used in prophylaxis after radiation exposure

Select Contraindications, Precautions, and Major Drug Interactions for Antithyroid Drugs (Also Called Thyroid Inhibitors)*

Drug	Contraindications/Precautions	Major Drug Interactions
Thioamides[†]		
methimazole	*Contraindications:* Hypersensitivity, breastfeeding, pregnancy *Precautions:* Bleeding disorders, bone marrow depression, immunocompromise, infection, hepatic disease *Pregnancy:* Definite fetal risks, but may be given despite risks in life-threatening conditions; can cause hypothyroidism, goiter and cretinism in fetus	Oral anticoagulants, antineoplastics, beta-adrenergic blockers, digitalis, digoxin, insulin, lithium, live vaccines, oral anticoagulants, oral antidiabetics, phenytoin, potassium iodide, theophylline

Select Contraindications, Precautions, and Major Drug Interactions for Antithyroid Drugs (Also Called Thyroid Inhibitors)—cont'd

Drug	Contraindications/Precautions	Major Drug Interactions
Thioamides		
propylthiouracil (PTU)	**Contraindications:** Hypersensitivity, pregnancy, breast-feeding, children, hepatitis, jaundice, agranulocytosis, clay-colored stools **Precautions:** Fever, bone marrow depression, infection, hepatic disease **Pregnancy:** Definite fetal risks, but may be given despite risks in life-threatening conditions; considered safer during 1st trimester than methimazole	Anticoagulants (oral), beta-adrenergic blockers, antineoplastics, digitalis glycosides, digoxin, insulin, lithium, oral antidiabetics, phenothiazines, phenytoin, potassium iodide, radiation, theophylline
Iodine		
potassium iodide	**Contraindications:** Hypersensitivity; hypersensitivity to iodide or iodine, pregnancy, breastfeeding, pulmonary edema, pulmonary TB, bronchitis **Precautions:** Cardiac/thyroid/kidney disease, hyperkalemia, tuberculosis, Addison disease, genetic muscle disorders, children **Pregnancy:** Definite fetal risks, but may be given despite risks in life-threatening conditions	ACE inhibitors, angiotensin-II receptor antagonists, antithyroid drugs (methimazole, propylthiouracil), lithium, potassium salts, potassium-sparing diuretics

*Pregnancy categories have been revised. See http://www.fda.gov/Drugs/DevelopmentApprovalProcess/DevelopmentResources/Labeling/ucm093307.htm for more information.
†Interfere with thyroid hormone synthesis (do not destroy thyroid tissue)

Adverse Effects/Side Effects
- Agranulocytosis (decreased white blood cells [WBCs]), leukopenia, thrombocytopenia; first signs may be sore throat and fever
- Angioneurotic edema: PTU
- Arthralgia: PTU
- Bruising or bleeding
- Decreased metabolism (decreased production of serum T_3, T_4)
- Dizziness, drowsiness
- Fever, flu-like symptoms
- Headache
- Insulin autoimmune syndrome
- Iodine—bitter taste, stains teeth (local oral effect on mucosa and teeth)
- Hematuria, hematochezia
- Hepatitis, hepatotoxicity/liver injury
- Hypothyroidism
- Jaundice, nausea, clay-colored stools
- Lymphadenopathy
- Nausea, vomiting (irritation of gastric mucosa), diarrhea
- Nephritis
- Paresthesias (PTU)
- Periarteritis, hypoprothrombinemia
- Propylthiouracil: liver injury in children
- Skin disturbances: rash, blistering, urticaria, pruritus, alopecia, hyperpigmentation

- Vertigo
- Weakness

Nursing Care of Clients with Hyperthyroidism

Assessment/Analysis

- Weight and vital signs to establish baseline (subsequently to assess for weight loss)
- Diaphoresis, diarrhea, insomnia, emotional lability, palpitations, peripheral edema, heat intolerance, dysrhythmias, severe tachycardia, fever, delirium, CNS irritability
- Eyes for exophthalmos, tearing, sensitivity to light (photophobia)
- Neck palpation for enlarged thyroid gland, enlarged lymph nodes

Planning/Implementation

- Establish climate for uninterrupted rest (e.g., decreased stimulation, back rub, prescribed medications); provide relaxing, calm environment
- Protect from stress-producing situations
- Keep room cool
- Provide diet high in calories, proteins, and carbohydrates with supplemental feedings between meals and at bedtime; vitamin and mineral supplements as prescribed
- Understand that client is upset by lability of mood and exaggerated response to environmental stimuli; explain disease processes involved; avoid rushing and surprises; prepare client for procedures
- Protect eyes (e.g., eye drops, patches, tinted eyeglasses, elevation of head of bed, cool compresses to eyes)
- Provide care before thyroidectomy
  - Teach importance of taking prescribed antithyroid medications to achieve euthyroid state
  - Teach deep-breathing exercises and use of hands to support neck to avoid strain on suture line after surgery
- Provide care after thyroidectomy
  - Observe for clinical findings of respiratory distress and laryngeal stridor caused by tracheal edema; explain a sore throat when swallowing is expected; keep tracheotomy set available
  - Assess for hoarseness which may result from endotracheal intubation or laryngeal nerve damage
  - Maintain in semi-Fowler position to reduce edema at surgical site
  - Observe for hemorrhage at operative site and back of neck and shoulders
  - Observe for thyrotoxicosis (e.g., high temperature, tachycardia, irritability, delirium, coma)
  - Notify health care provider immediately if clinical findings of thyrotoxicosis occur; administer propranolol (Inderal), iodine, propylthiouracil (PTU), and steroids as prescribed
  - Observe for signs of tetany (e.g., numbness or twitching of extremities, spasm of glottis, positive Chvostek and Trousseau signs) because hypocalcemia can occur after accidental trauma or removal of parathyroid glands; give calcium gluconate or calcium chloride (IV) as prescribed if tetany occurs
- Teach regarding radioactive iodine therapy
  - Client is mildly radioactive and should follow radiation precautions as advised (usually 7 days)
    - Increase clear fluid intake
    - Void hourly during first 8 to 12 hours
    - Flush toilet twice after use
    - Ensure thorough hand hygiene
    - Avoid contact with children; avoid close prolonged contact or sleeping with another person
    - Do not share dishes, utensils, food, or drink with another; avoid kissing and sexual contact until permitted

- Hospitalization in isolation may be required for several days if larger dose is used
- Clinical findings of hyperthyroidism may take 3 to 4 weeks to subside

Nursing Care of Patients Receiving Antithyroid Medications
- Instruct client to take antithyroid medications regularly and to report side effects, especially sore throat, jaundice, and fever
  - Avoid crowded places and potentially infectious situations
- Administer liquid iodine preparations diluted in a beverage; use straw to avoid staining teeth
- Assess for clinical findings of hypothyroidism as a result of treatment
- Assess for clinical findings of thyrotoxicosis or overmedication with thyroid hormone replacement therapy
- Instruct client to comply with periodic T_3, T_4, TSH studies to monitor hormone levels

Evaluation/Outcomes
- Maintains ideal body weight
- Establishes regular routine of activity and rest

VITAMIN D ANALOGUES

Hypoparathyroidism
- Insufficient amount of parathormone after thyroid surgery, parathyroid surgery, or radiation therapy of neck; idiopathic hypoparathyroidism is rare
- As level of parathormone drops, serum calcium level also drops, causing clinical findings of tetany; concomitant rise in serum phosphate level occurs

Therapeutic Interventions
- Calcium chloride or calcium gluconate given IV for emergency treatment of overt tetany
- Calcium salts administered orally: calcium carbonate, calcium gluconate; calcium citrate
- Vitamin D analogs
  - Mode of action, calcitriol: increases absorption of calcium from the GI tract; enhances calcium deposition into bone
  - Mode of action, cholecalciferol (vitamin D3): increases uptake of calcium by intestines
  - Mode of action, ergocalciferol: prohormone for hypoparathyroidism; increases absorption of calcium from the GI tract
- Parathormone injections
- High-calcium, low-phosphate diet
- Aluminum hydroxide to decrease absorption of phosphorus from the GI tract

Select Contraindications, Precautions, and Major Drug Interactions for Vitamin D Analogues*

Drug	Contraindications/Precautions	Major Drug Interactions
calcitriol	*Contraindications:* Hypersensitivity, hypercalcemia, hypervitaminosis D, hyperphosphatemia *Precautions:* Renal failure, dehydration, malabsorption syndrome, hypocalcemia, breastfeeding *Pregnancy:* Only given after risks to the fetus are considered	Barbiturates, calcium supplements, cardiac glycosides, digoxin, estrogen, cholestyramine, ketoconazole, lubricant laxatives, magnesium products, mineral oil, phenytoin, thiazide diuretics, verapamil

Continued

Select Contraindications, Precautions, and Major Drug Interactions for Vitamin D Analogues—cont'd

Drug	Contraindications/Precautions	Major Drug Interactions
cholecalciferol	**Contraindications:** Hypersensitivity, hypercalcemia, renal dysfunction, hyperphosphatemia, malabsorption syndrome, hypervitaminosis D **Precautions:** Renal failure, heart disease, electrolyte imbalance **Pregnancy:** Only given after risks to the fetus are considered	Anticonvulsants, calcium supplements/antacids, cholestyramine, colestipol, digoxin, diuretics, steroids
ergocalciferol	**Contraindications:** Hypersensitivity, hypercalcemia, renal dysfunction, hyperphosphatemia **Precautions:** Cardiovascular disease, kidney disease, renal calculi, breastfeeding, concurrent digoxin **Pregnancy:** Only given after risks to the fetus are considered	Antacids, cholestyramine, colestipol, digoxin, mineral oil, phenobarbital, phenytoin, thiazide diuretics, verapamil

*Pregnancy categories have been revised. See http://www.fda.gov/Drugs/DevelopmentApprovalProcess/DevelopmentResources/Labeling/ucm093307.htm for more information.

Adverse Effects/Side Effects
- Effects of hypercalcemia: anorexia, photophobia, dehydration, cardiac arrhythmias, decreased libido, hypertension, sensory disturbances, hypercalciuria, hypercalcemia, hyperphosphatemia
- After long-term use: hypertension, dysrhythmias, fatigue, weakness, dry mouth, headache, GI symptoms, polyuria, albuminuria, decreased bone growth, bone and muscle pain
- Ergocalciferol: hematuria, albuminuria, renal failure, seizures

Nursing Care of Clients with Hypoparathyroidism

Assessment/Analysis
- History of muscle spasms, numbness or tingling of extremities, visual disturbances, or seizures
- Neuromuscular irritability
- Status of respiratory functioning
- Heart rate and rhythm
- Serum calcium and phosphate levels
- Assess renal and nutritional status

Planning/Implementation
- Ask patient about any side effects
- Observe for respiratory distress; have emergency equipment available for tracheostomy and mechanical ventilation
- Maintain seizure precautions
- Reduce environmental stimuli
- Provide dietary instruction (encourage inclusion of dietary sources of calcium that are low in phosphorus)
  - Avoid other supplements unless directed by provider
  - Caution to avoid antacids and laxatives containing magnesium
- Teach clinical findings of hypocalcemia and hypercalcemia; instruct to contact health care provider immediately if either occurs

Evaluation/Outcomes

- Remains free from neuromuscular irritability
- Maintains respiratory functioning within acceptable limits

CALCITONIN AND CALCIMIMETICS

Hyperparathyroidism

- Hyperfunction of parathyroid glands; usually caused by adenoma; hypertrophy and hyperplasia of glands
- Increased reabsorption of calcium and excretion of phosphorus by kidneys
- Demineralization of bone occurs if dietary intake is not enough to meet calcium levels demanded by high levels of parathormone

Therapeutic Interventions

- Surgical excision of parathyroid tumor
- Restriction of dietary calcium intake
- Furosemide to increase renal excretion of calcium
- Pharmacology to decrease calcium level: calcitonin
  - Mode of action: calcitonin decreases serum calcium by binding at receptor sites on osteoclast; it inhibits osteoclasts
- Calcimimetics: cinacalcet
  - Mode of action: tricks parathyroid glands into releasing less parathyroid hormone by mimicking calcium in circulation
- Hormone replacement therapy for postmenopausal women with osteoporosis; may help bones retain calcium
- Bisphosphonates: alendronate, ibandronate, risedronate help prevent loss of calcium from bones
- After parathyroidectomy for parathyroid hyperplasia: autotransplant of a segment of parathyroid gland is placed in forearm or neck to prevent hypoparathyroidism

Select Contraindications, Precautions, and Major Drug Interactions for Calcitonin and Cinacalcet*

Drug	Contraindications/Precautions	Major Drug Interactions
calcitonin-salmon	*Contraindications:* Hypersensitivity, fish hypersensitivity, *Precautions:* Breastfeeding, children, geriatric, renal disease, osteogenic sarcoma, pernicious anemia *Pregnancy:* Only given after risks to the fetus are considered	Bisphosphonates, lithium
cinacalcet	*Contraindications:* Hypersensitivity, hypocalcemia *Precautions:* Breastfeeding, children, seizure disorders, hepatic disease, hyper or hypotension, heart disease, kidney disease *Pregnancy:* Only given after risks to the fetus are considered	CYP3A4 inhibitors, CYP2D6 substrates such as desipramine, metoprolol, carvedilol, and flecainide, and most TCAs

*Pregnancy categories have been revised. See http://www.fda.gov/Drugs/DevelopmentApprovalProcess/DevelopmentResources/Labeling/ucm093307.htm for more information.

Adverse Effects/Side Effects

- Allergic reactions
- Cramping, muscle pain
- Development of neutralizing antibodies
- Flushing
- GI symptoms (e.g., nausea and vomiting)
- Headache
- Hypocalcemia
- Hypotension
- Injection site reactions
- Seizures
- Tetany
- Urine sediment abnormalities
- Worsening heart failure or arrhythmia
- Intranasal calcitonin: nasal ulcers, malignancies

Nursing Care of Clients with Hyperparathyroidism

Assessment/Analysis

- GI disturbance or bone pain
- History of renal calculi or fractures
- Clinical findings of renal calculi (e.g., hematuria, flank pain)
- Use of thiazide diuretics or vitamin D, which can increase serum calcium level
- Serum calcium and phosphorus levels
- Baseline vital signs, particularly heart rate and rhythm
- Nutritional status

Planning/Implementation

- Strain urine for calculi
- Encourage fluid intake
- Assist with ambulation because weight-bearing helps prevent demineralization of bone
- Monitor I&O
- Instruct client
  - Avoid high-impact activities to prevent fractures, but continue moderate exercise to maintain bone health
  - Encourage foods with fiber to limit constipation
  - Limit intake of foods high in calcium, especially milk products
  - Take cinacalcet with or just after a meal; take it whole; do not divide it
- Provide cardiac monitoring if hypercalcemia is severe
- Recheck serum calcium 1 week and 2 months after starting cinacalcet
- Provide care after a parathyroidectomy: same nursing care as care after a thyroidectomy (see Nursing Care under Antithyroid Agents)

Evaluation/Outcomes

- Maintains skeletal integrity
- Remains free of urinary complications

APPLICATION AND REVIEW

6. A nurse is caring for a client who is experiencing an underproduction of thyroxine. Which client response is associated with an underproduction of thyroxine (T_4)?
   1. Myxedema
   2. Acromegaly
   3. Graves' disease
   4. Cushing disease

7. Propylthiouracil (PTU) is prescribed for a client diagnosed with hyperthyroidism. The client asks the nurse, "Why do I have to take this medication if I am going to get the atomic cocktail?" The nurse explains that the medication is being prescribed because it decreases the:
   1. vascularity of the thyroid gland.
   2. production of thyroid hormones.
   3. need for thyroid iodine supplements.
   4. amount of already formed thyroid hormones.

8. A nurse is caring for a client after radioactive iodine is administered for Graves' disease. What information about the client's condition after this therapy should the nurse consider when providing care?
   1. Not radioactive and can be handled as any other individual
   2. Highly radioactive and should be isolated as much as possible
   3. Mildly radioactive but should be treated with routine safety precautions
   4. Not radioactive but may still transmit some dangerous radiations and must be treated with precautions

9. A client with hyperthyroidism asks the nurse about the tests that will be ordered. Which diagnostic tests should the nurse include in a discussion with this client?
   1. T_4 and x-ray films
   2. TSH assay and T_3
   3. Thyroglobulin level and Po_2
   4. Protein-bound iodine and SMA

10. A nurse is caring for a client who just had a thyroidectomy. For which client response should the nurse assess the client when concerned about an accidental removal of the *para*thyroid glands during surgery?
    1. Tetany
    2. Myxedema
    3. Hypovolemic shock
    4. Adrenocortical stimulation

11. Levothyroxine 0.125 mg by mouth is prescribed for a client with hypothyroidism. The only tablets available contain 25 mcg per tablet. How many tablets should the nurse administer? **Record your answer using a whole number.**
    Answer: _____ tablets

12. For which client response should the nurse monitor when assessing for complications of hyperparathyroidism?
    1. Tetany
    2. Seizures
    3. Bone pain
    4. Graves' disease

See Answers on pages 275-279.

DIABETES MELLITUS

(See Chapter 12)

ALDOSTERONE ANTAGONIST

Adrenal Disorders: Primary Aldosteronism (Conn Syndrome)

- Excessive secretion of aldosterone, a mineralocorticoid, secreted in response to renin-angiotensin system and ACTH; causes kidneys to retain sodium and water and to excrete potassium and hydrogen
- Usually caused by adenoma of adrenal cortex; also may be caused by hyperplasia or carcinoma

Therapeutic Interventions

- Surgical removal of adrenal tumor
  - Bilateral adrenalectomy requires lifelong corticosteroid therapy

- Potassium-sparing diuretic to control blood pressure; e.g., spironolactone (See Chapter 8)
- Angiotensin-converting enzyme inhibitors (ACE-Is) and angiotensin receptor blockers (ARBs) are potential treatment options (See Chapter 8)
- Calcium channel blockers to reduce production of aldosterone (See Chapter 8)
- Thiazides to control blood pressure (See Chapter 8)
- Aldosterone antagonist to control blood pressure; e.g., eplerenone, a selective aldosterone receptor blocker
  - Mode of Action: binds to mineralocorticoid receptor and blocks the binding of aldosterone, thus normalizing serum potassium levels and blood pressure
  - Eplerenone is used as an antihypertensive and to treat heart failure

Select Contraindications, Precautions, and Major Drug Interactions for Aldosterone Antagonist*

Drug	Contraindications/Precautions	Major Drug Interactions
eplerenone	*Contraindications:* Hypersensitivity, increased serum creatinine, increased serum potassium, decreased creatinine clearance, hepatic disease, severe renal impairment, use of potassium-sparing diuretics or potassium supplements; in patients also receiving strong CYP3A4 inhibitors or clarithromycin, itraconazole, ketoconazole, nefazodone, nelfinavir, ritonavir, troleandomycin *Precautions:* Breastfeeding, children, geriatric, impaired renal/hepatic function, hyperkalemia, breastfeeding *Pregnancy:* No human studies available, but no adverse effects in animals	ACE inhibitors, angiotensin II antagonists, azole antifungals, CYP3A4 inhibitors, diuretics (potassium-sparing), erythromycin, fluconazole, lithium, NSAIDs, potassium supplements, verapamil

*Pregnancy categories have been revised. See http://www.fda.gov/Drugs/DevelopmentApprovalProcess/DevelopmentResources/Labeling/ucm093307.htm for more information.

Adverse Effects/Side Effects
- Hyperkalemia
- Abdominal pain
- Cough
- Diarrhea
- Dizziness
- Fatigue
- Flu-like syndrome
- Gynecomastia
- Myocardial infarction

Nursing Care of Clients with Primary Aldosteronism
Assessment/Analysis
- Vital signs, including blood pressure
- Electrolyte levels, especially serum potassium
- I&O, urine specific gravity
- Motor and sensory functions
- Cardiac dysrhythmias as result of hypokalemia

Planning/Implementation
- Regulate fluid intake
- Encourage continued health care supervision
- Provide care after bilateral adrenalectomy
  - Monitor vital signs, hemodynamic state, and blood glucose level

- Administer steroids with antacid, proton pump inhibitor (PPI), or H_2-blocker to prevent GI erosion
  - Protect from infection and stressful situations
  - Explain drugs and side effects
  - Instruct to carry medical alert identification card
  - Monitor fluid balance; blood pressure for hypotension
  - Monitor for emotional upset, which may require an increase in steroid medications
- Provide dietary instruction (e.g., encourage intake of foods high in potassium, avoidance of foods that contain sodium)
- Teach patients receiving eplerenone:
  - Avoid grapefruit juice and do not take potassium substitutes
  - Do not discontinue eplerenone abruptly
  - To continue to take the medication, even if they are feeling better

Evaluation/Outcomes
- Maintains blood pressure at an expected level
- Selects foods low in sodium and high in potassium
- Performs routine ADLs without fatigue

GLUCOCORTICOIDS AND MINERALOCORTICOIDS

- See *Adrenal Glands* section for descriptions of adrenocortical agents
- Indications include primary adrenal insufficiency (both glucocorticoids and mineralocorticoids); inflammatory (mainly glucocorticoids), allergic, and autoimmune disorders (such as rheumatoid arthritis); organ transplant recipients for immunosuppression (mainly glucocorticoids)

Addison Disease (Primary Adrenal Insufficiency)
- Hyposecretion of adrenocortical hormones
- Usually autoimmune destruction of cortex or idiopathic atrophy
  - Decreased levels of serum cortisol, 17-ketosteroids, and 17-hydroxysteroids; increased plasma ACTH level
- Addisonian crisis (acute adrenal insufficiency) precipitated by stresses (e.g., pregnancy, surgery, infection, dehydration, emotional turmoil); fatal if not treated
- Associated with endocrine disorders, sudden cessation of glucocorticoids, adrenalectomy, tuberculosis, acquired immunodeficiency syndrome (AIDS)

Therapeutic Interventions
- Replacement of adrenocorticoid hormones: glucocorticoids to correct metabolic imbalance; mineralocorticoids to correct electrolyte imbalance and hypotension
  - Available in oral, parenteral (intramuscular [IM], IV), inhalation, intraarticular, and topical (including ophthalmic) preparations
  - Glucocorticoid examples: Mode of action: decrease inflammation
    - Short-acting: hydrocortisone
    - Intermediate-acting: methylprednisolone
    - Long-acting: dexamethasone
  - Mineralocorticoid example: fludrocortisone
    - Mode of action: promotes increased reabsorption of sodium and loss of potassium, water, hydrogen from distal tubules

- Additional hormone replacement during illness or stress to prevent Addisonian crisis; e.g., hydrocortisone, fludrocortisones
  - Some glucocorticoids have weak mineralocorticoid actions, so they can be used individually in replacement; others must be combined with a mineralocorticoid
- Correction of fluid, electrolyte, and glucose imbalances
- High-carbohydrate, high-protein diet
- Prevention of osteoporosis, which may develop with use of steroid therapy that breaks down protein matrix in bones

Select Contraindications, Precautions, and Major Drug Interactions for Glucocorticoids*

Drug	Contraindications/Precautions	Major Drug Interactions
Short-Acting		
cortisone	*Contraindications:* Hypersensitivity, breastfeeding, infection, concurrent live vaccines, abrupt withdrawal *Precautions:* CHF, depression, diabetes, GI disorders, glaucoma, hypertension, liver/renal/thyroid disorder, myasthenia gravis, ocular herpes simplex, osteoporosis, tuberculosis, recent MI, amebiasis *Pregnancy:* Definite fetal risks, but may be given despite risks in life-threatening conditions	Antidiabetics, bupropion, aspirin, diuretics, insulin, oral antidiabetics, NSAIDs, and many others; refer to manufacturer's label
hydrocortisone	*Contraindications:* Hypersensitivity, fungal infection, varicella, serious infections such as septicemia, concurrent live vaccines *Precautions:* blood cell disorders, breastfeeding, cardiac/renal diseases, children, Cushing syndrome, diabetes mellitus, glaucoma, hepatic disease, hypothyroidism, infections, peptic ulcers and other GI diseases, mental health disorders, metastatic disease, myasthenia gravis, myocardial infarction (recent), osteoporosis, seizure disorders, septic shock, psychosis *Pregnancy:* Only given after risks to the fetus are considered	Acetaminophen, alcohol, anticoagulants, anticonvulsants, antidiabetics, aspirin barbiturates, calcium supplements, diuretics, insulin, oral antidiabetics, NSAIDs, salicylates, toxoids, vaccines, and many others; refer to manufacturer's label
Intermediate-Acting		
methylprednisone	*Contraindications:* Hypersensitivity, systemic fungal infections, intrathecal use, newborn infants, concurrent live vaccines, abrupt discontinuation *Precautions:* Breastfeeding, children, cardiac/renal disease, glaucoma, osteoporosis, ulcerative colitis, myasthenia gravis, esophagitis, peptic ulcer, infections, osteoporosis, Cushing syndrome *Pregnancy:* Only given after risks to the fetus are considered	Amphotericin B, aspirin, CYP3A4 inducers and inhibitors, NSAIDs, diuretics, estrogens, grapefruit juice, insulin, isoniazid, macrolide antibiotics, oral antidiabetics, oral contraceptives, oral anticoagulants, phenytoin, rifampin, vaccines
prednisolone	*Contraindications:* Hypersensitivity, fungal infections, abrupt discontinuation, concurrent live vaccines *Precautions:* Breastfeeding, children, cardiac/renal/hepatic disease, Cushing syndrome, diabetes mellitus, glaucoma, infections, osteoporosis, GI disorders, myasthenia gravis, hypertension, psychosis *Pregnancy:* Only given after risks to the fetus are considered	Alcohol, amphotericin B, anticholinesterases, anticoagulants, aspirin, barbiturates, contraceptives (oral), CYP3A4 inhibitors (e.g., ketoconazole), digitalis, NSAIDs, cyclosporine, diuretics, estrogens, immunosuppressants, insulin, oral antidiabetics, phenytoin, rifampin, toxoids, vaccines

Select Contraindications, Precautions, and Major Drug Interactions for Glucocorticoids—cont'd

Drug	Contraindications/Precautions	Major Drug Interactions
Intermediate-Acting		
prednisone	**Contraindications:** Hypersensitivity, untreated serious infections, varicella, fungal infection **Precautions:** Psychosis, cataracts, children, breastfeeding, Cushing syndrome, diabetes mellitus, renal disease, heart failure, myocardial infarction, glaucoma, hypertension, osteoporosis, cirrhosis, esophagitis, diverticulitis, recent MI, hypothyroidism, myasthenia gravis, ulcerative colitis, seizures, visual disturbances, GI disorders, ocular herpes simplex, abrupt discontinuation, peptic ulcer, ulcerative colitis **Pregnancy:** Immediate release: only given after risks to the fetus are considered; delayed release: definite fetal risks, but may be given despite risks in life-threatening conditions	Alcohol, amphotericin B, antiinfectives (macrolide), anticoagulants, antidiabetics (oral), aspirin, barbiturates, bupropion, CYP3A4 inhibitors (e.g., ketoconazole), cardiac glycosides, contraceptives (oral), cyclosporine, digoxin, diltiazem, diuretics, estrogens, immunosuppressants, insulin, isoniazid, NSAIDs, phenytoin, rifampin, salicylates
Long-Acting		
betamethasone	**Contraindications:** Hypersensitivity, intramuscular preparations in idiopathic thrombocytopenic purpura, concurrent live vaccines, breastfeeding **Precautions:** Cardiac/renal disorders, children, cirrhosis, GI disorders, glaucoma, hypertension, myasthenia gravis, osteoporosis, recent MI, infections, thyroid disorders, psychosis **Pregnancy:** Only given after risks to the fetus are considered	Alcohol, amphotericin B, antibiotics, anticholinesterases, aspirin, NSAIDs, carbamazepine, cholestyramine, cyclosporine, digitalis, diuretics, estrogens, insulin, isoniazid, oral antidiabetics, oral anticoagulants, oral contraceptives
dexamethasone	**Contraindications:** Hypersensitivity, fungal infection, live vaccines, abrupt discontinuation, breastfeeding **Precautions:** Cardiac/renal/hepatic disorders, diabetes, children, GI disorders, glaucoma, hypertension, myasthenia gravis, ocular herpes simplex, osteoporosis, recent MI, infections, thyroid disorders, psychosis **Pregnancy:** Only given after risks to the fetus are considered	Antacids, anti-*Pseudomonas* penicillin preparations, aspirin, barbiturates, estrogen, insulin, oral antidiabetics, NSAIDs, phenytoin, theophylline, rifampin,

*Pregnancy categories have been revised. See http://www.fda.gov/Drugs/DevelopmentApprovalProcess/DevelopmentResources/Labeling/ucm093307.htm for more information.

Adverse Effects/Side Effects

- Angioedema
- Avascular necrosis
- Cardiac arrest
- Cardiac arrhythmia
- Cardiomyopathy
- CHF
- Chronic therapy: adrenal suppression; Cushing syndrome
- CVA
- Exfoliative dermatitis
- Facial edema, fluid retention
- Fractures
- GI ulceration, bleeding and perforation
- Hyperglycemia, decreased glucose tolerance
- Hypertension

- Hypokalemia
- Increased ICP
- Leukopenia, decreased wound healing
- Lupus-like symptoms
- Mood alterations
- Ocular disease
- Osteoporosis
- Pancreatitis
- Pseudotumor cerebri

- Psychological disorders
- Pulmonary edema
- Seizures
- Septic arthritis
- Tendon rupture
- Thrombocytopenia
- Thromboembolism, thrombophlebitis
- Derivatives with 17-ketosteroid properties: masculinization in females

Select Contraindications, Precautions, and Major Drug Interactions for Mineralocorticoids*

Drug	Contraindications/Precautions	Major Drug Interactions
fludrocortisone	**Contraindications:** Hypersensitivity, children <2 yr, serious infections, fungal infections, amebiasis, psychosis, Cushing syndrome, concurrent live vaccine, abrupt discontinuation **Precautions:** Breastfeeding, children older than 2 yr, hypertension, diabetes, osteoporosis, cardiac/renal/hepatic disease, infections, GI disorders **Pregnancy:** Only given after risks to the fetus are considered	Amphotericin B, anticoagulants, barbiturates, digoxin, diuretics, estrogens, hydantoins, rifamycins, products containing sodium, salicylates, vaccines

*Pregnancy categories have been revised. See http://www.fda.gov/Drugs/DevelopmentApprovalProcess/DevelopmentResources/Labeling/ucm093307.htm for more information.

Adverse Effects/Side Effects

- Fluid imbalance
- Fluid overload/edema, CHF
- Flushing
- Glaucoma
- Hyperglycemia
- Hypertension
- Hypokalemia

- Increased intracerebral pressure
- Menstrual irregularities
- Metabolic alkalosis: GI symptoms, hypotension, cardiac rhythm changes, weakness, anorexia, and myalgia
- Skin rash, sweating
- Thrombophlebitis

Nursing Care of Clients with Addison Disease

Assessment/Analysis

- Baseline vital signs, weight, electrolytes, and serum glucose
- 24-hour urine specimens for diagnostic purposes (17-hydroxycorticosteroids and 17-ketosteroids)
- Assess for emaciation, appearance of skin
- Changes in energy or activity from history
- Assess for infection and potassium depletion

Planning/Implementation

- Monitor vital signs four times a day; identify increase in temperature (infection, dehydration), alterations in pulse rate and rhythm (hyperkalemia), and alterations in blood pressure
- Monitor for clinical findings of sodium and potassium imbalance

- Monitor I&O and weigh daily
- Collect 24-hour urine specimen
  - Teach foods and medications to be avoided before test
  - Have client void at beginning of the 24-hour time period and discard urine
  - Place urine from every voiding into collection container; ensure that appropriate preservative is used and container is kept refrigerated, if necessary
  - Have client void at end of the 24-hour time period and place urine in container
- Administer steroids as prescribed; give with antacid, PPI, or H_2-blocker to limit ulcerogenic factor effect
- Administer oral preparations with food, milk, or antacid
- Monitor serum electrolytes
- Assess for GI bleeding
- Monitor blood glucose level in people with diabetes
- Prevent exposure to others who may transmit infectious disease (e.g., provide a private room to prevent contact with other clients, limit number of visitors)
- Teach need for lifelong hormone replacement therapy with increased dosage during stress
- Review clinical findings of adrenal hypofunction and hyperfunction so client can identify need for adjustment of steroid dose
- Encourage diet consistent with U.S. Dietary Goals with emphasis on diet high in nutrient-dense foods and adequate salt (sodium)
- Administer antiemetics to prevent fluid and electrolyte loss by vomiting
- Encourage high protein diet for client receiving fludrocortisone
- Instruct client receiving adrenocorticoids to:
  - Avoid exposure to infections; notify health care provider if fever or sore throat occurs; avoid immunizations during therapy
  - Avoid using salt; encourage foods high in potassium
  - Look for signs of salt and water retention and hypokalemia
  - Take medications only as directed, and explain why; avoid missing, changing, or withdrawing drug suddenly
  - Avoid nonsteroidal antiinflammatory drugs (NSAIDs) and over-the-counter (OTC) medications
  - Carry medical alert card
  - Withdraw drug therapy gradually to permit adrenal recovery
  - Avoid physical and emotional stress

Evaluation/Outcomes
1. Maintains fluid balance
2. Maintains electrolyte balance

ADRENAL DISORDERS: CUSHING SYNDROME

- Excess secretion of adrenocortical hormones
  - Hyperglycemia, hypokalemia, elevated plasma cortisol level
  - Elevated levels of 17-hydroxycorticosteroids and 17-ketosteroids in urine
- Caused by hyperplasia or tumor of adrenal cortex; primary lesion may be in pituitary gland, causing excess production of ACTH
- *May be precipitated by administration of excess glucocorticoids or ACTH*

Therapeutic Interventions

- *Reduce dosage of externally administered corticoids*
- If lesion on pituitary is causing hypersecretion of ACTH: hypophysectomy or irradiation of pituitary; radiation in small doses over 6 weeks or stereotactic radiosurgery or gamma knife radiation may be given with a single high-dose intervention; radiation with cortisol–inhibiting drugs may help recovery
- Surgical excision of adrenal tumors (adrenalectomy)
- Adrenal enzyme inhibitors: ketoconazole, mitotane, metyrapone
- Potassium supplements
- High-protein diet with sodium restriction

Nursing Care of Clients with Cushing Syndrome

Assessment/Analysis

- Baseline vital signs, weight, blood glucose level, and electrolytes
- Physical appearance (Fig. 13.2)
- Changes in coping and sexuality from history

Planning/Implementation

- Monitor vital signs, daily weight, I&O, blood glucose level, and electrolyte level
- Protect from exposure to infections

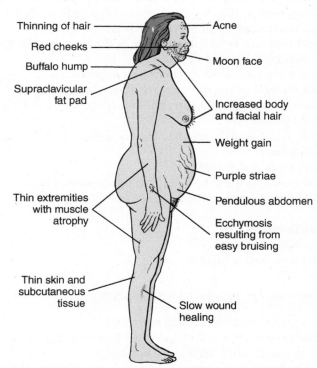

Thinning of hair — Acne
Red cheeks
Buffalo hump — Moon face
Supraclavicular fat pad
Increased body and facial hair
Weight gain
Purple striae
Thin extremities with muscle atrophy
Pendulous abdomen
Ecchymosis resulting from easy bruising
Thin skin and subcutaneous tissue
Slow wound healing

FIG. 13.2   Common characteristics of Cushing syndrome. (From Lewis, S.L., Bucher, L., Heitkemper, M.M., Harding, M.M., Kwong, J., Roberts, D. [2017]. *Medical-surgical nursing: Assessment and management of clinical problems* [10th ed.]. St. Louis: Elsevier.)

- Encourage ventilation of feelings by client and spouse because changes in body image and sex drive can influence spousal support
- Attempt to minimize stress in environment (e.g., limit visitors, explain procedures carefully)
- Provide instruction regarding diet and supplementation; encourage diet rich in nutrient-dense foods (e.g., fruits, vegetables, whole grains, legumes) to improve and maintain nutritional status and prevent drug-induced nutrient deficiencies
- Provide care after a bilateral adrenalectomy (see *Nursing Care of Clients with Primary Aldosteronism*)
- Provide care after a hypophysectomy (see *Nursing Care of Clients with Hyperpituitarism*)

Evaluation/Outcomes
- Maintains fluid balance
- Remains free of infection
- Discusses feelings regarding physical changes

ADRENAL DISORDERS: PHEOCHROMOCYTOMA

- Increased secretion of epinephrine and norepinephrine (catecholamines)
- Catecholamine-secreting tumor of the adrenal medulla; usually benign
  - Patient reports headache, visual disturbances, palpitations, anxiety, heat intolerance, and psychoneurosis
  - Hypertension, postural hypotension, tachycardia, diaphoresis, tremors, cardiac dysrhythmias, hyperglycemia, dilated pupils; brain attack or blindness may occur
  - Increased levels of plasma and urinary catecholamines; increased vanillylmandelic acid (VMA), a product of catecholamine breakdown
- Familial tendency; peak incidence 25 to 50 years of age

Therapeutic Interventions
- Surgical removal of tumor
- Antihypertensives and antidysrhythmics: nitroprusside, propranolol, phentolamine (See Chapter 8)

Nursing Care of Clients with Pheochromocytoma
Assessment/Analysis
- Blood pressures with client in upright and horizontal positions
- Clinical findings associated with hypertension
- 24-hour urine specimens for VMA and catecholamine studies

Planning/Implementation
- Instruct to avoid coffee, chocolate, beer, wine, citrus fruit, bananas, and vanilla before test for VMA
- Administer parenteral fluids and blood as ordered before and after surgery to maintain blood volume
- Decrease environmental stimulation
- Provide care after a bilateral adrenalectomy
  - Instruct regarding maintenance doses of steroids
  - Instruct to take antihypertensives as prescribed and to monitor blood pressure until it returns to expected range
- Emphasize importance of continued medical supervision and screening for other family members

Evaluation/Outcomes
1. Maintains blood pressure at expected level
2. Remains free of complications of hypertension

Nursing Care

See Nursing Care under *Aldosterone Antagonist*

APPLICATION AND REVIEW

13. A client is diagnosed with Cushing syndrome. Which clinical manifestation does the nurse expect to increase in a client with Cushing syndrome?
    1. Urine output
    2. Glucose level
    3. Serum potassium
    4. Immune response

14. Hydrocortisone is prescribed for a client with Addison disease. Before discharge, the nurse teaches the client about this medication. What did the nurse include as a therapeutic effect of the drug?
    1. Supports a better response to stress
    2. Promotes a decrease in blood pressure
    3. Decreases episodes of shortness of breath
    4. Controls an excessive loss of potassium from the body

15. A nurse is caring for a client with the clinical manifestation of hypotension associated with a diagnosis of Addison disease. Which hormone is impaired in its production as a result of this disease?
    1. Estrogens
    2. Androgens
    3. Glucocorticoids
    4. Mineralocorticoids

16. A nurse is caring for a client who had a hypophysectomy. For which complication specific to this surgery should the nurse assess the client for early clinical manifestations?
    1. Urinary retention
    2. Respiratory distress
    3. Bleeding at the suture line
    4. Increased intracranial pressure

17. A client is admitted to a medical unit with a diagnosis of Addison disease. The client is emaciated and reports muscular weakness and fatigue. Which disturbed body process does the nurse determine is the root cause of the client's clinical manifestations?
    1. Fluid balance
    2. Electrolyte levels
    3. Protein anabolism
    4. Masculinizing hormones

18. Which is an important intervention that the nurse should include in the plan of care that is specific for a client with Addison disease?
    1. Encouraging the client to exercise
    2. Protecting the client from exertion
    3. Restricting the client's fluid intake
    4. Monitoring the client for hypokalemia

19. A nurse is caring for a client who is scheduled for a bilateral adrenalectomy. Which medication should the nurse expect to be prescribed for this client on the day of surgery and in the immediate postoperative period?
    1. Methimazole
    2. Pituitary extract
    3. Regular insulin
    4. Hydrocortisone

20. A client who has just had an adrenalectomy is told about a death in the family and becomes very upset. What concern about the client requires the nurse to notify the health care provider?
    1. Analgesia and mild sedation will be required to ensure rest.
    2. Steroid replacement medication therapy will have to be reduced.
    3. There is a decreased ability to handle stress despite steroid therapy.
    4. Feelings of exhaustion and lethargy may result from the emotional stress.

21. Which information from the client's history does the nurse identify as a risk factor for developing osteoporosis?
    1. Receives long-term steroid therapy
    2. Has a history of hypoparathyroidism
    3. Engages in strenuous physical activity
    4. Consumes high doses of the hormone estrogen

22. A client with a head injury has been receiving dexamethasone. The health care provider plans to reduce the dexamethasone dosage gradually and to continue a lower maintenance dosage. Which effect associated with the gradual dosage reduction of the drug should the nurse explain to the client?
    1. Builds glycogen stores in the muscles
    2. Produces antibodies by the immune system
    3. Allows the increased intracranial pressure to return to normal
    4. Promotes return of cortisone production by the adrenal glands

23. A client with rheumatoid arthritis has been taking a steroid medication for the past year. For which complication of prolonged use of this medication should the nurse assess the client?
    1. Decreased white blood cells
    2. Increased C-reactive protein
    3. Increased sedimentation rate
    4. Decreased serum glucose levels

24. A client is scheduled for an adrenalectomy. Which nursing intervention should the nurse anticipate will be ordered for this client?
    1. Administer IV steroids.
    2. Provide a high-protein diet.
    3. Collect a 24-hour urine specimen.
    4. Withhold all medications for 48 hours.

25. A nurse is caring for a client newly admitted with a diagnosis of pheochromocytoma. Which clinical findings does the nurse expect when assessing this client? **Select all that apply**.
    1. Headache
    2. Palpitations
    3. Diaphoresis
    4. Bradycardia
    5. Hypotension

See Answers on pages 275-279.

ANSWER KEY: REVIEW QUESTIONS

1. **2 Desmopressin (DDAVP) replaces ADH, facilitating reabsorption of water and consequent return of a balanced fluid intake and urinary output.**

   1 The mechanisms that regulate pH are not affected. **3** DDAVP does not alter serum glucose levels; diabetes mellitus, not diabetes insipidus, results in hyperglycemia. **4** Although correction of tachycardia is consistent with correction of dehydration, the client is not dehydrated if the fluid intake is adequate; respirations are unaffected.

   Client Need: Pharmacologic and Parenteral Therapies; **Cognitive Level:** Application; **Nursing Process:** Evaluation/Outcomes

2. **3 Deficient antidiuretic hormone (ADH) from the posterior pituitary results in diabetes insipidus. This can be caused by head trauma; water is not conserved by the body and excess amounts of urine are produced.**

   1 Although increased serum glucose may cause polyuria, it is associated with diabetes mellitus, not diabetes insipidus. **2** Ineffective renal perfusion will cause decreased urine production. **4** Although excess amounts of IV fluids may cause dilute urine, it is unlikely that a client with head trauma will be receiving excess fluid because of the danger of increased intracranial pressure.

   Client Need: Physiologic Adaptation; **Cognitive Level:** Analysis; **Nursing Process:** Assessment/Analysis

> **Test-Taking Tip:** Reread the question if the answers do not seem to make sense, because you may have missed words such as *most* (like in this question), *only, not* or *except* in the statement.

3. **4 Reabsorption of sodium and water in the kidney tubules decreases urinary output and retains body fluids.**

   1 Serum osmolarity decreases. **2** Urine concentration increases. **3** There is no effect on filtration with ADH; ADH increases reabsorption in the tubules.
   Client Need: Physiologic Adaptation; **Cognitive Level:** Comprehension; **Nursing Process:** Assessment/Analysis

4. **Answers: 2, 4**

   2 Excessive levels of ADH cause inappropriate free water retention; for every liter of fluid retained, the client will gain approximately 2.2 lb. **4** Free water retention results in a hypoosmolar state with dilutional hyponatremia.

   1 Oliguria, not polyuria, occurs as antidiuretic hormone (ADH) acts on nephrons to cause water to be reabsorbed from the glomerular filtrate. **3** Because of water reabsorption, blood volume may increase, causing hypertension, not hypotension. **5** Specific gravity increases, not decreases, as a result of increased urine concentration.
   Client Need: Reduction of Risk Potential; **Cognitive Level:** Analysis; **Nursing Process:** Evaluation/Outcomes

5. **2 The hypophysis (pituitary gland) does not directly regulate insulin release. This is controlled by serum glucose levels. Because somatotropin release will stop after the hypophysectomy, any elevation of blood glucose level caused by somatotropin will also stop.**

   1 Sterility may be expected after a hypophysectomy because follicle-stimulating hormone and its releasing factor will no longer be present to stimulate spermatogenesis. **3** When adrenocorticotropic hormone (ACTH) is absent, cortisone will have to be administered. **4** Thyroid-stimulating hormone will not be present; extrinsic thyroxine will have to be taken.
   Client Need: Physiologic Adaptation; **Cognitive Level:** Analysis; **Integrated Process:** Teaching/Learning; **Nursing Process:** Evaluation/Outcomes

6. **1 Myxedema is the severest form of hypothyroidism. Decreased thyroid gland activity means reduced production of thyroid hormones.**

   2 Acromegaly results from excess growth hormone in adults once the epiphyses are closed. **3** Graves' disease results from an excess, not a deficiency, of thyroid hormones. **4** Cushing disease results from excess glucocorticoids.
   Client Need: Physiologic Adaptation; **Cognitive Level:** Comprehension; **Nursing Process:** Assessment/Analysis

7. **2 Propylthiouracil (PTU) is a thyroid hormone antagonist that inhibits thyroid hormone synthesis by decreasing the use of iodine in the manufacture of these hormones.**

   1 PTU does not affect the vascularity of the thyroid gland. **3** Iodine-containing agents are given for severe hyperthyroidism and before a thyroidectomy. **4** PTU does not affect the amount of already formed thyroid hormones.
   Client Need: Pharmacologic and Parenteral Therapies; **Cognitive Level:** Comprehension; **Nursing Process:** Planning/Implementation

8. **3 An individual treated for a thyroid problem by intake of radioactive iodine (^{131}I) becomes mildly radioactive, particularly in the region of the thyroid gland, which preferentially absorbs the iodine. Such clients should be treated with routine safety precautions for 48 hours (e.g., avoid prolonged contact or near-contact with others; flush toilet twice after using, because radioactive iodine is excreted via the urine; and thoroughly wash hands after toileting).**

   1 Because radioactive iodine is internalized, the client becomes the source of radioactivity. **2** The amount of radioactive iodine used is not enough to cause high radioactivity. **4** Because radioactive iodine is internalized, the client becomes the source of radioactivity.
   Client Need: Reduction of Risk Potential; **Cognitive Level:** Comprehension; **Nursing Process:** Evaluation/Outcomes

9. **2 A decreased TSH (thyroid stimulating hormone) assay together with an elevated T$_3$ (triiodothyronine) level may indicate hyperthyroidism.**

    1 X-ray results will not indicate thyroid disease, and elevation of T$_4$ (thyroxine) level might indicate hyperthyroidism. However, it may be a false reading because of the presence of thyroid-binding globulin (TBG) and is inadequate for diagnosis when used alone. **3** Po_2 is not specific to thyroid disease, and the thyroglobulin level is most useful to monitor for recurrence of thyroid carcinoma or response to therapy. **4** The results with the sequential multichannel autoanalyzer (SMA) are not specific to thyroid disease; the protein-bound iodine test is not definitive because it is influenced by the intake of exogenous iodine.

    Client Need: Reduction of Risk Potential; **Cognitive Level:** Application; **Integrated Process:** Teaching/Learning; **Nursing Process:** Planning/Implementation

10. **1 Parathyroid removal eliminates the body's source of parathyroid hormone (parathormone), which increases the blood calcium level. The resulting low body fluid calcium affects muscles, including the diaphragm, resulting in dyspnea, asphyxia, and death.**

    2 Loss of the thyroid gland will upset thyroid hormone balance and may cause myxedema. **3** The parathyroids are not involved in regulating plasma volume; the pituitary and adrenal glands are responsible. **4** The parathyroids do not regulate the adrenal glands.

    Client Need: Reduction of Risk Potential; **Cognitive Level:** Application; **Nursing Process:** Evaluation/Outcomes

11. **Answer: 5 tablets**

    First, convert 0.125 mg to its equivalent in mcg by multiplying by 1,000 (move the decimal 3 places to the right). Use the "Desire over Have" formula of ratio and proportion to solve this problem.

    $$\frac{\text{Desire}}{\text{Have}} \, \frac{125\,\text{mcg}}{25\,\text{mcg}} = \frac{x\,\text{tablets}}{1\,\text{tablet}}$$

    $$25\,x = 125$$

    $$x = 125 \div 25$$

    $$x = 5\,\text{tablets}$$

    Client Need: Pharmacologic and Parenteral Therapies; **Cognitive Level:** Application; **Nursing Process:** Planning/Implementation

12. **3 Hyperparathyroidism causes calcium release from the bones, leaving them porous, weak, and painful.**

    1 Tetany is the result of low calcium levels; in this condition the serum calcium level is increased. **2** Seizures are caused by increased neural activity, a condition not related to this disease. **4** Graves' disease is the result of increased thyroid, not parathyroid, activity.

    Client Need: Physiologic Adaptation; **Cognitive Level:** Application; **Nursing Process:** Assessment/Analysis

13. **2 As a result of increased cortisol levels, glucose metabolism is altered, which may contribute to an increase in blood glucose levels.**

    1 Increased mineralocorticoids will decrease urine output. **3** Sodium is retained by the kidneys, but potassium is excreted. **4** The immune response is suppressed.

    Client Need: Physiologic Adaptation; **Cognitive Level:** Analysis; **Nursing Process:** Assessment/Analysis

---

Study Tip: **C**ushing patients have high **C**ortisol levels. High cortisol levels can result in high blood glucose levels because cortisol is a stress hormone. You know that stress is bad for you. You know your body responds to stress by raising blood glucose. So don't stress yourself about cortisol! Take a few deep breaths as you remind yourself that Cushing patients have high cortisol levels and resultant high blood glucose levels.

14. **1 Hydrocortisone is a glucocorticoid that has antiinflammatory action and aids in metabolism of carbohydrates, fats, and proteins, causing elevation of the blood glucose level. Thus it enables the body to adapt to stress.**

    2 Hydrocortisone may promote fluid retention that results in hypertension and edema. 3 Shortness of breath (dyspnea) is caused by hypovolemia and decreased oxygen supply; neither is affected by hydrocortisone. 4 Hydrocortisone may cause potassium depletion.

    Client Need: Pharmacologic and Parenteral Therapies; **Cognitive Level:** Comprehension; **Integrated Process:** Teaching/Learning; **Nursing Process:** Planning/Implementation

15. **4 Mineralocorticoids such as aldosterone cause the kidneys to retain sodium ions. With sodium, water is also retained, elevating blood pressure. Absence of this hormone thus causes hypotension.**

    1 Estrogen is a female sex hormone produced by the ovaries; it does not affect blood pressure. 2 Androgens are produced by the adrenal cortex. Androgens have an effect similar to that of the male sex hormones; they do not affect blood pressure. 3 The major effect of glucocorticoids such as hydrocortisone is on glucose metabolism, not on sodium and water concentrations; absence of this hormone will not cause significant hypotension.

    Client Need: Physiologic Adaptation; **Cognitive Level:** Application; **Nursing Process:** Assessment/Analysis

16. **4 Because the pituitary gland is located in the brain, edema after surgery may result in increased intracranial pressure. Early signs include decreased visual acuity, papilledema, and unilateral pupillary dilation.**

    1 Urinary retention may follow any surgery because of the effects of anesthesia and is not a specific occurrence following cranial surgery. 2 Respiratory distress is a later, not early, sign of increased intracranial pressure; it is a decompensated response indicated by altered respiratory pattern, decreased respiratory rate, and finally respiratory arrest. This occurs because of increasing pressure on the medulla. 3 Bleeding at the suture line may occur with any surgery, not just a hypophysectomy.

    Client Need: Reduction of Risk Potential; **Cognitive Level:** Application; **Nursing Process:** Evaluation/Outcomes

17. **3 Glucocorticoids help maintain blood glucose and liver and muscle glycogen content. A deficiency of glucocorticoids causes hypoglycemia, resulting in breakdown of protein and fats as energy sources.**

    1 Muscular weakness and fatigue are related to fluid balance, but emaciation is not. 2 Emaciation results from diminished protein and fat stores and hypoglycemia, not from an alteration in electrolytes. 4 Masculinization does not occur in this disease.

    Client Need: Physiologic Adaptation; **Cognitive Level:** Analysis; **Nursing Process:** Assessment/Analysis

18. **2 Exertion, either physical or emotional, places additional stress on the adrenal glands, which may precipitate an Addisonian crisis.**

    1 Because of increased metabolic demands as a result of exercise, decreased levels of adrenocortical hormones will cause fatigue. 3 Restricting fluid intake is contraindicated because of the risk for hypovolemia. 4 The nurse should assess for hyperkalemia and hyponatremia.

    Client Need: Reduction of Risk Potential; **Cognitive Level:** Application; **Nursing Process:** Planning/Implementation

19. **4 Hydrocortisone is a glucocorticoid. A client undergoing bilateral adrenalectomy must be given adrenocortical hormones so that adjustment to the sudden lack of these hormones that occurs with this surgery can take place.**

    1 Methimazole is used to treat a client with hyperthyroidism, not a client with a bilateral adrenalectomy. 2 Because the surgery involves the adrenal glands, not the pituitary gland, secretion of pituitary hormones will not be affected. 3 Regular insulin is not necessary. Insulin is produced by the pancreas, and its function is not altered by this surgery.

    Client Need: Pharmacologic and Parenteral Therapies; **Cognitive Level:** Analysis; **Nursing Process:** Planning/Implementation

20. **3** Clients with adrenocortical insufficiency who are receiving steroid therapy usually require increased amounts of medication during periods of stress because they are unable to produce the increased levels of glucocorticoids needed by the body at this time.

    1 Although sedation may be prescribed, the major concern is the regulation of glucocorticoids in the presence of emotional or physiologic stress. **2** Increased stress requires increased glucocorticoids. **4** Although these symptoms may occur and may be minimized by an increase in glucocorticoids, the primary reason for an adjustment in dosage is to assist the body's ability to adapt to stress.

    Client Need: Reduction of Risk Potential; **Cognitive Level:** Comprehension; **Integrated Process:** Communication/Documentation; **Nursing Process:** Assessment/Analysis

21. **1 Increased levels of steroids will accelerate bone demineralization.**

    2 Hyperparathyroidism, not hypoparathyroidism, accelerates bone demineralization. **3** Weight-bearing that occurs with strenuous activity promotes bone integrity by preventing bone demineralization. **4** Although estrogen promotes deposition of calcium into bone, high levels will not be prescribed for osteoporosis; hormone replacement therapy is associated with an increased risk for breast cancer.

    Client Need: Pharmacologic and Parenteral Therapies; **Cognitive Level:** Analysis; **Nursing Process:** Assessment/Analysis

22. **4 Hormone therapy must be withdrawn slowly to allow the adrenal glands to adjust and resume production of their hormone.**

    1 Building glycogen stores in muscles is not the reason for the gradual withdrawal of dexamethasone. **2** Production of antibodies by the immune system is not the reason for the gradual withdrawal of dexamethasone. **3** Normalization of intracranial pressure is not the reason for the gradual withdrawal of dexamethasone.

    Client Need: Pharmacologic and Parenteral Therapies; **Cognitive Level:** Comprehension; **Integrated Processes:** Teaching/Learning; **Nursing Process:** Planning/Implementation

23. **1 Prolonged use of steroids may cause leukopenia as a result of bone marrow depression.**

    2 C-reactive protein elevates in acute inflammatory diseases; steroids help decrease it. **3** Sedimentation rate elevates in acute inflammatory diseases; steroids help decrease it. **4** Serum glucose levels increase with steroid use.

    Client Need: Pharmacologic and Parenteral Therapies; **Cognitive Level:** Application; **Nursing Process:** Evaluation/Outcomes

24. **1 Steroid therapy usually is instituted preoperatively and continued intraoperatively to prepare for the acute adrenal insufficiency that follows surgery.**

    2 The diet must supply ample, not high, protein and potassium; however, it must be low in calories, carbohydrates, and sodium to promote weight loss and reduce fluid retention. **3** A 24-hour urine specimen is unnecessary. **4** Glucocorticoids must be administered preoperatively to prevent adrenal insufficiency during surgery.

    Client Need: Pharmacologic and Parenteral Therapies; **Cognitive Level:** Analysis; **Nursing Process:** Planning/Implementation

25. **Answers: 1, 2, 3**

    1 A pounding headache is secondary to the severe hypertension associated with excessive amounts of catecholamines. **2** Palpitations are associated with stimulation of the sympathetic nervous system due to catecholamines (epinephrine and norepinephrine). **3** Diaphoresis is associated with stimulation of the sympathetic nervous system due to excessive catecholamines.

    4 Tachycardia, not bradycardia, is associated with stimulation of the sympathetic nervous system due to catecholamines. **5** Hypertension, not hypotension, is the principle clinical manifestation associated with pheochromocytoma because of stimulation of the sympathetic nervous system.

    Client Need: Physiologic Adaptation; **Cognitive Level:** Analysis; **Nursing Process:** Assessment/Analysis

14 Women's and Men's Health Drugs

INTRODUCTION TO REPRODUCTIVE SYSTEM DRUGS

Female Reproduction (Fig. 14.1)

Ovaries: Female Gonads

- Located behind and below fallopian tubes, anchored to uterus and broad ligaments; size and shape of large almonds
- At birth, contain several hundred thousand Graafian follicles (epithelial sacs in which ova develop) embedded in connective tissue
- Between menarche and menopause, one follicle matures each month, ruptures from ovarian surface, is expelled into pelvic cavity, and enters fallopian tube
- Functions
  - Oogenesis: formation of a mature ovum in Graafian follicle
  - Ovulation: expulsion of ovum from follicle into pelvic cavity
  - Release of ovarian hormones: maturing follicle produces estrogens (estradiol, estrone, and estriol); corpus luteum produces progesterone and estrogens
    - Estrogens: stimulate development of secondary sexual characteristics (e.g., breasts, pubic hair) and thickening of endometrium; accelerate protein anabolism; stimulate long bone calcification
    - Progesterone: prepares endometrium for implantation of fertilized ovum; inhibits uterine contractions during pregnancy; promotes development of alveoli of estrogen-primed breasts in preparation for lactation

Fallopian Tubes (Oviducts)

- Location: attached to upper, outer angles of uterus
- Structure: distal ends fimbriated and open into pelvic cavity; mucosal lining of tubes and peritoneal lining of pelvis in direct contact
- Function: ducts through which ova travel from ovaries to uterus; location of fertilization

Uterus

- Location: in pelvic cavity between bladder and rectum
- Structure
  - Shape and size: pear-shaped, approximate size of clenched fist
  - Corpus (body): upper, main portion; fundus is bulging upper area of corpus; two openings from fallopian tubes, one into cervix
  - Cervix: narrow, lower portion; internal os adjacent to uterus; external os adjacent to vagina; isthmus (lower uterine segment) separates corpus from cervix
  - Layers of uterus
    - Endometrium: inner layer
      - Myometrium: middle, muscular, thickest layer
      - Perimetrium: outer layer

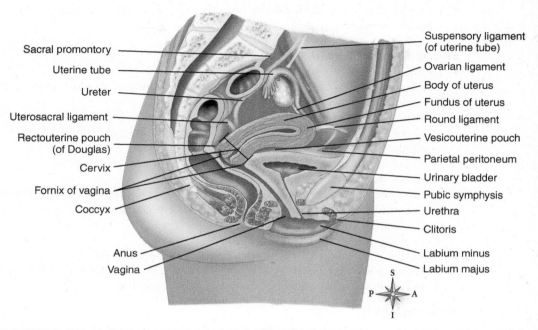

FIG. 14.1 Female reproductive organs. (From Patton, K.T., Thibodeau, G.A. [2016]. *Anatomy and physiology* [8th ed.]. St. Louis: Elsevier.)

- Location: over bladder in pelvic cavity; cervix joins vagina; ligaments (e.g., broad ligaments, uterosacral ligaments, posterior ligament, anterior ligament, round ligaments) maintain position of uterus
- Functions: menstruation, pregnancy, labor

Vagina
- Location: between rectum and urethra
- Structure: collapsible, musculomembranous tube, capable of distention; outlet to exterior covered by hymen (fold of mucous membrane)
- Functions
  - Receptacle for semen
  - Lower portion of birth canal
  - Excretory duct for uterine secretions and menstrual flow

Vulva (External Genitalia)
- Mons veneris: hairy, skin-covered pad of fat over symphysis pubis
- Labia majora: hairy, skin-covered folds
- Labia minora: small inner folds covered with modified skin
- Clitoris: small mound of erectile tissue, below junction of two labia minora
- Urinary meatus: opening into urethra; posterior to clitoris; anterior to vagina
- Vaginal orifice: posterior to urinary meatus; opening into vagina; hymen
- Skene glands: small mucous glands; ducts on each side of urinary meatus; prone to infection, especially gonococci

- Bartholin glands: two small glands; ducts on each side of vaginal orifice; prone to infection, especially gonococci

Breasts (Mammary Glands)
- Location: under skin, over pectoralis major
- Size: associated with deposits of adipose tissue, not amount of glandular tissue; glandular tissue approximately same in all females
- Structure
  - Internal: divided into lobes and lobules; excretory duct leads from each lobe to opening in nipple
  - External: nipples; areola (circular pigmented area surrounding nipples)
- Function: secrete milk (lactation)
  - Expulsion of placenta causes decrease in estrogens and progesterone that stimulates anterior pituitary to increase prolactin production; prolactin stimulates alveoli of breast to secrete milk
  - Suckling: controls lactation
- Stimulates release of prolactin, which stimulates milk production
- Stimulates posterior pituitary production of oxytocin causing release of milk from alveoli into ducts (let-down reflex), enabling removal of milk by suckling

Menstrual Cycle
- Periodic vaginal bleeding related to changes in uterus and ovaries; cyclical from time of menarche to menopause
- Length of cycle: measured from onset of uterine bleeding to onset of next period of bleeding; mean cycle length is 28 days; range of 21 to 45 days
- Regulated by hormonal communication between hypothalamus and pituitary gland (hypothalamic-pituitary cycle) and ovaries and uterine endometrium
- Ovarian activity: during each cycle several follicles begin maturation process; usually one reaches full maturity, expels its ovum, which enters a fallopian tube
- Menstrual cycle phases
  - First phase (menstrual or ischemic): shedding of spongiosum endometrium with discharge through vagina
    - Prostaglandin level in endometrium peaks causing vasoconstriction and myometrial contractions resulting in menstruation
    - Low estrogen and progesterone levels stimulate release of follicle-stimulating hormone (FSH)
    - FSH combines with low level of luteinizing hormone (LH) stimulating ovarian estrogen production
  - Second phase (follicular [ovary] or proliferative [endometrium])
    - Endometrium regenerates and thickens in preparation for possible implantation
    - Simultaneously, single dominant follicle develops from group of maturing follicles and approaches full maturation under influence of estradiol produced by ovarian follicles
    - Rising blood levels of estradiol exert negative feedback on FSH production and positive feedback on LH production
    - Estradiol's feedback effects are exerted on hypothalamic production of FSH-releasing hormone and LH-releasing hormone, which control hypophyseal production of FSH and LH
    - Resulting surge in LH level causes ovulation

- Ovulation usually occurs 14 days before menstruation; ovum remains viable for 24 to 36 hours
- Third phase (luteal [ovary] and secretory [endometrium])
  - Begins after ovulation; relatively finite time period of about 12 to 14 days
  - Continuing LH production forms temporary endocrine gland (corpus luteum) from ruptured follicle
  - Granulosa and thecal cells of follicle enlarge, divide into and occupy cavity of follicle, and produce progesterone and estrogen
  - Progesterone stimulates already proliferated endometrium to become glandular with a high glycogen-secreting potential (preparation for implantation)
  - Without fertilization corpus luteum becomes nonfunctional 10 to 12 days after ovulation; progesterone and estrogen blood levels drop
  - Negative feedback effect of estrogen on FSH ceases; first phase of menstrual cycle begins

Pregnancy

- Occurs when male sperm fertilizes female egg and it implants into uterine lining
- Causes: sexual intercourse, assistive reproductive methods
- Clinical findings
  - Presumptive signs: amenorrhea; fatigue; nausea and vomiting; breast changes; urinary frequency; darkening of pigmentation on face, breasts, and abdomen; quickening (feeling of movement at about 16 to 20 weeks)
  - Probable signs:
    - Uterine changes: uterine enlargement; Hegar sign (lower uterine segment softens), Goodell sign (cervix softens)
    - Vaginal change: Chadwick sign (color becomes purplish)
    - Fetal outline; ballottement
    - Pregnancy tests: urine and blood detects human chorionic gonadotropin (hCG)
    - Preparatory contractions (formerly called Braxton Hicks)
  - Positive signs: confirmation
    - Fetal heartbeat: heard with fetoscope, Doppler
    - Fetal outline and movement: felt by examiner
    - Ultrasonography: visualization of fetus and movement of fetal heart
    - Identification of singleton or multiple gestation (early determination vital because multiple gestation contributes to perinatal morbidity and mortality)
    - Estimating date of birth (EDB) and duration of pregnancy
      - Nägele rule: count back 3 months from first day of last menstrual period and add 7 days and 1 year
    - Fundal height: measurement from symphysis pubis to top of fundus; fundus rises about 1 cm per week up to 30 weeks; 20 weeks at umbilicus (McDonald rule), 36 weeks at xiphoid process
    - Ultrasonography: up to 11 weeks gestational age established by crown to rump measurement (must have full bladder to move uterus into abdominal cavity for visualization; instructed to drink quart of fluid before test); 11 weeks head measurements (biparietal diameter is 9.8 cm or more at term)
- Treatment: medical and self-care measures to maintain pregnancy until birth, miscarriage, abortion

Male Reproduction

Glands

- Testes: male sex glands (gonads)
  - Located in scrotum, one testis in each compartment
- Functions
  - Seminiferous tubules form spermatozoa (male sex cells or gametes); process called spermatogenesis (occurs at puberty)
  - Interstitial cells secrete testosterone, main androgen; increases protein synthesis, induces growth of secondary sex characteristics
  - Accessory glands
    - Seminal vesicles: secrete fluid that constitutes about 30% of semen
    - Prostate gland: secretes about 60% of semen; secretion is alkaline, which increases sperm motility; contains the enzyme acid phosphatase; this enzyme increases in metastasizing cancer of prostate
    - Bulbourethral glands (Cowper glands): secrete fluid that lubricates urethra before ejaculation

Ducts

- Epididymis: conducts semen from testes to vas deferens; sperm mature while semen is stored before ejaculation
- Vas deferens (seminal ducts): conduct sperm and fluid from each epididymis to an ejaculatory duct
- Ejaculatory ducts: ejaculate semen into urethra
- Urethra: disseminates semen and urine

Supporting Structures

- External: scrotum and penis (Fig. 14.2)
  - Scrotum: contains testes, epididymis, and first part of seminal duct; sperm develop at 2 to 3 degrees below body temperature (ideal for sperm development)
  - Penis: contains urethra; contains vascular spaces that when filled with blood cause erection
- Internal: fibrous tubes (spermatic cords) located in each inguinal canal; torsion of testes twists cords, destroys sperm, interrupts blood supply, and can result in cell death and gangrene

Reproductive System Pathogens

- *Haemophilus ducreyi:* gram-negative bacillus; causes venereal ulcer called chancroid (soft chancre)
- *Neisseria gonorrhoeae:* gram-negative diplococcus; causes gonorrhea; transmitted sexually
- *Treponema pallidum:* motile spirochete; causes syphilis; transmitted sexually
- *Chlamydia trachomatis:* parasite characterized as bacteria because of cell wall composition and process of reproduction; reproduce only within cells; causes genital infections in men and women; transmitted sexually
- *Trichomonas vaginalis:* flagellated protozoan; causes trichomonas vaginitis; transmitted sexually
- Human papillomavirus (genital or venereal warts [condylomata acuminata]): characterized by papillary or cauliflower-like masses in or on genitourinary structures; may be precursor to cancer of cervix; vaccine available

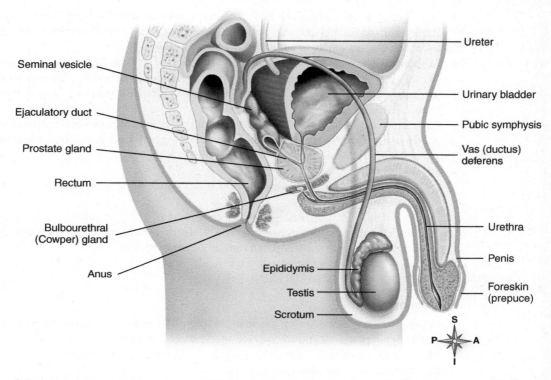

FIG. 14.2 Male reproductive organs. (From Patton, K.T., Thibodeau, G.A. [2016]. *Anatomy and physiology* [8th ed.]. St. Louis: Elsevier.)

Contraceptive Methods

- Oral contraceptives: inhibit ovulation; atrophic changes in endometrium prevent implantation; thickened cervical mucus inhibits sperm travel
- Intrauterine devices (IUDs): device inserted into uterus; prevents fertilization or implantation
- Diaphragm: shallow round rubber or latex device with flexible rim; fits over cervix; prevents sperm from entering cervical os; used with spermicide; fitted by health care provider
- Cervical cap: rubber thimble-like device; filled with a spermicide; fits over cervix; protects for up to 48 hours after insertion; fitted by health care provider
- Vaginal ring: hormonal control; worn for 3 weeks with a 1-week break; prescription required; fitting not required
- Female condom: latex vaginal elongated pouch with ring at each end; one ring covers cervix, other covers labia; available over-the-counter (OTC)
- Male condom: latex sheath covers penis; prevents semen from entering cervical os; OTC
- Spermicidal creams, jellies, foam tablets, and vaginal suppositories: spermicidal generally of low pH; inserted into vaginal canal by applicator immediately before coitus; may be used in conjunction with diaphragm and condom for added protection
- Coitus interruptus: withdrawal during sexual intercourse before ejaculation; least effective method

- Fertility awareness methods (FAM): contraceptive method depends on identifying beginning and end of fertile period and periodic abstinence during fertile period; multiple fertility awareness methods may be used concurrently
- Norplant system (implantable progestin): placement of six flexible rods of levonorgestrel under skin of upper arm; effective for 5 years; removal restores fertility; irregular periods may occur
- Medroxyprogesterone (Depo-Provera) intramuscular (IM) injection lasts 3 months; suppresses FSH and LH
- Emergency contraception (EC): used after unprotected intercourse ("morning after pill"); pharmacologic management with high dose of estrogen, progesterone, or testosterone; may be available OTC in some states
- Surgical sterilization
  - Male: bilateral vasectomy; vas deferens is ligated via small incision into scrotum; prevents ejaculation of sperm
  - Female: tubal ligation; interruption in continuity of fallopian tubes by surgical transection, electric cautery, or compression with soft clamp; performed via laparotomy, laparoscopy, or culdoscopy; prevents impregnation of ovum by sperm

MAJOR DISORDERS OF REPRODUCTIVE SYSTEM

Perimenopause

- Perimenopause (climacteric): gradual cessation of ovarian function and menstrual cycles; begins between age 40 and 60, average age 51; lasts 2 to 10 years
- Menopause: cessation of menstrual periods for 12 consecutive months
- Postmenopause: time after menopause
- Causes
  - Ovaries: loss of ability to respond to gonadotropic hormones; dramatic decrease in levels of circulating estradiol and progesterone
  - FSH gonadotropin blood level: increased because ovarian production is no longer inhibited; false-positive pregnancy test may occur
  - Atrophic changes in reproductive organs or hormonal stimulation of sympathetic nervous system
- Clinical findings
  - Early manifestations: dyspareunia, weight gain, facial hair growth, cardiac palpitations, hot flashes, profuse diaphoresis, constipation, pruritus, faintness, headache
  - Long-range manifestations: osteoporosis, cardiovascular disease
  - Emotional/behavioral responses: irritability; anxiety about loss of reproductive function, libido, feelings of womanliness
- Treatment
  - Hormone replacement therapy (HRT): eases transition through perimenopause (e.g., controls vasomotor instability, reduces atrophic genitourinary changes), reduces risk for cardiovascular disease, and prevents osteoporosis; used judiciously and on an individual basis because of cancer-causing potential
  - Alternative therapy: herbal supplements, diet management, relaxation modalities, exercise

Osteoporosis

- Metabolic bone disorder where bone formation declines resulting in decreased bone mass

- Cause: calcium deficiency, hormone imbalance, sedentary lifestyle, alcoholism, malnutrition, scurvy, prolonged steroid/heparin use, rheumatoid arthritis
- Clinical findings: bone fractures, height loss
  - X-ray, bone biopsy, CT scan, serum calcium/phosphorous/alkaline phosphatase
- Treatment: medications, supplements, supportive measures

Infertility/Sterility

- Infertility: inability to conceive after consistent attempts for a 1-year period; woman has never conceived; man has never impregnated a woman
  - Primary: couple has never had a child
  - Secondary: couple has conceived but woman is unable to sustain pregnancy or conceive again
- Sterility: unable to produce offspring; may be genetic, acquired, or elective
- Male infertility/sterility
  - Causes: coital difficulties, spermatozoal abnormalities, testicular abnormalities, varicocele, penis/urethra abnormalities, prostate/seminal vesicle abnormalities, epididymis/vas deferens abnormalities, severe nutritional deficiencies, STIs, excessive tobacco use, excessive marijuana use, excessive alcohol intake, in utero exposure to diethylstilbestrol (DES)/Agent Orange, decreased libido/impotence, frequent hot tub use
  - Clinical findings: inability to conceive
    - Semen analysis, blood studies
  - Treatment: medications, surgery, intrauterine insemination (IUI), in vitro fertilization, surrogate motherhood, adoption, education
- Female infertility/sterility
  - Causes: endocrine disorders, vaginal disorders, cervical/uterine/ovarian abnormalities, tubal disorders, coital factors, emotional issues, chronic illness, immunologic reaction to sperm, malnutrition, anorexia nervosa, in utero exposure to diethylstilbestrol (DES), teratogenic household cleaning products
  - Clinical findings: inability to conceive
    - Blood studies, serologic studies, urinalysis, hormone studies, ultrasonography, endometrial biopsy
  - Treatment: medications, surgery, intrauterine insemination (IUI), in vitro fertilization, surrogate motherhood, adoption, education

Low Testosterone

- Low testosterone is testosterone level below the required amount to maintain male sexual response
- Cause: testicular injury, testicular cancer, infection, hormonal disorders, HIV/AIDS, chronic renal/hepatic disorder, type 2 diabetes, obesity
- Clinical findings: low sex drive, difficulty achieving erection, low semen count, hair loss, muscle mass loss, fatigue, increased body fat, decreased bone mass, mood changes
  - Testosterone below 300 ng/dL
- Treatment: testosterone replacement

Erectile Dysfunction

- Erectile dysfunction is the inability to maintain an erection

- Cause: heart disease, atherosclerosis, hypertension, prostate cancer, obesity, diabetes, tobacco uses, alcoholism, sleep disorders, depression, stress, medications
- Clinical findings: small testes, penile plaques, prostate infection, hypertension
- Treatment: medications, self-care techniques, therapy to treat underlying psychologic symptoms

HORMONE REPLACEMENT THERAPY (HRT)

- Use of female hormones, estrogen and progesterone, to treat symptoms of menopause
- Symptoms of menopause may include hot flashes and vaginal dryness
- Lack of estrogen can lead to osteoporosis
- Estrogen controls use of calcium in the body and raises HDLs in the blood
- Estrogen therapy (low dose) is used in women who've had a hysterectomy
- Combination therapy—estrogen/progesterone/progestin—is used in women who still have their uterus
- Taking estrogen alone (in women who have their uterus) can cause increased risk for endometrial cancer
- Progesterone is used in combination therapy because it thins the endometrium, lowering the risk of endometrial cancer
- HRT can increase risk of breast cancer, heart disease, stroke, blood clots

APPLICATION AND REVIEW

1. A nurse is reviewing a postmenopausal client's history. It reveals that she previously received hormonal replacement therapy (HRT) as treatment for osteoporosis. For which problem does HRT increase the client's risk?
   1. Breast cancer
   2. Rapid weight loss
   3. Accelerated bone loss
   4. Vaginal tissue atrophy
2. What components of female reproduction are altered by the use of an oral contraceptive medication? **Select all that apply.**
   1. Ovulation
   2. Cervical os
   3. Fertilization
   4. Endometrium
   5. Cervical mucus

See Answers on pages 302-303.

WOMEN'S HEALTH DRUGS

Estrogen Replacement Agents

- Used to treat menopause, abnormal uterine bleeding, atrophic vaginitis, vulvar/vaginal atrophy; prevent osteoporosis
- Examples include estradiol, conjugated estrogens
- Available in PO, IM, IV, TOP preparations

Mode of Action

- Affects release of pituitary gonadotropins to ensure adequate function of female reproductive system

Contraindications, Precautions, and Drug Interactions of Estrogen Replacement Agents*

Drug	Contraindications/Precautions	Drug Interaction
estradiol, estradiol cypionate, estradiol gel, estradiol spray, estradiol topical emulsion, estradiol valerate, estradiol transdermal system, estradiol vaginal tablet/ring	*Contraindications:* Hypersensitivity, breastfeeding, reproductive cancer, genital bleeding, MI, angioedema, stroke, antithrombin deficiency *Precautions:* Cardiac/renal/hepatic/gallbladder/bone disease, hypertension, CHF, history of angioedema, asthma, blood dyscrasias, diabetes mellitus, seizures, depression, migraine headache, family history of reproductive cancer, uterine fibroids, vaginal infection, smoking *Pregnancy:* Absolute fetal abnormalities; not to be used at any time during pregnancy	Corticosteroids, tricyclics, cyclosporine, dantrolene, tamoxifen, anticoagulants, oral hypoglycemics, anticonvulsants, barbiturates, rifampin, calcium, phenylbutazone, DHEA, St. John's wort
conjugated estrogens, conjugated synthetic estrogens	*Contraindications:* Hypersensitivity, breastfeeding, reproductive cancer, genital bleeding, MI, stroke, thrombophlebitis *Precautions:* Cardiac/renal/hepatic/gallbladder/bone disease, hypertension, CHF, asthma, blood dyscrasias, diabetes mellitus, seizures, depression, dementia, migraine headache, family history of reproductive cancer, smoking, SLE, obesity, hypothyroidism *Pregnancy:* Absolute fetal abnormalities; not to be used at any time during pregnancy	Corticosteroids, tricyclics, cyclosporine, dantrolene, tamoxifen, anticoagulants, oral hypoglycemics, anticonvulsants, barbiturates, rifampin, bosentan, thyroid

*Pregnancy categories have been revised. See http://www.fda.gov/Drugs/DevelopmentApprovalProcess/DevelopmentResources/Labeling/ucm093307.htm for more information.

Adverse Effects

- Headache
- Dizziness
- Seizures
- Migraines
- Depression
- MI
- Stroke
- Pulmonary embolism
- Hypertension
- Edema
- Thromboembolism
- Chest pain
- Throat swelling
- Vision changes
- Nausea
- Vomiting
- Diarrhea
- Constipation
- Anorexia
- Increased appetite
- Increased weight
- Pancreatitis
- Jaundice
- Hepatic adenoma
- Increased risk of breast cancer
- Increased risk of endometrial cancer
- Libido changes
- Toxic shock
- Dysmenorrhea
- Breakthrough bleeding
- Rash

- Urticaria
- Acne

- Hirsutism
- Alopecia

- Hypercalcemia
- Hyperglycemia

Nursing Care
- Monitor cardiac/renal/hepatic function
- Monitor for mental status changes
- Monitor for hyperglycemia in diabetic patients
- Monitor I&O
- Encourage patient to stop smoking
- Teach patient to refrain from grapefruit products
- Teach patient to weigh weekly and report gain ≥5 lbs.
- Teach patient to report breast lumps/vaginal bleeding

Progestins

- Used to treat amenorrhea, premenstrual syndrome, abnormal uterine bleeding, endometrial hyperplasia prevention; used as a contraceptive
- Example includes progesterone
- Available in PO, IM, intravaginal preparations

Mode of Action
- Prevents follicular maturation, ovulation; fights endometrial tumors

Contraindications, Precautions, and Drug Interactions of Progestins*

Drug	Contraindications/Precautions	Drug Interaction
progesterone	**Contraindications:** Hypersensitivity, hypersensitivity to peanut products, cerebral hemorrhage, ectopic pregnancy, thromboembolic disorders, thrombophlebitis, reproductive cancers, genital bleeding, PID, STDs **Precautions:** Breastfeeding, cardiac/renal/hepatic/gallbladder/bone disease, hypertension, CHF, asthma, blood dyscrasias, diabetes mellitus, seizures, depression, migraine headache, family history of reproductive cancer **Pregnancy:** No adverse effects in animals; no human studies available	CYP3A4 inhibitors, phenytoin, barbiturates

*Pregnancy categories have been revised. See http://www.fda.gov/Drugs/DevelopmentApprovalProcess/DevelopmentResources/Labeling/ucm093307.htm for more information.

Adverse Effects
- Headache
- Dizziness
- Migraine
- Fatigue
- Depression
- Drowsiness
- Mood swings

- Dementia
- Angioedema
- Anaphylaxis
- Hypotension
- Edema
- MI
- Pulmonary embolism

- Stroke
- Thrombophlebitis
- Thromboembolism
- Hyperglycemia
- Vision changes
- Nausea
- Vomiting

- Constipation
- Anorexia
- Increased weight
- Jaundice
- Amenorrhea
- Dysmenorrhea

- Breakthrough bleeding
- Vaginal candidiasis
- Endometriosis
- Spontaneous abortion
- Ectopic pregnancy
- Rash

- Urticaria
- Acne
- Hirsutism
- Alopecia

Nursing Care
- Monitor cardiac/renal/hepatic function
- Monitor for mental status changes
- Monitor for hyperglycemia in diabetic patients
- Monitor I&O
- Encourage patient to stop smoking
- Teach patient to weigh weekly and report gain ≥5 lbs.
- Teach patient to report breast lumps/vaginal bleeding

Selective Estrogen Receptor Modulators (SERMs)
- Used to prevent osteoporosis
- Examples include raloxifene
- Available in PO preparations

Mode of Action
- Acts like estrogen on the bone, protecting its density

Contraindications, Precautions, and Drug Interactions of Selective Estrogen Receptor Modulators (SERMs)*

Drug	Contraindications/Precautions	Drug Interaction
raloxifene	*Contraindications:* Hypersensitivity, breastfeeding, thromboembolic disease *Precautions:* Women of childbearing age, cardiac/renal/hepatic disease, hypertriglyceridemia *Pregnancy:* Definite fetal risks, may be given in spite of risks if needed in life-threatening conditions	Bexarotene, tranexamic acid, lenalidomide, pomalidomide, thalidomide

*Pregnancy categories have been revised. See http://www.fda.gov/Drugs/DevelopmentApprovalProcess/DevelopmentResources/Labeling/ucm093307.htm for more information.

Adverse Effects
- Headache
- Dizziness
- Hot flashes

- Flushing
- Night sweats
- Pulmonary embolism

- DVT
- Rash
- Alopecia

Nursing Care
- Administer analgesics for bone pain
- Monitor blood counts
- Monitor for bleeding
- Monitor I&O

- Monitor for cardiac/respiratory distress
- Teach patient to stop smoking
- Teach patient DVT prevention
- Teach patient importance of maintaining ambulation

Hormone Contraceptives

- Used to prevent pregnancy
- Examples include ethinyl estradiol/desogestrel; ethinylestradiol/drospirenone; ethinyl estradiol/ethynodiol; ethinyl estradiol/levonorgestrel; ethinyl estradiol/norethindrone; ethinyl estradiol/norgestrel; mestranol/norethindrone; ethinyl estradiol/norgestimate; norethindrone; ethinyl estradiol/norethindrone acetate; levonorgestrel; etonogestrel; ethinyl estradiol/norelgestromin; medroxyprogesterone; levonorgestrel/ethinyl estradiol; levonorgestrel
- Available in PO, IM, SUBCUT, transdermal, intravaginal preparations

Mode of Action

- Prevent ovulation; maintain thin lining of uterus; maintain thick cervical mucous to prevent sperm implantation

Contraindications, Precautions, and Drug Interactions of Hormone Contraceptives*

Drug	Contraindications/Precautions	Drug Interaction
Oral Agents		
ethinyl estradiol/desogestrel; ethinyl-estradiol/drospirenone; ethinyl estradiol/ethynodiol; ethinyl estradiol/levonorgestrel; ethinyl estradiol/norethindrone; ethinyl estradiol/norgestrel; mestranol/norethindrone; ethinyl estradiol/norgestimate; nor-ethindrone; ethinyl estradiol/norethindrone acetate	*Contraindications:* Hypersensitivity, breast-feeding, women ≥40 yrs, hepatic disease, jaundice, MI, CAD, CVA, stroke, thrombophlebitis, reproductive cancer, breast cancer, vaginal bleeding *Precautions:* Hypertension, renal/gallbladder disease, depression, seizure, SLE, rheumatic disease, migraine headache, diabetes mellitus, sickle cell disease, acute mononucleosis, irregular menses, amenorrhea, heavy smoking *Pregnancy:* Absolute fetal abnormalities; not to be used at any time during pregnancy	Anticonvulsants, rifampin, analgesics, antibiotics, antihistamines, griseofulvin, St. John's wort
Intrauterine Agents		
levonorgestrel	*Contraindications:* Hypersensitivity, breast-feeding, women ≥40 yrs, hepatic disease, jaundice, MI, CAD, CVA, stroke, thrombophlebitis, reproductive cancer, breast cancer, vaginal bleeding *Precautions:* Hypertension, renal/gallbladder disease, depression, seizure, SLE, rheumatic disease, migraine headache, diabetes mellitus, sickle cell disease, acute mononucleosis, irregular menses, amenorrhea, heavy smoking *Pregnancy:* Absolute fetal abnormalities; not to be used at any time during pregnancy	Anticonvulsants, rifampin, analgesics, antibiotics, antihistamines, griseofulvin, St. John's wort

Contraindications, Precautions, and Drug Interactions of Hormone Contraceptives—cont'd

Drug	Contraindications/Precautions	Drug Interaction
Implant Agents		
etonogestrel	***Contraindications:*** Hypersensitivity, breast-feeding, women ≥40 yrs, hepatic disease, jaundice, MI, CAD, CVA, stroke, thrombophlebitis, reproductive cancer, breast cancer, vaginal bleeding ***Precautions:*** Hypertension, renal/gallbladder disease, depression, seizure, SLE, rheumatic disease, migraine headache, diabetes mellitus, sickle cell disease, acute mononucleosis, irregular menses, amenorrhea, heavy smoking ***Pregnancy:*** Absolute fetal abnormalities; not to be used at any time during pregnancy	Anticonvulsants, rifampin, analgesics, antibiotics, antihistamines, griseofulvin, St. John's wort
Vaginal Ring		
ethinyl/estradiol/etonogestrel	***Contraindications:*** Hypersensitivity, breast-feeding, women ≥40 yrs, hepatic disease, jaundice, MI, CAD, CVA, stroke, thrombophlebitis, reproductive cancer, breast cancer, vaginal bleeding ***Precautions:*** Hypertension, renal/gallbladder disease, depression, seizure, SLE, rheumatic disease, migraine headache, diabetes mellitus, sickle cell disease, acute mononucleosis, irregular menses, amenorrhea, heavy smoking ***Pregnancy:*** Absolute fetal abnormalities; not to be used at any time during pregnancy	Anticonvulsants, rifampin, analgesics, antibiotics, antihistamines, griseofulvin, St. John's wort
Transdermal		
ethinyl estradiol/norelgestromin	***Contraindications:*** Hypersensitivity, breast-feeding, women ≥40 yrs, hepatic disease, jaundice, MI, CAD, CVA, stroke, thrombophlebitis, reproductive cancer, breast cancer, vaginal bleeding ***Precautions:*** Hypertension, renal/gallbladder disease, depression, seizure, SLE, rheumatic disease, migraine headache, diabetes mellitus, sickle cell disease, acute mononucleosis, irregular menses, amenorrhea, heavy smoking ***Pregnancy:*** Absolute fetal abnormalities; not to be used at any time during pregnancy	Anticonvulsants, rifampin, analgesics, antibiotics, antihistamines, griseofulvin, St. John's wort

Continued

Contraindications, Precautions, and Drug Interactions of Hormone Contraceptives—cont'd

Drug	Contraindications/Precautions	Drug Interaction
Subcut/IM Agents		
medroxyprogesterone	***Contraindications:*** Hypersensitivity, breast-feeding, women ≥40 yrs, hepatic disease, jaundice, MI, CAD, CVA, stroke, thrombophlebitis, reproductive cancer, breast cancer, vaginal bleeding ***Precautions:*** Hypertension, renal/gallbladder disease, depression, seizure, SLE, rheumatic disease, migraine headache, diabetes mellitus, sickle cell disease, acute mononucleosis, irregular menses, amenorrhea, heavy smoking ***Pregnancy:*** Absolute fetal abnormalities; not to be used at any time during pregnancy	Anticonvulsants, rifampin, analgesics, antibiotics, antihistamines, griseofulvin, St. John's wort
Emergency (Morning After) Agents		
levonorgestrel/ethinyl estradiol; levonorgestrel	***Contraindications:*** Hypersensitivity, breast-feeding, women ≥40 yrs, hepatic disease, jaundice, MI, CAD, CVA, stroke, thrombophlebitis, reproductive cancer, breast cancer, vaginal bleeding ***Precautions:*** Hypertension, renal/gallbladder disease, depression, seizure, SLE, rheumatic disease, migraine headache, diabetes mellitus, sickle cell disease, acute mononucleosis, irregular menses, amenorrhea, heavy smoking ***Pregnancy:*** Absolute fetal abnormalities; not to be used at any time during pregnancy	Anticonvulsants, rifampin, analgesics, antibiotics, antihistamines, griseofulvin, St. John's wort

*Pregnancy categories have been revised. See http://www.fda.gov/Drugs/DevelopmentApprovalProcess/DevelopmentResources/Labeling/ucm093307.htm for more information.

Adverse Effects

- Anxiety
- Depression
- Fatigue
- Dizziness
- Nervousness
- Headache
- Cerebral hemorrhage
- Thrombosis
- Pulmonary embolism
- MI
- Edema
- Visual changes
- Photosensitivity
- Decreased glucose tolerance
- Nausea
- Vomiting
- Diarrhea
- Constipation
- Appetite change
- Weight change
- Jaundice
- Temporary infertility
- Amenorrhea
- Dysmenorrhea
- Breakthrough bleeding
- Vaginitis
- Breast changes
- Endocervical hyperplasia
- Increased clotting factor
- Increased fibrinogen
- Acne
- Rash
- Urticaria
- Pruritus
- Hirsutism
- Alopecia

BOX 14.1 Guidelines for Missed Doses of Oral Contraceptives

Combination Products
One Tablet
Take tablet as soon as realized.
Take next tablet as scheduled.
Two Tablets
Take two tablets as soon as realized and two tablets the next day.
Use backup method of contraception for rest of cycle.
Three Tablets
Discontinue present pack and allow for withdrawal bleeding. Start new package of tablets 7 days after last tablet taken. Use another form of contraception until tablets have been taken for 7 consecutive days.

Progestin-Only Products
One or More Tablets
Take tablet as soon as realized and follow with next tablet at regular time, PLUS use backup method of contraception for 48 hours.

From McCuistion, L., Vuljoin-DiMaggio, K., Winton, M.B., Yeager, J.J. (2018). *Pharmacology: A patient-centered nursing process approach* (9th ed.). St. Louis: Elsevier.

Nursing Care
- Monitor renal/hepatic function
- Monitor glucose levels
- Monitor for reproductive changes
- Advise patient to stop smoking
- Teach patient how to detect DVT
- Teach patient to wear sunscreen, protective clothing, sunglasses
- Teach patient to take medication at same time each day
- Teach patient to use alternative birth control method during first month of oral contraceptive use
- Teach patient to continue with preventative screenings (Pap smear, breast examination)
- Teach patient if dose is missed to take dose as soon as possible (Box 14.1)

APPLICATION AND REVIEW

3. A nurse is teaching a female client about the side effects of estrogen in an oral contraceptive. Which common side effect identified by the client indicates to the nurse that the teaching was effective?
   1. Nausea
   2. Lethargy
   3. Amenorrhea
   4. Hypomenorrhea
4. What assessment questions should the nurse ask a client in advance of the prescription of estrogen replacement therapy? **Select all that apply.**
   1. "Do you experience any break through vaginal bleeding?"
   2. "When did you have your last menstrual period?"
   3. "Have you ever been screened for osteoporosis?"
   4. "Are you interested in becoming pregnant?"
   5. "Are you experiencing vaginal dryness?"
5. What is the medical practice associated with the prescription of estrogen replacement therapy related to pregnancy?
   1. Not to be prescribed during pregnancy
   2. Safe to be prescribed during pregnancy
   3. Not to be prescribed during the first trimester
   4. Prescribed only when benefits and risks have been carefully assessed

6. What instructions should a nurse provide a client prescribed estrogen replacement therapy? **Select all that apply.**
   1. Follow a high protein diet
   2. Smoking is strongly discouraged
   3. Report a weekly weight gain >5 lbs.
   4. Avoid consuming any grapefruit products
   5. Report any signs/symptoms of depression
7. What classification of medications are prescribed to facilitate the release of hormones to trigger ovulation?
   1. Progestins
   2. Fertility agents
   3. Hormonal contraceptives
   4. Estrogen replacement agents
8. What assessments are particularly important for a client receiving oxytocics? **Select all that apply.**
   1. Fetal heart tones
   2. Urine retention
   3. Blood pressure
   4. Heart rate
   5. Skin
9. What is the primary focus for the prescription of a phosphodiesterase type 5 (PDES5) inhibitor?
   1. Treatment of erectile dysfunction
   2. Increased sperm production
   3. Elevate testosterone levels
   4. Increased weight

See Answers on pages 302-303.

Fertility Agents

- Used to treat female infertility
- Example is clomiphene
- Available in PO preparations

Mode of Action

- Cause release of hormones to trigger ovaries to produce eggs

Contraindications, Precautions, and Drug Interactions of Fertility Agents*

Drug	Contraindications/Precautions	Drug Interaction
clomiphene	**Contraindications:** Hypersensitivity, hepatic disease, adrenal/thyroid dysfunction, intracranial lesion, uterine bleeding, ovarian cysts, endometrial carcinoma **Precautions:** Hypertension, seizures, depression, diabetes mellitus, abnormal ovarian enlargement, ovarian hyperstimulation **Pregnancy:** Absolute fetal abnormalities; not to be used at any time during pregnancy	DHEA, soy

*Pregnancy categories have been revised. See http://www.fda.gov/Drugs/DevelopmentApprovalProcess/DevelopmentResources/Labeling/ucm093307.htm for more information.

Adverse Effects

- Dizziness
- Headache
- Insomnia
- Restlessness
- Anxiety
- Depression
- Fatigue
- Flushing
- Hot flashes
- Deep vein thrombosis
- Phlebitis
- Vision changes
- Nausea
- Vomiting
- Constipation

- Bloating
- Hepatitis
- Polyuria
- Urinary frequency
- Oliguria

- Birth defects
- Spontaneous abortion
- Breast pain
- Abnormal uterine bleeding
- Ovarian cyst

- Rash
- Urticaria
- Alopecia

Nursing Care
- Monitor renal/hepatic function
- Monitor for mental status changes
- Teach patient that multiple births are common
- Teach patient to report abdominal pain to prescriber
- Teach patient to report vision changes to prescriber
- Teach patient to double dose if previous dose is missed
- Teach patient how to determine when ovulation is occurring

Oxytocics
- Used to stimulate labor, missed/incomplete abortion; control postpartum bleeding
- Example includes oxytocin
- Available in IM, IV preparations

Mode of Action
- Stimulates uterine contractions and ejection of breast milk

Contraindications, Precautions, and Drug Interactions of Oxytocics*

Drug	Contraindications/Precautions	Drug Interaction
oxytocin	**Contraindications:** Hypersensitivity, active genital herpes, fetal distress, hypertonic uterus, prolapsed umbilical cord, cephalopelvic disproportion, serum toxemia **Precautions:** Uterine sepsis, cervical/uterine surgery, first/second stage of labor, primipara >35 yrs. **Pregnancy:** No adverse effects in animals; no human studies available	Vasopressors, ephedra

*Pregnancy categories have been revised. See http://www.fda.gov/Drugs/DevelopmentApprovalProcess/DevelopmentResources/Labeling/ucm093307.htm for more information.

Adverse Effects
- Seizures
- Hypo/hypertension
- Dysrhythmias
- Bradycardia
- Tachycardia
- PVC

- Anorexia
- Nausea
- Vomiting
- Constipation
- Water intoxication
- Tetanic contractions

- Abruptio placentae
- Decreased uterine blood flow
- Hyperbilirubinemia
- Rash
- Fetal distress

Nursing Care
- Monitor for cardiac/respiratory distress
- Monitor I&O
- Monitor contractions

- Monitor for water intoxication of the mother
- Monitor for fetal distress
- Teach patient to report increased blood loss, abdominal cramps, fever, foul-smelling lochia
- Teach patient that contractions will increase in intensity

APPLICATION AND REVIEW

10. A client has been receiving oxytocin (Pitocin) to augment labor. For what adverse reaction caused by a prolonged oxytocin (Pitocin) infusion should the nurse monitor the client?
    1. Change in affect
    2. Hyperventilation
    3. Water intoxication
    4. Elevated temperature

See Answers on pages 302-303.

Abortifacients

- Used to induce abortion of fetus
- Example includes mifepristone, misoprostol
- Available in PO, intravaginal preparations

Mode of Action

- Counteracts progesterone that is needed to maintain pregnancy

Contraindications, Precautions, and Drug Interactions of Abortifacients*

Drug	Contraindications/Precautions	Drug Interaction
mifepristone	**Contraindications:** Hypersensitivity, ectopic pregnancy **Precautions:** Breastfeeding, adrenal disorder, IUD **Pregnancy:** absolute fetal abnormalities; not to be used at any time during pregnancy	Corticosteroids, azole antifungals, macrolide antibiotics, carbamazepine, phenytoin, phenobarbital, antiplatelets, NSAIDs, anticoagulants, St. John's wort
misoprostol	**Contraindications:** Hypersensitivity, hypersensitivity to prostaglandins **Precautions:** Breastfeeding, children, geriatric patients, renal/CV/inflammatory bowel disease, sepsis, abnormal fetal position, C-section, ectopic pregnancy, fetal distress, vaginal bleeding, diarrhea, dehydration **Pregnancy:** Absolute fetal abnormalities; not to be used at any time during pregnancy	No known drug interactions

*Pregnancy categories have been revised. See http://www.fda.gov/Drugs/DevelopmentApprovalProcess/DevelopmentResources/Labeling/ucm093307.htm for more information.

Adverse Effects

- Dizziness
- Weakness
- Nausea
- Vomiting
- Diarrhea
- Constipation
- Abdominal pain
- Hypermenorrhea
- Menstrual disorders
- Cramps
- Spotting

Nursing Care

- Monitor patient for infection
- Teach patient that maximum drug concentrations are reached when taken with food
- Teach patient to avoid OTC preparations unless prescriber permits

MEN'S HEALTH DRUGS

Androgenic Anabolic Steroids

- Used to treat hypogonadism, impotence, low testosterone
- Examples include testosterone cypionate, testosterone enanthate, testosterone gel, testosterone pellets, testosterone transdermal, testosterone buccal, testosterone topical solution gel, testosterone nasal gel
- Available in PO, IM, transdermal, intranasal preparations

Mode of Action

- Builds body tissue to increase weight

Contraindications, Precautions, and Drug Interactions of Androgenic Anabolic Steroids*

Drug	Contraindications/Precautions	Drug Interaction
testosterone cypionate, testosterone enanthate, testosterone gel, testosterone pellets, testosterone transdermal, testosterone buccal, testosterone topical solution gel, testosterone nasal gel	**Contraindications:** Hypersensitivity, breast-feeding, cardiac/renal/hepatic disease, male breasts, prostate cancer, genital bleeding **Precautions:** CV disease, MI, diabetes mellitus, urinary tract disorder, prostate cancer, hypercalcemia **Pregnancy:** Absolute fetal abnormalities; not to be used at any time during pregnancy	ACTH, adrenal steroids, bupropion, oxyphenbutazone, anticoagulants

*Pregnancy categories have been revised. See http://www.fda.gov/Drugs/DevelopmentApprovalProcess/DevelopmentResources/Labeling/ucm093307.htm for more information.

Adverse Effects

- Headache
- Dizziness
- Fatigue
- Anxiety
- Insomnia
- Lability
- Paresthesias
- Flushing
- Sweating
- Hypertension
- Nasal congestion
- Nausea
- Vomiting
- Diarrhea
- Constipation
- Weight gain
- Jaundice
- Hematuria
- Decreased libido
- Decreased breast size
- Clitoral hypertrophy
- Testicular atrophy
- Gynecomastia
- Large prostate
- Polycythemia
- Rash
- Oily skin
- Acne
- Hirsutism
- Alopecia

Nursing Care

- Monitor renal/hepatic function
- Monitor for cardiac/respiratory distress
- Monitor I&O
- Monitor electrolytes

- Monitor for aggression
- Teach patient that changes in sex characteristics can occur
- Teach women to report menstrual irregularities to the prescriber

Phosphodiesterase Type 5 (PDE5) Inhibitors

- Used to treat erectile dysfunction
- Examples include alprostadil, avanafil, sildenafil, tadalafil, vardenafil
- Available in PO, intracavernosal, intraurethral preparations

Mode of Action
- Increase blood flow to the penis

Contraindications, Precautions, and Drug Interactions of Phosphodiesterase Type 5 Inhibitors*

Drug	Contraindications/Precautions	Drug Interaction
alprostadil	*Contraindications:* Hypersensitivity, respiratory distress syndrome, those at risk for priapism *Precautions:* Geriatric patients, respiratory disease *Pregnancy:* No adverse effects in animals; no human studies available	Alcohol, other PDE5 inhibitors
avanafil	*Contraindications:* Hypersensitivity, severe renal/hepatic disease, current nitrate/nitrite use, patients <18 yrs *Precautions:* Geriatric patients, renal/hepatic/CV disease, aortic stenosis, MI, stroke, sickle cell anemia, leukemia, multiple myeloma, bleeding disorders, HIV, active peptic ulcer, tinnitus, retinitis pigmentosa, visual disturbances, prolonged erection, anatomic penile deformities *Pregnancy:* No adverse effects in animals; no human studies available	CYP3A4 inhibitors, nitrites, nitrates, alcohol, other PDE5 inhibitors, alpha blockers, amlodipine
sildenafil	*Contraindications:* Hypersensitivity, hypersensitivity to nitrites *Precautions:* Geriatric patients, renal/hepatic/CV disease, multiproduct antihypertensive regimen, sickle cell anemia, leukemia, multiple myeloma, bleeding disorders, active peptic ulcer, retinitis pigmentosa, anatomic penile deformities *Pregnancy:* No adverse effects in animals; no human studies available	Nitrates, cimetidine, erythromycin, ketoconazole, itraconazole, antiretroviral protease inhibitors, tacrolimus, CYP-450 inducers, rifampin, bosentan, barbiturates, carbamazepine, dexamethasone, phenytoin, nevirapine, rifabutin, troglitazone, antacids, alpha blockers, alcohol, amlodipine, angiotensin II receptor blockers
tadalafil	*Contraindications:* Hypersensitivity, newborns, children, women, organic nitrate use, alpha adrenergic agonists *Precautions:* Renal/hepatic/CV disease, sickle cell anemia, leukemia, multiple myeloma, bleeding disorders, active peptic ulcer, anatomic penile deformities, prolonged erection *Pregnancy:* No adverse effects in animals; no human studies available	Nitrates, itraconazole, ketoconazole, ritonavir, alcohol, amlodipine, alpha blockers, enalapril, angiotensin II receptor blockers, bosentan, antacids

Contraindications, Precautions, and Drug Interactions of Phosphodiesterase Type 5 Inhibitors—cont'd

Drug	Contraindications/Precautions	Drug Interaction
vardenafil	**Contraindications:** Hypersensitivity, renal disease, QT prolongation, alpha blockers, nitrates **Precautions:** Women, newborns, children, renal/hepatic/CV disease, sickle cell anemia, leukemia, multiple myeloma, bleeding disorders, active peptic ulcer, retinitis pigmentosa, anatomic penile deformities **Pregnancy:** No adverse effects in animals; no human studies available	Nitrates, antiarrhythmics, clarithromycin, droperidol, procainamide, quinidine, quinolones, alpha blockers, protease inhibitors, metoprolol, nifedipine, alcohol, amlodipine, angiotensin II receptor blockers, azole fungals, erythromycin, cimetidine, antiretroviral protease inhibitors

*Pregnancy categories have been revised. See http://www.fda.gov/Drugs/DevelopmentApprovalProcess/DevelopmentResources/Labeling/ucm093307.htm for more information.

Adverse Effects

- Headache
- Dizziness
- Fatigue
- Flushing
- Seizures
- Ventricular dysrhythmias
- Sudden death
- MI
- CV collapse
- CV hemorrhage
- Postural hypotension
- Angina
- Tachycardia
- TIA
- Angioedema
- Sickle cell crisis
- Upper respiratory infection
- Pharyngitis
- Bronchitis
- Sinusitis
- Nausea
- Diarrhea
- Constipation
- Dyspepsia
- Jaundice
- Impotence
- Priapism
- Thrombocytopenia
- Vision changes
- Sudden hearing/vision loss
- Body aches/back pain
- Rash
- Urticaria
- Toxic epidermal necrolysis

Nursing Care

- Administer with food
- Administer 30 minutes before sexual activity
- Monitor renal/hepatic function
- Monitor urinary function
- Monitor for skin reactions
- Monitor for vision/hearing loss
- Teach patient not to drive or engage in hazardous activities
- Teach patient to rise slowly from sitting/lying positions
- Teach patient to avoid all OTC products unless approved by prescriber
- Teach patient to report to emergency care if erection persists longer than 4 hours
- Teach patient injection technique for intracavernosal/intraurethral preparations
- Teach patient to avoid grapefruit products
- Teach patient that high fat meal can block drug's efficacy
- Teach patient product does not protect against pregnancy, STIs, HIV

ANSWER KEY: REVIEW QUESTIONS

1 **There is a relationship between hormone replacement therapy (HRT) that combines estrogen and progesterone compounds and an increased incidence of invasive breast cancer.**

2 A side effect of HRT is weight gain with ankle and foot edema. 3 Bone loss is retarded with HRT. 4 Vaginal tissue maintains turgor and lubrication with HRT.

Clinical Area: Childbearing and Women's Health Nursing; **Client Needs:** Pharmacologic and Parenteral Therapies; **Cognitive Level:** Application; **Nursing Process:** Evaluation/Outcomes

> **Study Tip:** Take a moment and look for information on the Internet for the Women's Health Initiative study on HRT therapy. This huge randomized control trial was halted in 2002, 3½ years before its completion because of a large increase in breast cancer cases in women taking HRT. Then say this rhyming sentence to yourself "H-R-T is NOT [0]risk-free!"

2. **Answers: 1, 3, 4, 5**

   Oral contraceptives alters fertilization by inhibiting ovulation; atrophic changes in endometrium to prevent implantation; thickened cervical mucus inhibits sperm travel.

   2 A diaphragm covers the cervical os to prevent sperm from entering the uterus.

   Client Need: Pharmacologic and Parenteral Therapies; **Cognitive Level:** Analysis; **Nursing Process:** Assessment/Analysis

3. **1 Nausea is related to the amount of hormone in the contraceptive. There may be an excess of estrogen; this symptom usually can be controlled by reducing the dose or by changing to another oral contraceptive.**

   2 Lethargy can be related to excessive estrogen and progesterone, but they are not common side effects. 3 Amenorrhea is associated with pregnancy; breakthrough bleeding is a more common response to estrogen. 4 Hypomenorrhea is caused by estrogen deficiency.

   Clinical Area: Childbearing and Women's Health Nursing; **Client Needs:** Pharmacologic and Parenteral Therapies; **Cognitive Level:** Application; **Nursing Process:** Evaluation/Outcomes

4. **Answers: 1, 2, 3, 5**

   Estrogen replacement agents are used to treat menopause, abnormal uterine bleeding, atrophic vaginitis, vulvar/vaginal atrophy; prevent osteoporosis.

   4 Estrogen replacement agents are not used to alter the chance of a pregnancy occurring.

   Client Need: Pharmacologic and Parenteral Therapies; **Cognitive Level:** Analysis; **Nursing Process:** Assessment/Analysis

5. **1 Estrogen replacement agents are associated with fetal abnormalities and are not to be used at any time during pregnancy.**

   2 Estrogen replacement agents are associated with fetal abnormalities and are not to be used at any time during pregnancy. 3 Estrogen replacement agents are associated with fetal abnormalities and are not to be used at any time during pregnancy. 4 Estrogen replacement agents are associated with fetal abnormalities and are not to be used at any time during pregnancy.

   Client Need: Pharmacologic and Parenteral Therapies; **Cognitive Level:** Analysis; **Nursing Process:** Assessment/Analysis

6. **Answers: 2, 3, 4, 5**

   Clients prescribed estrogen replacement agents should be educated to avoid smoking and grapefruit, report a weekly weight gain greater than 5 lbs. and any changes in mental health status such as depression.

   1 A high fat diet is not associated with the use of estrogen replacement agents.

   Client Need: Pharmacologic and Parenteral Therapies; **Cognitive Level:** Analysis; **Integrated Process:** Teaching/Learning; **Nursing Process:** Planning/Implementation

7. **2 Fertility agents cause the release of hormones to trigger ovaries to produce eggs.**

   1 Progestins prevent ovulation by interfering with follicular maturation. **3** Hormonal contraceptives prevent ovulation. **4** Estrogen replacement agents release pituitary gonadotropins to treat menopause.

   Client Need: Pharmacologic and Parenteral Therapies; **Cognitive Level:** Analysis; **Nursing Process:** Assessment/Analysis

8. **Answers: 1, 3, 4, 5**

   A client receiving an oxytocics should be monitored for bradycardia as well as tachycardia, hypo and hypertension, and skin rashes.

   2 Urinary retention is not generally associated with adverse effects of this classification of medications.

   Client Need: Pharmacologic and Parenteral Therapies; **Cognitive Level:** Analysis; **Nursing Process:** Assessment/Analysis

9. **1 PDES5 is prescribed to increase blood flow to the penis for the purpose of managing erectile dysfunction.**

   2 PDES5 has no effect on sperm production. **3** Androgenic anabolic steroids are prescribed to increase testosterone levels by stimulating production. **4** Androgenic anabolic steroids are prescribed to increase weight through the production of body tissue.

   Client Need: Pharmacologic and Parenteral Therapies; **Cognitive Level:** Analysis; **Nursing Process:** Assessment/Analysis

 Study Tip: P D E S5 inhibitors help **P**enile **D**ysfunction of **E**rection.

10. **3 Oxytocin (Pitocin), a posterior pituitary hormone, has an antidiuretic effect, acting to reabsorb water from the glomerular filtrate.**

    1 Affect is not altered by oxytocin. **2** Hyperventilation is caused by inappropriate breathing patterns, not by prolonged use of oxytocin. **4** Fever occurs with infection or dehydration, not with prolonged use of oxytocin.

    Clinical Area: Childbearing and Women's Health Nursing; **Client Needs:** Pharmacologic and Parenteral Therapies; **Cognitive Level:** Application; **Nursing Process:** Evaluation/Outcomes

15 Respiratory Drugs

INTRODUCTION TO RESPIRATORY DISORDERS

Structures and Functions of the Respiratory System

- Upper portion of respiratory system filters, moistens, and warms air during inspiration
  - Nose: lining consists of ciliated mucosa; divided by septum; turbinates (conchae) projected from lateral walls; contains olfactory receptors for smell; aids in phonation
  - Paranasal sinuses drain into nose: frontal, maxillary, sphenoidal, ethmoidal; aid in phonation
  - Pharynx: nasopharynx, oropharynx, and laryngopharynx; composed of muscle with mucous lining; contains tonsils, adenoids, and other lymphoid tissue that help destroy incoming bacteria
  - Larynx: formed by cartilage including thyroid cartilage (Adam's apple), epiglottis (lid cartilage), cricoid (signet ring cartilage), and vocal cords (fibroelastic bands stretched across hollow interior of larynx); paired vocal cords (folds) and posterior arytenoid cartilages form the glottis; voice production—during expiration, air passing through larynx causes vocal cords to vibrate; short, tense cords produce a high pitch; long, relaxed cords, a low pitch
  - Trachea: smooth muscle walls contain C-shaped rings of cartilage that keep it open at all times; lined with ciliated mucosa; extends from larynx to bronchi; 10 to 12 cm long; furnishes open passageway for air going to and from lungs
  - Lower portion of respiratory system consists of lungs, which enable exchange of gases between blood and air to regulate arterial Po_2, Pco_2, and pH; left lung has two lobes and right lung has three lobes
  - Bronchi: right and left, formed by branching of trachea; right bronchus slightly larger and more vertical than left; each primary bronchus branches into segmental bronchi in each lung; primary and segmental bronchi contain C-shaped cartilage
  - Bronchioles: small branches off secondary bronchi, distinguished by lack of C-shaped cartilage and a duct diameter of about 1 mm; bronchi further branch into terminal bronchioles, respiratory bronchioles, and then alveolar ducts
  - Alveoli: microscopic sacs composed of a single layer of squamous epithelial cells (type I cell) enveloped by a network of pulmonary capillaries that allow for rapid gas exchange; type II cells produce surfactant to prevent alveolar collapse, and type III cells are macrophages that protect against bacteria by phagocytosis
  - Covering of lung: visceral layer of pleura that joins with parietal pleura lining the thorax and diaphragm; space between these two linings is the pleural space and contains a small amount of fluid to eliminate friction; negative pressure in pleural space relative to atmospheric pressure is essential for breathing

Physiology of Respiration

Mechanism of Breathing

- Following phrenic nerve stimulation, diaphragm and other respiratory muscles contract
- Thorax increases in size

- Intrathoracic and intrapulmonic pressures decrease
- Air rushes from positive pressure in atmosphere to negative pressure in alveoli
- Inspiration is completed with stimulation of stretch receptors
- Expiration occurs passively as a result of recoil of elastic lung tissue

Control of Respiration
- Alveolar stretch receptors respond to inspiration by sending inhibitory impulses to inspiratory neurons in brainstem that prevent lung overdistention (Hering-Breuer reflex)
- Central and peripheral chemoreceptors stimulate respirations in response to lowered pH, increased Pco_2, or decreased Po_2
- Medulla oblongata and pons control rate and depth of respirations

Amount of Air Exchanged in Breathing
- Directly related to gas pressure gradient between atmosphere and alveoli
- Inversely related to resistance that opposes airflow
- Positions such as orthopneic and semi- to high-Fowler lower abdominal organs and reduce pressure against diaphragm
- Influenced by lung volumes and capacities (pulmonary function evaluated with a spirometer)
  - Tidal volume: average amount expired after a regular inspiration; expected volume is approximately 500 mL
  - Expiratory reserve volume (ERV): largest additional volume of air that can be forcibly expired after a regular inspiration and expiration; expected volume is 1,000 to 1,200 mL
  - Inspiratory reserve volume (IRV): largest additional volume of air that can be forcibly inspired after a regular inspiration; expected volume is 3,000 mL
  - Residual volume: air that cannot be forcibly expired voluntarily from lungs; expected volume is 1,200 mL; increased in chronic obstructive pulmonary disease (COPD) as lungs lose elasticity and ability to recoil, resulting in air trapping
  - Vital capacity: amount of air that can be forcibly expired after forcible inspiration; varies with size of thoracic cavity, which is determined by various factors (e.g., size of rib cage, posture, volume of blood and interstitial fluid in lungs, size of heart); expected capacity is about 4,600 mL; decreased with COPD, neuromuscular disease, atelectasis
  - Forced expiratory volume (FEV): volume of air that can be forcibly exhaled within a specific time, usually 1 second; expected volume is decreased with increased airway resistance (e.g., bronchospasm, COPD)
  - Inspiratory capacity: largest amount of air that can be inspired after a regular exhalation; expected capacity is about 3,500 mL
  - Functional residual capacity: amount of air left in the lungs after a regular exhalation; expected capacity is about 2,300 mL; increased with COPD
  - Total lung capacity (Fig. 15.1): amount of air in lungs after maximum inhalation; equal to sum of tidal volume, residual volume, and inspiratory and expiratory reserve volumes; expected capacity is about 5,800 mL; increased with COPD; decreased with atelectasis and pneumonia

Diffusion of Gases Between Air and Blood
- Occurs across alveolar-capillary membranes (in lungs between air in alveoli and venous blood in lung capillaries); adequate diffusion depends on a balanced ventilation-perfusion (V/Q) ratio
- Direction of diffusion

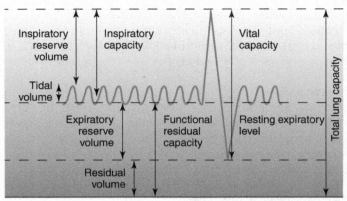

FIG. 15.1 Lung volumes and capacities (illustrated by spirography tracing). (From Monahan, F.D., Neighbors, M., Sands, J.K., Marek, J.F., Green, C.J. [2007]. *Phipps' medical-surgical nursing: Health and illness perspectives* [8th ed.]. St. Louis: Mosby.)

- Oxygen: net diffusion toward lower oxygen pressure gradient (from alveolar air to blood)
- Carbon dioxide: net diffusion toward lower carbon dioxide pressure gradient (from blood to alveolar air)
- V/Q ratios
  - Expected: balance between alveolar ventilation and capillary blood flow to facilitate gas exchange
  - Low V/Q ratio: alveoli are poorly ventilated, but capillary blood flow is adequate; blood is shunted past alveoli without adequate gas exchange (e.g., atelectasis, pneumonia)
  - High V/Q ratio: alveolar ventilation is adequate, but capillary blood flow is not; adequate gas exchange does not take place because of dead space (e.g., pulmonary embolism, cardiogenic shock)
  - Absence of ventilation and perfusion: causes a silent unit with no gas exchange (e.g., pneumothorax)
- Blood transports oxygen as a solute and primarily as oxyhemoglobin; oxygen saturation of hemoglobin (Sao_2) is 95% to 100%
- Blood transports carbon dioxide
  - Primarily as a bicarbonate ion (HCO_3^-) formed by ionization of carbonic acid; in lungs the molecule splits in the presence of carbonic anhydrase to form carbon dioxide (CO_2) and water (H_2O); CO_2 diffuses into the alveoli and the majority of water is retained
  - As a solute in plasma
  - In combination with hemoglobin (carboxyhemoglobin)

Normal Breath Sounds
- Bronchial sounds (over trachea, larynx): result of air passing through larger airways; sounds are loud, harsh, high-pitched; expiration longer than inspiration
- Vesicular sounds (over entire lung field except large airways): result of air moving in and out of alveoli; may reflect sound of air in larger passages that is transmitted through lung tissue; sounds are quiet, low-pitched; inspiration longer than expiration
- Bronchovesicular sounds (near main stem bronchi); result of air moving through smaller air passages; sounds are moderately pitched, breezy; inspiratory and expiratory phases equal

Adventitious Breath Sounds (Fig. 15.2)

- Fine crackles
  - Result of sudden opening of small airways and alveoli that contain fluid
  - Short, high-pitched bubbling sounds; sounds may be simulated by rubbing a few strands of hair between fingers next to the ear
  - Most common during height of inspiration
  - Associated with pneumonia and pulmonary edema
- Coarse crackles
  - Rush of air passing through airway intermittently occluded by mucus
  - Short, low-pitched bubbling sounds
  - Most common on inspiration and at times expiration
  - Associated with pneumonia, COPD, and pulmonary edema
- Wheezes
  - Result of air passing through narrowed small airways
  - Sounds are high-pitched and musical (sibilant wheezes), or low-pitched and rumbling (sonorous wheezes or rhonchi)
  - Most common on expiration
  - Associated with asthma and with conditions that cause partial obstruction of airway by mucus, foreign body, or tumor
- Pleural friction rub
  - Result of roughened pleural surfaces rubbing across each other
  - Sounds are crackling, grating
  - Most common during height of inspiration
  - Associated with conditions that cause inflammation of pleura

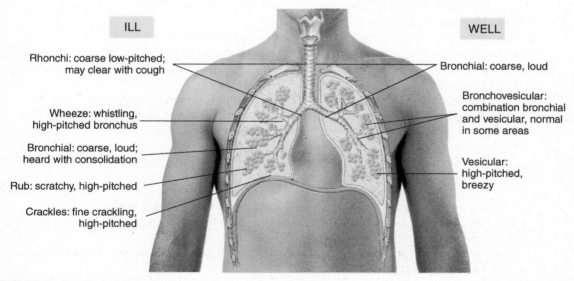

FIG. 15.2   Breath sounds in the ill and well client. (From Ball, J.W., Dains, J.E., Flynn, J.A., Solomon, B.S., Stewart, R.W. [2015]. *Seidel's guide to physical examination* [8th ed.]. St. Louis: Elsevier.)

Obstructive Airway Diseases

- Asthma: reversible bronchospasms, mucosal edema, and increased secretions that last an hour or more; severity classified as mild intermittent, mild persistent, moderate persistent, or severe persistent; status asthmaticus is an asthmatic attack that is difficult to control; asthma is no longer grouped with other diseases that comprise the broad classification of COPD, but it is an obstructive airway disease
- Chronic obstructive pulmonary disease (COPD): progressive airflow limitation associated with an inflammatory response; four stages classified as mild, moderate, severe, and very severe
- Chronic bronchitis: inflammation of bronchial walls with hypertrophy of mucous goblet cells; characterized by a chronic cough
- Emphysema: distended, inelastic, or destroyed alveolar walls that impair diffusion of gases through the alveolar capillary membrane that traps air, making exhalation difficult
- Traditionally, it was believed that clients with COPD become accustomed to an elevated residual carbon dioxide level and did not respond to high carbon dioxide concentrations as the respiratory stimulant; clients responded instead to a drop in oxygen concentration in the blood. Newer theories (e.g., Haldane effect) suggest the adverse effects of administering high concentrations of oxygen are caused by the inability of oxygen-saturated hemoglobin molecules to transport carbon dioxide, leading to increased hypercapnia; this oxygen sensitivity affects a small subset of clients
- May precipitate pulmonary hypertension, cor pulmonale, right ventricular heart failure, or pneumothorax

Asthma

- Chronic inflammatory disorder of airways
  - Reversible airflow limitation
  - Spasms of bronchi and bronchioles
  - Edema of mucous membranes
  - Increased secretions
  - Respiratory acidosis from accumulation of carbon dioxide
- Incidence: increasing rate of occurrence, severity, and mortality; most common chronic disease of childhood
- Risk factors
  - Immunologic exposure to antigen that is deposited on respiratory mucosa
  - Nonimmunologic stimuli (e.g., viral infections, physical and chemical substances)
- Primary cause of school absences; leading cause of pediatric hospitalizations
- Classification
  - Mild intermittent: symptoms two or fewer times each week; brief exacerbations; nighttime symptoms two or fewer times each month
  - Mild persistent: symptoms more than two times per week but less than once a day; exacerbations affect activity; nighttime symptoms more than twice per month
  - Moderate persistent: daily symptoms; frequent nighttime symptoms; limited physical activity
  - Severe persistent: continual symptoms; frequent exacerbations; frequent nighttime symptoms; limited physical activity
- Status asthmaticus: continued respiratory distress despite usual interventions; considered medical emergency

APPLICATION AND REVIEW

1. A client states that the health care provider said the tidal volume is slightly diminished and asks the nurse what this means. Which explanation should the nurse provide about the volume of air being measured to determine tidal volume?
   1. Exhaled after there is a normal inspiration
   2. Exhaled forcibly after a regular expiration
   3. Inspired forcibly above a typical inspiration
   4. Trapped in the alveoli after a maximum expiration

2. A client is scheduled for a pulmonary function test. The nurse explains that during the test one of the instructions the respiratory therapist will give the client is to breathe normally. What should the nurse teach is being measured when the client follows these directions?
   1. Tidal volume
   2. Vital capacity
   3. Expiratory reserve
   4. Inspiratory reserve

3. A nurse identifies that a client's hemoglobin level is decreasing and is concerned about tissue hypoxia. An increase in what diagnostic test result indicates an acceleration in oxygen dissociation from hemoglobin?
   1. pH
   2. Po_2
   3. Pco_2
   4. HCO_3

4. A nurse repositions a client who is diagnosed with emphysema to facilitate breathing. Which position facilitates maximum air exchange?
   1. Supine
   2. Orthopneic
   3. Low-Fowler
   4. Semi-Fowler

5. A client is admitted with suspected atelectasis. Which clinical manifestation does the nurse expect to identify when assessing this client?
   1. Slow, deep respirations
   2. Normal oral temperature
   3. Dry, unproductive cough
   4. Diminished breath sounds

6. A 5-year-old child is admitted to the pediatric intensive care unit with a diagnosis of acute asthma. A blood sample is obtained to measure the child's arterial blood gases. What finding does the nurse expect?
   1. High oxygen level
   2. Elevated alkalinity
   3. Decreased bicarbonate
   4. Increased carbon dioxide level

7. When planning discharge teaching for the parents of a child with asthma, what information should the nurse include?
   1. Avoid foods high in fat.
   2. Stay at home for 2 weeks.
   3. Increase the protein and calorie intake.
   4. Minimize exertion and exposure to cold.

8. When preparing a child with asthma for discharge, what must the nurse emphasize to the family? **Select all that apply.**
   1. Eliminate allergens in the home.
   2. Maintain a dry home environment.
   3. Avoid placing limits on the child's behavior.
   4. Continue the medications even if the child is asymptomatic.
   5. Prevent exposure to infection by having the child tutored at home.

9. A child with a history of asthma is brought to the emergency department experiencing an acute exacerbation of asthma. Which nursing assessments support this conclusion? **Select all that apply.**
   1. Fever
   2. Crackles
   3. Wheezing
   4. Tachycardia
   5. Hypotension

10. A child has been admitted to the pediatric unit with a severe asthma attack. What type of acid-base imbalance should the nurse expect the child to develop?
    1. Metabolic alkalosis caused by excessive production of acid metabolites
    2. Respiratory alkalosis caused by accelerated respirations and loss of carbon dioxide
    3. Respiratory acidosis caused by impaired respirations and increased formation of carbonic acid
    4. Metabolic acidosis caused by the kidneys' inability to compensate for increased carbonic acid formation

11. A client is admitted to the hospital with a diagnosis of an exacerbation of asthma. What should the nurse plan to do to **best** help this client?
    1. Determine the client's emotional state.
    2. Give prescribed drugs to promote bronchiolar dilation.
    3. Provide education about the effect of a family history.
    4. Encourage the client to use an incentive spirometer routinely.

12. A nurse is caring for a client experiencing an acute episode of bronchial asthma. What outcome should be achieved?
    1. Raising mucous secretions from the chest
    2. Curing the client's condition permanently
    3. Limiting pulmonary secretions by decreasing fluid intake
    4. Convincing the client that the condition is emotionally based

See Answers on pages 327-330.

UPPER RESPIRATORY TRACT AGENTS

Antitussives

- Used to suppress cough
- Two main categories: opioid and nonopioid
- Examples: codeine, benzonatate, hydrocodone
- Available in oral preparations

Mode of Action

- Inhibit cough reflex either by direct action on medullary cough center or by indirect action peripherally on sensory nerve endings

Contraindications, Precautions, and Drug Interactions of Antitussives*

Drug	Contraindications/Precautions	Drug Interaction
Opioid		
codeine	**Contraindications:** Hypersensitivity to opiates, respiratory depression, increased intracranial pressure, seizure disorders, severe respiratory disorders, breastfeeding	Alcohol, CNS depressants

Contraindications, Precautions, and Drug Interactions of Antitussives—cont'd

Drug	Contraindications/Precautions	Drug Interaction
Opioid		
	Precautions: Geriatric, cardiac dysrhythmias, bowel impaction, prostatic hypertrophy	
	Pregnancy: Only given after risks to the fetus are considered	
homatropine 1.5 mg and hydrocodone 5 mg	*Contraindications:* Hypersensitivity, abrupt discontinuation	Alcohol, antianxiety agents, antihistamines, antipsychotic agents, CNS depressants, narcotics, MAOIs, tricyclic antidepressants
	Precautions: Breastfeeding, neonates, addictive personality, psychosis, renal/hepatic disease	
	Pregnancy: Only given after risks to the fetus are considered	
Non-Opioid		
benzonatate	*Contraindications:* Hypersensitivity	Drugs that may cause drowsiness, CNS depressants
	Precautions: Asthma	
	Pregnancy: Only given after risks to the fetus are considered	

CNS, central nervous system; *MAOI,* monoamine oxidase inhibitor; *mg,* milligram.
*Pregnancy categories have been revised. See http://www.fda.gov/Drugs/DevelopmentApprovalProcess/DevelopmentResources/Labeling/ucm093307.htm for more information.

Adverse Effects/Side Effects
- Drowsiness
- Nausea, GI irritation
- Dry mouth (anticholinergic effect of antihistamine in combination products)

Nursing Care
- Provide adequate fluid intake
- Avoid offering fluids immediately after administering liquid preparations
- Encourage high-Fowler position
- Question if prescribed postoperatively, concurrently with CNS depressants, or for clients with a head injury or asthma
- Maintain safety precautions after administration; teach to avoid hazardous activity
- Teach patient to swallow benzonatate whole since it is an anesthetic that could impair epiglottis function if stuck in the throat

Decongestants
- Three main categories: adrenergics, anticholinergics, and corticosteroids

Adrenergic (Sympathomimetic) Decongestants
- Used for nasal congestion
- Examples: oxymetazoline, phenylephrine, pseudoephedrine, and tetrahydrozoline
- Available in tablets, capsules, liquid forms, intranasal sprays and drops

Mode of Action
- Stimulate alpha-adrenergic receptors causing vasoconstriction of the capillaries in the nasal mucosa

Contraindications, Precautions, and Drug Interactions of Adrenergic Decongestants*

Drug	Contraindications/Precautions	Drug Interaction
oxymetazoline	*Contraindications:* Narrow-angle glaucoma, uncontrolled cardiovascular disease, hypertension, diabetes, and hyperthyroidism *Precautions:* Breastfeeding, children, renal/hepatic insufficiency *Pregnancy:* Only given after risks to the fetus are considered; animal studies have shown adverse reactions; no human studies available	Caffeine, carbonic anhydrase inhibitors, MAOIs, ocular inhibitors, other sympathomimetic drugs, sulfonamides, thiazide diuretics
phenylephrine	*Contraindications:* Narrow-angle glaucoma, uncontrolled cardiovascular disease, hypertension, diabetes, and hyperthyroidism *Precautions:* Breastfeeding, children, renal/hepatic insufficiency *Pregnancy:* Only given after risks to the fetus are considered; animal studies have shown adverse reactions; no human studies available	Caffeine, carbonic anhydrase inhibitors, MAOIs, ocular inhibitors, other sympathomimetic drugs, sulfonamides, thiazide diuretics
pseudoephedrine	*Contraindications:* Narrow-angle glaucoma, uncontrolled cardiovascular disease, hypertension, diabetes, and hyperthyroidism *Precautions:* Breastfeeding, cardiac disorders, hyperthyroidism, diabetes mellitus, prostatic hypertrophy, hypertension *Pregnancy:* Only given after risks to the fetus are considered; animal studies have shown adverse reactions; no human studies available	Beta blockers, caffeine, MAOIs, other sympathomimetic drugs
tetrahydrozoline	*Contraindications:* Narrow-angle glaucoma, uncontrolled cardiovascular disease, hypertension, diabetes, and hyperthyroidism *Precautions:* Breastfeeding, children, renal/hepatic insufficiency *Pregnancy:* Only given after risks to the fetus are considered; animal studies have shown adverse reactions; no human studies available	Caffeine, MAOIs, other sympathomimetic drugs

MAOI, monoamine oxidase inhibitor.
*Pregnancy categories have been revised. See http://www.fda.gov/Drugs/DevelopmentApprovalProcess/DevelopmentResources/Labeling/ucm093307.htm for more information.

Adverse Effects/Side Effects
- Nervousness, restlessness
- Rebound nasal congestion
- Increased blood pressure
- Increased blood glucose

Nursing Care
- Assess for irritation of nasal mucosa before and during treatment
- Teach that stinging may occur when starting medication
- Teach to notify prescriber if irregular pulse, insomnia, dizziness, or tremors occur
- Teach proper technique to clean dropper to prevent infection

Anticholinergic Decongestants

- Used for nasal congestion
- Example: ipratropium
- Available in nasal spray, solution for inhalation

Mode of Action

- Inhibits interaction of acetylcholine at receptor sites on the bronchial smooth muscle, resulting in bronchodilation

Contraindications, Precautions, and Drug Interactions of Anticholinergic Decongestants*

Drug	Contraindications/Precautions	Drug Interaction
ipratropium	**Contraindications:** Hypersensitivity to ipratropium, atropine, bromide, soybean, or peanut products **Precautions:** Limit caffeine products **Pregnancy:** No human studies available, but no adverse effects in animals	Antihistamines, bronchodilators, disopyramide, phenothiazines

*Pregnancy categories have been revised. See http://www.fda.gov/Drugs/DevelopmentApprovalProcess/DevelopmentResources/Labeling/ucm093307.htm for more information.

Adverse Effects/Side Effects

- Anxiety
- Dizziness
- Headache
- Nausea, vomiting
- Cramps
- Cough
- Worsening of symptoms
- Bronchospasm

Nursing Care

- Monitor respiratory function
- Monitor for allergic reactions/bronchospasm; if either occur, withhold dose and notify healthcare provider
- Teach not to use OTC medications unless approved by healthcare provider
- Teach that ipratropium is used prophylactically
- Encourage consumption of fluids

Corticosteroid Decongestants

- Used for nasal congestion
- Examples: beclomethasone, budesonide, flunisolide, fluticasone, triamcinolone
- Available in tablets, capsules, liquid forms, intranasal sprays and drops

Mode of Action

- Antiinflammatory action to reduce inflammatory symptoms and improve patient comfort and air exchange

Contraindications, Precautions, and Drug Interactions of Corticosteroid Decongestants*

Drug	Contraindications/Precautions	Drug Interaction
beclomethasone	**Contraindications:** Hypersensitvity **Precautions:** Child <6 yr, untreated fungal infection, glaucoma, cataracts, nasal septum ulcer, nasal trauma/surgery, osteoporosis, hyperadrenocorticism **Pregnancy:** Only given after risks to the fetus are considered; animal studies have shown adverse reactions; no human studies available	aldesleukin, azathioprine, chemotherapy agents, cyclosporine, fluphenazine, mifepristone, omacetaxine
budesonide	**Contraindications:** Hypersensitivity **Precautions:** Breastfeeding, children, TB, fungal/viral/bacterial infections, ocular herpes simplex, nasal septal ulcer, hepatic disease, diabetes, GI disease, increased intraocular pressure **Pregnancy:** Only given after risks to the fetus are considered; animal studies have shown adverse reactions; no human studies available	Antiplatelet drugs, aldesleukin, dabigatran, mifepristone, NSAIDs, warfarin
flunisolide	**Contraindications:** Hypersensitivity **Precautions:** children <6 yr, geriatric patients, diabetes, CV disease, hypertension, hyperthyroidism, increased ICP, prostatic hypertrophy, glaucoma **Pregnancy:** Only given after risks to the fetus are considered; animal studies have shown adverse reactions; no human studies available	Corticosteroids, macrolide antibiotics, mifepristone
fluticasone	**Contraindications:** Hypersensitivity to this product or milk protein, primary treatment in status asthmaticus, acute bronchospasm **Precautions:** Breastfeeding, active infections, glaucoma, diabetes, immunocompromised patients, Cushing syndrome **Pregnancy:** Only given after risks to the fetus are considered; animal studies have shown adverse reactions; no human studies available	Amprenavir, atazanavir, CYP3A4 inhibitors, darunavir, delavirdine, lopinavir, nelfinavir, ritonavir, saquinavir
triamcinolone	**Contraindications:** Hypersensitivity, neonatal prematurity, epidural/intrathecal administration, systemic fungal infection **Precautions:** Breastfeeding, diabetes mellitus, glaucoma, osteoporosis, seizure disorders, ulcerative colitis, CHF, myasthenia gravis, renal disease, esophagitis, peptic ulcer, acne, cataracts, coagulopathy, head trauma, psychosis, fungal infections, AIDS, TB, adrenal insufficiency, Cushing syndrome, acute bronchospasm, MI, thromboembolism **Pregnancy:** Only given after risks to the fetus are considered; animal studies have shown adverse reactions; no human studies available	alcohol, amphotericin B, barbiturates, carbamazepine, cyclosporine, digoxin, diuretics, estrogens, indomethacin, oral contraceptives, macrolide antiinfectives, quinolones, salicylates, vaccines

d = day; max = maximum.
*Pregnancy categories have been revised. See http://www.fda.gov/Drugs/DevelopmentApprovalProcess/DevelopmentResources/Labeling/ucm093307.htm for more information.

Adverse Effects/Side Effects

- Mucosal irritation, dryness

Nursing Care

- Teach that stinging may occur when starting medication
- Teach patient that use of a humidifier may reduce drying of mucosa
- Demonstrate proper use of inhaler

Antihistamines

- Two main categories: first and second generation
- Relieve nasal decongestion associated with the common cold and allergies that are mediated by histamine
- Examples: azelastine, brompheniramine, cetirizine, chlorpheniramine, diphenhydramine, fexofenadine, levocetirizine, loratadine
- Available in oral and parenteral (IM, IV) preparations

Mode of Action

- Block action of histamine at H1 receptor sites via competitive inhibition; exert antiemetic, anticholinergic, and CNS depressant effects

Contraindications, Precautions, and Drug Interactions of Antihistamines*

Drug	Contraindications/Precautions	Drug Interaction
First Generation		
brompheniramine	***Contraindications:*** Hypersensitivity ***Precautions:*** Asthma, breastfeeding, diabetes, emphysema, glaucoma, heart problems, hypertension, hyperthyroidism, kidney/liver disease, seizures, stomach/intestinal problems, urinary retention ***Pregnancy:*** Only given after risks to the fetus are considered; animal studies have shown adverse reactions; no human studies available	Anti-Parkinson's agents, antispasmodics, beta-blockers, MAOIs, methyldopa, moclobemide, phenelzine, procarbazine, rasgiline, reserpine, scopolamine, selegiline, topical antihistamines, tricyclic antidepressants
chlorpheniramine	***Contraindications:*** Hypersensitivity ***Precautions:*** Breastfeeding, geriatric, increased intraocular pressure, renal/cardiac disease, hypertension, bronchial asthma, seizure disorder, hyperthyroidism, prostatic hypertrophy, GI obstruction, peptic ulcer disease, emphysema, hypersensitivity, lower respiratory tract disease, stenosed peptic ulcers, bladder neck obstruction, closed-angle glaucoma ***Pregnancy:*** No human studies available, but no adverse effects in animals; animal studies have shown adverse reactions; no human studies available	Alcohol, atropine, barbiturates, CNS depressants, haloperidol, MAOIs, opiates, phenothiazines, quinidine, sedative/hypnotics, tricyclics
diphenhydramine	***Contraindications:*** Acute asthma attack, severe liver disease, COPD, neonate ***Precautions:*** Narrow-angle glaucoma, prostatic hypertrophy, breastfeeding, urinary retention ***Pregnancy:*** No human studies available, but no adverse effects in animals; animal studies have shown adverse reactions; no human studies available	Alcohol, barbiturates, hypnotics, MAOIs, opioids

Continued

Contraindications, Precautions, and Drug Interactions of Antihistamines—cont'd

Drug	Contraindications/Precautions	Drug Interaction
First Generation		
levocetirizine	*Contraindications:* Hypersensitivity to beta-blockers, cardiogenic shock, heart block, sinus bradycardia, congestive heart failure, bronchial asthma *Precautions:* Breastfeeding, geriatric, diabetes, thyroid/renal/hepatic disease, chronic obstructive pulmonary disease, well-compensated heart failure, nonallergic bronchospasm, peripheral vascular disease *Pregnancy:* No human studies available, but no adverse effects in animals; animal studies have shown adverse reactions; no human studies available	Alcohol, antidiabetics, antihypertensives, beta-blockers, cimetidine, diuretics, lidocaine, MAOIs, NSAIDs, nitroglycerin, theophyllines, tricyclic antidepressants, verapamil
Second Generation		
azelastine	*Contraindications:* Hypersensitivity *Precautions:* Breastfeeding, children <5 yr *Pregnancy:* Only given after risks to the fetus are considered; animal studies have shown adverse reactions; no human studies available	Alcohol, CNS depressants, opioids, sedative/hypnotics
cetirizine	*Contraindications:* Hypersensitivity, breastfeeding, newborn or premature infants, severe hepatic disease *Precautions:* Asthma, bladder neck obstruction, closed-angle glaucoma, geriatric, prostatic hypertrophy, respiratory disease *Pregnancy:* Only given after risks to the fetus are considered; animal studies have shown adverse reactions; no human studies available	Alcohol, CNS depressants, MAOIs, opioids, ritonavir, sedative/hypnotics
fexofenadine	*Contraindications:* Breastfeeding, newborn or premature infants, hypersensitivity, severe hepatic disease *Precautions:* Asthma, bladder neck obstruction, closed-angle glaucoma, geriatric, prostatic hypertrophy, respiratory disease *Pregnancy:* Only given after risks to the fetus are considered; animal studies have shown adverse reactions; no human studies available	Aluminum, antacids, magnesium
loratadine	*Contraindications:* Hypersensitivity, acute asthma attacks, lower respiratory tract disease *Precautions:* Breastfeeding, bronchial asthma, hepatic/renal disease, increased intraocular pressure *Pregnancy:* No adverse effects in animals; no human studies available	Alcohol, antidepressants, other antihistamines, cimetidine, ketoconazole, macrolides, MAOIs, sedative-hypnotics

GI, gastrointestinal; *MAOI,* monoamine oxidase inhibitor; *NSAIDs,* nonsteroidal antiinflammatory drugs.
*Pregnancy categories have been revised. See http://www.fda.gov/Drugs/DevelopmentApprovalProcess/DevelopmentResources/Labeling/ucm093307.htm for more information.

Adverse Effects/Side Effects
- Drowsiness and dizziness particularly for first-generation antihistamines
- GI irritation
- Dry mouth
- Excitement
- Urinary retention

Nursing Care
- Question if prescribed concurrently with CNS depressants
- Teach to avoid engaging in hazardous activities
- Administer with food or milk to avoid GI irritation
- Offer gum or hard candy to promote salivation
- Teach to avoid using antihistamines as a hypnotic, especially older adults

Expectorants
- Liquefy secretions in respiratory tract, promoting a productive cough
- Examples: dextromethorphan, guaifenesin
- Available in liquids, syrups, capsules, gel capsules, extended release solutions, tablets, extended release tablets, oral solutions

Mode of Action
- Act indirectly to liquefy mucus by increasing respiratory tract secretions via oral absorption; available in oral preparations

Contraindications, Precautions, and Drug Interactions of Expectorants*

Drug	Contraindications/Precautions	Drug Interaction
dextromethorphan	*Contraindications:* Hypersensitivity *Precautions:* Asthma, bronchitis, heart failure, smoking, fever, hepatic disease, chronic cough *Pregnancy:* Only given after risks to the fetus are considered; animal studies have shown adverse reactions; no human studies available	Alcohol, amiodarone, antihistamines, antidepressants, furazolidone, linezolid, MAOIs, opiates, procarbazine, quinidine, sedative-hypnotics, serotonin receptor agonists
guaifenesin	*Contraindications:* Hypersensitivity, chronic persistent cough *Precautions:* Asthma, breastfeeding, CHF, emphysema, fever *Pregnancy:* Only given after risks to the fetus are considered; animal studies have shown adverse reactions; no human studies available	Alcohol, antihistamines

MAOI, monoamine oxidase inhibitor.
*Pregnancy categories have been revised. See http://www.fda.gov/Drugs/DevelopmentApprovalProcess/DevelopmentResources/Labeling/ucm093307.htm for more information.

Adverse Effects/Side Effects
- Gastrointestinal (GI) irritation (local effect)
- Skin rash (hypersensitivity)

Nursing Care
- Promote adequate fluid intake

- Encourage coughing and deep breathing
- Avoid offering fluids immediately after administering liquid expectorants
- Assess respiratory status
- Have suction apparatus available

Mucolytics

- Liquefy secretions in respiratory tract, promoting a productive cough
- Example: acetylcysteine
- Available in oral solutions, inhalation preparations

Mode of action

- Act directly to break up mucus plugs in tracheobronchial passages

Contraindications, Precautions, and Drug Interactions of Mucolytics*

Drug	Contraindications/Precautions	Drug Interaction
acetylcysteine	***Contraindications:*** Asthma, hypersensitivity, increased intracranial pressure ***Precautions:*** Alcoholism, anaphylactoid reactions, breastfeeding, bronchospasm, chronic obstructive pulmonary disease, CNS depression, fluid restriction, hypothyroidism, psychosis, renal/hepatic disease, seizure disorders, weight <40 kg ***Pregnancy:*** Only given after risks to the fetus are considered; animal studies have shown adverse reactions; no human studies available	Activated charcoal, iron, nitrates

*Pregnancy categories have been revised. See http://www.fda.gov/Drugs/DevelopmentApprovalProcess/DevelopmentResources/Labeling/ucm093307.htm for more information.

Adverse Effects/Side Effects

- Gastrointestinal (GI) irritation (local effect)
- Skin rash (hypersensitivity)
- Oropharyngeal irritation and bronchospasm

Nursing Care

- Promote adequate fluid intake
- Encourage coughing and deep breathing
- Avoid offering fluids immediately after administering liquid expectorants
- Assess respiratory status
- Have suction apparatus available

APPLICATION AND REVIEW

13. When a client exhibits severe bradycardia, which type of drug should the nurse be prepared to administer?
    1. Cardiac nitrate
    2. Anticholinergic
    3. Antihypertensive
    4. Cardiac glycoside

14. A client is receiving dexamethasone. For what side effect should the nurse monitor the client?
    1. Hyperkalemia
    2. Liver dysfunction
    3. Orthostatic hypotension
    4. Increased blood glucose

15. A client who recently started receiving oral corticosteroids for a severe allergic reaction is instructed that the dosage will be reduced gradually until all medication is stopped at the end of 2 weeks. What reason should the nurse provide for this gradual reduction in dosage?
    1. Discontinuing the drug too fast will cause the allergic reaction to reappear.
    2. Slow reduction of the drug will prevent a physiologic crisis because the adrenal glands are suppressed.
    3. The health care provider is attempting to determine the minimal dose that will be effective for the allergy.
    4. Sudden cessation of the drug will cause development of serious side effects, such as moon face and fluid retention.

16. A nurse administers beclomethasone, a corticosteroid, by inhalation to a client with asthma. The client asks why this medication is necessary. What should the nurse explain is the purpose of this pharmacologic therapy?
    1. Promotes comfort
    2. Decreases inflammation
    3. Stimulates smooth muscle relaxation
    4. Reduces bacteria in the respiratory tract

See Answers on pages 327-330.

LOWER RESPIRATORY TRACT AGENTS

Bronchodilators

- Reverse bronchoconstriction, thus opening air passages in lungs
- Three categories: xanthine derivatives, sympathomimetics, and anticholinergics
- Stimulate beta-adrenergic sympathetic nervous system receptors, relaxing bronchial smooth muscle, or inhibiting inflammation and reducing edema
- Available in oral, parenteral (intramuscular, subcutaneous, IV), rectal, and inhalation preparations

Nursing Care

- Question if prescribed for clients with hypertension, hyperthyroidism, and cardiovascular dysfunction
- Question if prescribed concurrently with CNS stimulants (adrenergics) and bronchoconstricting agents (beta blockers)
- Administer with food during waking hours
- Assess vital signs, breath sounds, oxygen saturation with pulse oximeter
- Assess I&O
- Teach use of metered-dose inhalers, spacers, and peak flow meters: rinse mouthpiece, cap, and mouth after each use; oropharyngeal fungal infections are common with inhaled steroids
- Explain importance of adhering to therapy to decrease need for short-acting beta agonists
- Explain that stimulants and some over-the-counter medications should be avoided because they may act as antagonists

Adverse Effects/Side Effects

- Dizziness
- Central nervous system stimulation
- Palpitations and hypertension
- Gastric irritation

Xanthines

- Used to dilate pulmonary and coronary vessels
- Examples: aminophylline, theophylline
- Available in oral and intravenous forms

Mode of Action

- Act directly on bronchial smooth muscle, decreasing spasm and relaxing smooth muscle of the vasculature

Contraindications, Precautions, and Drug Interactions of Xanthines*

Drug	Contraindications/Precautions	Drug Interaction
aminophylline	**Contraindications:** Hypersensitivity, tachydysrhythmias **Precautions:** Alcoholism, breastfeeding, children, congestive heart failure, cor pulmonale, diabetes, geriatric, hepatic disease, hypertension, hyperthyroidism, peptic ulcer disease, seizure disorder **Pregnancy:** Only given after risks to the fetus are considered; animal studies have shown adverse reactions; no human studies available	Allopurinol (high doses), barbiturates, benzodiazepines, beta-adrenergic blockers, beta-blockers, carbamazepine, cimetidine, clarithromycin, corticosteroids, disulfiram, diuretics (loop), diuretics, erythromycin, fluoroquinolones, fluvoxamine, halothane, influenza vaccines, interferon, isoniazid, ketoconazole, lithium, mexiletine, oral contraceptives, phenytoin, rifampin, sympathomimetics, tetracyclines,
theophylline	**Contraindications:** Hypersensitivity, tachydysrhythmias **Precautions:** Children, congestive heart failure, cor pulmonale, diabetes, hepatic disease, hypertension, hyperthyroidism, peptic ulcer disease, seizure disorder **Pregnancy:** Only given after risks to the fetus are considered; animal studies have shown adverse reactions; no human studies available	Barbiturates, beta-adrenergic agonist, beta blockers, carbamazepine, cimetidine, digitalis, propranolol, erythromycin, lithium, caffeine, nicotine

*Pregnancy categories have been revised. See http://www.fda.gov/Drugs/DevelopmentApprovalProcess/DevelopmentResources/Labeling/ucm093307.htm for more information.

Adverse Effects/Side Effects

- Anorexia
- Cardiac dysrhythmias
- Dizziness
- Gastric pain
- Headache
- Hyperreflexia
- Hypotension
- Intestinal bleeding
- Irritability
- Nausea and vomiting
- Nervousness
- Palpitations
- Seizures
- Tachycardia
- Toxicity

Nursing Care

- Monitor cardiovascular status
- Teach that smoking decreases serum levels of aminophylline and theophylline
- Teach that caffeine can increase central nervous system stimulation when combined with xanthines
- Teach that medications should be taken on a regular schedule
- Teach to report epigastric pain, nausea, tremors, headache

Sympathomimetics

- Used to cause bronchodilation and increase blood pressure
- Examples: albuterol, ephedrine, epinephrine, levalbuterol, salmeterol
- Available in oral, injection, intravenous, and inhalation forms

Mode of Action

- Increase cyclic adenosine monophosphate, causing bronchiole dilation

Contraindications, Precautions, and Drug Interactions of Sympathomimetics*

Drug	Contraindications/Precautions	Drug Interaction
albuterol	***Contraindications:*** Cardiac disease, heart block, hypersensitivity tachydysrhythmias ***Precautions:*** Breastfeeding, cardiac/renal disease, children, closed-angle glaucoma, diabetes mellitus, hypertension, hyperthyroidism, hypoglycemia, prostatic hypertrophy, seizures ***Pregnancy:*** Only given after risks to the fetus are considered; animal studies have shown adverse reactions; no human studies available	Adrenergics, atomoxetine, beta-agonists, bronchodilators, CNS stimulants, digoxin, MAOIs, oxytocics, selegiline, theophylline
ephedrine	***Contraindications:*** Hypersensitivity ***Precautions:*** Cardiovascular disease, children, diabetes, geriatric, glaucoma, hypertension, hyperthyroidism, increased intracranial pressure, prostatic hypertrophy ***Pregnancy:*** Only given after risks to the fetus are considered; animal studies have shown adverse reactions; no human studies available	Beta-agonists, MAOIs
epinephrine	***Contraindications:*** Closed-angle glaucoma, hypersensitivity ***Precautions:*** Breastfeeding, cardiac disorders, diabetes, hypertension, hyperthyroidism, labor, prostatic hypertrophy ***Pregnancy:*** Only given after risks to the fetus are considered; animal studies have shown adverse reactions; no human studies available	Antidepressants, beta-adrenergic blockers, MAOIs, other sympathomimetics

Continued

Contraindications, Precautions, and Drug Interactions of Sympathomimetics—cont'd

Drug	Contraindications/Precautions	Drug Interaction
levalbuterol	**Contraindications:** Bradycardia, bronchial asthma, cardiogenic shock, congestive heart failure, heart block, hypersensitivity **Precautions:** Breastfeeding, chronic obstructive pulmonary disease, coronary artery disease, diabetes, geriatric, major surgery, nonallergic bronchospasm, peripheral vascular disease, thyroid/renal/hepatic disease **Pregnancy:** Only given after risks to the fetus are considered; animal studies have shown adverse reactions; no human studies available	Alcohol, antidepressants, antidiabetics, antihypertensives, beta-blockers, diuretics, general anesthetics, lidocaine, MAOIs, NSAIDs, theophyllines, tricyclics, verapamil
salmeterol	**Contraindications:** Hypersensitivity, monotherapy treatment of asthma, severe cardiac disease, tachydysrhythmias **Precautions:** Acute asthma, breastfeeding, cardiac disorders, closed-angle glaucoma, diabetes, hypertension, hyperthyroidism, prostatic hypertrophy, QT prolongation, seizures **Pregnancy:** Only given after risks to the fetus are considered; animal studies have shown adverse reactions; no human studies available	Antidepressants, beta-adrenergic blockers, bronchodilators, MAOIs

CNS, central nervous system; *MAOI,* monoamine oxidase inhibitor; *NSAIDs,* nonsteroidal antiinflammatory drugs.
*Pregnancy categories have been revised. See http://www.fda.gov/Drugs/DevelopmentApprovalProcess/DevelopmentResources/Labeling/ucm093307.htm for more information.

Adverse Effects/Side Effects
- Anginal pain
- Anorexia
- Cardiac stimulation
- Headache
- Hyperglycemia
- Hypertension *or* hypotension
- Insomnia
- Restlessness
- Tremors

Nursing Care
- Administer long-acting formulations with glucocorticoid in asthma management
- Monitor respiratory status and function
- Monitor cardiac status and function
- Monitor I&O
- Teach to report side effects, including insomnia, heart palpitations, light-headedness
- Demonstrate proper use of inhaler

Anticholinergics
- Used for prevention of bronchospasm associated with chronic pulmonary disease
- NOT used for management of acute symptoms
- Examples: glycopyrrolate, tiotropium
- Available in oral, injection, intravenous, and inhalation forms

Mode of Action
- Inhibit action of acetylcholine at receptor sites on bronchial smooth muscle and prevent bronchospasm

Contraindications, Precautions, and Drug Interactions of Anticholinergics*

Drug	Contraindications/Precautions	Drug Interaction
glycopyrrolate	*Contraindications:* Children, GI/GU obstruction, hepatic disease, hypersensitivity, myasthenia gravis, myocardial ischemia, tachycardia, ulcerative colitis *Precautions:* Breastfeeding, congestive heart failure, coronary artery disease, geriatric, hypertension, hyperthyroidism, narrow-angle glaucoma, prostate enlargement, pulmonary/renal disease *Pregnancy:* Only given after risks to the fetus are considered; animal studies have shown adverse reactions; no human studies available	Other anticholinergics
tiotropium	*Contraindication:* Hypersensitivity *Precautions:* Bladder neck obstruction, breastfeeding, cardiac dysrhythmias, geriatric, lactose intolerance, narrow-angle glaucoma, renal impairment, prostate enlargement *Pregnancy:* Only given after risks to the fetus are considered; animal studies have shown adverse reactions; no human studies available	Cisapride, metoclopramide, parasympathomimetics, other anticholinergics, phenothiazines

*Pregnancy categories have been revised. See http://www.fda.gov/Drugs/DevelopmentApprovalProcess/DevelopmentResources/Labeling/ucm093307.htm for more information.

Adverse Effects/Side Effects
- Abdominal pain
- Chest pain
- Constipation
- Depression
- Dry mouth
- Dyspepsia
- Headache
- Insomnia
- Joint pain
- Peripheral edema
- Vomiting

Nursing Care
- Monitor respiratory function
- Monitor for allergic reactions/bronchospasm; if either occur, withhold dose and notify health care provider
- Teach not to use OTC medications unless approved by health care provider
- Encourage consumption of fluids
- Demonstrate proper use of inhaler

Antiinflammatories
- Used for decreasing pulmonary inflammation in asthma and chronic obstructive pulmonary disease

- Examples: montelukast, roflumilast, zafirlukast, zileuton
- Available in oral and extended release forms

Mode of Action
- Binds with receptors to inhibit smooth muscle contraction and inflammatory activity that cause bronchoconstriction

Contraindications, Precautions, and Drug Interactions of Antiinflammatories*

Drug	Contraindications/Precautions	Drug Interaction
montelukast	*Contraindications:* Acute bronchospasm, hypersensitivity, severe asthmatic attack *Precautions:* Alcoholism, breastfeeding, corticosteroid withdrawal, depression, hepatic disease, older adults, suicidal ideation *Pregnancy:* Only given after risks to the fetus are considered; animal studies have shown adverse reactions; no human studies available	Phenobarbital, rifampin, carbamazepine
roflumilast	*Contraindication:* Moderate to severe hepatic disease *Precautions:* Acute bronchospasm, anxiety, breastfeeding, children, depression, insomnia, suicidal ideation or behavior *Pregnancy:* Only given after risks to the fetus are considered; animal studies have shown adverse reactions; no human studies available	Alcohol, barbiturates, bexarotene, bosentan, carbamazepine, cimetidine, dalfopristin, delavirdine, dexamethasone, enoxacin, erythromycin, etravirine, fluvoxamine, fosamprenavir, indinavir, isoniazid, itraconazole, ketoconazole, metyrapone, modafinil, nevirapine, oral contraceptives, oxcarbazepine, phenobarbital, phenytoin, quinupristin, rifabutin, rifampin, ritonavir tipranavir
zafirlukast	*Contraindications:* Hepatic encephalopathy, hypersensitivity *Precautions:* Acute bronchospasm, breastfeeding, children, geriatric, hepatic disease *Pregnancy:* Only given after risks to the fetus are considered; animal studies have shown adverse reactions; no human studies available	Aspirin, erythromycin, theophylline, warfarin
zileuton	*Contraindications:* Hypersensitivity, liver disease *Precautions:* Alcoholism, breastfeeding, children <12 yr, geriatric, liver disease, not used for acute bronchospasm *Pregnancy:* Only given after risks to the fetus are considered; animal studies have shown adverse reactions; no human studies available	Leflunomide, lomitapide, mipomersen, pimozide, pseudoephedrine, terfenadine, teriflunomide, tizanidine, propranolol, theophylline, warfarin

*Pregnancy categories have been revised. See http://www.fda.gov/Drugs/DevelopmentApprovalProcess/DevelopmentResources/Labeling/ucm093307.htm for more information.

Adverse Effects/Side Effects

- Aggressive behavior
- Anaphylaxis
- Angioedema
- Bleeding, bruising
- Confusion
- Depression, suicidal ideation
- Dizziness
- Drowsiness
- Dyspepsia
- Edema
- Elevated liver enzymes
- Headache
- Restlessness, insomnia
- Seizures
- Stevens-Johnson syndrome

Nursing Care

- Teach that one dose may be taken 1 hour before exercise to reduce exercise-induced bronchospasm
- Teach that these medications are indicated for prevention of acute asthmatic attacks
- Instruct to take montelukast at night
- Teach to report any change in mood or emotions immediately

Lung Surfactants

- Used to prevent respiratory distress syndrome in premature neonates
- Example: lucinactant
- Available in oral solution

Mode of Action

- Synthetic surfactant designed to mimic human surfactant protein-B; lines the alveolar epithelium and serves to reduce surface tension, which facilitates alveoli expansion and allows gas exchange

Contraindications, Precautions, and Drug Interactions of Lung Surfactants

Drug	Contraindications/Precautions	Drug Interaction
lucinactant	*Precautions:* Not for use in adults	Not expected to interact with other drugs

Adverse Effects/Side Effects

- Bradycardia
- Endotracheal tube obstruction, reflux
- Hypotension
- Oxygen desaturation
- Pneumothorax
- Sepsis

Nursing Care

- Reposition neonate between doses
- Provide positive pressure ventilation when stable
- Frequently assess for lung compliance
- Monitor respiratory status

Opioid Antagonists

- Used to reverse opioid-induced respiratory depression
- Example: naloxone
- Available in injection, intravenous forms

Mode of Action
- Displace opioids at respiratory receptor sites via competitive antagonism

Contraindications, Precautions, and Drug Interactions of Opioid Antagonists*

Drug	Contraindications/Precautions	Drug Interaction
naloxone	**Contraindications:** Hypersensitivity	Opioid analgesics, tramadol
	Precautions: Breastfeeding, cardiovascular disease, children, hepatic disease, opioid dependency, seizure disorder	
	Pregnancy: Only given after risks to the fetus are considered; animal studies have shown adverse reactions; no human studies available	

*Pregnancy categories have been revised. See http://www.fda.gov/Drugs/DevelopmentApprovalProcess/DevelopmentResources/Labeling/ucm093307.htm for more information.

Adverse Effects/Side Effects
- Cardiac dysrhythmias
- Withdrawal symptoms
- Seizures
- Tachycardia
- Nausea, vomiting

Nursing Care
- Assess vital signs, especially respirations
- Have oxygen and emergency resuscitative equipment available
- Continue to monitor after effects of naloxone wear off because opioids have a longer duration of action

APPLICATION AND REVIEW

17. While receiving an adrenergic beta₂ agonist drug for asthma, the client complains of palpitations, chest pain, and a throbbing headache. What is the **most** appropriate nursing action?
    1. Withhold the drug until additional orders are obtained.
    2. Tell the client not to worry; these are expected side effects from the medicine.
    3. Ask the client to relax; then give instructions to breathe slowly and deeply for several minutes.
    4. Explain that the effects are temporary and will subside as the body becomes accustomed to the drug.
18. What is the **priority** goal for a client with asthma who is being discharged from the hospital?
    1. Is able to obtain pulse oximeter readings
    2. Demonstrates use of a metered-dose inhaler
    3. Knows the health care provider's office hours
    4. Can identify the foods that may cause wheezing

19. A client is receiving albuterol to relieve severe asthma. For which clinical indicators should the nurse monitor the client? **Select all that apply.**
    1. Tremors
    2. Lethargy
    3. Palpitations
    4. Visual disturbances
    5. Decreased pulse rate

20. A client receiving morphine is being monitored by the nurse for signs and symptoms of overdose. Which clinical findings support a conclusion of overdose? **Select all that apply.**
    1. Polyuria
    2. Lethargy
    3. Bradycardia
    4. Dilated pupils
    5. Slow respirations

21. A health care provider prescribes metaproterenol (a sympathomimetic) for a client who was recently admitted to the hospital. For what therapeutic effect should the nurse monitor the client?
    1. Induced sedation
    2. Relaxed bronchial spasm
    3. Decreased blood pressure
    4. Increased bronchial secretions

22. Which relationship does the nurse consider reflective of the relationship of naloxone to morphine sulfate?
    1. Aspirin to warfarin
    2. Amoxicillin to systemic infection
    3. Protamine sulfate to parenteral heparin
    4. Enoxaparin to dalteparin

23. A client receiving morphine by patient-controlled analgesia has a respiratory rate of 6 breaths/min. What intervention should the nurse anticipate?
    1. Nasotracheal suction
    2. Mechanical ventilation
    3. Naloxone administration
    4. Cardiopulmonary resuscitation

See Answers on pages 327-330.

ANSWER KEY: REVIEW QUESTIONS

1. **1 Tidal volume (TV) is defined as the amount of air exhaled after a normal inspiration.**
   2 The air exhaled forcibly after a regular expiration is the expiratory reserve volume (ERV). **3** The air inspired forcibly after a typical inspiration is the residual volume (RV). **4** The volume of air that can be forcibly inspired over and above a normal inspiration is the inspiratory reserve volume (IRV).
   Client Need: Physiologic Adaptation; **Cognitive Level:** Knowledge; **Integrated Process:** Teaching/Learning; **Nursing Process:** Planning/Implementation

2. **1 The tidal volume is the amount of air inhaled and exhaled while breathing normally.**
   2 The vital capacity is air that can be forcibly expired after maximum inspiration. **3** The expiratory reserve is the maximum amount of air that can be expired after a normal expiration. **4** The inspiratory reserve is the maximum amount of air that can be inspired after a normal inspiration.
   Client Need: Reduction of Risk Potential; **Cognitive Level:** Application; **Integrated Process:** Teaching/Learning; **Nursing Process:** Planning/Implementation

3. **3 The lower the Po_2 and the higher the Pco_2, the more rapidly oxygen dissociates from the oxyhemoglobin molecule.**
   1 The pH will decrease with an increase in CO_2 pressure. **2** An increase in Po_2 will not increase oxygen dissociation from hemoglobin. **4** Oxygen dissociation will decrease with an increase in HCO_3.
   Client Need: Reduction of Risk Potential; **Cognitive Level:** Analysis; **Nursing Process:** Assessment/Analysis

4. **2 The orthopneic position is a sitting position that permits maximum lung expansion for gaseous exchange; it also enables the client to press the lower chest or abdomen against the overbed table, which increases pressure on the diaphragm to help with exhalation, reducing residual volume.**

   1 The supine position does not permit the diaphragm to descend by gravity, and pressure of the abdominal organs against the diaphragm limits its movement. **3, 4** The low-Fowler and semi-Fowler positions do not maximize lung expansion to the same degree as the orthopneic position.

   Client Need: Physiologic Adaptation; **Cognitive Level:** Application; **Nursing Process:** Planning/Implementation

5. **4 Because atelectasis involves collapsing of alveoli distal to the bronchioles, breath sounds are diminished in the lower lobes.**

   1 The client will have rapid, shallow respirations to compensate for poor gas exchange. **2** Atelectasis results in an elevated temperature. **3** Atelectasis results in a loose, productive cough.

   Client Need: Physiologic Adaptation; **Cognitive Level:** Application; **Nursing Process:** Assessment/Analysis

6. **4 Gas exchange is limited because of narrowing and swelling of the bronchi; the carbon dioxide level increases.**

   1 The oxygen level will be decreased, not increased. **2** The pH will decrease; the child is in respiratory acidosis, not alkalosis. **3** The bicarbonate level will be increased to compensate for acidosis.

   Client Need: Reduction of Risk Potential; **Cognitive Level:** Application; **Nursing Process:** Assessment/Analysis

7. **4 Cold and exercise can precipitate bronchospasm, and increased exercise depletes oxygen.**

   1 Treatment of asthma does not involve a low-fat diet. **2** Asthma is a chronic condition. Return to usual activities after the acute stage is essential for growth and development. **3** Although increased protein and calories may be needed to support the child during a coexisting bacterial infection in the acute stage, a return to usual eating habits is indicated by the time of discharge.

   Client Need: Reduction of Risk Potential; **Cognitive Level:** Application; **Nursing Process:** Planning/Implementation

8. **Answers: 1, 4**

   1 Parents should be taught to limit allergens in the home that can precipitate asthma attacks (e.g., no carpets, no down pillows, wet-mop floors, vacuum when the child is not in the home, no scented household products). **4** Medications to control inflammation, including inhaled corticosteroids and long-acting beta$_2$ agonists, must be continued to suppress exacerbations of asthma.

   2 Environmental moisture is necessary for these children; in addition, cold environments should be avoided. **3** Consistent limits should be placed on the child's behavior regardless of the illness; a chronic illness does not eliminate the need for limit setting. **5** The child should return to school and continue to interact with schoolmates and friends.

   > **Test-Taking Tip:** Even if you think you are unfamiliar with the specific material, use your best judgment or "common" sense to evaluate each option. For this question, you would be able to eliminate choice 2 as incorrect just based on whether it seemed reasonable.

   Client Need: Health Promotion and Maintenance; **Cognitive Level:** Analysis; **Integrated Process:** Teaching/Learning; **Nursing Process:** Planning/Implementation

9. **Answers: 3, 4**

   3 Bronchial constriction with mucus production causes wheezing. **4** With the decrease in arterial oxygenation associated with asthma, the heart rate will increase.

   1 An elevated temperature is a characteristic of sepsis, not asthma. **2** Crackles are associated with pulmonary edema, not asthma. **5** Hypertension, not hypotension, may occur with asthma.

   Client Need: Physiologic Adaptation; **Cognitive Level:** Analysis; **Nursing Process:** Assessment/Analysis

10. **3 The restricted ventilation accompanying an asthma attack limits the body's ability to blow off carbon dioxide. As carbon dioxide accumulates in the body fluids, it reacts with water to produce carbonic acid; the result is respiratory acidosis.**

    1 The problem basic to asthma is respiratory, not metabolic. **2** Respiratory alkalosis is caused by exhaling large amounts of carbon dioxide; asthma attacks cause carbon dioxide retention. **4** Asthma is a respiratory problem, not a metabolic one; metabolic acidosis can result from an increase of nonvolatile acids or a loss of base bicarbonate.

    Client Need: Physiologic Adaptation; **Cognitive Level:** Analysis; **Nursing Process:** Assessment/Analysis

11. **2 Asthma involves spasms of the bronchi and bronchioles, as well as increased production of mucus. This decreases the size of the lumina, interfering with inhalation and exhalation. Bronchiolar dilation will reduce airway resistance and improve the client's breathing.**

    1 Although identifying and addressing a client's emotional state are important, maintaining airway and breathing are the priority. In addition, emotional stress is only one of many precipitating factors, which include allergens, temperature changes, odors, and chemicals. **3** Although recent studies indicate a genetic correlation along with other factors that may predispose a person to develop asthma, exploring this issue is not the priority. **4** Use of an incentive spirometer is not helpful because of mucosal edema, bronchoconstriction, and secretions, all of which cause airway obstruction.

    Client Need: Physiologic Adaptation; **Cognitive Level:** Analysis; **Nursing Process:** Assessment/Analysis

12. **1 In addition to dilation of bronchi, treatment is aimed at expectoration of mucus. Mucus interferes with gas exchange in the lungs.**

    2 A permanent cure is an unrealistic goal; asthma is a chronic illness. **3** Increased fluid intake helps liquefy secretions. **4** Asthma has a psychogenic factor, but this is not the only cause; it may occur as an allergic response to an antigen, such as dust.

    Client Need: Physiologic Adaptation; **Cognitive Level:** Analysis; **Nursing Process:** Assessment/Analysis

13. **2 An anticholinergic drug will block parasympathetic effects, causing an increased heart rate.**

    1 This will dilate coronary arteries, not increase the heart rate. **3** This will lower the blood pressure and may decrease the heart rate. **4** This will improve cardiac contractility but will decrease the heart rate.

    Client Need: Physiologic Adaptation; **Cognitive Level:** Analysis; **Nursing Process:** Assessment/Analysis

14. **4 Dexamethasone increases gluconeogenesis, which may cause hyperglycemia.**

    1 Hypokalemia, not hyperkalemia, is a side effect. **2** Liver dysfunction is not a side effect. **3** Hypertension, not hypotension, is a side effect.

    Client Need: Physiologic Adaptation; **Cognitive Level:** Application; **Nursing Process:** Assessment/Analysis

15. **2 The body's natural corticosteroid production has been suppressed during treatment; avoiding abrupt cessation of the drug will give the body time to adjust to less and less of the exogenous source and resume secretion of endogenous corticosteroid.**

    1 Not completing the course of therapy, rather than stopping it quickly, may cause signs and symptoms of the allergy to recur. **3** The health care provider has already determined the correct dosage, and it has been prescribed. **4** These side effects are associated with long-term steroid use, not with the cessation of therapy.

    Client Need: Physiologic Adaptation; **Cognitive Level:** Analysis; **Nursing Process:** Assessment/Analysis

16. **2 Beclomethasone reduces the inflammatory response in bronchial walls by suppression of polymorphonuclear leukocytes and fibroblasts and the reversal of capillary permeability.**

    1 Beclomethasone does not directly promote comfort. **3** Beclomethasone does not stimulate smooth muscle relaxation. **4** Beclomethasone is not an antibiotic.

17. **1 Adrenergic beta$_2$ agonists cause increased heart contraction (positive inotropic effect) and increased heart rate (positive chronotropic effect). If toxic levels are reached, side effects occur and the drug should be withheld until the health care provider is notified.**

2 Telling the client not to worry is false reassurance and a false statement. **3, 4** Controlled breathing may be helpful in allaying a client's anxiety; however, the drug may be producing adverse effects and should be withheld.

Client Need: Pharmacologic and Parenteral Therapies; **Cognitive Level:** Analysis; **Integrated Process:** Communication/Documentation; **Nursing Process:** Planning/Implementation

18. **2** Clients with asthma use metered-dose inhalers to administer medications prophylactically and/or during times of an asthma attack; this is an important skill to have before discharge.

1 Pulse oximetry is rarely conducted in the home; home management usually includes self-monitoring of the peak expiratory flow rate. **3** Although knowing the hours is important, it is not the priority; during a persistent asthma attack that does not respond to planned interventions, the client should go to the emergency department of the local hospital or call 911 for assistance. **4** Not all asthma is associated with food allergies.

Client Need: Pharmacologic and Parenteral Therapies; **Cognitive Level:** Application; **Nursing Process:** Planning/Implementation

19. **Answers: 1, 3**

1 Albuterol's (Proventil) sympathomimetic effect causes central nervous stimulation, precipitating tremors, restlessness, and anxiety. **3** Albuterol's (Proventil) sympathomimetic effect causes cardiac stimulation that may result in tachycardia and palpitations.

2 Albuterol may cause restlessness, irritability, and tremors, not lethargy. **4** Albuterol may cause dizziness, not visual disturbances. **5** Albuterol will cause tachycardia, not bradycardia.

Client Need: Pharmacologic and Parenteral Therapies; **Cognitive Level:** Analysis; **Nursing Process:** Evaluation/Outcomes

20. **Answers: 2, 3, 5**

2 The CNS depressant effect of morphine causes lethargy. **3** The CNS depressant effect of morphine causes bradycardia. **5** The CNS depressant effect of morphine causes bradypnea.

1 Morphine does not increase urine output. **4** Morphine causes constriction of pupils.

Client Need: Pharmacologic and Parenteral Therapies; **Cognitive Level:** Analysis; **Nursing Process:** Evaluation/Outcomes

> **Study Tip:** To understand this answer, remind yourself that mooooorphiiiine slooooows everythiiing dowwwnn; it depresses the CNS and causes bradycardia and bradypnea. (*Brady-* means "decreased" or "slower.")

21. **2** Metaproterenol stimulates beta receptors of the sympathetic nervous system, causing bronchodilation and an increased rate and strength of cardiac contractions.

1 Barbiturates and hypnotics produce sedation. **3** Antihypertensives and diuretics help decrease blood pressure. **4** Expectorants mobilize respiratory secretions.

Client Need: Pharmacologic and Parenteral Therapies; **Cognitive Level:** Analysis; **Nursing Process:** Evaluation/Outcomes

22. **3** Protamine sulfate is the antidote for heparin overdose and naloxone will reverse the effects of opioids such as morphine.

1 Aspirin and warfarin both interfere with coagulation. **2** While amoxicillin is used to treat some infections, an infection is not a medication, so amoxicillin cannot be considered an antidote. **4** Both enoxaparin and dalteparin are low molecular weight heparins.

Client Need: Pharmacologic and Parenteral Therapies; **Cognitive Level:** Analysis; **Nursing Process:** Planning/Implementation

23. **3** Naloxone is an opioid antagonist and will reverse respiratory depression caused by opioids.

1, 2, 4 Nasotracheal suction, mechanical ventilation, and cardiopulmonary resuscitation are not needed; naloxone will correct the respiratory depression.

Client Need: Pharmacologic and Parenteral Therapies; **Cognitive Level:** Analysis; **Nursing Process:** Planning/Implementation

Antiinfective Drugs

OVERVIEW OF IMMUNITY

- Nonspecific immune response: directed against invading microbes
- Body surface barriers: intact skin and mucosa, cilia, and mucus secretions
- Antimicrobial secretions: oil of skin, tears, gastric juice, and vaginal secretions
- Internal antimicrobial agents
  - Interferon: substance produced within cells in response to viral attack
  - Properdin (Factor P): protein agent in blood that destroys certain gram-negative bacteria and viruses
  - Lysozyme: destroys mainly gram-positive bacteria
  - Phagocytes (monocytes, macrophages): cells that ingest and destroy microbes; part of reticuloendothelial system
- Inflammatory response
  - First stage: release of histamine and chemical mediators (e.g., prostaglandin, bradykinin) leads to vascular dilation and increased capillary permeability, resulting in signs of inflammation (e.g., pain, heat, redness, edema, and loss of function)
  - Second stage: exudate production
  - Third stage: reparative phase
- Specific immune response: directed against a specific pathogen (foreign protein) or its toxin; may be cell-mediated or humoral
- Cell-mediated immunity
  - Occurs within cells of immune system
  - Involves T lymphocytes (e.g., T helper, T suppressor, T cytotoxic, lymphokines); each type plays a distinct role in immune response
  - Cluster designations: mature T cells carry markers on surface that permit them to be classified structurally (e.g., CD4 cells associated with acquired immunodeficiency syndrome [AIDS])
- Functions of cell-mediated immunity
  - Protect against most viral, fungal, protozoan, and slow-growing bacterial infections
  - Reject histoincompatible grafts
  - Cause skin hypersensitivity reactions (e.g., tuberculosis [TB] screening)
  - Assists with diagnosis of malignancies
- Humoral immunity: concerned with immune responses outside of cell; involves B lymphocytes that differentiate into plasma cells and secrete antibodies
  - Antigen: any substance, including allergen, that stimulates production of antibodies in body; typically, antigens are foreign proteins, most potent being microbial cells and their products
  - Antibody: immune substance produced by plasma cells; antibodies are gamma globulin molecules; commonly referred to as immunoglobulin (Ig)
  - Complement-fixation: group of blood serum proteins needed in certain antigen-antibody reactions; both complement and antibody must be present for reaction to occur
    - Types of immunoglobulins

- Immunoglobulin M (IgM) antibodies: first antibodies to be detected after exposure to antigen; protection from gram-negative bacteria
- Immunoglobulin G (IgG) antibodies: make up more than 75% of total immunoglobulins; highest increase in response to subsequent exposure to antigen; only immunoglobulin that passes placental barrier
- Immunoglobulin A (IgA) antibodies: present in blood, mucus, and human milk secretions; play important role against viral and respiratory pathogens
- Immunoglobulin E (IgE) antibodies: responsible for hypersensitivity and allergic responses; cause mast cells to release histamine; protection from parasites
- Immunoglobulin D (IgD) antibodies: help differentiate B lymphocytes
- Active immunity: antibodies formed in body
  - Natural active immunity: antibodies formed during course of disease; may provide lifelong immunity (e.g., measles, chickenpox, yellow fever, smallpox)
    - Artificial active immunity: vaccine or toxoid stimulate formation of homologous antibodies; revaccination (booster shot) often needed to sustain antibody titer (anamnestic effect)
    - Killed vaccines: antigenic preparations containing killed microbes (e.g., pertussis vaccine, typhoid vaccine)
    - Live vaccines: antigenic preparations containing weakened (attenuated) microbes; typically such vaccines are more antigenic than killed preparations (e.g., oral [Sabin] poliomyelitis vaccine, measles vaccine)
  - Toxoids: antigenic preparations composed of inactivated bacterial toxins (e.g., tetanus toxoids, diphtheria toxoids)
- Passive immunity: antibodies acquired from outside source produce short-term immunity
  - Natural passive immunity: passage of preformed antibodies from mother through placenta to fetus or though colostrum to neonate; during first few weeks of life newborn is immune to certain diseases to which mother has active immunity
  - Artificial passive immunity: injection of antisera derived from immunized animals or humans; provide immediate protection and also are of value in treatment (e.g., diphtheria antitoxin, tetanus antitoxin)

OVERVIEW OF INFECTIOUS PROCESS

- Infection: invasion of body by pathogenic microorganisms (pathogens) and reaction of tissues to their presence and to toxins generated by them
- Pathogenicity: ability of a microbe to cause disease
- Virulence: degree of pathogenicity
- Classifications
  - Extent of involvement
    - Local infection: limited to one locality (e.g., abscess), causing pain, swelling, and erythema; may have systemic repercussions such as fever, malaise, and lymphadenopathy
    - Systemic infection: infectious agent is spread throughout body (e.g., typhoid fever)
- Length of infectious process
  - Acute infection: one that develops rapidly, usually resulting in high fever and severe sickness; resolves in a short time
  - Chronic infection: one that develops slowly, with mild but longer-lasting clinical manifestation; sometimes an acute infection can become chronic
- Etiology of infectious process

- Primary infection: develops after initial exposure to pathogen, unrelated to other health problems
- Secondary infection: develops when pathogens take advantage of weakened defenses resulting from a primary infection (e.g., staphylococcal pneumonia as sequela of measles)
- Opportunistic infection: develops when host defenses are diminished because of disease process or therapeutic modalities (e.g., vaginal yeast infection following antibiotic therapy)
- Chain of infection
- Infectious agent
- Reservoir: source of almost all pathogens is human or animal
  - Persons exhibiting manifestations of disease
  - Carriers: persons who harbor pathogens in absence of discernible clinical disease
    - Healthy carriers: those who have never had the disease in question
    - Incubatory carriers: those in incubation phase of disease
    - Chronic carriers: those who have recovered from disease but continue to harbor pathogens
- Portals of exit: route by which microorganisms leave body; blood and body fluids, skin, mucous membranes; and respiratory, genitourinary, and GI tracts
- Mode of transmission
  - Contact transmission (e.g., *Staphylococcus aureus*)
    - Direct: contact between body surfaces
  - Indirect: contact between susceptible host and contaminated intermediate object (e.g., sink faucets)
  - Droplet transmission: droplets from infected individual are propelled short distance by coughing, sneezing, talking, or suctioning respiratory secretions (e.g., common cold)
  - Airborne transmission: small droplet nuclei (5 μm or smaller) or dust particles that contain pathogen remain suspended in air for extended period (e.g., *Mycobacterium tuberculosis*)
  - Common vehicle transmission: microorganisms are transmitted by contaminated food, water, or equipment (e.g., typhoid fever)
  - Vector-borne transmission: microorganisms transmitted by vectors such as mosquitoes, flies, ticks, and rats (e.g., Rocky Mountain spotted fever, Lyme disease)
- Portals of entry: same as portals of exit except skin; intact skin prevents infection
  - Susceptible host
  - Developmental level: extremes of age
    - Inadequate nutritional status
    - Coexisting disease
    - Decreased immune responses
    - Surgical client; client in intensive care unit (ICU); presence of invasive lines

Types of Pathogens

- Bacteria (Fig. 16.1)
  - Unicellular microbes without chlorophyll
- Capsule: material secreted by cell, protects it from phagocytosis and increases its virulence (e.g., *Streptococcus pneumoniae*)
- Spores: inactive resistant structures into which bacterial protoplasm can transform under adverse conditions; under favorable conditions spore germinates into active cell (e.g., *Clostridium tetani, Clostridium difficile*)
  - Examples of disease-producing bacteria

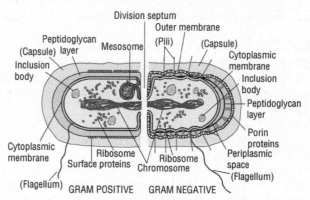

FIG. 16.1 General structure of bacteria. (From Huether, S.E., McCance, K.L., Brashers, V.L., Rote, N.S. [2012]. *Understanding pathophysiology* [5th ed.]. St. Louis: Mosby.)

- ▪ Eubacteriales: divided into five families based on shape, gram stain, and endospore formation
- Gram-positive cocci
  - Diplococci: occurring predominantly in pairs (e.g., *Streptococcus pneumoniae*)
  - Streptococci: may appear in pairs or chains (e.g., *Streptococcus pyogenes*)
  - Staphylococci: occurring predominantly in grapelike bunches (e.g., *S. aureus*)
- Gram-negative cocci include *Neisseria gonorrheae* and *Neisseria meningitidis*
- Gram-negative rods include enterobacteria such as Escherichia, Salmonella, and Shigella species
- Gram-positive rods that do not produce endospores include *Corynebacterium diphtheriae*
  - Gram-positive rods that produce endospores include *Bacillus anthracis, Clostridium botulinum,* and *Clostridium tetani*
- Actinomycetales (actinomycetes): mold-like microbes with elongated cells, frequently filamentous (e.g., *Mycobacterium tuberculosis, Mycobacterium leprae*)
- Spirochaetales (spirochetes): flexuous, spiral organisms (e.g., *Treponema pallidum*)
- Mycoplasmatales (mycoplasmas): delicate, nonmotile microbes displaying a variety of sizes and shapes
- Fungi
  - Saprophytic organisms that live on organic material
- Molds: fuzzy growths of interlacing filaments called hyphae; reproduce by spores
- Yeasts: organisms that usually are single-celled; usually reproduce by budding
  - Examples of disease-producing fungi
  - *Candida albicans,* a yeast: moniliasis ("thrush")
  - *Histoplasmosis capsulatum:* histoplasmosis
  - *Trichophyton rubrum:* tinea pedis ("athlete's foot")
  - Bactericidal effect: destroys bacteria at low concentrations
  - Bacteriostatic effect: slows reproduction of bacteria
  - Superinfection (secondary infection): emergence of microorganism growth when natural protective flora are destroyed by an antiinfective drug
  - Bacterial resistance: natural or acquired characteristic of an organism that prevents destruction by a drug to which it was previously susceptible

TABLE 16.1	Chemicals or Antimicrobials Identified that Prevent Growth of or Destroy Microorganisms
Mechanism of Action	**Agent**
Inhibits synthesis of cell wall	Penicillins, cephalosporins, monobactams, carbapenems, vancomycin, bacitracin, cycloserine, fosfomycin
Damages cytoplasmic membrane	Polymyxins, polyene antifungals, imidazoles
Alters metabolism of nucleic acid	Quinolones, rifampin, nitrofurans, nitroimidazoles
Inhibits protein synthesis	Aminoglycosides, tetracyclines, chloramphenicol, macrolides, clindamycin, spectinomycin, sulfonamides
Alters energy metabolism	Trimethoprim, dapsone, isoniazid

Modified from Ellner, P.D., Neu, H.C.P. (1992). *Understanding infectious disease*. St. Louis: Mosby.

Antibiotics *(Table 16.1)*

- Destroy bacteria or inhibit bacterial reproduction to control infection
- Antibiotic sensitivity tests: identify antibiotics that are effective against a particular organism
- Mechanism of action: interfere with or inhibit cell-wall synthesis of RNA or DNA of pathogen
- Include subclasses sulfonamides, penicillins, cephalosporins, macrolides, quinolones, aminoglycosides, tetracyclines, glycopeptides, nitroimidazoles
- Prevention of emergence of resistant strains of microorganisms (e.g., methicillin-resistant *Staphylococcus aureus* [MRSA]) by completing prescribed course of therapy

Antituberculars

- Used to treat tuberculosis (TB)
- Caused by *Mycobacterium tuberculosis*
- Drugs may need to be administered long-term over many months
- Associated problems: client noncompliance, bacterial resistance, drug toxicity
- Many TB strains have become drug-resistant
- Four drugs needed for initial treatment: isoniazid, rifampin, pyrazinamide, ethambutol, usually manufactured as combination therapy (i.e. rifampin/isoniazid)
- Preventative vaccine: Bacille Calmette-Guerin (BCG)
- Indicator for treatment: purified protein derivative (PPD), chest x-ray, acid-fast bacilli sputum cultures

Antifungals

- Destroy fungal cells (fungicidal) or inhibit reproduction of fungal cells (fungistatic)
- Treat systemic and localized fungal infections
- Include subclasses polyenes, imidazoles, triazoles, echinocandins

Sulfonamides

- Used to treat acute UTIs
- Examples include sulfamethoxazole/trimethoprim, sulfisoxazole, sulfasalazine
- Available in PO, IV preparations

Mode of Action

- Interferes with the bacterial biosynthesis of microorganisms by inhibiting folic acid production

Contraindications, Precautions, and Drug Interactions of Sulfonamides*

Drug	Contraindications/Precautions	Drug Interaction
sulfamethoxazole/trimethoprims	**Contraindications:** Hypersensitivity, hypersensitivity to trimethoprim or sulfonamides, breastfeeding, infants <2 months, pregnancy at term, megaloblastic anemia, decreased creatinine clearance **Precautions:** Infants, geriatric clients, renal/hepatic disease, G6PD deficiency, folate deficiency, severe allergy, bronchial asthma, porphyria, hyperkalemia, hypothyroidism, UV exposure **Pregnancy:** Only given after risks to the fetus are considered; animal studies have shown adverse reactions; no human studies available	Thiazide diuretics, potassium-sparing diuretics, potassium supplements, sulfonylurea agents, oral anticoagulants, dofetilide, methenamine, cyclosporine, methotrexate, phenytoin, CYP2C9, CYP3A4 inducers, oral contraceptives
sulfisoxazole	**Contraindications:** Hypersensitivity, hypersensitivity to sulfonamides, breastfeeding, pregnancy at term, megaloblastic anemia **Precautions:** Infants, geriatric clients, renal/hepatic disease, G6PD deficiency, severe allergy, bronchial asthma, anemia, diabetes mellitus **Pregnancy:** Only given after risks to the fetus are considered; animal studies have shown adverse reactions; no human studies available	Warfarin, methotrexate, chlorpropamide, glimepiride, glipizide, glyburide, tolazamide, tolbutamide
sulfasalazine	**Contraindications:** Hypersensitivity, hypersensitivity to salicylates or sulfonamides, children <2 yr, pregnancy at term, intestinal/urinary obstruction, porphyria **Precautions:** Breastfeeding, renal/hepatic disease, severe allergy, bronchial asthma, megoblastic anemia **Pregnancy:** No adverse effects in animals; no human studies available	Thiopurines, oral hypoglycemics, oral anticoagulants, cyclosporine, digoxin, folic acid, methotrexate

*Pregnancy categories have been revised. See http://www.fda.gov/Drugs/DevelopmentApprovalProcess/DevelopmentResources/Labeling/ucm093307.htm for more information.

Adverse Effects/Side Effects

- Headache
- Fatigue
- Anxiety
- Depression
- Insomnia
- Confusion
- Hallucinations
- Vertigo
- Seizures
- Aseptic meningitis
- Anaphylaxis
- SLE
- Cough
- SOB
- Allergic myocarditis
- Tinnitus
- Nausea
- Vomiting
- Diarrhea
- Abdominal pain
- Enterocolitis
- Anorexia
- Pseudomembranous colitis
- Stomatitis
- Glossitis
- Hepatitis
- Pancreatitis
- Renal failure
- Toxic nephrosis
- Crystalluria
- Increased BUN/creatinine
- Hyperkalemia
- Kernicterus
- Leukopenia
- Neutropenia
- Thrombocytopenia
- Agranulocytosis
- Hemolytic anemia
- Hypoprothrombinemia

- Methemoglobinemia
- Rash
- Dermatitis
- Urticaria
- Stevens-Johnson syndrome
- Photosensitivity
- Toxic epidermal necrolysis
- Erythema multiforme

Nursing Care
- Administer with full glass of water
- Administer on empty stomach 1 hour before meals/2 hours after meals
- Obtain culture and sensitivity before beginning therapy
- Monitor for cardiac/respiratory distress
- Monitor blood studies
- Monitor for CNS changes
- Monitor renal/hepatic function
- Monitor I&O
- Monitor for allergic reaction
- Advise client to complete full course to prevent superinfection
- Teach client to avoid sunlight and to use sunscreen/protective clothing/sunglasses
- Teach client to avoid aspirin and vitamin C
- Teach client to use additional contraception to oral contraceptives
- Teach client to notify prescriber of signs and symptoms of infection
- Teach client that urine, skin, contact lenses may turn yellow/orange

APPLICATION AND REVIEW

1. Which classification of medications is generally prescribed to treat acute urinary tract infections (UTIs)?
   1. Penicillins
   2. Quinolones
   3. Sulfonamides
   4. Aminoglycosides
2. What information should the nurse include in client education regarding a newly prescribed sulfonamide? **Select all that apply.**
   1. Take 1 hour before meals
   2. Avoid exposure to direct sunlight
   3. Report any changes in bowel habits
   4. Skin may temporarily turn yellow-orange
   5. Take medication with a full glass of water
   See Answers on pages 355-357.

Penicillins
- Used to treat gram-positive, gram-negative, anaerobic bacterial infections
- Examples include penicillin G benzathine, penicillin G potassium, penicillin G procaine, penicillin V, amoxicillin, amoxicillin/clavulanate, ampicillin, ampicillin/sulbactam, piperacillin/tazobactam
- Available in PO, IM, IV preparations

Mode of Action
- Interferes with cell wall synthesis and cell division of bacteria

Contraindications, Precautions, and Drug Interactions of Penicillins*

Drug	Contraindications/Precautions	Drug Interaction
penicillin G benzathine, penicillin G potassium, penicillin G procaine, penicillin V	**Contraindications:** Hypersensitivity to penicillins, corn **Precautions:** Breastfeeding, hypersensitivity to cephalosporins, severe renal disease, carbapenem, sulfites, GI disease, asthma **Pregnancy:** No adverse effects in animals; no human studies available	Aspirin, probenecid, heparin, methotrexate, oral contraceptives, typhoid vaccine, tetracyclines
amoxicillin	**Contraindications:** Hypersensitivity to penicillins **Precautions:** Children, geriatric clients, breastfeeding, neonates, hypersensitivity to cephalosporins/carbapenems, severe renal disease, mononucleosis, diabetes, phenylketonuria, asthma, colitis, dialysis, eczema, pseudomembranous colitis, syphilis **Pregnancy:** No adverse effects in animals; no human studies available	Allopurinol, probenecid, warfarin, methotrexate
amoxicillin/clavulanate	**Contraindications:** Hypersensitivity to penicillins, severe renal disease, dialysis **Precautions:** Breastfeeding, neonates, children, hypersensitivity to cephalosporins, renal/GI disease, asthma, colitis, diabetes, eczema, leukemia, viral infections, mononucleosis, phenylketonuria **Pregnancy:** No adverse effects in animals; no human studies available	Probenecid, warfarin, allopurinol
ampicillin	**Contraindications:** Hypersensitivity to penicillins **Precautions:** Breastfeeding, neonates, hypersensitivity to cephalosporins, renal disease, mononucleosis **Pregnancy:** No adverse effects in animals; no human studies available	Oral anticoagulants, probenecid, allopurinol, H2 antagonists, proton pump inhibitors
ampicillin/sulbactam	**Contraindications:** Hypersensitivity, hypersensitivity to penicillins **Precautions:** Breastfeeding, neonates, hypersensitivity to cephalosporins/carbapenems, renal disease, mononucleosis, viral infections, syphilis **Pregnancy:** No adverse effects in animals; no human studies available	Oral anticoagulants, allopurinol, probenecid, methotrexate
piperacillin/tazobactam	**Contraindications:** Hypersensitivity to penicillins, neonates, carbapenem allergy **Precautions:** Breastfeeding, renal insufficiency in neonates, hypersensitivity to cephalosporins, GI disease, seizures, electrolyte imbalances, biliary obstruction **Pregnancy:** No adverse effects in animals; no human studies available	Neuromuscular blockers, oral anticoagulants, methotrexate, aspirin, probenecid, tetracyclines, aminoglycosides

*Pregnancy categories have been revised. See http://www.fda.gov/Drugs/DevelopmentApprovalProcess/DevelopmentResources/Labeling/ucm093307.htm for more information.

Adverse Effects/Side Effects

- Anxiety
- Depression
- Lethargy
- Hallucinations
- Coma
- Seizures
- Twitching
- Hyperreflexia
- Anaphylaxis
- Respiratory distress
- Serum sickness
- Nausea
- Vomiting
- Diarrhea
- Abdominal pain
- Glossitis
- Colitis
- Pseudomembranous colitis
- Oliguria
- Proteinuria
- Hematuria
- Glomerulonephritis
- Renal tubular damage
- Vaginitis
- Moniliasis
- Anemia
- Increased prothrombin time
- Bone marrow suppression
- Granulocytopenia
- Hemolytic anemia
- Eosinophilia
- Hypo/hyperkalemia
- Alkalosis
- Hypernatremia
- Stevens-Johnson syndrome

Nursing Care

- Administer at equal intervals around the clock
- Monitor for allergies before initiating therapy
- Monitor for infection
- Monitor I&O
- Monitor renal/hepatic function
- Monitor blood studies
- Monitor for cardiac/respiratory distress
- Monitor for anaphylaxis
- Monitor for bowel changes
- Ensure emergency equipment is easily accessible
- Teach client that capsules may be opened and contents mixed with fluid/soft food
- Teach client to complete entire course of therapy to prevent antibiotic resistance
- Teach client to report signs and symptoms of infection

APPLICATION AND REVIEW

3. Ampicillin 250 mg po every 6 hours is prescribed for a client who is to be discharged. Which statement indicates to the nurse that the client understands the teaching about ampicillin?
   1. "I should drink a glass of milk with each pill."
   2. "I should drink at least six glasses of water every day."
   3. "The medicine should be taken with meals and at bedtime."
   4. "The medicine should be taken 1 hour before or 2 hours after meals."
4. A client has an anaphylactic reaction after receiving intravenous penicillin. What does the nurse conclude is the cause of this reaction?
   1. An acquired atopic sensitization occurred.
   2. There was passive immunity to the penicillin allergen.
   3. Antibodies to penicillin developed after a previous exposure.
   4. Potent antibodies were produced when the infusion was instituted.
5. Which statements made by a client prescribed an antibiotic demonstrate an understanding of the appropriate use of this classification of medications? **Select all that apply.**
   1. "This medication will destroy the bacteria causing my infection."
   2. "I need to complete the entire prescribed course of this medication."

Nitroimidazole Antibiotics

- Used to treat anaerobic bacterial and parasitic infections
- Examples include metronidazole, tinidazole
- Available in PO, IV preparations

Mode of Action

- Binds and disrupts DNA structure; inhibits bacterial nucleic acid synthesis

Contraindications, Precautions, and Drug Interactions of Nitroimidazole Antibiotics*

Drug	Contraindications/Precautions	Drug Interaction
metronidazole	**Contraindications:** Hypersensitivity, pregnancy first trimester, breastfeeding **Precautions:** Geriatric clients, blood dyscrasias, bone marrow suppression, CNS disorders, dental disease, candida infection, fungal infection, GI/renal/hepatic disease, heart failure, hematologic disease **Pregnancy:** No adverse effects in animals; no human studies available	Bortezomib, norfloxacin, zalcitabine, disulfiram, amprenavir, barbiturates, cholestyramine, alcohol, oral ritonavir, busulfan, cimetidine, lithium, CYP3A4 substrates, warfarin, phenytoin, lithium, fosphenytoin, azathioprine, fluorouracil
tinidazole	**Contraindications:** Hypersensitivity to this product or nitroimidazole derivative, breastfeeding **Precautions:** Geriatric clients, children, hepatic disease, CNS depression, blood dyscrasias, candidiasis, seizures, viral infection, alcoholism **Pregnancy:** Only given after risks to the fetus are considered; animal studies have shown adverse reactions; no human studies available	CYP3A inducers/inhibitors, anticoagulants, cyclosporine, tacrolimus, fluorouracil, hydantoins, lithium, cholestyramine, oxytetracycline

*Pregnancy categories have been revised. See http://www.fda.gov/Drugs/DevelopmentApprovalProcess/DevelopmentResources/Labeling/ucm093307.htm for more information.

Adverse Effects/Side Effects

- Dizziness
- Headache
- Seizures
- Peripheral neuropathy
- Malaise
- Fatigue
- Nausea
- Vomiting
- Increased AST/ALT
- Constipation
- Leukopenia
- Angioedema
- Pruritus

Nursing Care
- Monitor CBC, ESR, leukocyte counts
- Monitor amebic gel diffusion test
- Monitor ultrasound
- Monitor signs of infection, anemia
- Monitor bowel pattern before, during, after treatment
- Teach patient to take with food
- Teach patient to avoid alcohol
- Teach patient medication may leave an unpleasant taste in mouth

Cephalosporins
- Used to treat gram-positive, gram-negative bacterial infections
- Examples include cefadroxil, cefazolin, cephalexin, cefaclor, cefotetan, cefoxitin, cefprozil, cefuroxime, cefdinir, cefditoren pivoxil, cefepime, cefixime, cefotaxime, cefpodoxime, ceftazidime, ceftibuten, ceftriaxone
- Available in PO, IM, IV preparations

Mode of Action
- Inhibits bacterial cell wall synthesis

Contraindications, Precautions, and Drug Interactions of Cephalosporins*

Drug	Contraindications/Precautions	Drug Interaction
First Generation cefadroxil, cefazolin, cephalexin	**Contraindications:** Hypersensitivity to cephalosporins, infants <1 mo **Precautions:** Breastfeeding, hypersensitivity to penicillins, renal disease **Pregnancy:** No adverse effects in animals; no human studies available	Anticoagulants, aminoglycosides, loop diuretics, probenecid, oral contraceptives
Second Generation cefaclor, cefotetan, cefoxitin, cefprozil, cefuroxime	**Contraindications:** Hypersensitivity to cephalosporins, seizures **Precautions:** Breastfeeding, children, GI/renal disease, diabetes mellitus, coagulopathy, pseudomembranous colitis **Pregnancy:** No adverse effects in animals; no human studies available	Aminoglycosides, furosemide, probenecid, anticoagulants, thrombolytics, NSAIDs, antiplatelets, plicamycin, valproic acid, oral contraceptives, antacids, H2 blockers
Third/Fourth Generations cefdinir, cefditoren pivoxil, cefepime, cefixime, cefotaxime, cefpodoxime, ceftazidime, ceftibuten, ceftriaxone	**Contraindications:** Hypersensitivity to cephalosporins, seizures **Precautions:** Breastfeeding, children, GI/renal disease, diabetes mellitus, coagulopathy, pseudomembranous colitis **Pregnancy:** No adverse effects in animals; no human studies available	H2 blockers, antacids, cyclosporine, anticoagulants, thrombolytics, valproic acid, plicamycin, NSAIDs, aminoglycosides, furosemide, probenecid, iron

*Pregnancy categories have been revised. See http://www.fda.gov/Drugs/DevelopmentApprovalProcess/DevelopmentResources/Labeling/ucm093307.htm for more information.

Adverse Effects/Side Effects

- Headache
- Dizziness
- Fever
- Chills
- Seizures
- Paresthesia
- Anaphylaxis
- Serum sickness
- Dyspnea
- Nausea
- Vomiting
- Diarrhea
- Anorexia

- Glossitis
- Bleeding
- Pseudomembranous colitis
- Proteinuria
- Vaginitis
- Candidias
- Nephrotoxicity
- Renal failure
- Leukopenia
- Thrombocytopenia
- Agranulocytosis
- Anemia

- Neutropenia
- Lymphocytosis
- Eosinophilia
- Granulocytopenia
- Pancytopenia
- Hemolytic anemia
- Arthralgia
- Arthritis
- Rash
- Urticaria
- Dermatitis
- Stevens-Johnson syndrome

Nursing Care

- Monitor renal/hepatic function
- Monitor I&O
- Monitor electrolyte status
- Monitor blood studies
- Monitor for bowel changes
- Monitor for anaphylaxis
- Monitor for cardiac/respiratory distress
- Monitor for bleeding
- Monitor for infection

- Teach client to use birth control in addition to oral contraceptives
- Teach client to use yogurt/buttermilk to maintain intestinal flora
- Teach client not to abruptly discontinue drug to prevent superinfection
- Teach client to report signs and symptoms of infection to prescriber
- Teach diabetic clients to monitor blood sugar

APPLICATION AND REVIEW

7. What information should a nurse provide a client prescribed a cephalosporin medication?
   1. Using an electric razor
   2. Monitoring fluid intake
   3. Following a low fat diet
   4. Avoiding direct sunlight

See Answers on pages 355-357.

Macrolides

- Used to treat gram-positive, gram-negative bacterial infections
- Examples include erythromycin base, erythromycin ethylsuccinate, erythromycin lactobionate, erythromycin stearate, azithromycin, clarithromycin
- Available in PO, IV, ophthalmic preparations

Mode of Action

- Suppresses bacterial protein synthesis

Contraindications, Precautions, and Drug Interactions of Macrolides*

Drug	Contraindications/Precautions	Drug Interaction
erythromycin base, erythromycin ethylsuccinate, erythromycin lactobionate, erythromycin stearate	*Contraindications:* Hypersensitivity, preexisting hepatic disease *Precautions:* Breastfeeding, geriatric clients, hepatic/GI disease, QT prolongation, seizure, myasthenia gravis *Pregnancy:* No adverse effects in animals; no human studies available	Diltiazem, itraconazole, ketoconazole, nefazodone, pimozide, protease inhibitors, alfentanil, alprazolam, bromocriptine, buspirone, carbamazepine, cilostazol, clindamycin, clozapine, cyclosporine, diazepam, digoxin, disopyramide, ergots, felodipine, HMG-CoA reductase inhibitors, ibrutinib, methylprednisolone, midazolam, quinidine, rifabutin, sildenafil, tacrolimus, tadalafil, theophylline, triazolam, verapamil, warfarin, vinblastine, vardenafil
azithromycin	*Contraindications:* Hypersensitivity to azithromycin/erythromycin/macrolides, hepatitis, jaundice *Precautions:* Breastfeeding, geriatric clients, <2 yr for otitis media, <2 yr for pharyngitis, renal/hepatic/cardiac disease, tonsillitis, QT prolongation, ulcerative colitis, sunlight exposure, torsades de pointes, myasthenia gravis, sodium restriction, pseudomembranous colitis, hypokalemia, hypomagnesemia, contact lenses *Pregnancy:* No adverse effects in animals; no human studies available	Ergotamine, pimozide, amiodarone, quinidine, nilotinib, droperidol, methadone, propafenone, fluoroquinolones, lithium, paliperidone, antacids, triazolam, oral anticoagulants, digoxin, theophylline, methylprednisolone, cyclosporine, bromocriptine, disopyramide, triazolam, carbamazepine, phenytoin, tacrolimus, nelfinavir
clarithromycin	*Contraindications:* Hypersensitivity to macrolides, QT prolongation, torsades de pointes *Precautions:* Breastfeeding, geriatric clients, renal/hepatic disease *Pregnancy:* Only given after risks to the fetus are considered; animal studies have shown adverse reactions; no human studies available	Cisapride, pimozide, HMG-CoA reductase inhibitors, all CYP3A drugs, calcium channel blockers, midazolam, benzodiazepines, tacrolimus, class IA/III antidysrhythmics, zidovudine, rifampin, rifabutin, nevirapine, etravirine, alprazolam, buspirone, carbamazepine, cyclosporine, digoxin, disopyramide, ergots, felodipine, fluconazole, omeprazole, tacrolimus, theophylline

*Pregnancy categories have been revised. See http://www.fda.gov/Drugs/DevelopmentApprovalProcess/DevelopmentResources/Labeling/ucm093307.htm for more information.

Adverse Effects/Side Effects

- Seizures
- Anaphylaxis
- Dysrhythmias
- QT prolongation
- Torsades de pointes
- Hearing loss
- Tinnitus
- Anosmia
- Nausea
- Vomiting
- Diarrhea
- Anorexia
- Abdominal pain
- Heartburn
- Stomatitis
- Pseudomembranous colitis
- Esophagitis
- Hepatotoxicity
- Jaundice
- Vaginitis
- Moniliasis
- Thrombophlebitis
- Rash
- Urticaria
- Pruritus
- Stevens-Johnson syndrome
- Toxic epidermal necrolysis

Nursing Care
- Administer without food
- Administer at evenly spaced intervals around the clock
- Perform culture and sensitivity before beginning therapy
- Monitor for infection
- Monitor I&O
- Monitor renal/hepatic function
- Monitor cardiac rhythm
- Monitor for skin reactions
- Monitor for hearing loss
- Monitor for bowel changes
- Monitor for anaphylaxis
- Teach client to report signs and symptoms of infection
- Teach client not to take aluminum-magnesium containing antacids with the drug
- Teach client to report signs and symptoms of jaundice
- Teach client not to abruptly discontinue drug to prevent superinfection
- Teach client to use sunscreen, protective clothing, sunglasses

Quinolones
- Used to treat gram-negative infections (UTIs, upper respiratory tract infections, pneumonia, gonorrhea)
- Examples include ciprofloxacin, levofloxacin, gemifloxacin
- Available in PO, IV preparations

Mode of Action
- Interferes with DNA replication of bacteria

Contraindications, Precautions, and Drug Interactions of Quinolones*

Drug	Contraindications/Precautions	Drug Interaction
ciprofloxacin	**Contraindications:** Hypersensitivity to quinolones, myasthenia gravis **Precautions:** Breastfeeding, children, geriatric clients, renal/hepatic/CV disease, stroke, seizure, QT prolongation, colitis, hypokalemia **Pregnancy:** Only given after risks to the fetus are considered; animal studies have shown adverse reactions; no human studies available	Corticosteroids, cyclosporine, probenecid, warfarin, theophylline, CYP1A2 inhibitors, astemizole, droperidol, class IA/III antidysrhythmics, tricyclics, tetracyclines, local anesthetics, phenothiazines, haloperidol, riperidone, sertindole, ziprasidone, alfuzosin, arsenic trioxie, beta agonists, chloroquine, clozapine, cyclobenzaprine, dasatinib, dolasetron, droperidol, flecainide, macrolides, methadone, ondansetron, pentamidine, prpafenone, sunltinib, tacrolimus, terfenadine, vardenafil, antacids, warfarin
levofloxacin	**Contraindications:** Hypersensitivity to quinolones, myasthenia gravis **Precautions:** Breastfeeding, children, renal disease, acute MI, atrial fibrillation, QT prolongation, dehydration, diabetes colitis, myasthenia gravis, seizures, syphilis **Pregnancy:** Only given after risks to the fetus are considered; animal studies have shown adverse reactions; no human studies available	QT prolongation products, probenecid, NSAIDs, cyclosporine, foscarnet, antacids, sucralfate, zinc, iron, calcium, theophylline

Contraindications, Precautions, and Drug Interactions of Quinolones—cont'd

Drug	Contraindications/Precautions	Drug Interaction
gemifloxacin	**Contraindications:** Hypersensitivity to quinolones, myasthenia gravis **Precautions:** Breastfeeding, children, renal disease, acute MI, atrial fibrillation, QT prolongation, dehydration, diabetes colitis, myasthenia gravis, seizures, syphilis **Pregnancy:** Only given after risks to the fetus are considered; animal studies have shown adverse reactions; no human studies available	NSAIDs, probenecid, class IA/III dysrhythmics, tricyclics, amoxapine, phenothiazines, haloperidol, pimozide, risperidone, beta blockers, chloroquine, clozapine, dolasetron, droperidol, local anesthetics, methadone, erythromycin, telithromycin, ondansetron, pentamide, propafenone, tacrolimus, vardenafil, sucralfate, zinc, iron, antacids

*Pregnancy categories have been revised. See http://www.fda.gov/Drugs/DevelopmentApprovalProcess/DevelopmentResources/Labeling/ucm093307.htm for more information.

Adverse Effects/Side Effects
- Headache
- Confusion
- Hallucinations
- Dizziness
- Fatigue
- Insomnia
- Restlessness
- Seizures
- Anaphylaxis
- QT prolongation
- Nausea
- Vomiting
- Diarrhea
- Heartburn
- Dysphagia
- Pseudomembranous colitis
- Abdominal pain
- Pancreatitis
- Crystalluria
- Bone marrow depression
- Agranulocytosis
- Rash
- Pruritus
- Urticaria
- Toxic epidermal necrolysis
- Stevens-Johnson syndrome
- Tendon rupture

Nursing Care
- Monitor for infection
- Monitor renal/hepatic function
- Monitor heart rhythm
- Monitor for CNS changes
- Monitor I&O
- Monitor for anaphylaxis
- Teach client not to intake dairy, caffeine, alkaline foods/products
- Teach client to increase fluid intake
- Teach client not to take magnesium calcium products
- Teach client to report tendon pain
- Teach client to report signs and symptoms of rash

Aminoglycosides
- Used to treat gram-positive/gram-negative bacterial, mycobacterial, protozoal infections
- Examples include gentamicin, streptomycin, tobramycin
- Available in PO, IM, IV preparations

Mode of Action
- Interferes with protein synthesis of the bacteria, causing it to die

Contraindications, Precautions, and Drug Interactions of Aminoglycosides*

Drug	Contraindications/Precautions	Drug Interaction
gentamicin	**Contraindications:** Hypersensitivity to aminoglycosides **Precautions:** Breastfeeding, neonates, geriatric clients, pseudomembranous colitis **Pregnancy:** Definite fetal risks, may be given in spite of risks if needed in life-threatening conditions	Aminoglycosides, amphotericin B, polymyxin, vancomycin, furosemide, mannitol, cisplatin, cephalosporins, penicillins, cidofovir, acyclovir, foscarnet, cyclosporine, tacrolimus, digoxin, entecavir, neuromuscular blockers
streptomycin	**Contraindications:** Hypersensitivity to aminoglycosides **Precautions:** Breastfeeding, neonates, geriatric clients, renal disease, hearing disorders, dehydration, myasthenia gravis, cystic fibrosis, burns **Pregnancy:** Definite fetal risks, may be given in spite of risks if needed in life-threatening conditions	Live bacterial vaccines, amphotericin B, salicylates, NSAIDs, aminoglycosides, anesthetics, neuromuscular blocking agents
tobramycin	**Contraindications:** Hypersensitivity to aminoglycosides **Precautions:** Breastfeeding, neonates, geriatric clients, Parkinson's disease, myasthenia gravis, mild renal disease **Pregnancy:** Definite fetal risks, may be given in spite of risks if needed in life-threatening conditions	Aminoglycosides, amphotericin B, polymyxin, vancomycin, furosemide, mannitol, cisplatin, cephalosporins, penicillins, bacitracin, cisplatin, acyclovir, cidofovir

*Pregnancy categories have been revised. See http://www.fda.gov/Drugs/DevelopmentApprovalProcess/DevelopmentResources/Labeling/ucm093307.htm for more information.

Adverse Effects/Side Effects

- Headache
- Fever
- Lethargy
- Confusion
- Seizures
- Neurotoxicity
- Encephalopathy
- Apnea
- Anaphylaxis
- Ototoxicity
- Visual disturbances
- Nausea
- Vomiting
- Anorexia
- Hepatomegaly
- Hepatic necrosis
- Splenomegaly
- Oliguria
- Hematuria
- Renal damage/failure
- Nephrotoxicity
- Azotemia
- Agranulocytosis
- Thrombocytopenia
- Leukopenia
- Eosinophilia
- Rash
- Urticaria
- Alopecia
- Photosensitivity

Nursing Care
- Perform culture and sensitivity before beginning therapy
- Calculate dosage based on client's weight
- Monitor for CNS changes
- Monitor for hearing changes/ototoxicity
- Monitor hepatic/renal function
- Monitor I&O
- Monitor IV site
- Monitor for infection
- Teach client to drink 2 to 3 L fluids/day
- Teach client to report signs and symptoms of infection
- Teach client to report signs and symptoms of hearing changes/loss
- Teach client to avoid driving and other hazardous activities

Tetracyclines

- Used to treat infections caused by gram-positive/gram-negative bacteria, spirochetes, rickett-siae, mycoplasmas, chlamydia, gonorrhea, protozoa
- Examples include doxycycline, tetracycline, minocycline
- Available in PO, IM, IV preparations

Mode of Action

- Inhibits the growth or multiplication of bacteria

Contraindications, Precautions, and Drug Interactions of Tetracyclines*

Drug	Contraindications/Precautions	Drug Interaction
doxycycline	*Contraindications:* Hypersensitivity to tetracyclines, children <8 yr, esophageal ulceration *Precautions:* Breastfeeding, sulfite hypersensitivity, hepatic disease, ulcerative colitis, pseudomembranous colitis, excessive sunlight *Pregnancy:* Definite fetal risks, may be given in spite of risks if needed in life-threatening conditions	Anticoagulants, digoxin, methotrexate, penicillins, oral contraceptives, antacids, iron, kaolin/pectate, barbiturates, carbamazepine, phenytoin, cimetidine sucralfate, cholestyramine, colestipol, rifampin, bismuth, aluminum salts, calcium
tetracycline	*Contraindications:* Hypersensitivity to tetracyclines, children <8 yr, breastfeeding *Precautions:* Renal/hepatic disease, UV exposure *Pregnancy:* Definite fetal risks, may be given in spite of risks if needed in life-threatening conditions	Warfarin, digoxin, methoxyflurane, penicillins, cimetidine, antacids, sodium bicarbonate, alkali products, iron
minocycline	*Contraindications:* Hypersensitivity to tetracyclines, children <8 yr *Precautions:* Breastfeeding, hepatic disease *Pregnancy:* Definite fetal risks, may be given in spite of risks if needed in life-threatening conditions	Warfarin, digoxin, insulin, oral anticoagulants, theophylline, neuromuscular blockers, retinoids, antacids, sodium bicarbonate, alkali products, iron, kaolin/pectin, cimetidine, quinapril, sucralfate, barbiturates, carbamazepine, phenytoin, penicillins, calcium, oral contraceptives

*Pregnancy categories have been revised. See http://www.fda.gov/Drugs/DevelopmentApprovalProcess/DevelopmentResources/Labeling/ucm093307.htm for more information.

Adverse Effects/Side Effects

- Fever
- Headache
- Cough
- Pericarditis
- Angioedema
- Anaphylaxis
- Dysphagia
- Glossitis
- Oral candidas
- Tooth discoloration
- Nausea
- Vomiting
- Diarrhea
- Abdominal pain
- Anorexia
- Hepatotoxicity
- Neutropenia
- Eosinophilia
- Thrombocytopenia
- Hemolytic anemia
- Rash
- Urticaria
- Photosensitivity
- Stevens-Johnson syndrome
- Toxic epidermal necrolysis

Nursing Care

- Administer with full glass of water
- Take with food to prevent GI upset
- Monitor for infection
- Monitor I&O

- Monitor blood studies
- Monitor for signs and symptoms of allergic reaction
- Monitor IV site for phlebitis
- Teach client not to consume dairy products within 2 hours of drug administration
- Teach client not to consume alkali products
- Teach client not to consume antacids
- Teach client to avoid sun exposure
- Teach client not to abruptly discontinue medication to prevent superinfection
- Teach parents of clients that the teeth of young children will be permanently discolored

Glycopeptides

- Used to treat methicillin-resistant *S. aureus* infections; *C. difficile* infection
- Example includes vancomycin
- Available in PO, IV preparations

Mode of Action

- Inhibits bacterial wall synthesis

Contraindications, Precautions, and Drug Interactions of Glycopeptides*

Drug	Contraindications/Precautions	Drug Interaction
vancomycin	*Contraindications:* Hypersensitivity to glycopeptides, corn *Precautions:* Breastfeeding, neonates, geriatric clients, renal disease, hearing loss *Pregnancy:* *PO:* No adverse effects in animals; no human studies available *IV:* Only given after risks to the fetus are considered; animal studies have shown adverse reactions; no human studies available	Cholestyramine, colestipol, cidofovir, metformin, nondepolarizing muscle relaxants, aminoglycosides, cephalosporins, colistin, polymyxin, bacitracin, cisplatin, amphotericin B, methotrexate, NSAIDs, cyclosporine, acyclovir, adefovir, capreomycin, foscarnet, ganciclovir, pamidronate, IV pentamidine, streptozocin, tacrolimus, zoledronic acid

*Pregnancy categories have been revised. See http://www.fda.gov/Drugs/DevelopmentApprovalProcess/DevelopmentResources/Labeling/ucm093307.htm for more information.

Adverse Effects/Side Effects

- Headache
- Chills
- Fever
- Wheezing
- Dyspnea
- Cardiac arrest
- Vascular collapse
- Hypotension
- Peripheral edema
- Anaphylaxis
- Superinfection
- Ototoxicity
- Permanent deafness
- Tinnitus
- Nystagmus
- Nausea
- Pseudomembranous colitis
- Nephrotoxicity
- Fatal uremia
- Leukopenia
- Eosinophilia
- Neutropenia
- Rash
- Urticaria
- Pruritus
- Necrosis
- Back pain
- Red man syndrome

Nursing Care

- Administer at equal intervals around the clock
- Monitor for infection

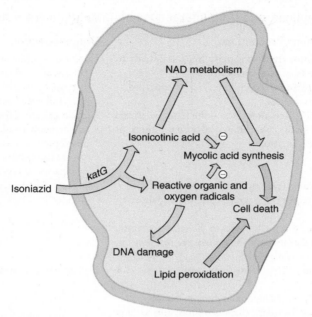

FIG. 16.2 Mechanism by which isoniazid kills tubercle bacilli. (From Wecker L., Crespo, L.M., Dunaway, G., Faingold, C. [2010]. *Brody's human pharmacology* [10th ed.]. Philadelphia: Mosby.)

- Monitor I&O
- Monitor blood levels
- Monitor auditory function
- Monitor for skin changes
- Teach client not to abruptly discontinue medication to prevent superinfection
- Teach client to report signs and symptoms of infection

Antituberculars

- Used to treat, prevent tuberculosis (TB)
- Examples include isoniazid, rifampin, pyrazinamide, ethambutol
- Available in PO, IM preparations

Mode of Action

- Inhibits biosynthesis of mycobacteria (Fig. 16.2)

Contraindications, Precautions, and Drug Interactions of Antituberculars*

Drug	Contraindications/Precautions	Drug Interaction
isoniazid	*Contraindications:* Hypersensitivity *Precautions:* Renal disease, cataracts, diabetic retinopathy, ocular defects, IV drug users, HIV, postpartum, neuropathy *Pregnancy:* Only given after risks to the fetus are considered; animal studies have shown adverse reactions; no human studies available	Alcohol, cycloserine, ethionamide, rifampin, carbamazepine, phenytoin, benzodiazepines, meperidine, SSRIs, SNRIs, BCG vaccine, ketoconazole, aluminum antacids

Continued

Contraindications, Precautions, and Drug Interactions of Antituberculars—cont'd

Drug	Contraindications/Precautions	Drug Interaction
rifampin	**Contraindications:** Hypersensitivity, hypersensitivity to rifamycins, active meningitis infection **Precautions:** Breastfeeding, children <5 yr, hepatic disease, blood dyscrasias **Pregnancy:** Only given after risks to the fetus are considered; animal studies have shown adverse reactions; no human studies available	Isoniazid, alcohol, acetaminophen, anticoagulants, antidiabetics, beta blockers, barbiturates, benzodiazepines, chloramphenicol, clofibrate, corticosteroids, cyclosporine, dapsone, digoxin, doxycycline, haloperidol, hormones, antifungals, nifedipine, oral contraceptives, phenytoin, protease inhibitors, theophylline, verapamil, zidovudine
pyrazinamide	**Contraindications:** Hypersensitivity **Precautions:** Breastfeeding, gout, renal/hepatic disease, diabetes **Pregnancy:** Only given after risks to the fetus are considered; animal studies have shown adverse reactions; no human studies available	Allopurinol, colchicine, probenecid, ethionamide
ethambutol	**Contraindications:** Hypersensitivity, optic neuritis, children <13 yr **Precautions:** Breastfeeding, renal disease, hepatic/hematopoietic disorders, diabetic retinopathy, ocular defects, cataracts, **Pregnancy:** No adverse effects in animals; no human studies available	Neurotoxics, aluminum salts

*Pregnancy categories have been revised. See http://www.fda.gov/Drugs/DevelopmentApprovalProcess/DevelopmentResources/Labeling/ucm093307.htm for more information.

Adverse Effects/Side Effects

- Dizziness
- Seizures
- Memory impairment
- Psychosis
- Dyspnea
- Toxic encephalopathy
- Angioedema
- Anaphylaxis
- Blurred vision
- Optic neuritis

- Nausea
- Vomiting
- Pseudomembranous colitis
- Pancreatitis
- Hematuria
- Acute renal failure
- Hemoglobinuria
- Hyperglycemia
- Jaundice
- Fatal hepatitis

- Agranulocytosis
- Hemolytic, aplastic anemia
- Thrombocytopenia
- Eosinophilia
- Leukopenia
- Methemoglobinemia
- Stevens-Johnson syndrome
- Toxic epidermal necrolysis

Nursing Care

- Monitor renal/hepatic function
- Monitor for CNS changes
- Monitor for respiratory distress
- Monitor for infection
- Monitor blood studies
- Monitor for skin changes/infection
- Monitor for bowel changes
- Teach client not to skip or double doses

- Teach client to avoid alcohol
- Teach diabetics to monitor blood glucose
- Teach client to report malaise, jaundice, skin/GI changes, flu-like symptoms
- Teach client that bodily fluids may be orange colored
- Teach client that contact lenses may become permanently stained

- Teach client to use nonhormonal form of birth control
- Teach client to avoid sun exposure

APPLICATION AND REVIEW

8. A nurse is caring for a female client who is receiving rifampin (Rifadin) for tuberculosis. Which statements indicate that the client understands the teaching about rifampin? **Select all that apply.**
   1. "Alcoholic drinks must be avoided while I'm on this drug."
   2. "I won't use the pill for contraception while I'm on this drug."
   3. "I cannot take an antacid within 2 hours before taking my medicine."
   4. "My doctor must be called immediately if my eyes and skin become yellow."
   5. "I won't open the capsule and mix the powder with applesauce if I can't swallow it."
9. A client is diagnosed with pulmonary tuberculosis, and the health care provider prescribes a combination medication, Rifamate, composed of rifampin (Rifadin) and isoniazid (INH). The nurse evaluates that the teaching regarding the drug is effective when the client says, "The **most** important thing I must do is:
   1. report any changes in vision."
   2. take the medicine with my meals."
   3. call my doctor if my urine or tears turn red-orange."
   4. continue taking the medicine even after I feel better."
10. Tuberculosis is confirmed and isoniazid (INH), rifampin (Rifadin), and pyridoxine (vitamin B_6) are prescribed for a client. The client says, "I've never had to take so many medicines for an infection before." What is the nurse's **best** reply?
    1. "Rifampin prevents side effects from INH."
    2. "This type of organism is difficult to destroy."
    3. "You'll need only one medication in a couple of months."
    4. "Aggressive therapy is needed because your infection is so advanced."

See Answers on pages 355-357.

Polyenes

- Used to treat invasive fungal infections
- Examples include amphotericin B, nystatin
- Available in PO, IV preparations

Mode of Action

- Alters cell membrane of fungi

Contraindications, Precautions, and Drug Interactions of Polyenes*

Drug	Contraindications/Precautions	Drug Interaction
amphotericin B	***Contraindications:*** Hypersensitivity ***Precautions:*** Breastfeeding, children, geriatric clients, anemia, cardiac disease, electrolyte imbalance, hematologic/hepatic/renal disease, hypotension ***Pregnancy:*** No adverse effects in animals; no human studies available	Nephrotoxic antibiotics, antineoplastics, cidofovir, corticosteroids, digoxin, loop diuretics, pentamidine, salicylates, skeletal muscle relaxants, tacrolimus, tenofovir, thiazides

Continued

Contraindications, Precautions, and Drug Interactions of Polyenes—cont'd

Drug	Contraindications/Precautions	Drug Interaction
nystatin	*Contraindications:* Hypersensitivity *Precautions:* Breastfeeding *Pregnancy:* Only given after risks to the fetus are considered; animal studies have shown adverse reactions; no human studies available	No known drug interactions

*Pregnancy categories have been revised. See http://www.fda.gov/Drugs/DevelopmentApprovalProcess/DevelopmentResources/Labeling/ucm093307.htm for more information.

Adverse Effects/Side Effects

- Headache
- Fever
- Chills
- Dizziness
- Seizures
- Peripheral neuropathy
- Paresthesias
- Bronchospasm
- Dyspnea
- Cardiac arrest
- Bradycardia
- Hypo/hypertension
- Deafness
- Vision changes
- Nausea
- Vomiting
- Diarrhea
- Hemorrhagic gastroenteritis
- Acute liver failure
- Jaundice
- Azotemia
- Renal tubular acidosis
- Permanent renal damage
- Anemia
- Thrombocytopenia
- Agranulocytosis
- Leukopenia
- Eosinophilia
- Toxic epidermal necrolysis
- Exfoliative dermatitis
- Sepsis
- Infection
- Infusion reactions

Nursing Care

- Monitor infusion and IV site
- Monitor I&O
- Monitor blood studies
- Monitor renal/hepatic function
- Monitor for infection
- Weigh client weekly
- Teach client that therapy may be long-term (several months)
- Teach client to notify prescriber of signs or symptoms of bleeding

Imidazoles

- Used to treat invasive fungal infections
- Examples include clotrimazole, ketoconazole, miconazole
- Available in PO, IV, topical, intravaginal preparations

Mode of Action

- Disrupts DNA function of amoebas, trichomonides

Contraindications, Precautions, and Drug Interactions of Imidazoles*

Drug	Contraindications/Precautions	Drug Interaction
clotrimazole	*Contraindications:* Hypersensitivity, ophthalmic use *Precautions:* Breastfeeding, children, hepatic impairment *Pregnancy:* No adverse effects in animals; no human studies available	Other imidazoles

Contraindications, Precautions, and Drug Interactions of Imidazoles—cont'd

Drug	Contraindications/Precautions	Drug Interaction
ketoconazole	*Contraindications:* Hypersensitivity, sulfite allergy *Precautions:* Breastfeeding, children *Pregnancy:* Only given after risks to the fetus are considered; animal studies have shown adverse reactions; no human studies available	Sulfites
miconazole	*Contraindications:* Hypersensitivity, hypersensitivity to imidazoles *Precautions:* Breastfeeding, children *Pregnancy:* Only given after risks to the fetus are considered; animal studies have shown adverse reactions; no human studies available	Other imidazoles

*Pregnancy categories have been revised. See http://www.fda.gov/Drugs/DevelopmentApprovalProcess/DevelopmentResources/Labeling/ucm093307.htm for more information.

Adverse Effects/Side Effects
- Headache
- Dizziness
- Confusion
- Seizures
- Aseptic meningitis
- Vision changes
- Nausea
- Vomiting
- Diarrhea
- Pseudomembranous colitis
- Pancreatitis
- Darkened urine
- Albuminuria
- Nephrotoxicity
- Thrombocytopenia
- Leukopenia
- Bone marrow depression
- Aplasia
- Eosinophilia
- Toxic epidermal neurolysis
- Stevens-Johnson syndrome

Nursing Care
- Monitor infusion and IV site
- Monitor I&O
- Monitor blood studies
- Monitor renal/hepatic function
- Monitor for infection
- Monitor for allergic reaction
- Monitor for vision changes
- Weigh client daily
- Teach client that urine may turn dark reddish-brown
- Teach client to avoid driving and other hazardous activities
- Teach client not to drink alcohol
- Teach client to avoid sun exposure

Triazoles
- Used to treat candidal infections
- Examples include fluconazole, itraconazole
- Available in PO, IV preparations

Mode of Action
- Causes damage to fungal cell membrane

Contraindications, Precautions, and Drug Interactions of Triazoles*

Drug	Contraindications/Precautions	Drug Interaction
fluconazole	*Contraindications:* Hypersensitivity to azoles *Precautions:* Breastfeeding, hepatic/renal disease, torsades de pointes *Pregnancy:* Definite fetal risks, may be given in spite of risks if needed in life threatening conditions	Calcium channel blockers, cyclosporine, ergots, glipizide, HMG-CoA reductase inhibitors, lovastatin, phenytoin, proton pump inhibitors, rifabutin sirolimus, simvastatin, tacrolimus, theophylline, warfarin, zidovudine, zolpidem

Continued

Contraindications, Precautions, and Drug Interactions of Triazoles—cont'd

Drug	Contraindications/Precautions	Drug Interaction
itraconazole	**Contraindications:** Hypersensitivity, fungal meningitis **Precautions:** Breastfeeding, children, cardiac/hepatic/renal disease, dialysis, hearing loss, cystic fibrosis neuropathy **Pregnancy:** Only given after risks to the fetus are considered; animal studies have shown adverse reactions; no human studies available	Pimozide, quinidine, dofetilide, levomethadyl, dronedarone, buspirone, busulfan, clarithromycin, digoxin, fentanyl, carbamazepine, nicardipine, phenytoin, quinidine, warfarin

*Pregnancy categories have been revised. See http://www.fda.gov/Drugs/DevelopmentApprovalProcess/DevelopmentResources/Labeling/ucm093307.htm for more information.

Adverse Effects/Side Effects

- Headache
- Seizures
- Angioedema
- Anaphylaxis
- QT prolongation
- Torsades de pointes
- Nausea
- Vomiting
- Diarrhea
- GI bleeding
- Hepatotoxicity
- Rhabdomyolysis
- Agranulocytosis
- Eosinophilia
- Leukopenia
- Neutropenia
- Thrombocytopenia
- Stevens-Johnson syndrome
- Exfoliative dermatitis
- Toxic epidermal necrolysis

Nursing Care

- Administer with food to decrease GI upset
- Monitor for infection
- Monitor renal/hepatic function
- Monitor for skin reactions
- Teach client that long-term therapy may be required
- Teach client to use alternative method of contraception
- Teach client to avoid grapefruit products

Echinocandins

- Used to treat invasive candidiasis infections
- Examples include caspofungin, micafungin
- Available in IV preparations

Mode of Action
- Targets fungal cell wall

Contraindications, Precautions, and Drug Interactions of Echinocandins*

Drug	Contraindications/Precautions	Drug Interaction
caspofungin	**Contraindications:** Hypersensitivity **Precautions:** Breastfeeding, children, geriatric clients, severe hepatic disease **Pregnancy:** Only given after risks to the fetus are considered; animal studies have shown adverse reactions; no human studies available	Carbamazepine, cyclosporine, dexamethasone, efavirenz, nelfinavir, nevirapine, phenytoin, rifampin, sirolimus, tacrolimus

Contraindications, Precautions, and Drug Interactions of Echinocandins—cont'd

Drug	Contraindications/Precautions	Drug Interaction
micafungin	*Contraindications:* Hypersensitivity *Precautions:* Breastfeeding, children, geriatric clients, severe hepatic disease, renal impairment, hemolytic anemia *Pregnancy:* Only given after risks to the fetus are considered; animal studies have shown adverse reactions; no human studies available	Itraconazole, sirolimus, nifedipine

*Pregnancy categories have been revised. See http://www.fda.gov/Drugs/DevelopmentApprovalProcess/DevelopmentResources/Labeling/ucm093307.htm for more information.

Adverse Effects/Side Effects
- Headache
- Dizziness
- Fever
- Chills
- ARDS
- Pleural effusions
- Anaphylaxis
- Hypertension
- Sinus tachycardia
- Atrial fibrillation
- Nausea
- Vomiting
- Diarrhea
- Anorexia
- Hepatitis
- Renal failure
- Thrombophlebitis
- Neutropenia
- Thrombocytopenia
- Leukopenia
- Anemia
- Stevens-Johnson syndrome

Nursing Care
- Monitor for infection
- Monitor renal/hepatic function
- Monitor for skin reactions
- Monitor blood studies
- Monitor infusion, IV site
- Monitor for anaphylaxis
- Monitor for bleeding
- Teach client to report symptoms of anaphylaxis, bleeding, infection

ANSWER KEY: REVIEW QUESTIONS

1. **3 Sulfonamides are used to treat acute UTIs by interfering with the bacteria biosynthesis of the causative microorganism.**
   1 Penicillins are used to treat gram-positive, gram-negative, anaerobic bacterial infections by interfering with cell wall synthesis and cell division of bacteria. **2** Quinolones are to treat UTIs, upper respiratory tract infections, pneumonia, and gonorrhea by interfering with DNA replication of the bacteria. **4** Aminoglycosides are used to treat gram-positive/gram-negative bacterial, mycobacterial, protozoal infections by interfering with DNA replication of the bacteria.
   Client Need: Pharmacologic and Parenteral Therapies; **Cognitive Level:** Analysis; **Nursing Process:** Assessment/Analysis

🔑 **Study Tip: SU**lfon**A**mides interfere with *bio***S**ynthesis of *b*acteria causing **A**cute **U**TIs. Even three examples all start with S-U: sulfamethoxazole/trimethoprim, sulfisoxazole, sulfasalazine. Think "**S:** bio**S**ynthesis interference" and "**U:** acute **U**TIs."

2. **Answers: 1, 2, 4, 5**

   Sulfonamides should be taken with a full glass of water and on an empty stomach (1 hour before or 2 hours after meals). Clients should be instructed to avoid direct sunlight and that skin, urine, and contact lenses may turn yellow-orange.

   3 Penicillins may alter bowel habits.

   Client Need: Pharmacologic and Parenteral Therapies; **Cognitive Level:** Analysis; **Nursing Process:** Assessment/Analysis

3. **4 Ampicillin is a form of penicillin that should be given on an empty stomach; food delays absorption.**

   1 Opaque liquids such as milk delay absorption of ampicillin. 2 It is not necessary to drink 6 glasses of water a day; however, it is appropriate with sulfonamides. 3 Ampicillin should not be taken with food; food delays absorption of this drug.

   Clinical Area: Medical-Surgical Nursing; **Client Needs:** Pharmacologic and Parenteral Therapies; **Cognitive Level:** Application; **Nursing Process:** Evaluation/Outcomes

---

Study Tip: Try a silly idea to help you remember that ampicillin should not be taken with food: "You wouldn't eat a stereo **amp,** right? So don't mix **amp**icillin [0]with food in your stomach!" Just picturing this idea—because it is ridiculous—will help you remember.

---

4. **3 Hypersensitivity results from the production of antibodies in response to exposure to certain foreign substances (allergens). Earlier exposure is necessary for the development of these antibodies.**

   1 An anaphylactic reaction is not a sensitivity reaction to penicillin; hay fever and asthma are atopic conditions. 2 An anaphylactic reaction is an active, not passive, immune response. 4 Antibodies developed when there was a prior, not current, exposure to penicillin.

   Client Need: Pharmacologic and Parenteral Therapies; **Cognitive Level:** Application; **Nursing Process:** Evaluation/Outcomes

5. **Answers: 1, 2, 4, 5**

   Antibiotics destroy bacteria or inhibit bacterial reproduction to control infection. Antibiotic sensitivity tests identify antibiotics that are effective against a particular organism. Mechanism of antibiotic action is to interfere with or inhibit cell-wall synthesis of RNA or DNA of pathogen. Prevent emergence of resistant strains of microorganisms (e.g., methicillin-resistant *Staphylococcus aureus* [MRSA]) by completing prescribed course of antibiotic therapy.

   3 Antituberculars rather than antibiotics are used to treat TB.

   Client Need: Pharmacologic and Parenteral Therapies; **Cognitive Level:** Analysis; **Integrated Process:** Teaching/Learning; **Nursing Process:** Evaluation/Outcomes

6. **1 Breastfeeding is a characteristic that is considered a precautionary factor for this classification of medication.**

   2 Infection (bacterial) is the reason this classification of medication is prescribed. 3 Anxiety is not a recognized precaution for the use of this classification of medication. 4 Eczema is not a recognized precaution for the use of this classification of medication.

   Client Need: Pharmacologic and Parenteral Therapies; **Cognitive Level:** Analysis; **Nursing Process:** Assessment/Analysis

7. **1 Cephalosporin medication classification of medications can trigger bleeding. Using an electric razor will minimize potential cuts.**

   2 Fluid intake is not a specific intervention for this classification of medications. 3 A low fat diet is not a specific intervention for this classification of medication. 4 Photosensitivity is not a recognized adverse reaction for this classification of medication.

   Client Need: Pharmacologic and Parenteral Therapies; **Cognitive Level:** Analysis; **Integrated Process:** Teaching/Learning; **Nursing Process:** Planning/Implementation

8. **Answers: 1, 2, 4**

   1 Alcohol may increase the risk of hepatotoxicity. **2** Rifampin (Rifadin) has teratogenic properties and also may reduce the effectiveness of oral contraceptives. **4** These are signs of hepatitis and should be reported immediately.

   3 An antacid may be taken 1 hour before taking the medication. **5** The capsule may be opened and the powder mixed with applesauce.

   Clinical Area: Medical-Surgical Nursing; **Client Needs:** Pharmacologic and Parenteral Therapies; **Cognitive Level:** Analysis; **Nursing Process:** Evaluation/Outcomes

9. **4 The medication should be taken for the full course of therapy; most regimens last from 6 to 9 months, depending on the state of the disease.**

   1 Visual changes are not side effects of this medication. **2** The medication should be taken 1 hour before meals or 2 hours after meals for better absorption. **3** Urine or tears turning orange is a side effect of rifampin (Rifadin); while this should be reported, it is not an adverse side effect.

   Clinical Area: Medical-Surgical Nursing; **Client Needs:** Pharmacologic and Parenteral Therapies; **Cognitive Level:** Application; **Nursing Process:** Evaluation/Outcomes

10. **2 Organism mutation commonly results in drug resistance when treatment is inadequate.**

    1 Rifampin decreases the replication of the *tubercle bacillus;* pyridoxine (vitamin B_6) is used to prevent neuropathy associated with INH. **3** It is inaccurate to state the drugs are necessary only for a couple of months. High concentrations of at least two antitubercular drugs are necessary for an extended period. **4** "Aggressive therapy is needed because your infection is so advanced" may raise anxiety and may not be true; aggressive combination drug therapy is always used for tuberculosis.

    Clinical Area: Medical-Surgical Nursing; **Client Needs:** Pharmacologic and Parenteral Therapies; **Cognitive Level:** Application; **Nursing Process:** Planning/Implementation

17 Antiviral Drugs

INTRODUCTION TO ANTIVIRAL DRUGS

Virus Replication

- Consists of a DNA or RNA strand stored in a capsule made of protein and covered with a lipid; it is not composed of cells like other organisms
- Cannot reproduce on their own; cause host cells to produce copies of themselves (Fig. 17.1)
  - Attaches to host cell
  - Releases viral genes/enzymes into host cell nucleus
  - Replicates viral components using host cell
  - Assembles viral components into complete viral particles
  - Releases viral particles to infect new host cells

MAJOR DISORDERS

Human Immunodeficiency Virus (HIV)/Acquired Immunodeficiency Syndrome (AIDS)

- Cause of HIV: contact with infected body fluids (e.g., blood, semen, vaginal secretions, blood-tinged saliva, tears, breast milk, and cerebrospinal fluid); virus not viable outside body
- Clinical findings: fever, fatigue, swollen lymph nodes, diarrhea, oral thrush, shingles
  - HIV positive confirmation: blood tests reveal HIV or antibodies to HIV
  - HIV is transmitted to others by HIV positive persons
  - Incubation period: ranges from 6 months to 10 years or longer
  - Antibodies first detected in blood 2 weeks to 3 months or longer after infection; test detects virus within 24 hours of exposure
- Treatment: antiretroviral therapy (ART), alternative therapies (yoga, herbal medicine, acupuncture), counseling
- Classification system for HIV infection according to CDC
  - T4/CD4 categories; each CD4 category has an A, B, or C clinical category
  - Category 1: 500 cells/μL or more
  - Category 2: 200 to 499 cells/μL
  - Category 3: Less than 200 cells/μL
- Clinical categories
  - Category A: categories B and C have not occurred; asymptomatic HIV infection; persistent generalized lymphadenopathy; acute (primary) HIV infection
  - Category B: category C has not occurred; conditions attributed to HIV infection; conditions that are complicated by HIV infection (e.g., oral candidiasis, pelvic inflammatory disease, oral hairy leukoplakia, idiopathic thrombocytopenia purpura, herpes zoster, peripheral neuropathy)
  - Category C: includes all clinical conditions listed as advanced HIV disease or AIDS; once classified in category C, person remains in this category (e.g., recurrent bacterial pneumonia; candidiasis of esophagus, bronchi, trachea, lungs; cytomegalovirus disease;

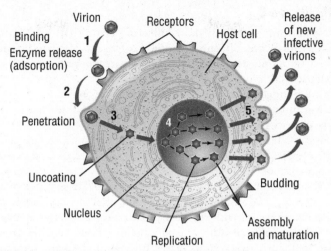

FIG. 17.1 Stages of viral infection of a host cell. (From Huether, S.E., McCance, K.L., Brashers, V.L., Rote, N.S. [2012]. *Understanding pathophysiology* [5th ed.]. St. Louis: Mosby.)

encephalopathy; Kaposi sarcoma; pulmonary or extrapulmonary tuberculosis; *Pneumocystis jiroveci* infection; wasting syndrome)
- Classification according to World Health Organization
  - Categories 1 through 4 progress from primary HIV infection to advanced HIV/AIDS
  - CD4 cell counts not included; testing may be unavailable or too costly in some environments
- Cause of AIDS: human immunodeficiency virus (HIV), a retrovirus; most commonly caused by HIV-1; other strains include HIV-2 and HIV-3
  - HIV infects helper T lymphocytes (T4/CD4 cells), B lymphocytes, macrophages, promyelocytes, fibroblasts, and epidermal Langerhans cells
  - When T4/CD4 cell count falls below 200/μL opportunistic infections occur because of severely depressed immune system
- Clinical findings: anorexia, fatigue, dyspnea, chills, sore throat, night sweats, enlarged lymph nodes, wasting syndrome, HIV encephalopathy
  - Positive test result for HIV antibodies: ELISA (enzyme-linked immunosorbent assay) for screening; Western blot used to confirm positive ELISA result
  - Positive test result for HIV; polymerase chain reaction (PCR); HIV RNA provides evidence of viral load
  - Decreased T4/CD4 cells to less than 200/μL
  - Decreased ratio of T4 cell (helper cell) to T8 cell (suppressor cell)
- Treatment: highly active antiretroviral therapy (HAART), alternative therapies (yoga, herbal medicine, acupuncture), counseling
- Opportunistic infections and disorders associated with AIDS
  - Protozoal: *Pneumocystis jiroveci* pneumonia, toxoplasmosis, cryptosporidiosis
  - Fungal: candidiasis, cryptococcosis, histoplasmosis, tinea
  - Bacterial: *Mycobacterium avium-intracellulare complex, Mycobacterium tuberculosis* (MTB)
  - Viral: herpes simplex, varicella-zoster, cytomegalovirus, molluscum contagiosum, human papillomavirus, Epstein-Barr
  - Malignant: Kaposi sarcoma, B-cell lymphomas, non-Hodgkin lymphoma

Hepatitis B and C

- Causes: contact with body fluids/infected persons; virus shed in all body fluids
  - Hepatitis B: bloodborne, parenteral route, sexual, maternal-neonate
    - Commonly associated with health care workers
  - Hepatitis C: bloodborne, parenteral route
- Clinical findings: anorexia, jaundice, hepatomegaly
  - Liver function studies show hepatitic injury and necrosis
- Three stages of viral hepatitis
  - Prodromal: fever, fatigue, anorexia, weight loss, malaise, headache, nausea/vomiting, weakness, depression, muscle/joint pain, photophobia, changes in taste/smell, dark-colored urine, clay-colored stools
  - Clinical: begins 1 to 2 weeks after prodromal stage; phase of acute illness
    - Itching, abdominal tenderness/pain, appetite loss, indigestion, jaundice
  - Recovery: begins with recovery of jaundice; lasts 2 to 6 weeks
    - Poor prognosis if hepatic encephalopathy and edema develop
- Treatment: antivirals, rest, increased protein intake, parenteral nutrition
- Vaccines can prevent virus

Influenza A and B

- Causes: close proximity to/contact with infected persons
  - Influenza A: H1N1
  - Influenza B: H3N2
- Clinical findings: productive cough, dyspnea, sore throat, runny/stuffy nose, cyanosis, high fever, chills, headache, myalgia, moist crackles on auscultation
  - Severe cases can lead to pneumonia
- Treatment: antivirals, treating underlying symptoms
- The number one preventative treatment for influenza is frequent and effective hand washing
- Flu vaccine is effective in preventing the virus

Herpes

- Cause: herpes simplex type 2 (herpes virus hominis type 2); may be caused by type 1, which is most often associated with mouth lesions ("cold sores")
- Lesions occur 3 to 7 days after infection and may last several weeks (Fig. 17.2)
- Once resolved, virus lies dormant in spinal root ganglia and is capable of repeatedly causing lesions; stress may precipitate recurrence (called reactivation)
- Transmitted through sexual contact when active lesions are present; newborn may be infected during vaginal birth; therefore, cesarean birth is advocated when infection is active (i.e., lesions are visible)
- May cause aseptic meningitis, proctitis, and prostatitis; associated with higher rate of cervical cancer
- Clinical findings: dysuria, flulike clinical findings, tingling sensation before vesicles appear, genital itching and pain
  - Leukorrhea, vaginal bleeding, vesicles and papules on genitalia, urinary retention, culture reveals herpesvirus type 2
- Treatment: no cure; antivirals; sedation for severe pain; topical alcohol to dry lesions

Cytomeglavirus

- Cause: contact with infected body fluids (e.g., blood, semen, vaginal secretions, blood-tinged saliva, urine, tears, breast milk, and cerebrospinal fluid)

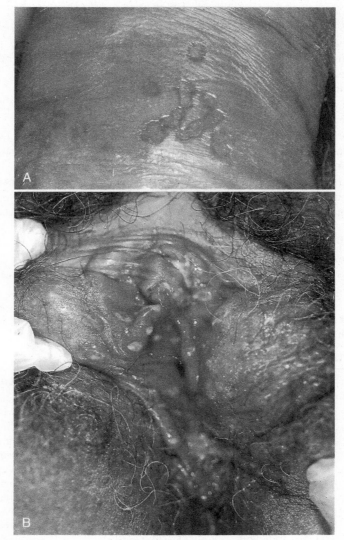

FIG. 17.2 Herpes simplex virus type 2, in male (A) and female (B) clients. (From Nugent, P.M., Green, J.S., Hellmer Saul, M.A., Pelikan, P.K. [2012]. *Mosby's comprehensive review of nursing for the NCLEX-RN examination* [20th ed.]. St Louis: Mosby.)

- Cytomeglavirus is relation to herpes virus
- Most common sites: lungs, adrenal glands, blood, eyes, CNS, GI tract, male GU tract
- Clinical findings: fever, sore throat, fatigue, malaise, swollen glands, muscle aches, loss of appetite, weight loss
  - Severe: blindness, blurred vision, floaters, dyspnea, dry nonproductive cough, pneumonia, diarrhea, seizures, bleeding esophageal ulcers, encephalitis, hepatomegaly, splenomegaly
- Treatment: antivirals; treatment of symptoms

ANTIVIRAL AGENTS

- Treat viral infections, not bacterial ones
- Most antivirals are used for specific viral infections: HIV/AIDs, hepatitis B and C, influenza A and B, herpes and cytomegalovirus
- Don't kill virus cells but inhibit viral replication
- Block virus from host cell
- Prevent virus from releasing genetic material
- Prevent virus' genetic material from being spliced into host cell's DNA
- Highly specific antiviral drugs target enzymes and proteins that infected host cell use to assemble new virus particles; prevent them from functioning
- Other agents target the virus indirectly, increasing efficiency of host's immune system to fight virus
- Antivirals can be combined with other antivirals or other drug classes to fight viruses

Nucleoside Reverse Transcriptase Inhibitors (NRTIs)

- Used to treat advanced HIV infection
- Examples include zidovudine, didanosine, telbivudine, stavudine, abacavir, lamivudine
- Available in PO, IV preparations

Mode of Action
- Inhibit DNA replication of HIV

Contraindications, Precautions, and Drug Interactions of NRTIs*

Drug	Contraindications/Precautions	Drug Interaction
zidovudine	**Contraindications:** Hypersensitivity **Precautions:** Breastfeeding, children, obesity, severe renal disease, granulocyte count <1,000 mm³ **Pregnancy:** Only given after risks to the fetus are considered; animal studies have shown adverse reactions; no human studies available	Dapsone, interferons, NRTIs, doxorubicin, ribavirin, stavudine, antineoplastics, radiation, ganciclovir, valganciclovir, acyclovir, methadone, atovaquone, fluconazole, probenecid, trimethoprim, valproic acid, pentamidine isethionate, flucytosine, vincristine, vinblastine, salicylates, acetaminophen, cimetidine, lorazepam,
didanosine	**Contraindications:** Hypersensitivity, pancreatitis, lactic acidosis, phenylketonuria **Precautions:** Breastfeeding, children, CHF, hypertension, peripheral neuropathy, hyperuricemia, gout, renal disease, sodium-restricted diet, elevated amylase **Pregnancy:** No adverse effects in animals; no human studies available	Gatifloxacin, gemifloxacin, levofloxacin, moxifloxacin, norfloxacin, antiretrovirals, tetracyclines, allopurinol, tenofovir, stavudine, ketoconazole, itraconazole, dapsone, fluoroquinolones, magnesium/aluminum antacids, delavirdine, fluoroquinolones, zalcitabine
telbivudine	**Contraindications:** Hypersensitivity, breastfeeding **Precautions:** Children, organ transplant, anemia, dialysis, obesity, alcoholism, renal disease, HIV, Hispanic or African ethnicity **Pregnancy:** No adverse effects in animals; no human studies available	Any renal drugs, pegylated interferon alpha-2a, corticosteroids, hydrochloroquine, erythromycin, cyclosporine, ZDV, zidovudine, niacin, azole antifungals, HMG-CoA reductase inhibitors, fibric acid derivatives, penicillamine

Contraindications, Precautions, and Drug Interactions of NRTIs—cont'd

Drug	Contraindications/Precautions	Drug Interaction
stavudine	**Contraindications:** Hypersensitivity, hypersensitivity to zidovudine, severe peripheral neuropathy, lactic acidosis **Precautions:** Breastfeeding, renal/hepatic disease, osteoporosis, obesity, advanced HIV infection, bone marrow suppression, pancreatitis, peripheral neuropathy **Pregnancy:** Only given after risks to the fetus are considered; animal studies have shown adverse reactions; no human studies available	Didanosine, zalcitabine, lithium, dapsone, probenecid, methadone, zidovudine, myleosuppressants, chloramphenicol, ethambutol, vincristine, zalcitabine, phenytoin, hydralazine
abacavir	**Contraindications:** Hypersensitivity, severe hepatic disease, lactic acidosis **Precautions:** Breastfeeding, children <3 months, severe renal disease, MI, obesity, black/Caucasian/Asian ethnicities, polymyositis, low granulocyte/hemoglobin count **Pregnancy:** Only given after risks to the fetus are considered; animal studies have shown adverse reactions; no human studies available	Abacavir-containing products, interferon, ribavirin, methadone, alcohol, tipranavir
lamivudine	**Precautions:** Breastfeeding, children, geriatric patients, pancreatitis, renal disease, peripheral neuropathy, low granulocyte/hemoglobin counts **Pregnancy:** Only given after risks to the fetus are considered; animal studies have shown adverse reactions; no human studies available	Emtricitabine, interferons, zalcitabine, amiloride, metformin, trospium, procainamide, dofetilide, entecavir, memantine, trimethoprin-sulfamethoxazole

*Pregnancy categories have been revised. See http://www.fda.gov/Drugs/DevelopmentApprovalProcess/DevelopmentResources/Labeling/ucm093307.htm for more information.

Adverse Effects/Side Effects

- Anaphylaxis
- Wheezing
- Dyspnea
- Cough
- CHF
- Pancreatitis
- Lactic acidosis
- Fever
- Headache
- Malaise
- Insomnia
- Dizziness
- Diaphoresis
- Chills
- Tremors
- Confusion
- Depression
- Vertigo
- Hearing loss
- Photophobia
- Taste change
- Nausea
- Vomiting
- Diarrhea
- Anorexia
- Constipation
- Dysphagia
- Rectal bleeding
- Dysuria
- Polyuria
- Urinary hesitancy/frequency
- Myalgia
- Arthralgia
- Rash
- Granulocytopenia
- Anemia
- Hepatomegaly

Nursing Care

- Administer on an empty stomach
- Administer antiemetic or antidiarrheal, if indicated
- Monitor renal/hepatic function
- Monitor blood counts
- Monitor for infection
- Monitor patient's mental status when giving IV drugs
- Monitor I&O
- Teach patient to avoid alcohol
- Teach patient to report signs and symptoms of anemia, infection, bleeding
- Teach patient to report numbness/tingling in extremities
- Teach patient alopecia may occur during treatment
- Teach patient safety techniques for mental status changes

Nonnucleoside Reverse Transcriptase Inhibitors (NNRTIs)

- Used to treat HIV infection
- Examples include rilpivirine, etravirine, delavirdine, nevirapine, efavirenz
- Available in PO preparations

Mode of Action

- Prevents HIV replication by binding to reverse transcriptase enzyme

Contraindications, Precautions, and Drug Interactions of NNRTIs*

Drug	Contraindications/Precautions	Drug Interaction
rilpivirine	**Contraindications:** Hypersensitivity **Precautions:** Breastfeeding, neonates, infants, children, adolescents, QT prolongation, torsades de pointes, hepatic disease, HIV, antimicrobial resistance, pancreatitis, immune reconstitution syndrome, coinfection of hepatitis B or C and HIV, hyperlipidemia, depression, suicidal ideation **Pregnancy:** No adverse effects in animals; no human studies available	Antidysrhythmics, phenothiazines, tricyclics, pentamidine, CYP3A4 inducers, CYP3A4 inhibitors, CYP3A4 substrates, chloroquine, haloperidol, droperidol, fluconazle, voriconazole, proton pump inhibitors, H2 receptor agonists, antacids, efavirenz, ritonavir, nevirapine, aminoglutethimide, bexarotene, flutamide
etravirine	**Contraindications:** Hypersensitivity, breastfeeding **Precautions:** Children, geriatric patients, hepatic disease, hepatitis, antimicrobial resistance, immune reconstitution syndrome, hypercholesterolemia, hypertriglycerides **Pregnancy:** No adverse effects in animals; no human studies available	Atazanavir, carbamazepine, delavirdine, fosamprenavir, phenytoin, phenobarbital, rifampin, tipranavir, rilpivirine, cyclosporine, tacrolimus, sirolimus, HMG-CoA reductase inhibitors, CYP3A4 inducers, CYPA3A4 inhibitors, methadone, diazepam, warfarin, rifampin, voriconazole, dexamethasone, darunavir, tipranavir, saquinavir, disopyramide, efavirenz, nevirapine, ritonavir, St. John's wort

Contraindications, Precautions, and Drug Interactions of NNRTIs—cont'd

Drug	Contraindications/Precautions	Drug Interaction
delavirdine	*Contraindications:* Hypersensitivity *Precautions:* Breastfeeding, children, hepatic disease, hepatitis, antimicrobial resistance, immune reconstitution syndrome, exfoliative dermatitis *Pregnancy:* Only given after risks to the fetus are considered; animal studies have shown adverse reactions; no human studies available	Nevirapine, efavirenz, rilpivirine, amphetamines, benzodiazepines, ergots, calcium channel blockers, antidysrhythmics, alprazolam, opiates, sedative hypnotics, sildenafil, pimozide, astemizole, midazolam, triazolam, fluoxetine, ketoconazole, warfarin, quinidine, clarithromycin, didanosine, anticonvulsants, antacids, rifamycins, protease inhibitors, H2 blockers, PPIs, atorvastatin, simvastatin, CYP3A4/2D6 inhibitors
nevirapine	*Contraindications:* Hypersensitivity, hepatic disease *Precautions:* Breastfeeding, children, Hispanic ethnicity, renal disease *Pregnancy:* No adverse effects in animals; no human studies available	Macrolide antiinfectives, cimetidine, anticonvulsants, diazepam, clonazepam, warfarin, rifamycins, protease inhibitors, oral contraceptives, methadone, itraconazole, ketoconazole, St. John's wort
efavirenz	*Contraindications:* Hypersensitivity, moderate/severe hepatic disease *Precautions:* Breastfeeding, children <3 yr, renal/hepatic disease, seizures, depression, myelosuppression *Pregnancy:* Definite fetal risks, may be given in spite of risks if needed in life-threatening conditions	Benzodiaepines, ergots, midazolam, triazolam, pimozide, boceprevir, saquinavir, delavirdine, rilpivirine, telaprevir, indinavir, amprenavir, lopinavir, oral contraceptives, ketoconazole, itraconazole, posaconazole, voriconazole, cyclosporine, tacrolimus, sirolimus, alcohol, antidepressants, bupropion, sertraline, opioids, antihistamines, anticonvulsants, estrogens, ritonavir, warfarin, statins, CYP3A4 inducers, CYP3A4 inhibitors, St John's wort

*Pregnancy categories have been revised. See http://www.fda.gov/Drugs/DevelopmentApprovalProcess/DevelopmentResources/Labeling/ucm093307.htm for more information.

Adverse Effects/Side Effects

- Headache
- Dizziness
- Asthenia
- Anxiety
- Confusion
- Seizure
- Stroke
- Tremor
- Atrial fibrillation
- Hypertension
- MI
- Bronchospasm
- Blurred vision
- Fatigue
- Nausea
- Vomiting
- Diarrhea
- Constipation
- GERD
- Anorexia
- Hepatitis
- Pancreatitis
- Renal failure
- Glomerulonephritis
- Hypercholesterolemia
- Hyperbilirubinemia
- Neutropenia
- Thrombocytopenia
- Depression
- Suicidal ideation/attempts
- Rash

Nursing Care

- Administer an antiemetic or antidiarrheal, if indicated
- Administer after meals

- Assess and monitor patient for suicidal ideation
- Monitor renal/hepatic function
- Monitor for bleeding
- Monitor for infection
- Monitor I&O
- Teach patient to report signs and symptoms of infection
- Teach patient to avoid grapefruit juice
- Teach patient to use contraception during treatment
- Teach patient safety techniques for mental status changes
- Teach patient to report suicidal ideation

Protease Inhibitors

- Used to treat HIV infection
- Examples include atazanavir, boceprivir, darunavir, fosamprenavir, indinavir, lopinavir/ritonavir, nelfinavir, ritonavir, simeprevir, tipranavir
- Available in PO preparations

Mode of Action

- Act against HIV enzyme protease, preventing cell division

Contraindications, Precautions, and Drug Interactions of Protease Inhibitors*

Drug	Contraindications/Precautions	Drug Interaction
atazanavir	*Contraindications:* Hypersensitivity *Precautions:* Breastfeeding, children, geriatric patients, females, hepatic disease, dialysis, pancreatitis, alcoholism, AV block, hypercholesterolemia, lactic acidosis, drug resistance, diabetes, hemophilia, immune reconstitution syndrome, serious rash *Pregnancy:* No adverse effects in animals; no human studies available	NSAIDs, antiinflammatories, alcohol, corticosteroids, antacids, ACE inhibitors, beta blockers, loop diuretics, thrombolytics, anticoagulants, penicillins, oral hypoglycemics, insulin, sulfonamides, plicamycin, cefamandole, ticlopidine, clopidogrel, tirofiban, eptifibatide, methotrexate, phenytoin, valproic acid, urinary acidifiers, ammonium chloride, nizatidine, nitroglycerin, ginko
boceprevir	*Contraindications:* Hypersensitivity, male partners of women who are pregnant *Precautions:* Breastfeeding, neonates, infants, children, adolescents, hepatic/liver disease, organ transplantation, anemia, neutropenia, thrombocytopenia, HIV *Pregnancy:* Absolute fetal abnormalities; not to be used at any time during pregnancy	Ergots, cisapride, pimozide, alfuzosin, lovastatin, simvastatin, ezetimibe, midazolam, triazolam, sildenafil, tadalafil, PDE5 inhibitors, acetaminophen, alprazolam, amiodarone, drospirenone, CYP3A4 inhibitors, methadone, efavirenz, ritonavir, atazanavir, lopinavir, amitriptyline, amlodipine, atorvastatin, buspirone, clopidogrel, doxorubicin, hydrocodone, trazodone, St. John's wort
darunevir	*Contraindications:* Hypersensitivity *Precautions:* Breastfeeding, children, geriatric patients, renal/hepatic disease, diabetes, hypercholesterolemia, pancreatitis, bleeding, antimicrobial resistance, immune reconstitution syndrome *Pregnancy:* No adverse effects in animals; no human studies available	Sulfonamides, ergots, midazolam, rifampin, pimozide, triazolam, HMG-CoA reductase inhibitors, CYP3A4 inducers, CYP3A4 inhibitors, CYP3A4 substrates, clarithromycin, zidovudine, telapravir, rilpivarine, rifamycins, fluconazole, nevirapine, efavirenz, tenofovir, oral contraceptives, St. John's wort

Contraindications, Precautions, and Drug Interactions of Protease Inhibitors—cont'd

Drug	Contraindications/Precautions	Drug Interaction
fosamprenavir	*Contraindications:* Hypersensitivity to protease inhibitors *Precautions:* Breastfeeding, geriatric patients, hepatic disease, hemolytic anemia, diabetes, autoimmune disease with immune reconstitution disease *Pregnancy:* Only given after risks to the fetus are considered; animal studies have shown adverse reactions; no human studies available	Sulfas, ergots, warfarin, amiodarone, calcium channel blockers, lidocaine, pimozide, midazolam, triazolam, flecainide, lovastatin, simvastatin, propafennone, HMG-CoA reductase inhibitors, aripiprazole, ributin, ketoconazole, itraconazole, sildenafil, vardenafil, oral contraceptives, nevirapine, efavirenz, saquinavir, rantidine, carbamazepine, phenytoin, barbiturates, proton pump inhibitors, antacids, H2-receptor antagonists, dexamethasone, St. John's wort
indinavir	*Contraindications:* Hypersensitivity, breast-feeding *Precautions:* Children, renal/hepatic disease, diabetes, hypercholesterolemia, hemophilia, autoimmune disease, immune reconstitution syndrome *Pregnancy:* Only given after risks to the fetus are considered; animal studies have shown adverse reactions; no human studies available	Ergots, statins, CYP3A4 inducers, CYP3A4 inhibitors, CYP3A4 substrates, phosphodiesterase-5 inhibitors, midazolam, rifampin, triazolam, amiodarone, pimozide, alfazosin, clarithromycin, zidovudine, isoniazid, anticonvulsants, oral contraceptives, St. John's wort
lopinavir/ritonavir	*Contraindications:* Hypersensitivity, hypersensitivity to polyoxyethylated castor oil *Precautions:* Breastfeeding, neonates, children, elderly patients, hepatic disease, AV block, cardiomyopathy, congenital long-QT prolongation, hypercholesterolemia, pancreatitis, diabetes, hemophilia, hypokalemia, immune reconstitution syndrome, Graves' disease, Guillain-Barre syndrome, HBV/HCV coinfection *Pregnancy:* Only given after risks to the fetus are considered; animal studies have shown adverse reactions; no human studies available	CYP3A4 metabolized products, antidysrhythmics, antifungals, benzodiazepines, HMG-CoA reductase inhibitors, interleukins, amiodarone, avanafil, bupropion, clozapine, desipramine, dihydroergotamine, ergotamine, meperidine, midazolam, quinidine, saquinavir, triazolam, zolpidem, phenothiazines, tricyclics, haloperidol, droperidol, CYP3A4 inhibitors, CYP3A4 substrates, fluconazole, clarithromycin, anticoagulants
ritonavir	*Contraindications:* Hypersensitivity *Precautions:* Breastfeeding, neonates, infants, hepatic disease, AV block, cardiomyopathy, hypercholesterolemia, pancreatitis, diabetes, hemophilia, immune reconstitution syndrome *Pregnancy:* No adverse effects in animals; no human studies available	Amiodarone, antifungals, benzodiazepines, bupropion, clozapine, ergotamine, interleukins, HMG-CoA reductase inhibitors, midazolam, quinidine, saquinavir, triazolam, zolpidem, CYP2D6 inhibitors, antidysrhythmics, phenothiazines, beta-agonists, tricyclics, haloperidol, CYP3A4 inhibitors, CYP3A4 substrates, fluconazole, clarithromycin, bosentan, rifamycins, nevirapine, barbiturates, phenytoin, anticoagulants, theophylline, zidovudine *Continued*

Contraindications, Precautions, and Drug Interactions of Protease Inhibitors—cont'd

Drug	Contraindications/Precautions	Drug Interaction
simeprevir	**Contraindications:** Hypersensitivity, male-mediated teratogenicity **Precautions:** Breastfeeding, children, liver transplant, hepatic disease, UV exposure, serious rash, Asian ethnicity **Pregnancy:** Only given after risks to the fetus are considered; animal studies have shown adverse reactions; no human studies available	CYP3A4 inducers, CYP3A4 inhibitors, bromocriptine, chloramphenicol, cimetidine, fluoxetine, isoniazid, octreotide, erythromycin, protease inhibitors, amiodarone, atorvastatin, digoxin, quinidine, calcium channel blockers, rosuvastatin, PDE5-inhibitors, St John's wort
tipranavir	**Contraindications:** Hypersensitivity, hepatic disease **Precautions:** Breastfeeding, children, renal disease, hemophilia, diabetes mellitus, pancreatitis, alcoholism, surgery, trauma, infection, immune reconstitution syndrome **Pregnancy:** Only given after risks to the fetus are considered; animal studies have shown adverse reactions; no human studies available	Sulfas, amiodarone, cisapride, ergots, midazolam, quinidine, rifampin, triazolam, HMG-CoA reductase inhibitors, ketoconazole, clarithromycin, zidovudine, rifamycins, fluconazole, nevirapine, efavirenz, oral contraceptives, St. John's wort

*Pregnancy categories have been revised. See http://www.fda.gov/Drugs/DevelopmentApprovalProcess/DevelopmentResources/Labeling/ucm093307.htm for more information.

Adverse Effects/Side Effects

- Seizures
- Suicidal ideation
- Headache
- Dizziness
- Anxiety
- Fatigue
- Blurred vision
- Dry mouth
- Acid reflux
- Angioedema
- Nausea
- Vomiting
- Diarrhea
- Constipation
- Hepatotoxicity
- Hypo/hyperglycemia
- Pancreatitis
- Parathesias
- Night sweats
- Insomnia
- Anemia
- Neutropenia
- Thrombocytopenia
- Bleeding gums
- Muscle weakness
- Alopecia
- Rash

Nursing Care

- Administer medication at same time each day
- Monitor renal/hepatic function
- Monitor for mental status changes
- Monitor I&O
- Monitor for signs and symptoms of infection, anemia, sexually transmitted diseases
- Monitor viral load
- Monitor cholesterol, lipid panel throughout treatment
- Teach patient to use nonhormonal birth control
- Teach patient to take as prescribed and not to miss doses
- Teach patient that accumulation/redistribution of body fat may occur
- Teach patient to contact prescriber before taking OTC medications (Box 17.1)

Drug Interactions with HAART

Drug interaction associated with HAART is a challenging issue facing providers who treat patients with HIV. Medications used as initial treatment are associated with significant drug interactions. Concurrent treatment of comorbid disease states and therapies for preventing and/or treating opportunistic infections further increase the risk of drug interactions.

Nucleoside Reverse Transcriptase Inhibitors (NRTIs)

Drug interactions associated with NRTIs are minimal because these medications are not metabolized by the CYP450 system. Nevertheless, drug interactions may still occur within the class.

Non-Nucleoside Reverse Transcriptase Inhibitors (NNRTIs)

Drugs in this class are prone to interactions because they are extensively metabolized via CYP3A4 and can act as either inducers or inhibitors of CYP3A4. Efavirenz and nevirapine are inducers of CYP3A4, and delavirdine is an inhibitor.

Protease Inhibitors (PIs)

All PIs are potent inhibitors of CYP3A4 and result in drug interactions. Levels of medications also metabolized by the same system have the potential to be markedly increased, leading to an increased incidence of adverse effects. The protease inhibitor ritonavir is the most potent inhibitor of CYP3A4 in this class.

CCR5 Antagonists

CCR5 antagonists are a substrate of CYP3A. Concentrations are significantly increased in the presence of strong CYP3A inhibitors and reduced with CYP3A inducers. Dosage adjustments are necessary when used with these agents.

Integrase Inhibitors

Integrase inhibitor raltegravir is primarily eliminated by glucuronidation mediated by UDP-glucuronosyltransferase enzymes (UGTIA1). Strong inducers of UGTIA1 enzymes can significantly decrease the concentration of raltegravir.

From Kee, J.L., Hayes, E.R., McCuistion, L.E. (2015). *Pharmacology: A patient-centered nursing process approach* (8th ed.). St. Louis: Saunders.

Fusion Inhibitors

- Used to treat HIV
- Example includes enfuvirtide
- Available in SUBCUT preparations

Mode of Action
- Inhibits HIV from entering cells

Contraindications, Precautions, and Drug Interactions of Fusion Inhibitors*

Drug	Contraindications/Precautions	Drug Interaction
enfuvirtide	*Contraindications:* Hypersensitivity, breastfeeding *Precautions:* Children, liver disease, myelosuppression, infections *Pregnancy:* No adverse effects in animals; no human studies available	New drug; no known interaction at this time

*Pregnancy categories have been revised. See http://www.fda.gov/Drugs/DevelopmentApprovalProcess/DevelopmentResources/Labeling/ucm093307.htm for more information.

Adverse Effects/Side Effects

- Anxiety
- Nausea
- Constipation
- Anorexia
- Pancreatitis

- Glomerulonephritis
- Renal failure
- Guillain-Barre syndrome
- Insomnia
- Depression

- Thrombocytopenia
- Neutropenia
- Pneumonia
- Rash

Nursing Care

- Monitor for infection
- Monitor renal function
- Monitor blood counts
- Teach patient how to administer subcutaneous injection

APPLICATION AND REVIEW

1. Which classification of antiviral drugs are used to inhibit DNA replication of the HIV virus?
   1. Nucleoside Reverse Transcriptase Inhibitors (NRTIs)
   2. Nonnucleoside Reverse
   3. Protease Inhibitors
   4. Fusion Inhibitors
2. Which client is the best candidate for NRTIs therapy?
   1. A male adolescent
   2. A breastfeeding mother
   3. A client in the early stages of HIV infection
   4. A client diagnosed with advanced HIV infection
3. Which instruction concerning the administration of NNRTIs antiviral medications should be included in client education?
   1. Avoid grapefruit juice
   2. Take the medication at bedtime
   3. Take the medication on an empty stomach
   4. Remain upright for 30 minutes after taking the medication
4. When considering the ABCs, which adverse effect associated with NNRTI antiviral medications should be given priority when identified?
   1. Anxiety
   2. Asthenia
   3. Anorexia
   4. Atrial fibrillation
5. What instruction should be provided to a client prescribed a protease inhibitor?
   1. Acidic juices should be avoided
   2. Lay flat for 15 minutes after taking medication
   3. Take the medication at the same time each day
   4. Medication should be taken on an empty stomach

See Answers on pages 383-384.

CCR5-RECEPTOR ANTAGONISTS

- Used to treat HIV
- Examples include maraviroc
- Available in PO preparations

Mode of Action
- Inhibits fusion of HIV and the cell membrane

Contraindications, Precautions, and Drug Interactions of CCR5-Receptor Antagonists

Drug	Contraindications/Precautions	Drug Interaction
maraviroc	*Contraindications:* Hypersensitivity, dialysis, renal impairment *Precautions:* Breastfeeding, children, geriatric patients, renal/hepatic/cardiac disease, dehydration, electrolyte imbalance, MI, orthostatic hypotension, immune reconstitution disease, Graves' disease, Guillan Barre syndrome, polymyositis	CYP3A4 inducers, CYP3A4 inhibitors, St. John's wort

Adverse Effects/Side Effects
- Dizziness
- Depression
- Cough
- Upper respiratory tract infection
- Sinitis
- Bronchitis
- Bronchospasm
- Dyspnea
- Respiratory obstruction
- Pneumonia
- Viral meningitis
- Peripheral neuropathy
- Paresthesia
- Fever
- Dysethesia
- MI
- Cardiac ischemia
- Orthostatic hypotension
- Visual changes
- Gingival hyperplasia
- Diarrhea
- Constipation
- Hepatotoxicity
- Joint pain
- Muscle cramps
- Rash
- Urticaria
- Pruritus
- Herpes virus

Nursing Care
- Monitor renal function
- Monitor electrolytes and fluid balance
- Monitor for infection
- Monitor renal/hepatic function
- Teach patient to take as prescribed and not to miss doses
- Teach patient to report signs and symptoms of infection
- Teach patient to avoid all OTC products unless approved by prescriber
- Teach patient to change positions slowly
- Teach patient to avoid driving and other hazardous activities

Integrase Inhibitors
- Used to treat HIV
- Examples include raltegravir, dolutegravir, elvitegravir, tenofovir
- Available in PO preparations

Mode of Action
- Inhibits HIV integrase needed for replication

Contraindications, Precautions, and Drug Interactions of Integrase Inhibitors*

Drug	Contraindications/Precautions	Drug Interaction
raltegravir	*Contraindications:* Hypersensitivity, breastfeeding *Precautions:* Children, geriatric patients, hepatic disease, hepatitis, lactase deficiency, immune reconstitution syndrome, antimicrobial resistance *Pregnancy:* Only given after risks to the fetus are considered; animal studies have shown adverse reactions; no human studies available	H2 blockers proton pump inhibitors, UGT1A1 inhibitors, fibric acid derivatives, HMG-CoA reductase inhibitors, rifampin, efavirenz, tenofovir, tipranavir/ritonavir
dolutegravir	*Contraindications:* Hypersensitivity, breastfeeding *Precautions:* Children, geriatric patients, hepatic disease, hepatitis, lactase deficiency, immune reconstitution disorder, antimicrobial resistance *Pregnancy:* Only given after risks to the fetus are considered; animal studies have shown adverse reactions; no human studies available	Antacids, laxatives, sucralfate, oral iron, oral calcium, buffered products, rifampin, efavirenz, tenofovir, tipranavir/ritonavir, St. John's wort
elvitegravir	*Contraindications:* Hypersensitivity, severe hepatic disease *Precautions:* Breastfeeding, children, geriatric patients *Pregnancy:* Only given after risks to the fetus are considered; animal studies have shown adverse reactions; no human studies available	Creatinine products
tenofovir	*Contraindications:* Hypersensitivity, severe hepatic disease *Precautions:* Breastfeeding, children, geriatric patients *Pregnancy:* Only given after risks to the fetus are considered; animal studies have shown adverse reactions; no human studies available	Creatinine products

*Pregnancy categories have been revised. See http://www.fda.gov/Drugs/DevelopmentApprovalProcess/DevelopmentResources/Labeling/ucm093307.htm for more information.

Adverse Effects/Side Effects

- Suicidal ideation
- Fatigue
- Fever
- Dizziness
- Headache
- Asthenia
- MI
- Nausea
- Vomiting
- Diarrhea
- Gastritis
- Hyperglycemia
- Hepatitis
- Anemia
- Neutropenia
- Oliguria
- Proteinuria
- Hematuria
- Acute renal failure
- Glomerulonephritis
- Renal tubular necrosis
- Hyperamylasia
- Hyperglycemia
- Myopathy
- Rhabdomyolysis
- Immune reconstitution syndrome
- Rash
- Urticaria
- Pruritus
- Unusual sweating
- Alopecia

Nursing Care

- Monitor for suicidal ideation
- Monitor renal/hepatic function
- Monitor I&O
- Monitor blood counts
- Monitor for infection
- Monitor cholesterol levels
- Teach patient to take as prescribed and not to miss doses
- Teach patient to report signs and symptoms of infection

Nucleotide Reverse Transcriptase Inhibitors

- Used to treat HBV
- Examples include adefovir
- Available in PO preparations

Mode of Action

- Causes viral death of HBV DNA

Contraindications, Precautions, and Drug Interactions of Nucleotide Reverse Transcriptase Inhibitors*

Drug	Contraindications/Precautions	Drug Interaction
adefovir	**Contraindications:** Hypersensitivity **Precautions:** Breastfeeding, children, geriatric patients, females, labor, renal/hepatic disease, dialysis, obesity, organ transplant **Pregnancy:** Only given after risks to the fetus are considered; animal studies have shown adverse reactions; no human studies available	Emtricitabine/tenofovir, emtricitabine/rilpivirine, emtricitabine/efavirenz/tenofovir, aminoglycosides, NNRTIs, NRTIs, antiretroviral protease inhibitors, memantine, emtricitabine, efavirenz, dofetilide, digoxin, cyclosporine, amiloride, quinine, quinidine, procainamide, pemetrexed, midodrine, metformin, NSAIDs, morphine, ranitidine, vancomycin, cimetidine, trospium, tenofovir, triamterene, tacrolimus

*Pregnancy categories have been revised. See http://www.fda.gov/Drugs/DevelopmentApprovalProcess/DevelopmentResources/Labeling/ucm093307.htm for more information.

Adverse Effects/Side Effects

- Fever
- Headache
- Cough
- Dyspepsia
- Nausea
- Vomiting
- Diarrhea
- Weakness
- Weight loss
- Lactic acidosis
- Pancreatitis
- Hepatomegaly
- Nephrotoxicity
- Hematuria
- Glycosuria
- Renal failure
- Rash

Nursing Care

- Monitor patient for infection
- Monitor for respiratory distress
- Monitor I&O
- Monitor renal/hepatic function

- Teach patient to notify prescriber of decreased urinary output
- Teach patient not to stop medication abruptly

Interferons

- Used to HBV, HCV
- Examples include interferon alfa-2b, interferon alfacon-1
- Available in SUBCUT, IM, IV preparations

Mode of Action

- Induce antiviral immune response to inhibit HBV replication

Contraindications, Precautions, and Drug Interactions of Interferons*

Drug	Contraindications/Precautions	Drug Interaction
interferon alfa-2b	**Contraindications:** Hypersensitivity, auto-immune disorders, infections, ischemic disorders, neuropsychiatric disorders **Precautions:** Breastfeeding, children, mental illness, thrombocytopenia **Pregnancy:** Only given after risks to the fetus are considered; animal studies have shown adverse reactions; no human studies available	CNS depressants, theophylline, aminophylline, live virus vaccine, radiation
interferon alfacon-1	**Contraindications:** Hypersensitivity, hypersensitivity to alpha interferons, hypersensitivity to products from *Escherichia coli,* decompensated hepatic disease, autoimmune hepatitis **Precautions:** Breastfeeding, children, geriatric patients, hepatitic disease, hepatitis, cardiac disease, autoimmune disease, infection, seizure disorder, thyroid disorders, myelosuppression, alcoholism, depression **Pregnancy:** Only given after risks to the fetus are considered; animal studies have shown adverse reactions; no human studies available	Elflornithine, NRTI, myelosuppressives, aldesleukin, IL-2 elflornithine, theophylline, antiretrovirals

*Pregnancy categories have been revised. See http://www.fda.gov/Drugs/DevelopmentApprovalProcess/DevelopmentResources/Labeling/ucm093307.htm for more information.

Adverse Effects/Side Effects

- Headache
- Fever
- Insomnia
- Dizziness
- Depression
- Agitation
- Nervousness
- Anxiety
- Anaphylaxis
- Angioedema
- Upper respiratory infection
- Cough
- Sinusitis
- Epistaxis
- Dyspnea
- Bronchitis
- Tachycardia
- Hypertension
- Palpitation
- Eye pain
- Ear pain

- Tinnitus
- Nausea
- Vomiting
- Diarrhea
- Constipation
- Dyspepsia
- Abdominal pain

- Hemorrhoids
- Decreased salivation
- Granulocytopenia
- Thrombocytopenia
- Leukopenia
- Aplastic anemia
- Dysmenorrhea

- Vaginitis
- Menstrual disorders
- Bone pain
- Alopecia
- Pruritus
- Rash

Nursing Care

- Administer analgesics to combat flu-like symptoms
- Monitor for infection
- Monitor for depression/suicidal ideation
- Monitor renal/hepatic function
- Teach patient to report signs and symptoms of infection
- Teach patient to report signs and symptoms of depression/suicidal ideation
- Teach patient how to self-administer injection

Antiretroviral Nucleoside Reverse Transcriptase Inhibitor

- Used to treat HBV
- Example includes entecavir
- Available in PO preparations

Mode of Action

- Causes viral HBV DNA death

Contraindications, Precautions, and Drug Interactions of Antiretroviral Nucleoside Reverse Transcriptase Inhibitor*

Drug	Contraindications/Precautions	Drug Interaction
entecavir	**Contraindications:** Hypersensitivity **Precautions:** Breastfeeding, children, geriatric patients, renal disease, liver transplant **Pregnancy:** Only given after risks to the fetus are considered; animal studies have shown adverse reactions; no human studies available	Platelets, albumin

*Pregnancy categories have been revised. See http://www.fda.gov/Drugs/DevelopmentApprovalProcess/DevelopmentResources/Labeling/ucm093307.htm for more information.

Adverse Effects/Side Effects

- Headache
- Fatigue
- Dizziness
- Insomnia
- Nausea

- Vomiting
- Diarrhea
- Dyspepsia
- Hyperglycemia
- Elevated liver function enzymes

- Lactic acidosis
- Severe hepatomegaly
- Alopecia
- Rash

Nursing Care

- Do not administer with food
- Monitor renal/hepatic function

- Monitor I&O
- Teach patient to avoid high fat meal
- Teach patient to take medication exactly as prescribed
- Teach patient not to discontinue medication abruptly
- Teach patient to report hematuria and decreased urinary output

Nucleotide Analog Polymerase Inhibitor

- Used to treat HCV
- Examples include sofosbuvir, simeprevir
- Available in PO preparations

Mode of Action

- Inhibits HCV RNA synthesis

Contraindications, Precautions, and Drug Interactions of Nucleotide Analog Polymerase Inhibitor*

Drug	Contraindications/Precautions	Drug Interaction
sofosbuvir	**Precautions:** Breastfeeding, children, hepatic/renal disease **Contraindications:** Hypersensitivity, male-mediated teratogenicity **Pregnancy:** No adverse effects in animals; no human studies available	Carbamazepine, phenobarbital, phenytoin, rifampin, oxcarbazepine, rifabutin, rifapentine, tipranavir, amiodarone, carvedilol, cobicistat, St. John's wort
Simeprevir	**Contraindications:** Hypersensitivity, male-mediated teratogenicity **Precautions:** Breastfeeding, children, Asian patients, liver transplant, UV exposure, hepatic disease, serious rash **Pregnancy:** Only given after risks to the fetus are considered; animal studies have shown adverse reactions; no human studies available	CYP3A4 inducers/inhibitors, bromocriptine, chloramphenicol, cimetidine, fluoxetine, protease inhibitors, digoxin, quinidine

*Pregnancy categories have been revised. See http://www.fda.gov/Drugs/DevelopmentApprovalProcess/DevelopmentResources/Labeling/ucm093307.htm for more information.

Adverse Effects/Side Effects

- Headache
- Chills
- Fever
- Weakness
- Insomnia
- Fatigue
- Dyspnea
- Blurred vision
- Conjunctivitis
- Diarrhea
- Nausea
- Hyperbilirubinemia
- Neutropenia
- Anemia
- Myalgia
- Rash
- Pruritus
- Photosensitivity

Nursing Care

- Monitor renal/hepatic function
- Monitor I&O
- Monitor electrolytes

- Monitor for infection and allergic reaction
- Teach patient not to stop medication abruptly
- Teach patient not to use other medications unless approved by prescriber
- Teach patient to notify prescriber if pregnancy is planned or occurs
- Teach patient to report signs and symptoms to the prescriber

Virus Proliferation Inhibitors

- Used to treat HBV, HCV
- Example includes peginterferon alfa-2a, peginterferon alfa-2b
- Available in SUBCUT, IM preparations

Mode of Action

- Stimulates genes to inhibit viral replication of HBV, HCV

Contraindications, Precautions, and Drug Interactions of Virus Proliferation Inhibitors*

Drug	Contraindications/Precautions	Drug Interaction
peginterferon alfa-2a, peginterferon alfa-2b	*Contraindications:* Hypersensitivity to interferons, neonates, infants, benzyl alcohol, sepsis, *Escherichia coli* protein *Precautions:* Breastfeeding, children, mental illness, thrombocytopenia *Pregnancy:* Only given after risks to the fetus are considered; animal studies have shown adverse reactions; no human studies available	Theophylline, myelosuppressives, NNRTIs, NRTIs, protein inhibitors

*Pregnancy categories have been revised. See http://www.fda.gov/Drugs/DevelopmentApprovalProcess/DevelopmentResources/Labeling/ucm093307.htm for more information.

Adverse Effects/Side Effects

- Suicidal ideation
- Homicidal ideation
- Headache
- Dizziness
- Insomnia
- Anxiety
- Nervousness
- Lability
- Hostility
- Mania
- Psychosis
- Relapse of drug addiction
- Fatigue
- Poor concentration
- Depression
- Ischemic CV events
- Nausea
- Vomiting
- Diarrhea
- Anorexia
- Dry mouth
- Fatal colitis
- Fatal pancreatitis
- Cough
- Dyspnea
- Diabetes
- Hypothyroidism
- Thrombocytopenia
- Neutropenia
- Anemia
- Lymphopenia
- Myalgia
- Arthralgia
- Alopecia
- Pruritus
- Rash

Nursing Care

- Monitor for neuropsychiatric symptoms
- Monitor renal/hepatic studies
- Monitor for infection

- Monitor for colitis/pancreatitis
- Monitor for cardiac and respiratory distress
- Teach patient to use two forms of contraception during treatment and for 6 months after
- Teach patient to avoid driving and other hazardous activities
- Teach patient to report adverse effects to the prescriber

Neuramidase Inhibitors

- Used to treat influenza A, influenza B
- Examples include oseltamivir, zanamivir, peramivir
- Available in PO, IV preparations

Mode of Action

- Inhibits influenza virus neuraminidase action of virus release

Contraindications, Precautions, and Drug Interactions of Miscellaneous Neuramidase Inhibitors*

Drug	Contraindications/Precautions	Drug Interaction
oseltamivir	*Contraindications:* Hypersensitivity *Precautions:* Breastfeeding, neonates, infants, children, geriatric patients, renal/hepatic/pulmonary/cardiac disease, viral infection, psychosis *Contraindications:* Hypersensitivity *Pregnancy:* Only given after risks to the fetus are considered; animal studies have shown adverse reactions; no human studies available	H1N1 virus vaccine, intranasal influenzae vaccine
zanamivir	*Contraindications:* Hypersensitivity *Precautions:* Breastfeeding, children, geriatric patients, angioedema, respiratory disease, Reye's syndrome, milk protein sensitivity *Contraindications:* Hypersensitivity *Pregnancy:* Only given after risks to the fetus are considered; animal studies have shown adverse reactions; no human studies available	Separate from intranasal influenzae vaccine by ≥48 hr; do not restart antiviral products for ≥2 wk
peramivir	*Contraindications:* Hypersensitivity *Precautions:* Breastfeeding, infants, children, infection, renal disease, dialysis, psychosis *Pregnancy:* Only given after risks to the fetus are considered; animal studies have shown adverse reactions; no human studies available	H1N1 vaccines, intranasal influenza vaccines

*Pregnancy categories have been revised. See http://www.fda.gov/Drugs/DevelopmentApprovalProcess/DevelopmentResources/Labeling/ucm093307.htm for more information.

Adverse Effects/Side Effects

- Headache
- Dizziness
- Fatigue
- Insomnia
- Delirium
- Seizures

- Nausea
- Throat infections
- Vomiting
- Diarrhea
- Abdominal pain
- Bronchospasm

- Cough
- Hyperglycemia
- Stevens-Johnson syndrome
- Erythema multiforme

Nursing Care

- Monitor for infection
- Monitor for respiratory distress
- Teach patient to report mental status changes
- Teach patient to avoid driving and other hazardous activities
- Teach patients with asthma or COPD to carry fast-acting inhaled bronchodilator
- Teach patient to take as soon as symptoms appear and to complete therapy even if feeling better
- Teach patient that product should not be substituted for flu shot
- Teach patient to avoid other medications unless approved by prescriber

Nucleoside Analogs

- Used to treat HSV, CMV
- Examples include acyclovir, cidofovir, famciclovir, ganciclovir, valacyclovir, valganciclovir
- Available in PO, IV preparations

Mode of Action

- Interferes with DNA synthesis

Contraindications, Precautions, and Drug Interactions of Nucleoside Analogs*

Drug	Contraindications/Precautions	Drug Interaction
acyclovir	**Contraindications:** Hypersensitivity **Precautions:** Breastfeeding, renal/hepatic/neurologic disease, hypersensitivity to famciclovir/ganciclovir/penciclovir/valganciclovir, dehydration, electrolyte imbalance, obesity **Pregnancy:** No adverse effects in animals; no human studies available	Zidovudine, aminoglycosides, probenecid, valproic acid, hydantoins, entecavir, tenofovir, pemetrexed
cidofovir	**Contraindications:** Hypersensitivity, hypersensitivity to probenecid/sulfas; direct intraocular injection **Precautions:** Breastfeeding, children, geriatric patients, dehydration, renal disease, preexisting cytopenias, thrombocytopenia **Pregnancy:** Only given after risks to the fetus are considered; animal studies have shown adverse reactions; no human studies available	NSAIDs, salicylates, foscarnet, aminoglycosides, amphotericin B, pentamidine IV

Continued

Contraindications, Precautions, and Drug Interactions of Nucleoside Analogs—cont'd

Drug	Contraindications/Precautions	Drug Interaction
famciclovir	*Contraindications:* Hypersensitivity, hypersensitivity to penciclovir/acyclovir/ganciclovir/valacyclovir/valganciclovir *Precautions:* Breastfeeding, renal disease *Pregnancy:* No adverse effects in animals; no human studies available	Probenecid, zoster vaccine
ganciclovir	*Contraindications:* Hypersensitivity, hypersensitivity to acyclovir/ganciclovir *Precautions:* Breastfeeding, children, geriatric patients, dehydration, renal disease, preexisting cytopenias, radiation, hypersensitivity to famciclovir/penciclovir/valacyclovir/galganciclovir *Pregnancy:* Only given after risks to the fetus are considered; animal studies have shown adverse reactions; no human studies available	Zidovudine, antineoplastics, aminoglycosides, radiation, didanosine, imipenem/cilastatin, cyclosporine, adriamcyin, flucytosine, amphotericin B, dapsone, pentamidine, doxorubicin, probenecid, vinblastine, vincristine, NSAIDs, tenofovir, mycophenolate, tacrolimus, nucleoside analogs
valganciclovir	*Contraindications:* Hypersensitivity, hypersensitivity to valacyclovir/ganciclovir, breastfeeding, neutropenia, thrombocytopenia, liver transplantation, hemodialysis *Precautions:* Children, geriatric patients, dehydration, renal disease, hypersensitivity to famciclovir/penciclovir/acyclovir *Pregnancy:* Only given after risks to the fetus are considered; animal studies have shown adverse reactions; no human studies available	Immunosuppressants, zidovudine, antineoplastics, radiation, mycophenolate, imipenem-cilastatin, didanosine, probenecid, valganciclovir, dapsone, flucytosine, pentamidine, vinblastine, vincristine, doxorubicin, adriamycin, cyclosporine, amphotericin B, nucleoside analogs

*Pregnancy categories have been revised. See http://www.fda.gov/Drugs/DevelopmentApprovalProcess/DevelopmentResources/Labeling/ucm093307.htm for more information.

Adverse Effects/Side Effects

- Coma
- Headache
- Confusion
- Lethargy
- Dizziness
- Seizures
- Tremors
- Nausea
- Vomiting
- Diarrhea
- Dyspnea
- Dysrhythmias
- Hypo/Hypertension
- Colitis
- Gingival hyperplasia
- Thrombic thrombocytopenia purpura
- Hemolytic uremic syndrome
- Hemorrhage
- Granulocytopenia
- Thrombocytopenia
- Anemia
- Neutropenia
- Oliguria
- Proteinuria
- Hematuria
- Acute renal failure
- Glomerulonephritis
- Nephrotoxicity
- Pancreatitis
- Stevens-Johnson syndrome
- Rash
- Urticaria
- Pruritus
- Unusual sweating
- Alopecia

Nursing Care

- Monitor for infection
- Monitor for anemia
- Monitor for respiratory distress
- Monitor renal/hepatic function
- Monitor electrolytes
- Monitor neurologic status (herpes encephalitis)
- Monitor I&O
- Teach patient to report signs and symptoms of infection
- Teach patient oral product may be taken before infection occurs
- Teach patient to seek dental care to prevent gingival hyperplasia
- Teach patient to wear condoms during sexual intercourse to prevent spread of infection
- Teach patient not to touch lesions to prevent spread of infection
- Teach women about risk of developing cervical cancer and to participate in regular screening

Pyrophosphate Analogs

- Used to treat CMV retinitis, acyclovir-resistant HSV infections
- Examples include foscarnet
- Available in IV preparations

Mode of Action

- Prevents viral replication by inhibiting DNA polymerase

Contraindications, Precautions, and Drug Interactions of Pyrophosphate Analogs*

Drug	Contraindications/Precautions	Drug Interaction
foscarnet	*Contraindications:* Hypersensitivity, impaired creatinine clearance *Precautions:* Breastfeeding, children, geriatric patients, severe anemia, seizure disorders *Pregnancy:* Only given after risks to the fetus are considered; animal studies have shown adverse reactions; no human studies available	Acyclovir, cidofovir, cisplatin, penicillamine, tenofovir, tacrolimus, aminoglycosides, gold compounds, vancomycin, amphotericin B, cyclosporine, lithium, NSAIDs

*Pregnancy categories have been revised. See http://www.fda.gov/Drugs/DevelopmentApprovalProcess/DevelopmentResources/Labeling/ucm093307.htm for more information.

Adverse Effects/Side Effects

- Headache
- Fever
- Dizziness
- Fatigue
- Seizures
- Malaise
- Confusion
- Anxiety
- Depression
- Neuropathy
- Paresthesia
- Encephalopathy
- Cardiomyopathy
- Cardiac arrest
- Atrial fibrillation
- CHF
- Sinus tachycardia
- Coughing
- Dyspnea
- Pneumonia
- Hemoptysis

- Pneumothorax
- Nausea
- Vomiting
- Diarrhea
- Anorexia
- Pancreatitis
- Acute renal failure
- Increased serum creatinine

- Diabetes insipidus
- Renal tubular disorders
- Anemia
- Granulocytopenia
- Leukopenia
- Thrombocytopenia
- Thrombosis
- Neutropenia

- Rash
- Pruritus
- Sweating
- Hypokalemia
- Hypocalcemia
- Hypomagnesemia
- Hypophosphatemia

Nursing Care

- Administer IV infusions slowly, over at least 1 hour using an infusion pump
- Monitor for infection
- Monitor renal/hepatic function
- Monitor blood counts
- Monitor electrolyte balance
- Monitor I&O
- Teach patient to report signs and symptoms of infection
- Teach patient to report tingling, numbness, parathesias
- Teach patient not to take OTC medications without notifying prescriber

APPLICATION AND REVIEW

6. Regarding HIV treatment therapy, which mode of action is associated with CCR5-Receptor Antagonists?
   1. Induce antiviral immune response to inhibit HBV replication
   2. Inhibit HIV integrase needed for replication
   3. Inhibit the fusion of HIV and the cell membrane
   4. Cause viral death of HBV DN

7. A client prescribed a CCR5-ReceptorAntagonist should be regularly monitored for which complication? **Select all that apply.**
   1. Gastrointestinal bleeding
   2. Electrolyte imbalance
   3. Renal failure
   4. Infection
   5. Cough

8. A client prescribed an Antiretroviral Nucleoside Reverse Transcriptase Inhibitor should be given what instruction concerning the administration of the medication?
   1. Take on an empty stomach
   2. Limit seafood while on medication
   3. Take medication with a high fat meal
   4. Drink an 8-ounce glass of water with each dose

9. Which action by a nurse administering a pyrophosphate analog medication indicates a need for further instruction regarding the intravenous administration of this medication?
   1. Administers the IV infusion slowly
   2. Requires the client to remain in bed during the infusion
   3. Uses an infusion pump to regulate the flow of medication
   4. Administers the medication over a minimum of 60 minutes

10. Which statement by a nurse administering a nucleotide analog polymerase inhibitor indicates a need for further instruction regarding client assessment and monitoring?
    1. "I need to see if the client's temperature is remaining stable."
    2. "I've asked the client to let me know each time they urinate."
    3. "I need to see if the client's electrolyte results are back yet."
    4. "The client denies any allergies to eggs, ragweed, or flower pollen."

See Answers on pages 383-384.

ANSWER KEY: REVIEW QUESTIONS

1. **1 NRTIs are used to inhibit DNA replication of the HIV virus.**
   2 NNRTIs prevent HIV replication by binding to reverse transcriptase enzyme. **3** Protease Inhibitors act against HIV enzyme protease, preventing cell division. **4** Fusion Inhibitors interfere with HIV from entering cells.
   Client Need: Pharmacologic and Parenteral Therapies; **Cognitive Level:** Analysis; **Nursing Process:** Assessment/ Analysis

> **Study Tip: N**RTIs i**N**hibit d**N**a replicatio**N**. Knowing that NRTI stands for nucleoside reverse transcriptase inhibitors helps you know that they interfere with replication; noticing all the n's will help you remember it!

2. **4 NRTIs are used to treat advanced HIV infection.**
   1 Children are prescribed NRTIs only after all risks and benefits are evaluated. **2** Breastfeeding is considered a precautionary situation. NRTIs are prescribed only after all risks and benefits are evaluated. **3** NRTIs are not prescribed for early HIV infection.
   Client Need: Pharmacologic and Parenteral Therapies; **Cognitive Level:** Analysis; **Nursing Process:** Assessment/ Analysis

3. **1 Grapefruit juice should be avoided when prescribed NNRTI therapy.**
   2 It is not necessary to schedule NNRTIs at bedtime. **3** NNRTIs need to be taken after meals. **4** An upright position is not required after taking an NRTI.
   Client Need: Pharmacologic and Parenteral Therapies; **Cognitive Level:** Application; **Integrated Process:** Teaching/ Learning; **Nursing Process:** Planning/Implementation

4. **4 Considering the ABCs, the cardiac issues presented by atrial fibrillation should be given priority care.**
   1 Although anxiety requires treatment, it does not present dramatic an acute risk for the client as the cardiac issues associated with atrial fibrillation. **2** Asthenia, extreme fatigue, does not present the acute risks to health presented by atrial fibrillation. **3** Although anorexia requires treatment, it does not present as dramatic an acute risk for the client as the cardiac issues associated with atrial fibrillation.
   Client Need: Pharmacologic and Parenteral Therapies; **Cognitive Level:** Analysis; **Nursing Process:** Assessment/Analysis

5. **3 Protease inhibitors should be taken at the same time each day.**
   1 Protease inhibitors are not known to be affected by acidic juices. **2** Protease inhibitors do not require a flat position postadministration. **4** The effectiveness of protease inhibitors does not seem to be effected by the presence of food in the stomach.
   Client Need: Pharmacologic and Parenteral Therapies; **Cognitive Level:** Application; **Nursing Process:** Assessment/ Analysis

6. **3 CCR5-Receptor Antagonists inhibit the fusion of HIV and the cell membrane.**
   1 Interferons induce antiviral immune response to inhibit HBV replication. **2** Integrase Inhibitors inhibit HIV integrase needed for replication. **4** Nucleotide Reverse Transcriptase Inhibitors cause viral death of HBV DNA.
   Client Need: Pharmacologic and Parenteral Therapies; **Cognitive Level:** Analysis; **Nursing Process:** Assessment/ Analysis

7. **Answers: 2, 3, 4, 5**

Adverse effects of CCR5-Receptor Antagonists include fluid and electrolyte imbalances, renal failure, infections, and cough.

1 GI bleeding is not associated with the adverse reactions to CCR5-Receptor Antagonist therapy. **2** Integrase Inhibitors inhibit HIV integrase needed for replication. **4** Nucleotide Reverse Transcriptase Inhibitors cause viral death of HBV DNA.

Client Need: Pharmacologic and Parenteral Therapies; **Cognitive Level:** Application; **Nursing Process:** Assessment/Analysis

> **Study Tip:** Write "C C R Five rEceptor Antagonists" in block letters, using the Capital letters shown. Then write "Adverse" down from the "A" of "Antagonists". Write "Cough" down, using the first "C". Write "infeCtions" using the second "C". Write "Renal" using the "R" and "Failure" using the 'f' of "Five." Write "fluid and Electrolyte imbalances" using the "E" of rEceptor. You now have a word diagram of the adverse effects of CCR5-Receptor Antagonists.

8. **1 Antiretroviral Nucleoside Reverse Transcriptase Inhibitors should not be administered with food.**

2 Antiretroviral Nucleoside Reverse Transcriptase Inhibitor therapy does not require restriction on dietary seafood. **3** Clients should be instructed to adhere to a low fat diet while on an Antiretroviral Nucleoside Reverse Transcriptase Inhibitor. **4** Although not discouraged, administration of an Antiretroviral Nucleoside Reverse Transcriptase Inhibitor does not require drinking 8 ounces of water with each dose.

Client Need: Pharmacologic and Parenteral Therapies; **Cognitive Level:** Application; **Integrated Process:** Teaching/Learning; **Nursing Process:** Planning/Implementation

9. **2 Pyrophosphate analog medication does not require the client to remain in bed during the infusion.**

1 Pyrophosphate analog medication should be infused slowly. **3** An infusion pump should be used to ensure safe administration of the medication. **4** Pyrophosphate analog medication should be infused slowly, over at least 1 hour.

Client Need: Pharmacologic and Parenteral Therapies; **Cognitive Level:** Analysis; **Integrated Process:** Teaching/Learning; **Nursing Process:** Evaluation/Outcomes

10. **4 The safe administration of a nucleotide analog polymerase inhibitor is not affected by allergies to eggs, ragweed or flower pollens.**

1 Adverse effects of a nucleotide analog polymerase inhibitor includes fever and infection. Monitoring the client's temperature would be appropriate. **2** Adverse effects of a nucleotide analog polymerase inhibitor includes impaired renal function. Monitoring the client's urinary output would be appropriate. **3** Adverse effects of a nucleotide analog polymerase inhibitor includes electrolyte imbalances. Monitoring the client's electrolyte results would be appropriate.

Client Need: Pharmacologic and Parenteral Therapies; **Cognitive Level:** Analysis; **Integrated Process:** Teaching/Learning; **Nursing Process:** Evaluation/Outcome

Antineoplastic Drugs 18

INTRODUCTION TO ANTINEOPLASTIC DRUGS

- Cancer cells look, grow, and function differently than normal cells; have no cellular boundaries
- Most common cancer type is solid tumor that responds poorly to chemotherapy and requires surgery
- Most common cancers: breast, lung, colorectal, prostate, cervical, skin
- Cancer develops at molecular level
  - Stage 1: Initiation
    - Environmental exposures cause irreversible changes in cell DNA
    - Causative factors: cigarette smoke, chemicals (asbestos, uranium), radiation, breast implants, UV light (Box 18.1)
  - Stage 2: Promotion
    - More changes in DNA, decreased differentiation, tumor development
    - Causative factors: cigarette smoke, alcohol, high fat/calorie diet, hormones, prolonged stress
  - Stage 3: Progression
    - Changes in DNA result in malignant tumor
    - Characteristics: tumor grows quickly and into surrounding tissue; tumor cells metastasize to other tissues/organs
- Metastasis: cancer cells travel via lymph or blood to other tissues and organs
- Metastasis occurs when tumor cells travel via lymph or blood to other tissues and organs
- Immune system: key role in controlling growth of cancer cells (Table 18.1)
  - Recognize pathogen as foreign
  - Coordinate response to eliminate pathogen
  - T-cell lymphocytes, macrophages, antigens, NK cells recognize and destroy cancer cells
- Warning signs of cancer
  - Change in bowel/bladder habits
  - Unusual bleeding/discharge anywhere in body
  - Indigestion/difficulty swallowing
  - Persistent cough/hoarseness
  - Sore that won't heal
  - Solid lump anywhere in body
  - Change in wart/mole
  - Unexplained weight loss
- Treatment: radiation, chemotherapy, biotherapy, bone marrow transplant, surgical removal of tumor
- Cancer prevention: tobacco and alcohol cessation, early detection, screening

CLASSIFICATION OF NEOPLASMS

- Benign neoplasia
  - Cells adhere to one another; growth remains circumscribed

BOX 18.1 Environmental, Infective, and Dietary Influences on Cancer Development

Environmental
Tobacco
Gastric cancers and cancer of the bladder, cervix, colon, esophagus, head and neck, kidney and ureter, liver, lung, pancreas, trachea and bronchus, and acute myeloid leukemia
Asbestos
Lung cancer
Benzene
Acute myelogenous leukemia
Formaldehyde
Cancer of the nose, throat, and trachea
Vinyl Chloride
Sarcoma, leukemia
Arsenic
Cancer of the lung and skin, sarcoma
Ionizing Radiation
Leukemia; cancer of the thyroid, breast
Ultraviolet Rays
Skin cancer
Aflatoxin
Liver cancer

Infective
Herpes Simplex 2 Virus (Genital Herpes)
Cervical and penile cancer
Hepatitis B and C Viruses
Cancer of the liver
Epstein-Barr Virus
Non-Hodgkin lymphoma, Hodgkin disease, nasopharyngeal cancers
Human Papillomavirus (HPV)
Cancer of the cervix, vulva, vagina, anus, penis, head and neck
Human Immunodeficiency Virus (HIV)
Kaposi sarcoma, non-Hodgkin lymphoma, cervical cancer
Human T-Cell Lymphotropic Virus
T-cell leukemia
Helicobacter pylori
Cancer of the stomach, gastric mucosa-associated lymphoid tissue (MALT) lymphoma

Diet
Animal Fat
Cancer of the colon, rectum, breast, uterus, prostate, ovary
Heterocyclic Amines (found in some smoked meats)
Cancer of the stomach, colon, rectum, pancreas, breast
Alcohol
Cancer of the mouth, throat, esophagus, liver, breast

From McCuistion, L., Vuljoin-DiMaggio, K., Winton, M.B., Yeager, J.J. (2018). *Pharmacology: A patient-centered nursing process approach* (9th ed.). St. Louis: Elsevier.

TABLE 18.1	Cells of the Immune System	
Cell Type	**Synonyms**	**Primary Immune-Related Actions**
Major Cell Types		
B lymphocytes	B cells	• Produce antibodies
Cytolytic T lymphocytes (CTLs)	Cytolytic T cells, cytotoxic T cells, CD8 cells	• Lyse target cells
Helper T lymphocytes	Helper T cells, CD4 cells	• Promote proliferation and differentiation of B cells and CTLs • Initiate delayed-type hypersensitivity
Macrophages		• Promote proliferation and differentiation of helper T cells and CTLs by serving as antigen-presenting cells • Participate in delayed-type hypersensitivity • Phagocytize cells tagged with antibodies • Phagocytize cells in the effector stage of delayed-type hypersensitivity
Dendritic cells		• Promote proliferation of CTLs and helper T cells by serving as antigen-presenting cells
Accessory Cells		
Mast cells		• Mediate immediate hypersensitivity reactions
Basophils		• Mediate immediate hypersensitivity reactions
Neutrophils	Polymorphonuclear leukocytes	• Phagocytize foreign particles (e.g., bacteria), especially those tagged with IgG • Mediate inflammation
Eosinophils		• Attack helminths and foreign particles that have been coated with IgE • Contribute to immediate hypersensitivity reactions

IgE, immunoglobulin E; *IgG,* immunoglobulin G.
From Burchum, J.R., Rosenthal, L.D. (2016). *Lehne's pharmacology for nursing* (9th ed.). St. Louis: Saunders.

- Generally not life-threatening unless they occur in restricted area (e.g., skull)
- Classified according to tissue involved (e.g., glandular tissue [adenoma], bone [osteoma], nerve cells [neuroma], fibrous tissue [fibroma])
- Malignant neoplasia
  - Cells are undifferentiated (anaplasia) and rapidly dividing
  - Cells infiltrate surrounding tissue
  - May spread (metastasize) by direct extension, lymphatic permeation and embolization; diffusion of cancer cells can occur by mechanical means and produce secondary lesions
  - Membranes of malignant cells contain specific proteins (tumor-specific antigens)
- Tumors are classified according to tissue involved (e.g., glandular epithelial tissue [adenocarcinoma], epithelial surface tissue [carcinoma], connective tissue [sarcoma], melanocytes [melanoma])

- Tumors are often classified by universal system of staging classification, TNM system
  - T designates primary tumor
  - N designates lymph node involvement
  - M designates metastasis
- A number (0–4) after any of the previously discussed letters designates degree of involvement
  - 0: cancer in situ
  - I: limited to tissue of origin; localized
  - II: limited local spread
  - III: extensive local and regional spread
  - IV: metastasis
- TIS designates carcinoma in situ or one that has not infiltrated

ANTINEOPLASTIC AGENTS

- Destroy malignant cells by interfering with reproduction of cancer cell (Fig. 18.1)
- Act at specific points in cycle of cell division (cell-cycle specific) or at any phase in cycle of cell division (cell-cycle nonspecific)
- Affect any rapidly dividing cell within body, thus having potential for toxicity development in healthy, functional tissue (e.g., bone marrow, hair follicles, GI mucosa); combination therapy often is used to reduce possibility of toxicity and maximize therapeutic effect (e.g., CHOP: cyclophosphamide (Cytoxan), DOXOrubicin, vinCRIStine, prednisone)

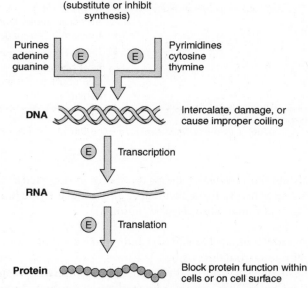

FIG. 18.1 Basic mechanisms by which antineoplastic drugs selectively kill tumor cells. *E* stands for enzymes, some of which are inhibited by these drugs. Inhibition of DNA or RNA synthesis or replication, production of miscoded nucleic acids, and formation of modified proteins are key mechanisms of action for many of these drugs. (From Wecker L., Crespo, L.M., Dunaway, G., Faingold, C. [2010]. *Brody's human pharmacology* [10th ed.]. Philadelphia: Mosby.)

- Biologic response modifiers (BRMs), also called immunotherapies, restore the body's immune system in the presence of cancer
  - Targeted therapy: target cancer cells directly
  - Indirect therapy: stimulates immune system but does not directly target cancer cells
  - Include interferons (alpha, beta, gamma), colony-stimulating factors, interleukins, and monoclonal antibodies

Alkylating Agents

- Used in the treatment of childhood and adult cancers, and aplastic anemia
- Examples include cyclophosphamide, busulfan, carmustine, lomustine, dacarbazine, procarbazine, thiotepa, cisplatin
- Available in PO, IV preparations

Mode of Action
- Damages deoxyribonucleic acid (DNA) by halting the replication process; cross links DNA strands

Contraindications, Precautions, and Drug Interactions of Alkylating Agents*

Drug	Contraindications/Precautions	Drug Interaction
cyclophosphamide	**Contraindications:** Hypersensitivity, prostatic hypertrophy, bladder neck obstruction **Precautions:** Children, geriatric patients, radiation therapy, cardiac disease, anemia, dysrhythmias, heart failure, leukopenia **Pregnancy:** Definite fetal risks, may be given in spite of risks if needed in life-threatening conditions	Succinylcholine, warfarin, digoxin, corticosteroids, live virus vaccines, CYP3A4 inducers/inhibitors
busulfan	**Contraindications:** Hypersensitivity, breastfeeding **Precautions:** Women of childbearing age, anemia, leucopenia, liver/kidney toxicity, radiation, chemotherapy, seizures, hyperkalemia, hyperphosphatemia, hypocalcemia, hyperuricemia **Pregnancy:** Definite fetal risks, may be given in spite of risks if needed in life-threatening conditions	Anticoagulants, salicylates, acetaminophen, phenytoin, live virus vaccines
carmustine	**Contraindications:** Hypersensitivity, breastfeeding, leukopenia, thrombocytopenia **Precautions:** Dental disease, females, infection, renal disease **Pregnancy:** Definite fetal risks, may be given in spite of risks if needed in life-threatening conditions	Aspirin, anticoagulants, platelet inhibitors, cimetidine, radiation, digoxin, phenytoins, live vaccines

Continued

Contraindications, Precautions, and Drug Interactions of Alkylating Agents—cont'd

Drug	Contraindications/Precautions	Drug Interaction
lomustine	*Contraindications:* Hypersensitivity, breastfeeding, bacterial/fungal/viral infection, leucopenia *Precautions:* Respiratory disease *Pregnancy:* Definite fetal risks, may be given in spite of risks if needed in life-threatening conditions	Radiation, anticoagulants, live virus vaccines
dacarbazine	*Contraindications:* Hypersensitivity, breastfeeding *Precautions:* Renal disease, infection *Pregnancy:* Definite fetal risks, may be given in spite of risks if needed in life-threatening conditions	Salicylates, anticoagulants, NSAIDs, live virus vaccines, aminoglycosides, loop diuretics, phenytoin, phenobarbital
procarbazine	*Contraindications:* Hypersensitivity, breastfeeding, bone marrow depression, thrombocytopenia *Precautions:* Parkinson's disease, seizure disorder, bipolar disorder, cardiac/renal/hepatic disease, radiation, anemia *Pregnancy:* Definite fetal risks, may be given in spite of risks if needed in life-threatening conditions	Meperidine, alcohol, SSRIs, SNRIs, MAOIs, tricyclics, levodopa, methyldopa, reserpine, caffeine, barbiturates, antihistamines, opioids, phenothiazines, NSAIDs, anticoagulants, platelet inhibitors, thrombolytics
thiotepa	*Contraindications:* Hypersensitivity, breastfeeding, liver/kidney disease *Precautions:* Infections, radiation *Pregnancy:* Definite fetal risks, may be given in spite of risks if needed in life-threatening conditions	Aspirin, salicylates, NSAIDs, corticosteroids, live virus vaccinations
cisplatin	*Contraindications:* Hypersensitivity, breastfeeding *Precautions:* Geriatric patients, infections, peripheral neuropathy, radiation *Pregnancy:* Definite fetal risks, may be given in spite of risks if needed in life-threatening conditions	Aspirin, NSAIDs, salicylates, alcohol, furosemide, live virus vaccines

*Pregnancy categories have been revised. See http://www.fda.gov/Drugs/DevelopmentApprovalProcess/DevelopmentResources/Labeling/ucm093307.htm for more information.

Adverse Effects/Side Effects
- Headache
- Syndrome of inappropriate antidiuretic hormone (SIADH)
- Nausea
- Vomiting
- Diarrhea
- Hepatotoxicity
- Thrombocytopenia
- Leukopenia
- Myelosuppression
- Anemia
- Stomatitis
- Reversible hair loss
- Hyperuricemia
- Serotonin syndrome

Nursing Care
- Administer chemotherapy agents according to policies and procedures
- Keep epinephrine, corticosteroids, and antihistamines on hand during drug administration
- Monitor I&O
- Monitor liver/kidney function

- Monitor pulmonary function
- Monitor for bleeding
- Monitor for cold, cough, fever
- Teach patient to rinse mouth with water TID
- Teach patient to use a sponge brush to clean teeth
- Teach patient to avoid foods with citric acid
- Teach patient to avoid aspirin, ibuprofen, razors, commercial mouthwash

Antimetabolites

- Used to treat cancers
- Examples include methotrexate, gemcitabine, fluorouracil, cytarabine, mercaptopurine
- Available in PO, IM, IV preparations

Mode of Action
- Inhibits DNA and RNA synthesis

Contraindications, Precautions, and Drug Interactions of Antimetabolites*

Drug	Contraindications/Precautions	Drug Interaction
methotrexate	*Contraindications:* Hypersensitivity, leukopenia, thrombocytopenia, anemia, alcoholism, AIDS, renal disease *Precautions:* Breastfeeding, children *Pregnancy:* Absolute fetal abnormalities; not to be used anytime during pregnancy	Proton pump inhibitors, salicylates, NSAIDs, sulfas, radiation, alcohol, probenecid, penicillins, theophylline, cholestyramine, anticoagulants, digoxin
gemcitabine	*Contraindications:* Hypersensitivity, breastfeeding *Precautions:* Children, geriatric patients, myelosuppression, radiation, renal/hepatic disease, alcoholism, dental disease, infection *Pregnancy:* Definite fetal risks, may be given in spite of risks if needed in life-threatening conditions	NSAIDs, salicylates, alcohol, anticoagulants, live virus vaccines
fluorouracil	*Contraindications:* Hypersensitivity, breastfeeding, poor nutritional status, infection, dihydropyrimidine *Precautions:* Children, renal/hepatic disease, angina, stomatitis, diarrhea, sunlight exposure, vaccination, occlusive dressing *Pregnancy:* Absolute fetal abnormalities; not to be used anytime during pregnancy	Anticoagulants, antineoplastics, irinotecan, live virus vaccines metronidazole, NSAIDS, platelet inhibitors, thrombolytics
cytarabine	*Contraindications:* Hypersensitivity *Precautions:* Breastfeeding, children, renal/hepatic disease, tumor lysis syndrome, infection, hyperkalemia, hyperphosphatemia, hyperuricemia, hypocalcemia *Pregnancy:* Definite fetal risks, may be given in spite of risks if needed in life-threatening conditions	Live virus vaccines, do not use within 24 hours of chemotherapy, immunosuppressants, methotrexate, radiation, anticoagulants, platelet inhibitors, salicylates, NSAIDs, thrombolytics

Continued

Contraindications, Precautions, and Drug Interactions of Antimetabolites—cont'd

Drug	Contraindications/Precautions	Drug Interaction
mercaptopurine	**Contraindications:** Hypersensitivity, breast-feeding, patients with prior product resistance **Precautions:** Renal/hepatic disease, tumor lysis syndrome, dental disease, herpes, radiation, leukopenia, thrombocytopenia, anemia, infection, hypocalcemia, hyperuricemia, hyperphosphatemia, hyperkalemia **Pregnancy:** Definite fetal risks, may be given in spite of risks if needed in life-threatening conditions	Salicylates, NSAIDs, allopurinol, radiation, immunosuppressants, anticoagulants, thrombolytics, platelet inhibitors, live virus vaccines

*Pregnancy categories have been revised. See http://www.fda.gov/Drugs/DevelopmentApprovalProcess/DevelopmentResources/Labeling/ucm093307.htm for more information.

Adverse Effects/Side Effects
- Weakness
- Nausea
- Vomiting
- Diarrhea
- Pulmonary toxicity
- Hyperglycemia
- Stomatitis
- Hepatotoxicity
- Pancreatitis
- Renal failure
- Hematuria
- Thrombocytopenia
- Leukopenia
- Myelosuppression
- Anemia
- Rash
- Urticaria
- Alopecia

Nursing Care
- Monitor renal/hepatic function
- Monitor for fever
- Monitor I&O
- Monitor for extravasation with IV administration
- Monitor for bleeding
- Teach patient proper and protective oral hygiene
- Teach patient to avoid foods with citric acid
- Teach patient to maintain hydration
- Teach patient to report signs and symptoms of anemia, bleeding, infection

Antineoplastic Antibiotics
- Used to treat cancer
- Examples include daunorubicin, doxorubicin, bleomycin, mitomycin, mitoxantrone
- Available in IV, IM, SUBCUT preparations

Mode of Action
- Insert themselves between adjacent pairs of DNA molecules, resulting in mutant DNA molecules that result in cell death

Contraindications, Precautions, and Drug Interactions of Antineoplastic Antibiotics*

Drug	Contraindications/Precautions	Drug Interaction
daunorubicin	*Contraindications:* Hypersensitivity, breastfeeding, systemic infections, cardiac disease, bone marrow suppression *Precautions:* Tumor lysis syndrome, MI, infection, thrombocytopenia, renal/hepatic disease, gout *Pregnancy:* Definite fetal risks, may be given in spite of risks if needed in life-threatening conditions	Clarithromycin, antidysrhythmics, erythromycin, tricyclic antidepressants, NDSAIDs, salicylates, anticoagulants, platelet inhibitors, thrombolytics
doxorubicin	*Contraindications:* Hypersensitivity, breastfeeding, systemic infections, cardiac disorders, severe myelosuppression, hepatic disease *Precautions:* Cardiac disease, dental work, electrolyte imbalance, infection, hyperuricemia *Pregnancy:* Definite fetal risks, may be given in spite of risks if needed in life-threatening conditions	Progesterone, calcium channel blockers, cyclosporine, mercaptopurine, cyclophosphamide, phenytoin, digoxin, black cohosh, St. John's wort, live virus vaccine
bleomycin	*Contraindications:* Hypersensitivity, breastfeeding, prior idiosyncratic reaction *Precautions:* children, geriatric patients, renal/hepatic disease, respiratory disease *Pregnancy:* Definite fetal risks, may be given in spite of risks if needed in life-threatening conditions	Live virus vaccines, radiation, general anesthesia, filgrastim, sargramostim, phenytoin, digoxin
mitomycin	*Contraindications:* Hypersensitivity, coagulation disorders *Precautions:* Accidental exposure, children, acute bronchospasm, anemia, dental work/disease, extravasation, females, infection, radiation, renal/respiratory disease *Pregnancy:* Definite fetal risks, may be given in spite of risks if needed in life-threatening conditions	Radiation, NSAIDs, anticoagulants, vaccines
mitoxantrone	*Contraindications:* Hypersensitivity *Precautions:* Breastfeeding, children, myelosuppression, renal/cardiac/hepatic disease, gout *Pregnancy:* Definite fetal risks, may be given in spite of risks if needed in life-threatening conditions	Radiation, live virus vaccines, NSAIDs, anticoagulants, digoxin, phenytoin

*Pregnancy categories have been revised. See http://www.fda.gov/Drugs/DevelopmentApprovalProcess/DevelopmentResources/Labeling/ucm093307.htm for more information.

Adverse Effects/Side Effects

- Headache
- Confusion
- Fever
- Chills
- Nausea
- Vomiting

- Myelosuppression
- MI
- Stroke
- Cardiomyopathy
- Nausea
- Vomiting

- Stomatitis
- Hemolytic-uremic syndrome
- Pulmonary toxicity
- Anaphylaxis

Nursing Care

- Monitor for pulmonary toxicity
- Monitor for anaphylaxis
- Monitor for fever
- Monitor renal/hepatic function
- Teach patient to rinse mouth with water TID
- Teach patient some drugs may change the color of urine
- Teach patient to report respiratory changes
- Teach patient to avoid citric acid
- Teach patient to report bleeding

Mitotic Inhibitors

- Used to treat cancer
- Examples include vinblastine, vincristine, vinorelbine
- Available in IV preparations

Mode of Action

- Inhibits mitosis (cell division)

Contraindications, Precautions, and Drug Interactions of Miotic Inhibitors*

Drug	Contraindications/Precautions	Drug Interaction
vinblastine	**Contraindications:** Hypersensitivity, breastfeeding, infants, leukopenia, granulocytopenia, bone marrow suppression, infection, intrathecal use **Precautions:** Renal/hepatic disease, tumor lysis syndrome **Pregnancy:** Definite fetal risks, may be given in spite of risks if needed in life-threatening conditions	Bleomycin, mitomycin, erythromycin, radiation, NSAIDs, anticoagulants, thrombolytics, antiplatelets, antineoplastics, methotrexate, phenytoin, live virus vaccines, CYP3A4 inducers/inhibitors
vincristine	**Contraindications:** Hypersensitivity, breastfeeding, infants, radiation, intrathecal use **Precautions:** Renal/hepatic disease, hypertension, neuromuscular disease **Pregnancy:** Definite fetal risks, may be given in spite of risks if needed in life-threatening conditions	Vaccines, toxoids, digoxin, radiation, mitomycin, calcium channel blockers, CYP3A4 inducers/inhibitors
vinorelbine	**Contraindications:** Hypersensitivity, breastfeeding, infants, granulocyte count <1,000 cells/mm³ pretreatment **Precautions:** Children, geriatric patients, renal/hepatic/pulmonary/neurologic disease, anemia, bone marrow suppression **Pregnancy:** Definite fetal risks, may be given in spite of risks if needed in life-threatening conditions	NSAIDs, anticoagulants, fluconazole, barbiturates, carbamazepine, rifampin, CYP3A4 inducers/inhibitors

*Pregnancy categories have been revised. See http://www.fda.gov/Drugs/DevelopmentApprovalProcess/DevelopmentResources/Labeling/ucm093307.htm for more information.

Adverse Effects/Side Effects

- Paresthesias
- Peripheral neuropathy
- Depression
- Headache
- Seizures
- Tachycardia
- Nausea
- Vomiting
- Constipation
- Stomatitis
- Alopecia
- Hepatotoxicity
- Renal failure
- Thrombocytopenia
- Leukopenia
- Anemia
- Rash
- SIADH

Nursing Care

- Give an antiemetic before administering drug
- Prepare medication per policies and procedures
- If extravasation occurs, stop infusion immediately and notify prescriber
- Do not repeat dosage more frequently than every 7 days due to possible development of severe leukopenia.
- Monitor for bleeding, jaundice, bronchospasm, neuropathy, stomatitis
- Teach patient to maintain adequate fluid intake to promote excretion of uric acid
- Teach patient to restrict fluids in presence of SIADH

Other Inhibitors

- Used to treat cancer
- Examples include cetuximab, panitumumab, lenvatinib, erlotinib, imatinib, dasatinib, nilotinib, sunitinib, bortezomib
- Available in PO, IV preparations

Mode of Action

- Blocks epidermal growth factor, tyrosine, protease, various proteins, and vascular endothelial growth factor that help tumors grow and metastasize

Contraindications, Precautions, and Drug Interactions of Other Inhibitors*

Drug	Contraindications/Precautions	Drug Interaction
cetuximab	**Contraindications:** Hypersensitivity, murine products **Precautions:** Breastfeeding, children, geriatric patients, CV/renal/hepatic, ocular disorders, pulmonary disorders **Pregnancy:** Only given after risks to the fetus are considered; animal studies have shown adverse reactions; no human studies available	Anti-EGFR antibodies
panitumumab	**Contraindications:** Hypersensitivity **Precautions:** Breastfeeding, children, hepatic disease, bronchospasm, hypomagnesemia, diarrhea, hypotension, pulmonary fibrosis, sepsis, soft tissue toxicities **Pregnancy:** Only given after risks to the fetus are considered; animal studies have shown adverse reactions; no human studies available	Antineoplastics

Continued

Contraindications, Precautions, and Drug Interactions of Other Inhibitors—cont'd

Drug	Contraindications/Precautions	Drug Interaction
lenvatinib	*Contraindications:* Hypersensitivity *Precautions:* Breastfeeding, children *Pregnancy:* Only given after risks to the fetus are considered; animal studies have shown adverse reactions; no human studies available	Antineoplastics, CYP3A4 inducers/inhibitors
erlotinib	*Contraindications:* Hypersensitivity, breastfeeding *Precautions:* Children, geriatric patients, diverticulitis, pulmonary/renal/hepatic/otic disorders *Pregnancy:* Definite fetal risks, may be given in spite of risks if needed in life-threatening conditions	Warfarin, NSAIDs, CYP3A4 inhibitors, CYP3A4 inducers, metoprolol, HMG-CoA reductase-inhibitors, proton pump inhibitors, St. John's wort
imatinib	*Contraindications:* Hypersensitivity, breastfeeding *Precautions:* Breastfeeding, children, geriatric patients, cardiac/renal/hepatic/dental disease, bone marrow suppression, immunosuppression, infection, thrombocytopenia, neutropenia, GI bleeding *Pregnancy:* Definite fetal risks, may be given in spite of risks if needed in life-threatening conditions	Acetaminophen, CYP3A4 inducers, CYP3A4 inhibitors, simvastatin, calcium channel blockers, ergots, warfarin, St. John's wort
dasatinib	*Contraindications:* Hypersensitivity *Precautions:* Breastfeeding, children, geriatric patients, QT prolongation, infection, edema, infertility, thrombocytopenia, neutropenia *Pregnancy:* Definite fetal risks, may be given in spite of risks if needed in life-threatening conditions	CYP3A4 substrates, CYP3A4 inhibitors, CYP3A4 inducers, simvastatin, HMG-CoA reductase inhibitors, antidysrhythmics, H2 blockers, proton pump inhibitors
nilotinib	*Contraindications:* Hypersensitivity, breastfeeding *Precautions:* Children, females, geriatric patients, anemia, infection, infertility, thrombocytopenia, neutropenia, pancreatitis, gelatin hypersensitivity, bone marrow suppression *Pregnancy:* Definite fetal risks, may be given in spite of risks if needed in life-threatening conditions	Phenothiazines, pimozide, ziprasidone, antidysrhythmics, local anesthetics, tricyclics, CYP3A4 inhibitors, CYP3A4 substrates, acetaminophen, ketoconazole, erythromycin, clarithromycin, simvastatin, calcium channel blockers, warfarin, dexamethasone, phenytoin, carbamazepine, rifampin, phenobarbital, St. John's wort
sunitinib	*Contraindications:* Hypersensitivity, breastfeeding *Precautions:* Children, females, geriatric patients, QT prolongation, stroke, heart failure, infection, *Pregnancy:* Definite fetal risks, may be given in spite of risks if needed in life-threatening conditions	Bevacizumab, antidysrhythmics, phenothiazines, local anesthetics, tricyclics, CYP3A4 inhibitors, CYP3A4 substrates, acetaminophen, simvastatin, calcium channel blockers, warfarin, dexamethasone, phenytoin, carbamazepine, rifampin, phenobarbital, St. John's wort

CHAPTER 18 Antineoplastic Drugs   **397**

Contraindications, Precautions, and Drug Interactions of Other Inhibitors—cont'd

Drug	Contraindications/Precautions	Drug Interaction
bortezomib	**Contraindications:** Hypersensitivity, breastfeeding **Precautions:** Children, geriatric patients, CV/hepatic disease, hypotension, diabetes mellitus, intracranial bleeding, peripheral neuropathy, tumor lysis syndrome, infection, bone marrow suppression, thrombocytopenia **Pregnancy:** Definite fetal risks, may be given in spite of risks if needed in life-threatening conditions	Oral hypoglycemics, anticoagulants, NSAIDs, salicylates, thrombolytics, platelet inhibitors, antihypertensives, amiodarone, cisplatin, colchicine, cyclosporine, phenytoin, vinblastine, vincristine, statins, CYP3A4 inducers, CYP3A4 inhibitors, oral contraceptives, St. John's wort

*Pregnancy categories have been revised. See http://www.fda.gov/Drugs/DevelopmentApprovalProcess/DevelopmentResources/Labeling/ucm093307.htm for more information.

Adverse Effects/Side Effects

- Headache
- Insomnia
- Aseptic meningitis
- Cardiac arrest
- Nausea
- Vomiting
- Leukopenia
- Anemia
- Neutropenia
- Myelosuppression
- Thrombosis
- Angioedema
- Rash
- Pruritus
- Renal toxicity
- Liver toxicity
- Infusion reactions
- Lung disease
- Pulmonary embolus
- Respiratory arrest
- Anaphylaxis
- Sepsis
- Infection

Nursing Care

- Administer IV infusions slowly, at least over 30 minutes
- Monitor electrolytes and fluid balance
- Monitor for infection
- Monitor renal/hepatic function
- Protect unopened vials of the drug from light
- Teach the patient to report respiratory or cardiac distress immediately
- Advise patient to use contraception during treatment
- Advise patient to wear sunscreen and limit sun exposure
- Teach female patients to avoid pregnancy and breastfeeding
- Teach the patient not to eat grapefruit
- Teach patient to avoid crowds, persons with known infections

APPLICATION AND REVIEW

1. What is the mode of action associated with antineoplastic agents known as alkylating agents?
   1. Inserting themselves between pairs of DNA molecules, causing mutant DNA molecules
   2. Damaging DNA by halting the replication process and cross linking DNA strands
   3. Inhibiting both DNA and RNA synthesis
   4. Inhibiting mitosis or cell division

2. What information should a pregnant woman be given regarding the use of an alkylating agent for the treatment of her cancerous tumor?
   1. There are no known fetal risks
   2. Fetal risks exist, but treatment may be warranted
   3. Fetal risks have been identified in animal studies only
   4. Fetal risks are severe and inevitable, so the medication is contraindicated

3. Which drug intervention poses a potential risk for drug interaction when administered with most antineoplastic agents?
   1. Proton pump inhibitors
   2. Live virus vaccines
   3. Beta blockers
   4. Salicylates

4. When considering adverse effects of miotic inhibitors, which nursing intervention is appropriate? **Select all that apply.**
   1. Screening for depression
   2. Medication for nausea
   3. Seizure precautions
   4. Assess for insomnia
   5. I&O

5. Which type of antineoplastic therapy requires at least 7 days between doses to minimize the risk of developing severe leukopenia?
   1. Antimetabolites
   2. Miotic inhibitors
   3. Alkylating agents
   4. Antineoplastic antibiotics

See Answers on pages 407-409.

Hormones and Hormone Modulators

- Used to treat hormone dependent tumors found in the prostate, breast, and endometrium
- Examples include exemestane, anastrozole, letrozole, tamoxifen citrate, toremifene citrate, fulvestrant, testosterone enanthate, flutamide, medroxyprogesterone acetate, megestrol acetate, goserelin acetate, leuprolide acetate
- Available in PO, IM, SUBCUT, transdermal preparations

Mode of Action
- Alters growth of tumors found in sexual organs

Contraindications, Precautions, and Drug Interactions of Hormones and Hormone Modulators*

Drug	Contraindications/Precautions	Drug Interaction
exemestane	*Contraindications:* Hypersensitivity, breastfeeding, premenopausal women *Precautions:* Children, geriatric patients, renal/hepatic disease, osteoporosis, vitamin D deficiency *Pregnancy:* Absolute fetal abnormalities; not to be used at any time during pregnancy	Estrogens, CYP3A4 inducers

Contraindications, Precautions, and Drug Interactions of Hormones and Hormone Modulators—cont'd

Drug	Contraindications/Precautions	Drug Interaction
anastrozole	*Contraindications:* Hypersensitivity, breastfeeding *Precautions:* Children, geriatric patients, premenopausal women, osteoporosis, hepatic/cardiac disease *Pregnancy:* Absolute fetal abnormalities; not to be used at any time during pregnancy	Oral contraceptives, estrogen, tamoxifen, DHEA, androstene-dione
letrozole	*Contraindications:* Hypersensitivity, premenopausal women *Precautions:* Respiratory/hepatic disease, osteoporosis *Pregnancy:* Definite fetal risks, may be given in spite of risks if needed in life-threatening conditions	Estrogens, oral contraceptives
tamoxifen citrate	*Contraindications:* Hypersensitivity, breastfeeding *Precautions:* Women of childbearing age, leukopenia, thrombocytopenia, cataracts *Pregnancy:* Definite fetal risks, may be given in spite of risks if needed in life-threatening conditions	Paroxetine, anticoagulants, bromocriptine, cytotoxics, CYP34A inhibitors, aminoglutethimide, rifamycin, letrozole, CYP2D6 inhibitors (antidepressants)
fulvestrant	*Contraindications:* Hypersensitivity, breastfeeding, children *Precautions:* Hepatic disease, jaundice, thrombocytopenia, biliary tract disease, coagulopathy *Pregnancy:* Definite fetal risks, may be given in spite of risks if needed in life-threatening conditions	Anticoagulants
testosterone enanthate	*Contraindications:* Hypersensitivity, breastfeeding, severe cardiac/renal/hepatic disease, genital bleeding, male breast/prostate cancer *Precautions:* Diabetes mellitus, cardiovascular disease, MI, urinary tract disorders, prostate cancer, hypercalcemia *Pregnancy:* Absolute fetal abnormalities; not to be used at any time during pregnancy	Adrenal steroids, ACTH, bupropion, oxyphenbutazone, anticoagulants, insulin, antidiabetics
flutamide	*Contraindications:* Hypersensitivity *Precautions:* G6PD deficiency, hemoglobinopathy, lactase deficiency, polycystic ovary syndrome, tobacco smoking *Pregnancy:* Definite fetal risks, may be given in spite of risks if needed in life-threatening conditions	Warfarin, leuprolide
medroxyprogesterone acetate	*Contraindications:* Hypersensitivity, reproductive cancer, genital bleeding, missed abortion, stroke, cerebrovascular disease, cervical/uterine/vaginal cancer, hepatic disease *Precautions:* Breastfeeding, children, hypertension, asthma, blood dyscrasias, gallbladder disease, CHF, diabetes mellitus, bone disease, depression, migraine headache, seizure disorder, renal/hepatic disease, bone loss, ocular disorders, HIV/AIDS, alcoholism, hyperlipidemia *Pregnancy:* Absolute fetal abnormalities; not to be used at any time during pregnancy	Anticoagulants, corticosteroids, aminoglutethimide, carbamazepine, phenytoins, phenobarbital, rifampin

Continued

Contraindications, Precautions, and Drug Interactions of Hormones and Hormone Modulators—cont'd

Drug	Contraindications/Precautions	Drug Interaction
megestrol acetate	*Contraindications:* Hypersensitivity *Precautions:* Diabetes, thrombosis, adrenal insufficiency *Pregnancy:* Definite fetal risks, may be given in spite of risks if needed in life-threatening conditions	Dofetilide, antidiabetics
goserelin acetate	*Contraindications:* Hypersensitivity, breastfeeding, children, vaginal bleeding, LHRH-agonist analogs *Precautions:* Renal disease, spinal cord decompression, bone loss, hyperglycemia, diabetes mellitus, cardiovascular disease *Pregnancy:* Absolute fetal abnormalities; not to be used at any time during pregnancy	Oral contraceptives, antidiabetic agents
leuprolide acetate	*Contraindications:* Hypersensitivity, breastfeeding, children, vaginal bleeding, thromboembolic disorders *Precautions:* Hepatic disease, hypertension, CVA, MI, CHF, seizures, edema, depression, diabetes mellitus, osteoporosis, spinal cord compression, urinary tract obstruction *Pregnancy:* Absolute fetal abnormalities; not to be used at any time during pregnancy	Flutamide, megestrol, black cohosh

*Pregnancy categories have been revised. See http://www.fda.gov/Drugs/DevelopmentApprovalProcess/DevelopmentResources/Labeling/ucm093307.htm for more information.

Adverse Effects/Side Effects
- Thrombophlebitis
- Myocardial infarction
- CVA
- Deep vein thrombosis
- Pulmonary embolism
- Dizziness
- Fever
- Pharyngitis
- Nausea
- Anorexia
- Hot flashes
- Urinary tract infection
- Vaginal bleeding
- Vaginal dryness
- Alopecia
- Pruritus
- Increased sweating
- Muscle/joint aches

Nursing Care
- Administer after meals
- Do not administer with estrogen-containing drugs
- Administer only to postmenopausal women
- Administer analgesics for pain
- Monitor patient for Stevens-Johnson syndrome
- Teach patient that vaginal bleeding, pruritus, hot flashes decrease after drug discontinuation
- Teach patient to take calcium and vitamin D to prevent bone loss

Monoclonal Antibodies
- Used to treat cancer
- Examples include rituximab, nivolumab, trastuzumab, dinutuximab
- Available in IV preparations

Mode of Action
- Bind to cancer cells causing tumor death; trigger immune system to attack cancer cells

Contraindications, Precautions, and Drug Interactions of Monoclonal Antibodies*

Drug	Contraindications/Precautions	Drug Interaction
rituximab	*Contraindications:* Hypersensitivity, murine proteins *Precautions:* Breastfeeding, children, geriatric patients, cardiac/pulmonary/renal disease *Pregnancy:* Only given after risks to the fetus are considered; animal studies have shown adverse reactions; no human studies available	Antihypertensives, cisplatin, anticoagulants, vaccines, toxoids
nivolumab	*Contraindications:* Hypersensitivity, murine proteins *Precautions:* Breastfeeding, children, geriatric patients, cardiac/pulmonary/renal disease *Pregnancy:* Only given after risks to the fetus are considered; animal studies have shown adverse reactions; no human studies available	Vaccines, toxoids
trastuzumab	*Contraindications:* Hypersensitivity, Chinese hamster ovary cell protein *Precautions:* Breastfeeding, children, geriatric patients, pulmonary disease, anemia, leukopenia *Pregnancy:* Definite fetal risks, may be given in spite of risks if needed in life-threatening conditions	Warfarin, anthracyclines, cyclophosphamide, vaccines, toxoids
dinutuximab	*Contraindications:* Hypersensitivity *Precautions:* Breastfeeding, children, geriatric patients, cardiac/pulmonary/renal disease *Pregnancy:* Only given after risks to the fetus are considered; animal studies have shown adverse reactions; no human studies available	Vaccines, toxoids

*Pregnancy categories have been revised. See http://www.fda.gov/Drugs/DevelopmentApprovalProcess/DevelopmentResources/Labeling/ucm093307.htm for more information.

Adverse Effects/Side Effects

- Dysrhythmia
- Heart failure
- Hypertension
- MI
- GI obstruction/perforation
- Renal failure
- Leukopenia
- Neutropenia
- Thrombocytopenia
- Infection
- Nausea
- Vomiting
- Rash
- Bronchospasm

Nursing Care

- Monitor patient for infection
- Monitor fluid intake
- Teach patient to use contraception during and for 12 months after therapy
- Teach patient to avoid crowds, those with infection
- Teach patient to avoid OTC products

Podophyllotoxins

- Used to treat cancer
- Examples include etoposide, teniposide
- Available in PO, IV preparations

Mode of Action
- Inhibits DNA/RNA synthesis in tumor cells

Contraindications, Precautions, and Drug Interactions of Podophyllotoxins*

Drug	Contraindications/Precautions	Drug Interaction
etoposide	**Contraindications:** Hypersensitivity, breastfeeding **Precautions:** Children, renal/hepatic disease, gout, neutropenia, thrombocytopenia **Pregnancy:** Definite fetal risks, may be given in spite of risks if needed in life-threatening conditions	Antineoplastics, radiation, immunosuppressives, anticoagulants, NSAIDs, salicylates, thrombolytics, platelet inhibitors, sargramostim, filgrastim, voriconazole, cyclosporine, imatinib, telithromycin, CYP3A4 inhibitors
teniposide	**Contraindications:** Hypersensitivity, breastfeeding **Precautions:** Children, renal/hepatic disease, gout, neutropenia, thrombocytopenia **Pregnancy:** Definite fetal risks, may be given in spite of risks if needed in life-threatening conditions	Sodium salicylate, sulfamethizole, tolbutamide, methotrexate, vincristine, vaccines

*Pregnancy categories have been revised. See http://www.fda.gov/Drugs/DevelopmentApprovalProcess/DevelopmentResources/Labeling/ucm093307.htm for more information.

Adverse Effects/Side Effects
- Headache
- Fever
- Nausea
- Vomiting
- Peripheral neuropathy
- MI
- Dysrhythmia
- Hepatotoxicity
- Nephrotoxicity
- Thrombocytopenia
- Leukopenia
- Myelosuppression
- Anemia
- Alopecia
- Rash
- Bronchospasm
- Anaphylaxis

Nursing Care
- Monitor patient for infection, jaundice, bleeding
- Administer IV infusions slowly, at least over 30 minutes
- Stop infusion if patient experiences hypotension
- Teach patient to store capsules in the refrigerator
- Teach patient to report signs of respiratory distress
- Teach patient metallic taste may occur
- Teach patient hair loss is possible but reversible after treatment
- Teach patient to avoid grapefruit juice

Interferons
- Used to treat cancer
- Examples include interferon alfa-2a, alfa-2b, and alfa-n3
- Available in SUBCUT, IM, IV preparations

Mode of Action
- Slows the rate of cell proliferation in cancer tumors

Contraindications, Precautions, and Drug Interactions of Interferons*

Drug	Contraindications/Precautions	Drug Interaction
alpha-2a, alpha 2-b, alpha-n3	*Contraindications:* Hypersensitivity, autoimmune disorders, infections, ischemic disorders, neuropsychiatric disorders *Precautions:* Breastfeeding, children, mental illness, thrombocytopenia *Pregnancy:* Only given after risks to the fetus are considered; animal studies have shown adverse reactions; no human studies available	CNS depressants, theophylline, aminophylline, live virus vaccine, radiation
beta-1b	*Contraindications:* Hypersensitivity, hypersensitivity to human albumin, hamster protein, rotavirus vaccine *Precautions:* Breastfeeding, children, mental disorders, depression, seizure disorder, chronic progressive MS, latex allergy, autoimmune disorders, hepatotoxicity, alcoholism, chickenpox, herpes zoster, bone marrow suppression, cardiac disease *Pregnancy:* Only given after risks to the fetus are considered; animal studies have shown adverse reactions; no human studies available	Antiretrovirals, antineoplastics, zidovudine
gamma-1b	*Contraindications:* Hypersensitivity, hypersensitivity to interferon *Precautions:* Breastfeeding, children <1 yr, cardiac disease, seizure disorders, myelosuppression, CNS disorders *Pregnancy:* Only given after risks to the fetus are considered; animal studies have shown adverse reactions; no human studies available	Myelosuppressive agents, theophylline, aminophylline, protease inhibitors, NRTIs, NNRTIs

*Pregnancy categories have been revised. See http://www.fda.gov/Drugs/DevelopmentApprovalProcess/DevelopmentResources/Labeling/ucm093307.htm for more information.

Adverse Effects/Side Effects

- Hematotoxicity
- Kidney failure
- Nausea
- Diarrhea
- Anorexia
- Fever
- Fatigue
- Headache
- Chills
- Joint pain
- Muscle pain
- Hypotension
- Edema
- Coughing
- Shortness of breath
- Depression
- Suicidal thoughts

Nursing Care

- Administer at night to decrease daytime drowsiness
- Administer with acetaminophen to decrease flulike symptoms
- Monitor for signs of bleeding
- Monitor intake of fluids
- Refrigerate medication
- Teach the patient to report respiratory or cardiac distress
- Teach female patients they may experience dysmenorrheal or breast pain
- Teach patient to use sunscreen and avoid the sun

Colony-Stimulating Factors

- Used to treat cancer-associated anemia
- Examples include epoetin alpha, darbepoetin alfa, sargramostim, filgrastim
- Available in SUBCUT, IV preparations

Mode of Action

- Increase bone marrow stem cells to aid in treatment of cancer

Contraindications, Precautions, and Drug Interactions of Colony-Stimulating Factors*

Drug	Contraindications/Precautions	Drug Interaction
epoetin alfa	**Contraindications:** Hypersensitivity, autoimmune disorders, infections, ischemic disorders, neuropsychiatric disorders **Precautions:** Breastfeeding, children, mental illness, thrombocytopenia **Pregnancy:** Only given after risks to the fetus are considered; animal studies have shown adverse reactions; no human studies available	Androgens, other colony-stimulating factors
darbepoetin alfa	**Contraindications:** Hypersensitivity, autoimmune disorders, infections, ischemic disorders, neuropsychiatric disorders **Precautions:** Breastfeeding, children, mental illness, thrombocytopenia **Pregnancy:** Only given after risks to the fetus are considered; animal studies have shown adverse reactions; no human studies available	Androgens, other colony-stimulating factors
sargramostim	**Contraindications:** Hypersensitivity, mannitol hypersensitivity, neonates, leukemic myeloid blast in bone marrow/peripheral blood **Precautions:** Breastfeeding, children, lung/cardiac/hepatic/renal disease, peripheral edema, pericardial effusions, leukocytosis, **Pregnancy:** Only given after risks to the fetus are considered; animal studies have shown adverse reactions; no human studies available	Corticosteroids, lithium
filgrastim	**Contraindications:** Hypersensitivity, hypersensitivity to proteins of *Escherichia coli* **Precautions:** Breastfeeding, children, myeloid malignancies, respiratory disease, radiation, sepsis, chemotherapy, sickle cell disease **Pregnancy:** Only given after risks to the fetus are considered; animal studies have shown adverse reactions; no human studies available	Antineoplastics, lithium

*Pregnancy categories have been revised. See http://www.fda.gov/Drugs/DevelopmentApprovalProcess/DevelopmentResources/Labeling/ucm093307.htm for more information.

Adverse Effects/Side Effects

- Angioedema
- Bronchospasm
- MI
- Seizure
- Stroke
- Thromboembolism
- Hypertension
- Heart failure
- Encephalopathy
- Myalgia
- Arthralgia
- Cephalgia
- Cough
- Nausea
- Vomiting
- Pruritus
- Urticaria
- Dizziness
- Fever
- Insomnia
- Anemia
- Hypokalemia

Nursing Care

- Monitor hematologic, renal, hepatic studies
- Monitor fluid status
- Monitor for infection
- Monitor for blood clots
- Teach patient not to come into contact with semen of patient taking these drugs
- Teach patient that volume of ejaculate may be decreased during treatment

Interleukins

- Used to improve immune response to cancer
- Example includes aldesleukin
- Available in SUBCUT, IV preparations

Mode of Action

- Stimulates immunologic reaction against tumor

Contraindications, Precautions, and Drug Interactions of Interleukins*

Drug	Contraindications/Precautions	Drug Interaction
aldesleukin	**Contraindications:** Hypersensitivity, cardiac/respiratory/renal disease, MI, cardiac arrhythmias, cardiac tamponade, tachycardia, angina, GI bleed/perforation, psychosis, organ transplant, seizures **Precautions:** Breastfeeding, children, mental illness, thrombocytopenia **Pregnancy:** Only given after risks to the fetus are considered; animal studies have shown adverse reactions; no human studies available	Dexamethasone, NSAIDs, vancomycin, cyclosporine, methotrexate, beta blockers, calcium channel blockers, vaccines

*Pregnancy categories have been revised. See http://www.fda.gov/Drugs/DevelopmentApprovalProcess/DevelopmentResources/Labeling/ucm093307.htm for more information.

Adverse Effects/Side Effects

- Shortness of breath
- Stomatitis
- Nausea
- Vomiting
- Anemia
- Thrombocytopenia
- Leukopenia
- Acidosis
- Hypomagnesemia
- Urinary retention
- Hypertension
- Hypocalcemia

Nursing Care

- Monitor hematologic, renal, hepatic studies
- Monitor for cardiac and respiratory distress
- Teach patient to report adverse effects to the prescriber

Miscellaneous Antineoplastics

- Used to treat cancer or associated related disorders
- Examples include hydroxyurea
- Available in PO preparations

Mode of Action

- Impedes DNA/RNA synthesis of cancer cells

Contraindications, Precautions, and Drug Interactions of Miscellaneous Antineoplastics*

Drug	Contraindications/Precautions	Drug Interaction
hydroxyurea	**Contraindications:** Hypersensitivity, breastfeeding, leukopenia, thrombocytopenia, anemia **Precautions:** Geriatric patients, infection, bone marrow suppression, anemia, renal/dental disease, HIV, hyperkalemia, hypocalcemia, hyperuricemia, infertility, tumor lysis syndrome, vaccinations **Pregnancy:** Definite fetal risks, may be given in spite of risks if needed in life-threatening conditions	Didanosine, stavudine, antineoplastics, radiation, NSAIDs, anticoagulants, thrombolytics, salicylates, platelet inhibitors, sargramostim, filgrastim, probenecid, sulfinpyrazone

*Pregnancy categories have been revised. See http://www.fda.gov/Drugs/DevelopmentApprovalProcess/DevelopmentResources/Labeling/ucm093307.htm for more information.

Adverse Effects/Side Effects

- Headache
- Dizziness
- Confusion
- Seizures
- Coma
- Nausea
- Vomiting
- Diarrhea
- Stomatitis
- Pancreatitis
- Hepatotoxicity
- Angina
- Anemia
- Thrombocytopenia
- Leukopenia
- Megaloblastic erythropoiesis
- Myelosuppression
- Rash
- Urticaria
- Pruritus

Nursing Care

- Monitor hematologic, renal, hepatic studies
- Monitor for respiratory/cardiac distress
- Monitor I&O
- Monitor for electrolyte imbalance and acidosis
- Monitor for infection, bone marrow suppression
- Monitor for bleeding
- Warn the patient that alopecia occurs in majority of patients
- Teach patient to rinse mouth with water 2 to 3 times daily
- Teach patient to report signs and symptoms of anemia, bleeding, infection
- Teach patient to avoid foods with citric acid

APPLICATION AND REVIEW

6. What is the mode of action associated with antineoplastic agents known as hormone modulators?
   1. Inhibits DNA/RNA synthesis in tumor cells
   2. Alters growth of tumors found in sexual organs
   3. Slows the rate of cell proliferation in cancer tumors
   4. Binds to cancer cells triggering the immune system to attack those cells

7. What information should a pregnant woman be given regarding the use of monoclonal antibodies for the treatment of her cancerous tumor? **Select all that apply.**
   1. There are no known fetal risks
   2. No human studies are available
   3. Fetal risk is low after first trimester
   4. Given only after risks to the fetus are considered
   5. Medication is contraindicated at all stages of pregnancy

8. When considering adverse effects of interleukins, which nursing intervention is appropriate? **Select all that apply.**
   1. Assess for orthostatic hypotension
   2. Access to supplemental oxygen
   3. Seizure precautions
   4. Frequent oral care
   5. I&O

9. Which female client is a good candidate for hormonal modulator therapy with the drug exemestane?
   1. A breastfeeding mother
   2. A premenopausal woman
   3. The client with a diagnosis of osteoporosis
   4. A woman with a diagnosis of chronic depression

10. Which medical diagnosis is considered a contraindication for the administration of interleukin therapy? **Select all that apply.**
    1. Angina
    2. Seizures
    3. Psychosis
    4. Renal disease
    5. Sickle cell anemia

See Answers on pages 407-409.

ANSWER KEY: REVIEW QUESTIONS

1. **2 Alkylating agents damage deoxyribonucleic acid (DNA) by halting the replication process and cross linking DNA strands.**
   1 Antineoplastic antibiotics insert themselves between adjacent pairs of DNA molecules, causing mutant DNA molecules. 3 Antimetabolites inhibit both DNA and RNA synthesis. 4 Mitotic inhibitors prevent mitosis or cell division.
   Client Need: Pharmacologic and Parenteral Therapies; **Cognitive Level:** Analysis; **Nursing Process:** Assessment/Analysis

> **Study Tip:** When you think of the word "alkylating," imagine an 'h' at the beginning: halkylating because that will help you see the word "halt" in it: **hal**kyla**t**ing to help you recall that alkylating agents' mode of action is to *halt* the replication of DNA.

2. **2 Definite fetal risks exist but alkylating agents may be given in spite of risks if needed in life-threatening conditions.**
   1 Fetal risks are definitely known to exist with the administration of alkylating agents. 3 Fetal risks are definitely known to exist with the administration of alkylating agents. 4 Definite fetal risks exist but alkylating agents may be given in spite of risks if needed in life-threatening conditions.

Client Need: Pharmacologic and Parenteral Therapies; **Cognitive Level:** Analysis; **Integrated Process:** Teaching/Learning; **Nursing Process:** Planning/Implementation

3. **2 Live virus vaccines pose a risk for drug interaction when administered during most forms of antineoplastic medication therapy.**

1 Proton pump inhibitors pose a risk for drug interaction with only a few specific antineoplastic medications. **3** Beta blocks pose a risk for drug interaction with only a few specific antineoplastic medications. **4** Salicylates pose a risk for drug interaction with only a few specific antineoplastic medications.

Client Need: Pharmacologic and Parenteral Therapies; **Cognitive Level:** Analysis; **Nursing Process:** Assessment/Analysis

4. **Answers: 1, 2, 3, 5**

Adverse effects of miotic inhibitor therapy include depression, nausea, seizures, and renal failure.

4 Insomnia is not generally acknowledged as an adverse effect of miotic inhibitors.

Client Need: Pharmacologic and Parenteral Therapies; **Cognitive Level:** Analysis; **Nursing Process:** Planning/Implementation

5. **2 Miotic inhibitor therapy requires at least 7 days between doses in order to help prevent the development of severe leukopenia.**

1 Leukopenia is not associated with possible adverse reactions to antimetabolites therapy. **3** Although leukopenia is recognized as a possible adverse reaction to alkylating agents, the 7 days between dose schedule is not required. **4** Leukopenia is not associated with possible adverse reactions to antineoplastic antibiotic therapy.

Client Need: Pharmacologic and Parenteral Therapies; **Cognitive Level:** Analysis; **Nursing Process:** Planning/Implementation

> **Study Tip:** Here's a silly sentence to help you remember the 7-day gap between doses of miotic inhibitor therapy: "I like to keep at least 7 days between **m(i)**yself and **tic**(k)s."

6. **2 Hormone modulators alter growth of tumors found in sexual organs.**

1 Podophyllotoxins inhibit DNA/RNA synthesis in tumor cells. **3** Interferons slow the rate of cell proliferation in cancer tumors. **4** Monoclonal antibodies bind to cancer cells triggering the immune system to attack those cells.

Client Need: Pharmacologic and Parenteral Therapies; **Cognitive Level:** Analysis; **Nursing Process:** Assessment/Analysis

7. **Answers: 2, 4**

Monoclonal antibiotics are prescribed only after risks to the fetus are considered as animal studies involving monoclonal antibodies have shown adverse reactions but no human studies available.

1 Animal research studies confirm fetal risks exist with the administration of monoclonal antibodies. **3** Animal research studies confirm fetal risks exist with the administration of monoclonal antibodies regardless of trimester. **5** Monoclonal antibiotics are prescribed only after risks to the fetus are considered.

Client Need: Pharmacologic and Parenteral Therapies; **Cognitive Level:** Analysis; **Integrated Process:** Teaching/Learning; **Nursing Process:** Planning/Implementation

8. **Answers: 2, 4, 5**

Adverse effects of interleukins therapy include shortness of breath, stomatitis, and urinary retention.

1 Hypertension not hypotension is an adverse reaction to interleukin therapy. **3** Seizures are not associated with adverse reactions to interleukin therapy.

Client Need: Pharmacologic and Parenteral Therapies; **Cognitive Level:** Analysis; **Nursing Process:** Planning/Implementation

9. **4 Chronic depression is neither a precaution or contraindication for hormonal modulator therapy.**

   1 Breastfeeding is a contraindication for hormonal modulator therapy. **2** Being premenopausal is a contraindication for hormonal modulator therapy. **3** Osteoporosis is a precautionary condition that must be evaluated when considering hormonal modulator therapy.

   Client Need: Pharmacologic and Parenteral Therapies; **Cognitive Level:** Analysis; **Nursing Process:** Assessment/Analysis

10. **Answers: 1, 2, 3 4**

    Contraindications to interleukin therapy include angina, seizures, psychosis, and renal disease.

    5 Sickle cell anemia is not a contraindication to interleukin therapy.

    Client Need: Pharmacologic and Parenteral Therapies; **Cognitive Level:** Analysis; **Process:** Assessment/Analysis

Immunomodulating and Immunosuppressant Drugs

REVIEW OF PHYSIOLOGY (IMMUNITY)

Nonspecific Immune Response

- Directed against invading microbes
- Body surface barriers: intact skin and mucosa, cilia, and mucus secretions
- Antimicrobial secretions: oil of skin, tears, gastric juice, and vaginal secretions
- Internal antimicrobial agents
  - Interferon: substance produced within cells in response to viral attack
  - Properdin (Factor P): protein agent in blood that destroys certain gram-negative bacteria and viruses
  - Lysozyme: destroys mainly gram-positive bacteria
- Phagocytes (monocytes, macrophages): cells that ingest and destroy microbes; part of reticuloendothelial system
- Inflammatory response
  - First stage: release of histamine and chemical mediators (e.g., prostaglandin, bradykinin) leads to vascular dilation and increased capillary permeability, resulting in signs of inflammation (e.g., pain, heat, redness, edema, and loss of function)
  - Second stage: exudate production
  - Third stage: reparative phase

Specific Immune Response

- Directed against a specific pathogen (foreign protein) or its toxin
- May be cell-mediated or humoral
- Cell-mediated immunity
  - Occurs within cells of immune system
  - Involves T lymphocytes (e.g., T helper, T suppressor, T cytotoxic, lymphokines); each type plays a distinct role in immune response
  - Cluster designations: mature T cells carry markers on surface that permit them to be classified structurally (e.g., CD4 cells associated with acquired immunodeficiency syndrome [AIDS])
  - Functions of cell-mediated immunity
    - Protect against most viral, fungal, protozoan, and slow-growing bacterial infections
    - Reject histoincompatible grafts
    - Cause skin hypersensitivity reactions (e.g., tuberculosis [TB] screening)
    - Assists with diagnosis of malignancies
- Humoral immunity: concerned with immune responses outside of cell; involves B lymphocytes that differentiate into plasma cells and secrete antibodies
  - Antigen: any substance, including allergen, that stimulates production of antibodies in body; typically, antigens are foreign proteins, most potent being microbial cells and their products
  - Antibody: immune substance produced by plasma cells; antibodies are gamma globulin molecules; commonly referred to as immunoglobulin (Ig)

- Complement-fixation: group of blood serum proteins needed in certain antigen-antibody reactions; both complement and antibody must be present for reaction to occur
- Types of immunoglobulins
  - Immunoglobulin M (IgM) antibodies: first antibodies to be detected after exposure to antigen; protection from gram-negative bacteria
  - Immunoglobulin G (IgG) antibodies: make up more than 75% of total immunoglobulins; highest increase in response to subsequent exposure to antigen; only immunoglobulin that passes placental barrier
  - Immunoglobulin A (IgA) antibodies: present in blood, mucus, and human milk secretions; play important role against viral and respiratory pathogens
  - Immunoglobulin E (IgE) antibodies: responsible for hypersensitivity and allergic responses; cause mast cells to release histamine; protection from parasites
  - Immunoglobulin D (IgD) antibodies: help differentiate B lymphocytes

Types of Immunity

- Active immunity: antibodies formed in body
  - Natural active immunity: antibodies formed during course of disease; may provide lifelong immunity (e.g., measles, chickenpox, yellow fever, smallpox)
  - Artificial active immunity: vaccine or toxoid stimulate formation of homologous antibodies; revaccination (booster shot) often needed to sustain antibody titer (anamnestic effect)
    - Killed vaccines: antigenic preparations containing killed microbes (e.g., pertussis vaccine, typhoid vaccine)
    - Live vaccines: antigenic preparations containing weakened (attenuated) microbes; typically such vaccines are more antigenic than killed preparations (e.g., oral [Sabin] poliomyelitis vaccine, measles vaccine)
    - Toxoids: antigenic preparations composed of inactivated bacterial toxins (e.g., tetanus toxoids, diphtheria toxoids)
    - Current vaccination schedules for the United States can be found at: https://www.cdc.gov/vaccines/schedules/hcp/imz/child-adolescent.html
- Passive immunity: antibodies acquired from outside source produce short-term immunity
  - Natural passive immunity: passage of preformed antibodies from mother through placenta to fetus or though colostrum to neonate; during first few weeks of life, newborn is immune to certain diseases to which mother has active immunity
  - Artificial passive immunity: injection of antisera derived from immunized animals or humans; provide immediate protection and also are of value in treatment (e.g., diphtheria antitoxin, tetanus antitoxin)

APPLICATION AND REVIEW

1. A senior high school student whose immunization status is current asks the school nurse which immunizations will be included in the precollege physical. Which vaccine should the nurse tell the student to expect to receive?
    1. Hepatitis C (HepC)
    2. Influenza type B (HIB)
    3. Measles, mumps, rubella (MMR)
    4. Diphtheria, tetanus, pertussis (TDaP)

2. A 70-year-old client with the diagnosis of heart failure and chronic obstructive pulmonary disease (COPD) is admitted to a unit in a long-term care facility for a cardiopulmonary rehabilitation program. Pneumococcal and flu vaccines are administered. The client asks the nurse if the pneumococcal vaccine has to be taken every year like the flu vaccine. How should the nurse respond?
   1. "You need to receive the pneumococcal vaccine every other year."
   2. "The pneumococcal vaccine should be received in early autumn every year."
   3. "You should get the flu and pneumococcal vaccines at your annual physical examination."
   4. "It is unnecessary to have any follow-up injections of the pneumococcal vaccine after this dose."

3. A nurse is caring for a client with an impaired immune system. Which blood protein associated with the immune system is important for the nurse to consider?
   1. Albumin
   2. Globulin
   3. Thrombin
   4. Hemoglobin

4. A client who was exposed to hepatitis A asks why an injection of gamma globulin is needed. Before responding, what should the nurse consider about how it provides passive immunity?
   1. It increases production of short-lived antibodies.
   2. It accelerates antigen-antibody union at the hepatic sites.
   3. The lymphatic system is stimulated to produce antibodies.
   4. The antigen is neutralized by the antibodies that it supplies.

5. A client is admitted to the emergency department with a contaminated wound. The client is a poor historian, and the nurse realizes that it is impossible to determine whether the client is immunized against tetanus. Which medication does the nurse expect the health care provider to prescribe because it will produce passive immunity for several weeks with minimal danger of an allergic reaction?
   1. Tetanus toxoid
   2. Equine tetanus antitoxin
   3. Human tetanus antitoxin
   4. Diphtheria, tetanus, pertussis vaccine

6. A client who is suspected of having tetanus asks a nurse about immunizations against tetanus. Before responding, what should the nurse consider about the benefits of tetanus antitoxin?
   1. It stimulates plasma cells directly.
   2. A high titer of antibodies is generated.
   3. It provides immediate active immunity.
   4. A long-lasting passive immunity is produced.

7. A client is seeking treatment for seasonal pollen triggered allergies. Medication prescribed will focus on the functions of which immunoglobulin antibodies?
   1. M (IgM)
   2. A (IgA)
   3. E (IgE)
   4. D (IgD)

8. Medication prescribed for the management of seasonal pollen allergies will focus on the first stage of the inflammatory response with the purpose of initially interpreting with what process?
   1. Exudate production
   2. Release of histamine
   3. Vascular constriction
   4. Decreasing capillary permeability

See Answers on pages 426–429.

SELECTED DISORDERS TREATED WITH IMMUNOMODULATORS

Rheumatoid Arthritis (RA)

- Altered immune response
  - Enzymes destroy collagen
  - Synovial membrane proliferates, forming pannus, which destroys cartilage and bone
  - HLA-DR4 antibody usually present
- Other effects: fever, weight loss, anemia, Raynaud phenomenon, arteritis, neuropathy, pericarditis, ankylosis, and Sjögren syndrome
- Etiology unclear; apparent genetic predisposition; incidence higher in women

Multiple Sclerosis

- Destruction of myelin in the CNS by sensitized T and B lymphocytes, causing randomly scattered plaques of sclerotic tissue on demyelinated axons; frequently affected areas include optic nerves, cerebrum, brainstem, cerebellum, and spinal cord
- Considered a chronic, debilitating, progressive disease with periods of remission and exacerbation
- Types
  - Relapsing-remitting (RR): acute episodes with almost a complete recovery between attacks
  - Primary progressive (PP): steady degenerative progression without exacerbation
  - Secondary progressive (SP): initially RR followed by steady deterioration later in disease process
  - Progressive-relapsing (PR); progressive but with periodic acute exacerbations
- Cause unknown; viral, environmental, and immunologic causes are implicated
- Onset in early adult life (20 to 40 years); higher incidence in females, Caucasians, those living in temperate climates, and those with trigeminal neuralgia
- Fatigue, stress, and heat tend to increase symptoms

Neoplastic Disease

- See Chapter 18

IMMUNOMODULATING DRUGS

Interleukin Receptor Agonists

- Used to treat metastatic renal cancer and metastatic melanoma
- Examples: aldesleukin (IL-2)
- Available in intravenous form

Mode of Action

- Binds to receptor sites on T cells, which stimulates the T cells to multiply

Contraindications, Precautions, and Drug Interactions of Interleukin Receptor Agonists*

Drug	Contraindications/Precautions	Drug Interaction
aldesleukin (IL-2)	**Contraindications:** Angina, cardiac arrhythmias, cardiac disease, cardiac tamponade, coma, gastrointestinal bleeding, gastrointestinal perforation, myocardial infarction, organ transplant, psychosis, pulmonary disease, renal failure, respiratory insufficiency, seizures, ventricular tachycardia **Precautions:** Cardiac disease, central nervous system impairments, diabetes, electrolyte imbalance, hepatic disease, hyperglycemia, metabolic and respiratory acidosis, pulmonary disease, renal disease **Pregnancy:** Only given after risks to the fetus are considered	Antihypertensives, beta blockers, calcium channel blockers, corticosteroids, cyclosporine, drugs known to cause such kidney/liver toxicity, ethanol, isoniazid, methotrexate, nonsteroidal antiinflammatory drugs, vaccines, vancomycin *Many other drugs can cause potential interaction.*

*Pregnancy categories have been revised. See http://www.fda.gov/Drugs/DevelopmentApprovalProcess/DevelopmentResources/Labeling/ucm093307.htm for more information.

Adverse Effects/Side Effects

- Abdominal pain
- Antibody formation
- Capillary leak syndrome
- Cephalgia
- Diarrhea
- Disorders
- Electrolyte imbalances
- Elevated liver function tests
- Fever/chills
- Hypotension
- Malaise
- Myalgia
- Nausea/vomiting
- Pancytopenia
- Peripheral edema
- Pruritus
- Rash
- Renal impairment
- Respiratory
- Tachycardia
- Weakness
- Weight gain/anorexia

Nursing Care

- Assess for drug allergy
- Assess thallium cardiac stress test
- Assess liver function studies
- Monitor pulmonary function tests
- Monitor vital signs and breath and heart sounds
- Document any history of respiratory and/or cardiac disorders
- Monitor weight daily during treatment (for capillary leak syndrome)

Monoclonal Antibodies for Immunomodulation

- Used to treat various cancers
- Examples: alemtuzumab, bevacizumab, cetuximab, ibritumomab tiuxetan, panitumumab, rituximab, trastuzumab
- Available in intravenous forms

Mode of Action (Fig. 19.1)

- Binds to specific target antigens on the cancer cell to inactivate or destroy the cell

Contraindications, Precautions, and Drug Interactions of Monoclonal Antibodies for Immunomodulation*

Drug	Contraindications/Precautions	Drug Interaction
alemtuzumab	*Contraindications:* Active systemic infections and immuno-deficiency conditions *Precautions:* Breastfeeding, cardiovascular disease, children, geriatric *Pregnancy:* Only given after risks to the fetus are considered	
bevacizumab	*Contraindications:* Hypersensitivity *Precautions:* Cardiovascular disease, gastrointestinal obstruction/perforation, glaucoma, hypersensitivity, hypertension, nephrotic syndrome, renal disease, serious bleeding, wound dehiscence *Pregnancy:* Definite fetal risks, may be given despite risks in life-threatening conditions	Daunorubicin, doxo-rubicin, epirubicin, irinotecan, suni-tinib
cetuximab	*Contraindications:* Hypersensitivity *Precautions:* Breastfeeding, cardiovascular disease, child, geriatric, hepatic disease, ocular disease, pulmonary disorders, renal disease *Pregnancy:* Only given after risks to the fetus are considered	
ibritumomab tiuxetan	*Contraindications:* Hypersensitivity *Precautions:* Breastfeeding, cardiac conditions, children, geriatric, immunizations *Pregnancy:* Definite fetal risks, may be given despite risks in life-threatening conditions	
panitumumab	*Contraindication:* Hypersensitivity *Precautions:* Acute bronchospasm, breastfeeding, children, diarrhea, hepatic disease, hypomagnesemia, sepsis, pulmonary fibrosis, hypotension *Pregnancy:* Only given after risks to the fetus are considered	Antineoplastics
rituximab	*Contraindications:* Hepatitis B, hypersensitivity *Precautions:* Breastfeeding; infection; pulmonary fibrosis; renal, liver, and/or cardiac disease *Pregnancy:* Only given after risks to the fetus are considered	Antihypertensives, drugs that cause bone marrow sup-pression, vaccines
trastuzumab	*Contraindications:* Hypersensitivity *Precautions:* Anemia, breastfeeding, children, geriatric, leukopenia, pulmonary disease *Pregnancy:* Definite fetal risks, may be given despite risks in life-threatening conditions	Anthracyclines, cyclo-phosphamide, vaccines/toxoids, warfarin

*Pregnancy categories have been revised. See http://www.fda.gov/Drugs/DevelopmentApprovalProcess/DevelopmentResources/Labeling/ucm093307.htm for more information.

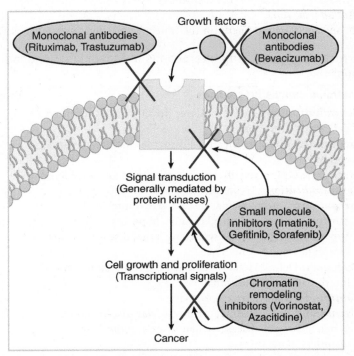

FIG. 19.1   Biologics and signal transduction inhibitors. New generation anticancer drugs and immunomodulators are based on interruption of extra- and intracellular signaling. These newer agents bind to growth factors, growth factor receptors, signal transduction protein kinases, or factors responsible for regulating gene expression (chromatin and DNA modifiers). (From Kester, M., Karpa, K.D., Vrana, K.E. [2012]. *Elsevier's integrated review pharmacology* [2nd ed.]. Philadelphia: Saunders.)

Adverse Effects/Side Effects

- Anemia
- Constipation
- Cough
- Deep vein thrombosis
- Depression
- Diarrhea
- Dyspnea
- Electrolyte disturbances
- Fatigue
- Fever/chills
- Gastrointestinal bleeding
- Hyper/hypotension
- Infusion-related events
- Insomnia
- Nausea/vomiting
- Neutropenia
- Pruritus
- Rash
- Reaction at injection site
- Respiratory infection
- Urinary tract infection

Nursing Care

- Assess history of allergic reactions
- Monitor for signs of infection
- Establish baseline vital signs
- Review patient history for presence of any immune deficiencies
- Perform thorough neurologic assessment
- Assess any existing cardiopulmonary disease

Interferons

- Used to treat hairy-cell leukemia, Kaposi sarcoma, malignant melanoma, non-Hodgkin lymphoma, hepatitis B and C viruses; human papillomavirus, and relapsing-remitting multiple sclerosis

- Three main categories: alfa, beta, and gamma
- Examples: interferon alfa-2b, interferon beta-1b, interferon gamma-1b
- Available in injectable, intravenous forms

Mode of Action
- Induce biologic responses and have antiviral, antiproliferative, and immunomodulatory effects

Contraindications, Precautions, and Drug Interactions of Interferons*

Drug	Contraindications/Precautions	Drug Interaction
interferon alfa-2b	**Contraindications:** Autoimmune hepatitis, creatinine clearance <50 mL/min, decompensated liver disease, hemoglobinopathies, hypersensitivity **Precautions:** Alcoholism, autoimmune disorders, bone marrow suppression, breastfeeding, cardiac disease, chickenpox, children <18 yr, chronic progressive multiple sclerosis, depression, hepatotoxicity, herpes zoster, latex allergy, mental disorders, seizure disorders **Pregnancy:** Only given after risks to the fetus are considered	Antiretroviral protease inhibitors, barbiturates, chemotherapy, colchicine, CYP3A4 inhibitors, CYP3A4 substrates, eflornithine, hydroxyurea, nonnucleoside reverse transcriptase inhibitors, theophylline
interferon beta-1b	**Contraindications:** Hypersensitivity **Precautions:** Alcoholism, autoimmune disorders, bone marrow suppression, breastfeeding, cardiac disease, chickenpox, children <18 yr, chronic progressive multiple sclerosis, depression, hepatotoxicity, herpes zoster, latex allergy, mental disorders, seizure disorders **Pregnancy:** Only given after risks to the fetus are considered	Antineoplastics, antiretrovirals, zidovudine
interferon gamma	**Contraindications:** Hypersensitivity **Precautions:** Breastfeeding, cardiac disease, central nervous system disorders, children <1 yr, myelosuppression, seizure **Pregnancy:** Only given after risks to the fetus are considered	Aminophylline, myelosuppressive agents, nonnucleoside reverse transcriptase inhibitors, nucleoside reverse transcriptase inhibitors, protease inhibitors, theophylline

min, minute; *mL*, milliliter.
*Pregnancy categories have been revised. See http://www.fda.gov/Drugs/DevelopmentApprovalProcess/DevelopmentResources/Labeling/ucm093307.htm for more information.

Adverse Effects/Side Effects
- Abdominal pain
- Alopecia
- Amenorrhea
- Cephalgia
- Chest pain
- Chills
- Cough
- Depression
- Diarrhea
- Dizziness
- Drowsiness/fatigue
- Dyspnea
- Fever
- Insomnia
- Irritability
- Myalgia
- Nausea/vomiting
- Pancytopenia
- Paresthesia
- Pharyngitis
- Skin rash
- Tachycardia
- Xerostomia

Nursing Care
- Monitor complete blood count
- Perform chest radiography
- Monitor liver function tests
- Monitor triglycerides
- Monitor thyroid function
- Assess for headache, fatigue
- Assess for multiple sclerosis symptoms
- Assess mental status (depression, depersonalization, suicidal thoughts, insomnia)
- Monitor gastrointestinal status: diarrhea or constipation, vomiting, abdominal pain
- Monitor cardiac status; perform regular electrocardiography

Miscellaneous Immunomodulators
- Used to treat rheumatoid arthritis, ankylosing spondylitis, relapsing multiple sclerosis, some cancers (see following section for details)
- Examples: abatacept, etanercept, leflunomide, mitoxantrone, thalidomide, tretinoin
- Available in injection, intravenous forms, tablets

Mode of Action
- Varies by drug

Contraindications, Precautions, and Drug Interactions of Miscellaneous Immunomodulators*

Drug	Contraindications/Precautions	Drug Interaction
abatacept	*Contraindications:* Hypersensitivity *Precautions:* Breastfeeding, children, chronic obstructive pulmonary disease, geriatric, immunosuppression, neoplastic disease, recurrent infections, respiratory infection, tuberculosis, viral hepatitis *Pregnancy:* Only given after risks to the fetus are considered	Adalimumab, anakinra, atropine, corticosteroids, etanercept, halothane, immunosuppressives, infliximab, scopolamine, vaccines
etanercept	*Contraindications:* Sepsis *Precautions:* Breastfeeding, children <4 yr, congestive heart failure, geriatric, latex hypersensitivity, malignancies, multiple sclerosis, seizures *Pregnancy:* No human studies available, but no adverse effects in animals	Anakinra, cyclophosphamide, immunizations, live vaccines, rilonacept, sulfasalazine
leflunomide	*Contraindications:* Breastfeeding, hepatic disease, hypersensitivity, jaundice, lactase deficiency, pregnancy *Precautions:* Alcoholism, children, immunosuppression, infection, renal disorders, vaccinations *Pregnancy:* Definite fetal abnormalities; do not use during pregnancy	Activated charcoal, cholestyramine, hepatotoxic agents, live virus vaccines, methotrexate, nonsteroidal antiinflammatory drugs, rifampin

Contraindications, Precautions, and Drug Interactions of Miscellaneous Immunomodulators—cont'd

Drug	Contraindications/Precautions	Drug Interaction
mitoxan-trone	*Contraindications:* Hypersensitivity *Precautions:* Breastfeeding, cardiac disease, children, hepatic disease, myelosuppression, renal disease, gout *Pregnancy:* Definite fetal risks, may be given despite risks in life-threatening conditions	Anticoagulants, antineoplastics, digoxin, live virus vaccines, nonsteroidal antiinflammatory drugs, phenytoin, radiation, trastuzumab
thalidomide	*Contraindications:* Hypersensitivity, pregnancy *Precautions:* Breastfeeding, children, hepatic/renal disease *Pregnancy:* Definite fetal abnormalities; do not use during pregnancy	Alcohol, alpha/beta-adrenergic blockers, amiodarone, antianxiety agents, antihistamines, antipsychotics, beta blockers, bortezomib, calcium channel blockers, cisplatin, digoxin, disulfiram, docetaxel, erythropoietic agents, H2 blockers, hormonal contraceptives, lithium, metronidazole, neuromuscular blockers, opioids, paclitaxel, phenytoin, tricyclic antidepressants, vincristine, warfarin
tretinoin	*Contraindications:* Hypersensitivity *Precautions:* Breastfeeding, eczema, sunburn, sun exposure *Pregnancy:* Definite fetal risks, may be given despite risks in life-threatening conditions	Alcohol, aminocaproic acid, aprotinin, diuretics (thiazide), ketoconazole, phenothiazines, quinolones, resorcinol, retinoids, sulfonamides, sulfonylureas, sulfur, tetracyclines, tranexamic acid

*Pregnancy categories have been revised. See http://www.fda.gov/Drugs/DevelopmentApprovalProcess/DevelopmentResources/Labeling/ucm093307.htm for more information.

Adverse Effects/Side Effects
- Albuminuria
- Hematuria
- Hepatotoxicity
- Proteinuria
- Renal failure

Nursing Care
- Assess past and present medical conditions
- Assess allergies
- Assess current medications (prescription, over-the-counter, herbal supplements, etc.)
- Assess for current infection
- Assess complete blood count, and monitor complete blood count during therapy
- Teach regarding frequency of dosing (e.g., weekly instead of daily)

APPLICATION AND REVIEW

9. A client who had an organ transplant is receiving cyclosporine. For what should the nurse monitor to identify a serious adverse effect of cyclosporine?
   1. Skin for hirsutism
   2. Stools for constipation
   3. Heart rhythm for dysrhythmias
   4. Creatinine level for an increase

10. Three weeks after a kidney transplant, a client develops leukopenia. Which factor should the nurse conclude is the **most** probable cause of the leukopenia?
    1. Bacterial infection
    2. High creatinine levels
    3. Rejection of the kidney
    4. Antirejection medications

11. A client who weighs 176 pounds is being immunosuppressed by daily maintenance doses of cyclosporine to prevent organ transplant rejection. The dose prescribed is 8 mg/kg each day. How many milligrams should the nurse administer each day? **Record your answer using a whole number.**

    Answer: _____ mg

12. A client has been prescribed interleukin receptor agonist therapy for a diagnosis of metastatic renal cancer. When asked what the medication will do, which response demonstrates the client's medication knowledge?
    1. "It will cause my body to make more T cells."
    2. "The medication works well in treating metastatic renal cancer."
    3. "It will help me fight off infections during my chemotherapy treatments."
    4. "It is available in intravenous form so it will work quickly to kill the cancer cells."

13. When counseling a client prescribed the interleukin medication aldesleukin (IL-2), which Black Box Warnings should the nurse address? **Select all that apply.**
    1. Angina
    2. Seizures
    3. Severe infections
    4. Capillary Leak Syndrome
    5. Cardiopulmonary disease

14. The nurse is providing care for a client prescribed interleukin receptor agonist therapy for diagnosis of metastatic melanoma. Which gastrointestinal adverse effects should the nurse monitor the client for frequently?
    1. Diarrhea
    2. Constipation
    3. Tarry stools
    4. Bright red streaked stools

15. The nurse is providing care for a client prescribed a monoclonal antibody medication for the treatment of cancer. When asked by the client, what explanation about its mode of action should the nurse provide?
    1. It stimulates the multiplication of T cells
    2. It binds to specific target antigens on the cell itself
    3. It prevents the cancer cells from acquiring nutrients
    4. It supports the primary cancer killing medications being prescribed

16. Considering the Black Box Warnings for the monoclonal antibody medication ibritumomab tiuxetan which specific assessment for which condition should the nurse provide?
    1. Gastrointestinal bleeding
    2. Respiratory infections
    3. Depression
    4. Delirium

See Answers on pages 426–429.

IMMUNOSUPPRESSANT DRUGS

T-Cell Suppressors

- Used to prevent organ rejection, reduce frequent relapses of relapsing-remitting multiple sclerosis
- Examples: azathioprine, cyclosporine, fingolimod, glatiramer, mycophenolate, sirolimus, tacrolimus

Mode of Action (Fig. 19.2)

- Selectively suppress various T-lymphocyte lines

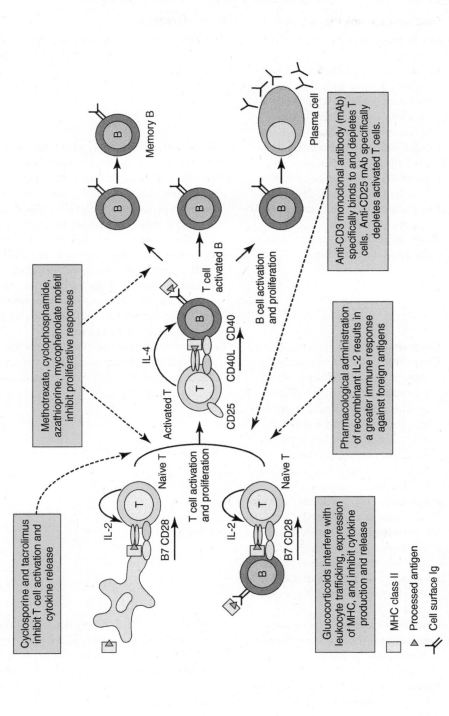

Memory B

Plasma cell

Anti-CD3 monoclonal antibody (mAb) specifically binds to and depletes T cells. Anti-CD25 mAb specifically depletes activated T cells.

Methotrexate, cyclophosphamide, azathioprine, mycophenolate mofetil inhibit proliferative responses

T cell activated B

IL-4

B cell activation and proliferation

Activated T

CD40L   CD40

CD25

Pharmacological administration of recombinant IL-2 results in a greater immune response against foreign antigens

Cyclosporine and tacrolimus inhibit T cell activation and cytokine release

Naïve T

IL-2

B7 CD28

T cell activation and proliferation

Naïve T

IL-2

B7 CD28

Glucocorticoids interfere with leukocyte trafficking, expression of MHC, and inhibit cytokine production and release

☐ MHC class II
△ Processed antigen
⅄ Cell surface Ig

FIG. 19.2 Primary mechanisms of action of immunosuppressive drugs. (From Wecker L., Crespo, L.M., Dunaway, G., Faingold, C. [2010]. *Brody's human pharmacology* [10th ed.]. Philadelphia: Mosby.)

Contraindications, Precautions, and Drug Interactions of T-Cell Suppressors*

Drug	Contraindications/Precautions	Drug Interaction
azathio-prine	*Contraindications:* Breastfeeding, hypersensitivity *Precautions:* Geriatric, severe renal/hepatic disease, infection *Pregnancy:* Definite fetal risks, may be given despite risks in life-threatening conditions	ACE inhibitors, allopurinol, antineoplastics, cyclosporine, sulfamethoxazole-trimethoprim, toxoids, vaccines, warfarin
cyclospo-rine	*Contraindications:* Breastfeeding, eye infections, hypersensitivity, methotrexate, psoriasis, rheumatoid arthritis in renal disease *Precautions:* Geriatric, severe renal/hepatic disease *Pregnancy:* Only given after risks to the fetus are considered	Allopurinol, amiodarone, amphotericin B, androgens, anticonvulsants, antifungals (azole), beta-blockers, bromocriptine, calcium channel blockers, carvedilol, cimetidine, colchicine, contraceptives (oral), corticosteroids, digoxin, diuretics, etoposide, fluoroquinolones, foscarnet, HMG-CoA reductase inhibitors, imipenem-cilastatin, live virus vaccines, macrolides, melphalan, methotrexate, metoclopramide, nafcillin, NSAIDs, orlistat, phenobarbital, phenytoin, rifamycins, selective serotonin reuptake inhibitors, sirolimus, tacrolimus, terbinafine, ticlopidine, trimethoprim/sulfamethoxazole
fingolimod	*Contraindications:* Hypersensitivity *Precautions:* Breastfeeding, cardiac disease, children, chronic obstructive pulmonary disease, diabetes mellitus, dysrhythmias, heart failure, hepatic disease, human immunodeficiency virus, hypertension, immunosuppression, leukemia, lymphoma, respiratory insufficiency, syncope, uveitis *Pregnancy:* Only given after risks to the fetus are considered	Antineoplastics, class Ia/III antidysrhythmics, immune modulating therapies, immunosuppressants, inactive vaccines, ketoconazole, live vaccines, toxoids
glatiramer	*Contraindications:* Hypersensitivity *Precautions:* Breastfeeding, children, immune disorders, renal disease *Pregnancy:* No human studies available, but no adverse effects in animals	Natalizumab
mycophe-nolate	*Contraindications:* Hypersensitivity *Precautions:* Anemia, breastfeeding, lymphomas, neutropenia, renal disease *Pregnancy:* Definite fetal risks, may be given despite risks in life-threatening conditions	Acyclovir, antacids, anticoagulants, azathioprine, cholestyramine, contraceptives (oral), cyclosporine, ganciclovir, immunosuppressives, live attenuated vaccines, NSAIDs, phenytoin, probenecid, rifamycin, salicylates, theophylline, thrombolytics, valacyclovir

Contraindications, Precautions, and Drug Interactions of T-Cell Suppressors—cont'd

Drug	Contraindications/Precautions	Drug Interaction
sirolimus	**Contraindications:** Breastfeeding, hypersensitivity **Precautions:** Children <13 yr, diabetes mellitus, hyperkalemia, hyperlipidemia, hypertension, hyperuricemia, interstitial lung disease, cardiac/renal/hepatic disease, infection **Pregnancy:** Only given after risks to the fetus are considered	ACE inhibitors, angiotensin II receptor antagonists, antifungal agents, bromocriptine, calcium channel blockers, carbamazepine, cephalosporins, cimetidine, cyclosporine, danazol, erythromycin, human immunodeficiency virus protease inhibitors, iodine-containing radiopaque contrast media, live virus vaccines, metoclopramide, neuromuscular blockers, NSAIDs, penicillins, phenobarbital, phenytoin, rifamycin, rifapentine, salicylates, thrombolytics
tacrolimus	**Contraindications:** Hypersensitivity long-term use (topical) **Precautions:** Acute bronchospasm, African descent, breastfeeding, children, diabetes mellitus, heart failure, hyperkalemia, hypertension, hyperuricemia, lymphomas, QT prolongation, seizures, severe renal/hepatic disease **Pregnancy:** Only given after risks to the fetus are considered	Aminoglycosides, antifungals, arsenic trioxide, beta-agonists, calcium channel blockers, carbamazepine, chloroquine, cimetidine, cisplatin, class IA/III antidysrhythmics, cyclosporine, CYP3A4 inhibitors, CYP3A4 substrates, danazol, droperidol, erythromycin, haloperidol, ibuprofen, levomethadyl, live virus vaccines, local anesthetics, mycophenolate, pentamidine, phenobarbital, phenothiazines, phenytoin, rifamycin, tricyclics

ACE, angiotensin converting enzyme; *NSAID,* nonsteroidal antiinflammatory drug.
*Pregnancy categories have been revised. See http://www.fda.gov/Drugs/DevelopmentApprovalProcess/DevelopmentResources/Labeling/ucm093307.htm for more information.

Adverse Effects/Side Effects

- Albuminuria
- Gum hyperplasia
- Headache
- Hematuria
- Hepatotoxicity
- Leukopenia
- Nausea and vomiting
- Oral candida infection
- Proteinuria
- Renal failure
- Secondary infection
- Thrombocytopenia
- Tremors

Nursing Care

- Monitor blood urea nitrogen, creatinine at least monthly during treatment, 3 mo after treatment
- Monitor alkaline phosphatase, AST, ALT, bilirubin
- Monitor serum drug levels during treatment
- Assess for dark urine, jaundice, itching, light-colored stools (signs of hepatoxicity)
- Teach to report fever, chills, sore throat, fatigue
- Evaluate for absence of rejection

Interleukin Receptor Antagonists

- Used to reduce the signs and symptoms of moderate to severe active rheumatoid arthritis
- Example: anakinra
- Available in prefilled syringes

Mode of Action

- Blocks the activity of interleukin 1, resulting in decreased inflammation, bone resorption

Contraindications, Precautions, and Drug Interactions of Interleukin Receptor Antagonists*

Drug	Contraindications/Precautions	Drug Interaction
anakinra	*Contraindications:* Known drug allergy *Precautions:* Asthma, breastfeeding, children, geriatric, immunosuppression, infections, neoplastic disease, renal impairment, sepsis *Pregnancy:* No human studies available, but no adverse effects in animals	Etanercept, rilonacept, TNF-blocking agents

TNF, tumor necrosis factor.
*Pregnancy categories have been revised. See http://www.fda.gov/Drugs/DevelopmentApprovalProcess/DevelopmentResources/Labeling/ucm093307.htm for more information.

Adverse Effects/Side Effects

- Headache
- Local reactions at injection site
- Respiratory tract infections

Nursing Care

- Assess joint pain, stiffness, swelling, range of motion
- Assess for local reaction at injection site
- Assess for infections; do not start if patient has active infection
- Update vaccinations before beginning drug

Monoclonal Antibodies for Immunosuppression

- Used to prevent the body from mounting an immune response (transplanted organs, rheumatoid arthritis)
- Examples: basiliximab, muromonab CD-3, and tocilizumab
- Available as a powder or solution for injection

Mode of Action

- Inhibit cytotoxic T killer cell function

Contraindications, Precautions, and Drug Interactions of Monoclonal Antibodies for Immunosuppression*

Drug	Contraindications/Precautions	Drug Interaction
basiliximab	*Contraindications:* Breastfeeding, exposure to viral infections, hypersensitivity *Precautions:* Geriatric, human antimurine antibody *Pregnancy:* No human studies available, but no adverse effects in animals	Immunosuppressants
muromonab CD-3	*Contraindications:* Epilepsy, hypersensitivity, uncompensated heart failure, uncontrolled arterial hypertension *Precautions:* Breastfeeding, exposure to viral infections *Pregnancy:* Only given after risks to the fetus are considered	Immunosuppressants

Contraindications, Precautions, and Drug Interactions of Monoclonal Antibodies for Immunosuppression—cont'd

Drug	Contraindications/Precautions	Drug Interaction
tocilizumab	*Contraindications:* Hypersensitivity *Precautions:* Hepatic disease, breastfeeding, demyelinating disorders, risk for gastrointestinal perforation, severe neutropenia/thrombocytopenia *Pregnancy:* Only given after risks to the fetus are considered	Cyclosporine, disease-modifying antirheumatic drugs, CYP3A4 substrates, immunosuppressives, live virus vaccines, theophylline, TNF modifiers, warfarin

TNF, tumor necrosis factor.
*Pregnancy categories have been revised. See http://www.fda.gov/Drugs/DevelopmentApprovalProcess/DevelopmentResources/Labeling/ucm093307.htm for more information.

Adverse Effects/Side Effects
- Anaphylaxis
- Aseptic meningitis
- Bleeding/platelet disorders (thrombosis, thrombocytopenia, anemia, neutropenia, leukopenia)
- Cardiac arrest
- Capillary leak syndrome
- Cytokine release syndrome
- Diabetes mellitus
- Encephalopathy
- Leukopenia
- Lymphoproliferative disorders
- Malignancy
- Opportunistic infection
- Respiratory arrest
- Seizures
- Sepsis
- Thrombocytopenia
- Weakness

Nursing Care
- Monitor renal/hepatic function tests
- Monitor drug-blood levels during treatment
- Monitor hemoglobin, white blood cell count, platelets every month
- Assess for hepatotoxicity

APPLICATION AND REVIEW

17. What is the primary focus of T-cell suppressor therapy?
    1. Decreasing inflammation
    2. Prevention of organ rejection
    3. Blocking the activity of interleukin 1
    4. Targeting the antigen of specific cancer cells

18. Assessment for which condition has highest priority for a client prescribed monoclonal antibodies therapy?
    1. Hepatotoxicity
    2. Injection site reaction
    3. Respiratory infections
    4. Joint swelling and pain

See Answers on pages 426–429.

ANSWER KEY: REVIEW QUESTIONS

1. **3 Individuals born after 1957 should receive one additional dose of measles, mumps, and rubella (MMR) vaccine if they are students in postsecondary educational institutions.**

   1 Currently there is no vaccine for hepatitis C. **2** The influenza B (HIB) immunization is unnecessary. **4** If the student received an additional tetanus/diphtheria vaccine (DTaP) at age 12, it is not necessary. A booster dose of tetanus toxoid (Td) should be received every 10 years.
   Client Need: Health Promotion and Maintenance; **Cognitive Level:** Comprehension; **Integrated Process:** Teaching/Learning; **Nursing Process:** Planning/Implementation

2. **4 The Centers for Disease Control and Prevention recommend that adults be immunized with pneumococcal vaccine at age 65 or older with a single dose of the vaccine; if the pneumococcal vaccine was received before 65 years of age or if there is the highest risk of fatal pneumococcal infection, revaccination should occur 5 years after the initial vaccination.**

   1 The pneumococcal vaccine should not be administered every 2 years. **2, 3** The pneumococcal vaccine should not be administered annually.
   Client Need: Health Promotion and Maintenance; **Cognitive Level:** Application; **Integrated Process:** Communication/Documentation; **Nursing Process:** Planning/Implementation

3. **2 The gamma-globulin fraction in the plasma is the fraction that includes the antibodies.**

   1 Albumin helps regulate fluid shifts by maintaining plasma oncotic pressure. **3** Thrombin is involved with clotting. **4** Hemoglobin carries oxygen.
   Client Need: Physiologic Adaptation; **Cognitive Level:** Comprehension; **Nursing Process:** Assessment/Analysis

4. **4 Gamma globulin, which is an immune globulin, contains most of the antibodies circulating in the blood. When injected into an individual, it prevents a specific antigen from entering a host cell.**

   1, 3 Gamma globulin does not stimulate antibody production. **2** accelerating antigen-antibody union at the hepatic sites does not affect antigen-antibody function.
   Client Need: Health Promotion and Maintenance; **Cognitive Level:** Comprehension; **Nursing Process:** Assessment/Analysis

5. **3 Human tetanus antitoxin (tetanus immune globulin [TIG]) provides antibodies against tetanus; it is used for the individual who may be infected and has never received tetanus toxoid or has not received it for more than 10 years. It confers passive immunity.**

   1 Administration of the tetanus toxoid (Td) will produce active, not passive, immunity. **2** Although equine tetanus antitoxin provides passive immunity, the risk for a hypersensitivity reaction is high and therefore TIG is preferred. **4** Diphtheria, tetanus, pertussis (DTaP) vaccine produces active, not passive, immunity; in addition, DTaP usually is not given to adults.
   Client Need: Health Promotion and Maintenance; **Cognitive Level:** Analysis; **Nursing Process:** Planning/Implementation

> **Study Tip:** Be sure you understand the difference between how a vaccination works versus how the administration of human tetanus antitoxin works. A vaccination stimulates your immune system to make its own antibodies. Human tetanus antitoxin contains the antibodies premade. That is why it confers passive immunity; your body isn't doing the active work of making the antibodies.

6. **2 Tetanus antitoxin provides antibodies, which confer immediate passive immunity.**

   1 Antitoxin does not stimulate production of antibodies. **3** Antitoxin provides passive, not active, immunity. **4** Passive immunity, by definition, is not long-lasting.

   Client Need: Health Promotion and Maintenance; **Cognitive Level:** Application; **Nursing Process:** Planning/Implementation

7. **3 Immunoglobulin E (IgE) antibodies are responsible for hypersensitivity and allergic responses; cause mast cells to release histamine; protection from parasites.**

   1 Immunoglobulin M (IgM) antibodies are the first antibodies to be detected after exposure to antigen; protection from gram-negative bacteria. **2** Immunoglobulin A (IgA) antibodies are present in blood, mucus, and human milk secretions; play important role against viral and respiratory pathogens. **4** Immunoglobulin D (IgD) antibodies help differentiate B lymphocytes.

   Client Need: Health Promotion and Maintenance; **Cognitive Level:** Analysis; **Nursing Process:** Assessment/Analysis

8. **2 The first stage of the inflammation process involves the release of histamine.**

   1 Immunoglobulin M (IgM) antibodies are the first antibodies to be detected after exposure to antigen; protection from gram-negative bacteria. **3** The first stage of the inflammation process involves vascular dilation. **4** The first stage of the inflammation process involves increased capillary permeability.

   Client Need: Pharmacologic and Parenteral Therapies; **Cognitive Level:** Analysis; **Nursing Process:** Assessment/Analysis

9. **4 A life-threatening effect of cyclosporine is nephrotoxicity. Therefore creatinine and blood urea nitrogen (BUN) levels should be monitored.**

   1 Although abnormal hairiness (hirsutism) is an effect of cyclosporine, it is not life-threatening. **2** Diarrhea, not constipation, is a response to cyclosporine. **3** Cyclosporine does not cause cardiovascular life-threatening effects.

   Client Need: Health Promotion and Maintenance; **Cognitive Level:** Application; **Nursing Process:** Assessment/Analysis

   > **Study Tip:** Print the word *cyclosporine*. Then intersect the word *nephrotoxicity* (as if on an infinite crossword) as many times as possible by overlapping the same letters in cyclosporine. So you could write nephrotoxicity starting with the "n" of cyclosporine, and again overlapping one of the o's, and again overlapping the i's, and so on. Then draw a kidney shape around your diagram to reinforce this potential adverse effect.

10. **4 Immunosuppressants such as azathioprine and cyclosporine are given to prevent rejection and therefore depress WBCs.**

    1 An increased WBC level is associated with bacterial infection. **2** High creatinine levels do not cause leukopenia; increased creatinine levels are caused by kidney failure. **3** Rejection of the kidney does not cause leukopenia; signs of rejection include decreased urine output, increased serum creatinine, hypertension, and edema.

    Client Need: Health Promotion and Maintenance; **Cognitive Level:** Comprehension; **Nursing Process:** Assessment/Analysis

11. **Answer: 360 mg per day.**

    First compute the client's weight in kilograms and then compute the dosage. Use the "Desired over Have" formula of ratio and proportion to solve this problem.

    $$\frac{\text{Desired}}{\text{Have}} \quad \frac{176\,\text{lb}}{2.2\,\text{lb}} = \frac{x\,\text{kg}}{1\,\text{kg}}$$

    $$2.2x = 176$$
    $$x = 176 \div 2.2$$
    $$x = 80\,\text{kg}$$

$$\frac{\text{Desired}}{\text{Have}} \quad \frac{80\,\text{kg}}{1\,\text{kg}} = \frac{\text{x}\,\text{mg}}{8\,\text{mg}}$$

$$1\text{x} = 80 \times 8$$

$$\text{x} = 640\,\text{mg}$$

Client Need: Health Promotion and Maintenance; **Cognitive Level:** Application; **Nursing Process:** Planning/Implementation

12. **1 Interleukin receptor agonist therapy binds to receptor sites on T cells, which stimulates the T cells to multiply.**

2 Although it is true that interleukin receptor agonist therapy is used to treat metastatic renal cancer, the statement doesn't address its action in doing so. **3** Interleukin therapy is not directed toward infection control but rather the stimulation of T cells. **4** Although it is true that interleukin receptor agonist therapy is administered via the intravenous route, the statement doesn't address its action related to cancer treatment.

Client Need: Pharmacologic and Parenteral Therapies; **Cognitive Level:** Analysis; **Integrated Process:** Teaching/Learning; **Nursing Process:** Assessment/Analysis

13. **Answers: 3, 4, 5**

Black Box Warnings for aldesleukin (IL-2) include cardiopulmonary disease, Capillary Leak Syndrome, and severe infections.

1 Black Box Warnings for aldesleukin (IL-2) do not include angina. Angina is a contraindication for this medication. **2** Black Box Warnings for aldesleukin (IL-2) do not include seizures. Seizures are a contraindication for this medication.

Client Need: Pharmacologic and Parenteral Therapies; **Cognitive Level:** Analysis; **Integrated Process:** Teaching/Learning; **Nursing Process:** Assessment/Analysis

14. **1 Diarrhea may occur as an adverse effect of this medication therapy.**

2 Constipation is not generally identified as an adverse effect of this medication therapy. **3** Tarry stools result from an upper GI bleed; such bleeding is not generally identified as an adverse effect of this medication therapy. **4** Bright red streaked stools usually result from lower GI tract bleeding; such bleeding is not generally identified as an adverse effect of this medication therapy.

Client Need: Pharmacologic and Parenteral Therapies; **Cognitive Level:** Analysis; **Nursing Process:** Assessment/Analysis

15. **2 Monoclonal antibody medication acts by binding to specific target antigens on the cancer cell to inactivate or destroy the cell.**

1 Interleukin receptor agonists work by binding to receptor sites on T cells, which stimulates the T cells to multiply. **3** Interleukin receptor agonists are not involved in starving cancer cells. **4** Interleukin receptor agonists are primary chemotherapy; they are not adjunct therapies.

Client Need: Pharmacologic and Parenteral Therapies; **Cognitive Level:** Analysis; **Integrated Process:** Teaching/Learning; **Nursing Process:** Planning/Evaluation; **Reference:** Monoclonal Antibodies for Immunomodulation

16. **3 Clients receiving the monoclonal antibody medication ibritumomab tiuxetan should be regularly assessed for depression as this is the focus of a Black Box Warning.**

1 GI bleeding is not a focus of a Black Box Warning for the monoclonal antibody medication ibritumomab tiuxetan. **2** Respiratory infections are not a focus of a Black Box Warning for the monoclonal antibody medication ibritumomab tiuxetan. **4** Delirium is not a focus of a Black Box Warning for the monoclonal antibody medication ibritumomab tiuxetan.

Client Need: Pharmacologic and Parenteral Therapies; **Cognitive Level:** Analysis; **Nursing Process:** Planning/Evaluation

17. **2 T-Cell suppressors are used to prevent organ rejection.**

1 The action of interleukin receptor antagonists result in decreased inflammation. **3** Interleukin receptor antagonists block the activity of interleukin 1. **4** Monoclonal antibodies bind to specific target antigens on the cancer cell.

Client Need: Pharmacologic and Parenteral Therapies; **Cognitive Level:** Analysis; **Nursing Process:** Assessment/Analysis

18. **1 Clients prescribed monoclonal antibodies therapy require regular assessment for hepatotoxicity.**
2 Interleukin receptor antagonists therapy places clients at a high risk for the development of injection site reactions. 3 Interleukin receptor antagonists therapy places clients at a high risk for the development of respiratory infections. 4 Interleukin receptor antagonists therapy places clients at a high risk for the development of joint swelling and pain.
Client Need: Pharmacologic and Parenteral Therapies; **Cognitive Level:** Analysis; **Nursing Process:** Assessment/Analysis

20 Gastrointestinal Drugs

INTRODUCTION TO GASTROINTESTINAL DISORDERS

Structures and Functions of the Gastrointestinal System

Structures *(Fig. 20.1)*

- Mouth: lips and cheeks; hard palate; soft palate; gums; teeth; tongue; tonsils; salivary glands
  - Moistens and masticates food; moves food to esophagus
- Esophagus: secretes mucous; facilitates movement of food
- Stomach: secretes gastric juice; food storage and liquefaction (chyme)
  - Small intestine: digestion and absorption; enzymes include sucrase, lactase, and maltase; cholecystokinin stimulates release of bile from gallbladder
  - Large intestine: water and sodium ion absorption; temporary storage of fecal matter; defecation
- Liver: carbohydrate, protein, fat, and vitamin metabolism; ketogenesis; fat storage; synthesis of triglycerides, phospholipids, cholesterol, and B complex factor choline; secretes bile
- Gallbladder: concentrates and stores bile
- Pancreas: digests carbohydrates, proteins, and fats; secretes glucagon and insulin

Functions

- Digestion: Changes to food in alimentary canal occur so it can be absorbed and metabolized
  - Mechanical digestion: movements of alimentary tract that change physical state of foods; propel food along alimentary tract
  - Chemical digestion: series of hydrolytic processes dependent on specific enzymes and chemicals; an additional substance may be necessary to act as a catalyst to facilitate the process
- Absorption: passage of small molecules from food sources through intestinal mucosa into blood or lymph
  - Majority occurs in small intestine; most water is absorbed from large intestine
- Metabolism: sum of all chemical reactions engaged in energy production and expenditure
  - Anabolism: synthesis of various compounds from simpler compounds
  - Catabolism: metabolic process in which complex substances are broken down into simple compounds; energy is liberated for use in movement, energy storage, and heat production
- Metabolism of carbohydrates: insulin promotes transport of glucose and amino acids through cell membranes
  - Glycogenesis: conversion of glucose to glycogen for storage in liver and muscle cells
  - Glycogenolysis: glycogen is converted to glucose in muscle cells; glucagon and epinephrine accelerate liver glycogenolysis
  - Glycolysis: breakdown of one glucose molecule into two pyruvic acid molecules, with conversion of about 5% of energy stored in glucose to heat and ATP molecules
  - Gluconeogenesis: chemical reaction that converts protein or fat compounds into glucose; occurs in liver cells

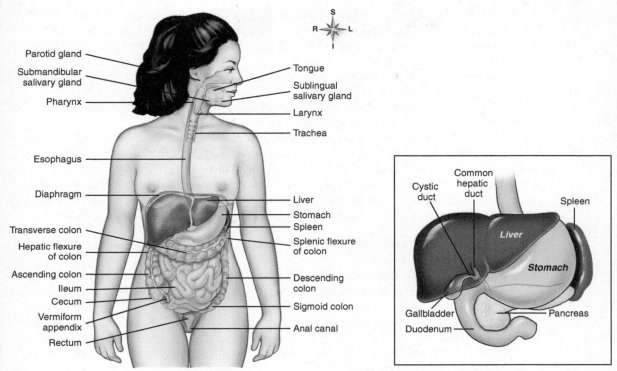

FIG. 20.1 Structures of the digestive system. (From Patton, K.T. , Thibodeau, G.A. [2016]. *Anatomy and physiology* [8th ed.]. St. Louis: Elsevier.)

Sources of Energy

- Carbohydrates: help provide basic fuel for energy
- Food sources: sugars, honey, fruit, milk, syrups, potatoes, rice, legumes, and products made with flour from grain (e.g., bread, cereal, pasta, crackers, cake, and cookies)
- Proteins: necessary for body growth, development, and healthy functioning; maintains nitrogen balance
  - Food sources: meat, fish, poultry, dry beans, eggs, nuts, milk, and cheese
- Fats: contribute to cellular transport; dietary source of fuel and fuel reserve; vitamin absorption and transport; insulation and protection afforded by adipose tissue
  - Food sources: animal fat, coconut and palm oil, dairy products, whole milk, vegetable oils, butter, margarine, mayonnaise, salad dressings, and baked goods and snacks that contain significant fat
- Vitamins: catalyze metabolic processes; essential for growth, development, and maintenance of body processes
  - Types: A, D, E, K, C, B-complex
- Minerals: help build body tissues
  - Types: calcium, sodium, potassium, iron, iodine, and fluorine

Types of Diets

- MyPlate dietary guidelines: recommended by the U.S. Department of Agriculture, Center for Nutrition Policy and Promotion; includes food groups appropriate for a healthy diet (Fig. 20.2)
- Clear liquid diet: minimizes stimulation of gastrointestinal (GI) tract; for clients with nausea and vomiting
  - Permitted: clear broth, bouillon, clear juices, plain gelatin, fruit-flavored water, ices, ginger ale, black coffee, tea
- Full liquid diet: for client with GI disturbance or inability to tolerate solid or semisolid food; may follow clear liquid diet postoperatively
  - Permitted: all foods on clear liquid diet plus milk and items made with milk, such as cream soups, milk drinks, sherbet, ice cream, puddings, custard, yogurt
- Soft diet: for clients who have difficulty chewing or swallowing
  - Permitted: all foods on clear and full liquid diets plus soft, refined cereals; pasta; rice; white bread and crackers; eggs; cheese; shredded or chopped meat; potatoes; cooked vegetables; soft cake; bread pudding; cooked fruits; and a few soft, ripe, plain fruits without membranes or skins
- Regular diet: full, well-balanced diet of all foods as desired and tolerated; generally 2000 calories or as ordered by health care provider
- Low-residue diet; minimizes fecal volume and residue; used for severe diarrhea, partial bowel obstruction, and during acute episode of inflammation of bowel; can be used in progression to regular diet
  - Excluded: milk and milk products; food with seeds, nuts, grains, and raw or dried vegetables and fruits
- High-fiber diet: foods high in fiber resist digestion, causing bulky stool that increases peristalsis; increases water content of stool
  - Sources: whole grain foods, bran, root vegetables and their skins, prunes, nuts, fruits, beans

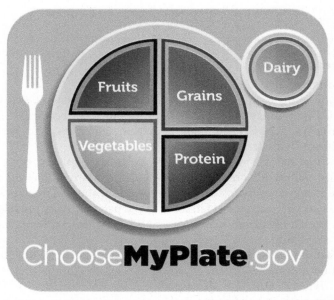

FIG. 20.2   MyPlate. (From U.S. Department of Agriculture, Center for Nutrition Policy and Promotion; available at www.choosemyplate.gov.)

- Restrictive diets: individually designed to meet specific needs of client
- Low-sodium diet (e.g., 2 g sodium): limits sodium/salt intake
  - Permitted: fresh fish, meat and poultry, fresh or frozen vegetables, pasta, unsalted butter, cooking oil, coffee, tea, lemonade, unflavored gelatin, jam, jelly, honey and maple syrup, unsalted nuts and popcorn, unsalted canned foods
  - Excluded: salt, monosodium glutamate, soy sauce, milk, cheese, processed luncheon meats and bacon, snack foods (e.g., chips, pretzels, etc.), baked goods containing salt, bouillon, canned or packaged soup, rice/noodles, pickles, olives, sauerkraut, tomato juice, mustard, most bottled and canned drinks, canned vegetables unless low-sodium type, salad dressings, smoked or salted meat or fish, corned beef, powdered milk drinks, buttermilk, highly processed convenience foods, meat extracts, meat tenderizers, sugar substitutes containing sodium, and sauces such as catsup, tartar, horseradish, Worcestershire, and teriyaki
- Low-fat diet: to reduce saturated fat, reduce cholesterol, and prevent coronary heart disease
  - Excluded: candy, ice cream, cake, cookies, and fried foods
  - Strategies to reduce dietary fat: grill, bake, broil, or microwave food; eat less meat; eat leaner cuts of meat; remove fat from meat and skin/fat from poultry before cooking; use skim milk; use less butter or margarine; eat more fish, lima beans, and navy beans for protein
- Calorie restriction: calories are restricted to reduce weight
- Renal diet: low sodium, potassium, protein, and possibly fluid restriction; specific restrictions indicated by health care provider
- Nonallergic diet: food causing the allergic response is eliminated from diet
- Diabetic diet: recommended by the American Diabetic Association to control weight and nutritional intake; balances proteins, carbohydrates, and fats
- Consistency modifications (e.g., mechanical soft): foods may be cut up, chopped, or pureed to make them easier for client to ingest

Review of Microorganisms

- Bacterial pathogens
  - *Escherichia coli:* small, gram-negative bacilli; part of normal flora of large intestine; certain strains cause urinary tract infections and diarrhea
  - *Clostridium difficile:* anaerobic, spore-forming bacterial pathogen; produces toxins that affect bowel mucosa; major cause of agency acquired diarrhea
  - *Salmonella:* genus of gram-negative, rod-shaped bacteria; origin: raw foods of animal origin (e.g., poultry, eggs, dairy products, beef); also vegetables and fruit when irrigated or washed with contaminated water or packed with contaminated ice for transport
  - *Shigella:* gram-negative bacilli, similar to Salmonella; *Shigella dysenteriae* causes bacillary dysentery or shigellosis
- Protozoal pathogens
  - *Balantidium coli:* ciliated protozoan; causes enteritis
  - *Entamoeba histolytica:* an amoeba; causes amebiasis (amoebic dysentery)
  - *Giardia lamblia:* flagellated protozoan; causes enteritis
- Parasitic pathogens
  - Nematodes (roundworms): include *Necator americanus* (hookworm), *Ascaris lumbricoides, Enterobius vermicularis* (pinworm), *Trichuris trichiura* (whipworm), all may be found in intestine
  - Cestodes (tapeworm): may be found in adult form in intestine; larval stage (hydatid) of some forms may develop and form cysts in liver, lungs, and kidneys
  - Trematodes (flukes): may be found in lungs, liver, and abdominal cavity

MAJOR DISORDERS OF THE GASTROINTESTINAL SYSTEM

- Peptic ulcer disease (PUD) (Table 20.1)
  - Cause: *Campylobacter pylori* or *H. pylori*, Zollinger-Ellison syndrome, aspirin/steroids/NSAIDs, smoking
  - Clinical findings: heartburn, nausea, epigastric pain, bleeding (tarry stools)
  - Therapeutic interventions: restrict irritating substance, small meals of bland foods, medications, smoking cessation
- Gastroesophageal reflux disease (GERD)
  - Cause: backflow of gastric contents into esophagus, gradually breaking down esophageal mucosa
  - Clinical findings: dyspepsia, dysphagia, heartburn (pyrosis), regurgitation, hoarseness, chronic cough
  - Therapeutic interventions: small meals of bland foods, medications, weight reduction, smoking cessation, endoscopic therapy
- Irritable bowel syndrome (IBS)
  - Cause: serotonin associated with neurologic hormonal regulation, infection, genetics
  - Clinical findings: abdominal pain, dyspepsia, abdominal cramps, constipation, diarrhea, abdominal distension
  - Therapeutic interventions: avoidance of trigger foods, medications, high-fiber diet
- Crohn's disease
  - Cause: ulceration and thickening of small bowel, autoimmune response, genetics
  - Clinical findings: nausea, diarrhea, cramping, abdominal pain, fever, increased WBC count
  - Therapeutic interventions: bland, low-residue, low-fat diet; medications; fluid and electrolyte balance; surgery to correct fistula/obstruction

TABLE 20.1 Predisposing Factors for Peptic Ulcer Disease

Predisposing Factors	Effects
Mechanical disturbances	Hypersecretion of acid and pepsin; inadequate GMB mucous secretion; impaired GMB resistance; hypermotility of the stomach; incompetent (defective) cardiac or pyloric sphincter
Genetic influences	Increased number of parietal cells in the stomach; susceptibility of mucosal lining to acid penetration; susceptibility to excess acetylcholine and histamine; excess hydrochloric acid caused by external stimuli
Environmental influences	Foods and liquids containing caffeine; fatty, fried, and highly spiced foods; alcohol; nicotine, especially from cigarette smoking; stressful situations; pregnancy; massive trauma; major surgery
Helicobacter pylori	A gram-negative bacterium, *H. pylori*, infects gastric mucosa and can cause gastritis, gastric ulcer, and duodenal ulcer. If not eradicated, peptic ulcer may return as frequently as every year. *H. pylori* can lead to atrophic gastritis in some patients. Serology and special breath tests can detect the presence of *H. pylori*.
Drugs	NSAIDs, including aspirin and aspirin compounds, ibuprofen, and indomethacin; corticosteroids; potassium salts; antineoplastic drugs

GMB, Gastric mucosal barrier; *NSAIDs*, nonsteroidal antiinflammatory drugs.

- Ulcerative colitis
  - Cause: bacterial infection, autoimmune response, genetics, emotional stress
  - Clinical findings: anorexia, nausea, abdominal cramps, fever, dehydration, hypocalcemia
  - Therapeutic interventions: low-residue diet, avoidance of dairy, medications, fluid/electrolyte replacement, surgical interventions

ACID CONTROLLING AGENTS

Systemic Antibiotics

- Used in the treatment of peptic ulcers caused by the bacteria *H. pylori*
- Examples include amoxicillin, clarithromycin, metronidazole, tetracycline
- Available in PO preparations

Mode of Action

- Systemic antibiotics are absorbed by the gastrointestinal tract and block acid production in the stomach; decreasing excess stomach acid allows the ulcer to heal

Contraindications, Precautions, and Drug Interactions of Systemic Antibiotics*

Drug	Contraindications/Precautions	Drug Interaction
amoxicillin	*Contraindications:* Hypersensitivity, severe renal disease, dialysis *Precautions:* Breastfeeding, neonates, children, hypersensitivity to cephalosporins, renal/GI disease, asthma, colitis, diabetes, eczema, leukemia, mononucleosis, viral infections, phenylketonuria *Pregnancy:* No adverse effects in animals; no human studies available	Probenecid, anticoagulants, allopurinol
clarithromycin	*Contraindications:* Hypersensitivity, hypersensitivity to macrolide antibiotics, torsades de pointes, QT prolongation *Precautions:* Breastfeeding, geriatric patients, renal/hepatic disease *Pregnancy:* Only given after risks to the fetus are considered; animal studies have shown adverse reactions; no human studies available	Cisapride, pimozide, alprazolam, buspirone, carbamazepine, cyclosporine, digoxin, omeprazole, antidiabetics, calcium channel blockers, grapefruit juice
metronidazole	*Contraindications:* Hypersensitivity, pregnancy first trimester, breastfeeding *Precautions:* Geriatric patients, *Candida* infections, heart failure, bone marrow suppression, GI/renal/hepatic disease, blood dyscrasias, CNS disorders	Anticoagulants, zalcitabine, bortezomib, norfloxacin, disulfiram
tetracycline	*Contraindications:* Hypersensitivity, pregnancy (D), breastfeeding, children <8 yr *Precautions:* Renal/hepatic disease, UV exposure *Pregnancy:* Definite fetal risks, may be given in spite of risks if needed in life-threatening conditions	Digoxin; methoxyflurane; anticoagulants; dairy products

*Pregnancy categories have been revised. See http://www.fda.gov/Drugs/DevelopmentApprovalProcess/DevelopmentResources/Labeling/ucm093307.htm for more information.

Adverse Effects/Side Effects

- Rash
- Urticaria
- Pruritus
- Hearing loss
- Nausea
- Vomiting
- Abdominal cramps
- Diarrhea
- Abnormal tastes
- Pericarditis
- Hemolytic anemia
- Flushing
- Headache

Nursing Care

- Keep patient head of bed elevated
- Administer with water
- Administer with or without food as prescribed
- Monitor patient for anemia
- Monitor patient for allergic reactions (rash, itching, pruritus, angioedema)
- Teach patient to eat small meals of bland foods
- Teach patient to avoid fats, chocolate, citric juices, coffee, alcohol
- Teach patient not to crush, chew, break extended release product
- Teach patient to avoid smoking

Histamine$_2$-receptor Antagonists

- Used to promote healing of duodenal and gastric ulcers
- Examples include cimetidine, famotidine, nizatidine, ranitidine
- Available in PO, IM, IV preparations

Mode of Action

- H$_2$-receptor antagonists block histamine from stimulating the acid-secreting parietal cells of the stomach

Contraindications, Precautions, and Drug Interactions of H$_2$-receptor Antagonists*

Drug	Contraindications/Precautions	Drug Interaction
cimetidine	*Contraindications:* Hypersensitivity, H$_2$-blockers, benzyl alcohol *Precautions:* Breast feeding, children <16 yr, geriatric patients, organic brain syndrome, renal/hepatic disease *Pregnancy:* No adverse effects in animals; no human studies available	Antacids, anticoagulants, carmustine, benzodiazepines, beta blockers, calcium channel blockers
famotidine	*Contraindications:* Hypersensitivity *Precautions:* Breastfeeding, children <12 yr, geriatric patients, severe renal/hepatic disease *Pregnancy:* No adverse effects in animals; no human studies available	Antacids, ketoconazole, itraconazole, cefpodoxime, cefditoren
nizatidine	*Contraindications:* Hypersensitivity *Precautions:* Breastfeeding, renal/hepatic impairment *Pregnancy:* No adverse effects in animals; no human studies available	Antacids, nifedipine, mefloquine, ketoconazole, gefitinib
ranitidine	*Contraindications:* Hypersensitivity *Precautions:* Breastfeeding, children <12 yr, renal/hepatic disease *Pregnancy:* No adverse effects in animals; no human studies available	Antacids, nifedipine, sulfonylureas, benzodiazepines, calcium channel blockers

*Pregnancy categories have been revised. See http://www.fda.gov/Drugs/DevelopmentApprovalProcess/DevelopmentResources/Labeling/ucm093307.htm for more information.

Adverse Effects/Side Effects

- Confusion
- Nausea
- Dizziness
- Malaise

- Anxiety
- Diarrhea
- Constipation
- Rash

- Itching
- Muscle pain
- Headache
- Seizures

Nursing Care

- Administer at bedtime
- Administer with a snack
- Do not administer within 1 hour of antacids
- Monitor for internal bleeding (black tarry stools)
- Monitor for confusion, diarrhea, rash
- Monitor for hepatic/renal impairment
- Teach patient not to stop the drug suddenly
- Teach patient to consult prescriber before taking OTC products, herbal remedies
- Teach patient to avoid smoking

APPLICATION AND REVIEW

1. Famotidine (Pepcid) 20 mg IVPB is prescribed for a client with a duodenal ulcer. The medication is diluted in 50 mL of 5% dextrose and is to infuse over 15 minutes. At what rate should the infusion control device be set? **Record your answer using a whole number.**
   Answer: _____ mL/hr

   See Answers on pages 456-458.

Antacids

- Used adjunctively to relieve pain in peptic ulcer disease; relieve symptoms of acid indigestion, heartburn, dyspepsia, gastroesophageal reflux disease (GERD)
- Examples include calcium carbonate, magnesium hydroxide, aluminum hydroxide, simethicone, aluminum hydroxide gel
- Available in PO preparations

Mode of Action

- Neutralize gastric acid in the stomach, which reduces total amount of acid in GI tract, allowing peptic ulcers to heal; allows more rapid movement of stomach contents into duodenum

Contraindications, Precautions, and Drug Interactions of Antacids*

Drug	Contraindications/Precautions	Drug Interaction
calcium carbonate	**Contraindications:** Hypersensitivity, hypercalcemia **Precautions:** Breastfeeding, geriatric patients, fluid restriction, decreased GI motility, GI obstruction, dehydration, renal disease, hyperparathyroidism, bone tumors **Pregnancy:** Only given after risks to the fetus are considered; animal studies have shown adverse reactions; no human studies available	Digoxin, quinidine, amphetamines, thiazide diuretics, calcium supplements, calcium channel blockers, phenytoin

Continued

Contraindications, Precautions, and Drug Interactions of Antacids—cont'd

Drug	Contraindications/Precautions	Drug Interaction
magnesium hydroxide	**Contraindications:** Hypersensitivity, abdominal pain, nausea/vomiting, obstruction, rectal bleeding, heart block, impaired renal function **Precautions:** Renal/cardiac disease **Pregnancy:** No risk demonstrated to the fetus in any trimester; no adverse effects in animals; no human studies available	Antihypertensives, calcium channel blockers, digoxin
aluminum hydroxide	**Contraindications:** Hypersensitivity, hypophosphatemia **Precautions:** Breastfeeding, geriatric patients, fluid restriction, decreased GI motility, GI obstruction, dehydration, GI bleeding, hypokalemia, sodium-restricted diet, renal disease **Pregnancy:** Only given after risks to the fetus are considered; animal studies have shown adverse reactions; no human studies available	Digoxin, allopurinol, corticosteroids, gabapentin, phenothiazines
simethicone	**Contraindications:** Hypersensitivity **Precautions:** Breastfeeding, geriatric patients **Pregnancy:** Only given after risks to the fetus are considered; animal studies have shown adverse reactions; no human studies available	Aluminum, magnesium, lanthanum
aluminum hydroxide gel	**Contraindications:** Hypersensitivity, hypophosphatemia **Precautions:** Breastfeeding, geriatric patients, fluid restriction, decreased GI motility, GI obstruction, dehydration, GI bleeding, hypokalemia, sodium-restricted diet, renal disease **Pregnancy:** Only given after risks to the fetus are considered; animal studies have shown adverse reactions; no human studies available	Digoxin, allopurinol, corticosteroids, gabapentin, phenothiazines

*Pregnancy categories have been revised. See http://www.fda.gov/Drugs/DevelopmentApprovalProcess/DevelopmentResources/Labeling/ucm093307.htm for more information.

Adverse Effects/Side Effects

- Nausea
- Vomiting
- Diarrhea
- Constipation
- Headache
- Confusion
- Electrolyte imbalance
- Alkalosis
- Osteoporosis
- Reduced absorption of calcium, iron, most medications

Nursing Care

- Administer antacids at least 2 hours from other medications
- Do not administer calcium carbonate with milk or other vitamin D foods
- Shake suspension well before administering
- Monitor for signs and symptoms of hypophosphatemia (anorexia, weakness, fatigue, bone pain, hyporeflexia)
- Monitor for white stools
- Teach patient measures to avoid constipation: increase fluids, fiber, exercise
- Teach patient on sodium-restricted diet to monitor sodium intake (most antacids contain sodium)

Proton Pump Inhibitors

- Used to treat active gastric, duodenal, and peptic ulcers; erosive esophagitis; GERD; Zollinger-Ellison syndrome
- Examples include esomeprazole, omeprazole, pantoprazole, lansoprazole, dexlansoprazole
- Available in PO and IV preparations

Mode of Action

- Block gastric acid secretion by combining with hydrogen, potassium, and adenosine triphosphate in parietal cells of stomach

Contraindications, Precautions, and Drug Interactions of Proton Pump Inhibitors*

Drug	Contraindications/Precautions	Drug Interaction
esomeprazole	*Contraindications:* Hypersensitivity to proton pump inhibitors *Precautions:* Breastfeeding, children, geriatric patients, hypomagnesemia, osteoporosis *Pregnancy:* No adverse effects in animals; no human studies available	Digoxin, diazepam, penicillins, warfarin, citalopram
omeprazole	*Contraindications:* Hypersensitivity to proton pump inhibitors *Precautions:* Breastfeeding, children, hypomagnesemia *Pregnancy:* Only given after risks to the fetus are considered; animal studies have shown adverse reactions; no human studies available	Warfarin, digoxin, diazepam, citalopram
pantoprazole	*Contraindications:* Hypersensitivity to proton pump inhibitors or benzimidazole *Precautions:* Breastfeeding, children, hypomagnesemia *Pregnancy:* Only given after risks to the fetus are considered; animal studies have shown adverse reactions; no human studies available	Warfarin, diazepam, phenytoin
lansoprazole	*Contraindications:* Hypersensitivity to proton pump inhibitors *Precautions:* Breastfeeding, children, osteoporosis, hypomagnesemia *Pregnancy:* No adverse effects in animals; no human studies available	Warfarin, sucralfate, loop/thiazide diuretics, dasatinib, delavirdine
dexlansoprazole	*Contraindications:* Hypersensitivity *Precautions:* Breastfeeding, children, proton pump hypersensitivity, gastric cancer, hepatic disease, colitis, vitamin B_{12} deficiency *Pregnancy:* No adverse effects in animals; no human studies available	CYP2C19 inhibitors, 3A4 inhibitors, sucralfate, ketoconazole, itraconazole, iron, delavirdine, ampicillin, calcium carbonate

*Pregnancy categories have been revised. See http://www.fda.gov/Drugs/DevelopmentApprovalProcess/DevelopmentResources/Labeling/ucm093307.htm for more information.

Adverse Effects/Side Effects

- Abdominal pain
- Flatulence
- Diarrhea
- Nausea
- Vomiting
- Headache
- Dizziness
- Dry mouth
- Hepatitis
- Heart failure
- Pneumonia
- Osteoporosis
- *c. difficile*

Nursing Care

- Administer 30 minutes before meals
- Do not crush or chew tablets
- Capsules may be opened and mixed with juice or soft food
- Monitor patient for electrolyte imbalances
- Teach patient signs and symptoms of adverse effects
- Teach patient to report signs of internal bleeding (black, tarry stools)
- Teach patient to avoid alcohol, salicylates, NSAIDs
- Teach patient to consult prescriber before taking OTC products, herbal remedies

Prokinetic Agents

- Used to treat acid reflux, GERD
- Examples include bethanechol, metoclopramide
- Available in PO preparations

Mode of Action

- Stimulates gastric motility, increases lower esophageal sphincter pressure

Contraindications, Precautions, and Drug Interactions of Prokinetic Agents*

Drug	Contraindications/Precautions	Drug Interaction
bethanechol	**Contraindications:** Hypersensitivity, severe bradycardia, asthma, severe hypotension, hyperthyroidism, peptic ulcer, parkinsonism, seizure disorders, CAD, COPD **Precautions:** Breastfeeding, children <8 yr, hypertension **Pregnancy:** Only given after risks to the fetus are considered; animal studies have shown adverse reactions; no human studies available	Ganglionic blockers, cholinergic agonists, anticholinesterase agents
metoclopramide	**Contraindications:** Hypersensitivity, procaine, procainamide, seizure disorder, pheochromocytoma, GI obstruction **Precautions:** Breastfeeding, GI hemorrhage, CHF, Parkinson's disease **Pregnancy:** No adverse effects in animals; no human studies available	MAOIs, haloperidol, phenothiazines, anticholinergics, opiates

*Pregnancy categories have been revised. See http://www.fda.gov/Drugs/DevelopmentApprovalProcess/DevelopmentResources/Labeling/ucm093307.htm for more information.

Adverse Effects/Side Effects

- Anxiety
- Depression
- Drowsiness
- Fatigue
- Dizziness
- Headache
- Malaise
- Bradycardia
- Muscle spams
- Tardive dyskinesia
- Circulatory collapse

Nursing Care

- Monitor for change in blood pressure, pulse
- Monitor for mental status changes
- Teach patient to avoid driving and other hazardous activities
- Teach patient to avoid alcohol and other CNS depressants

2. Which classification of acid-controlling medications block acid production in the stomach thus decreasing excess stomach acid allowing the ulcer to heal?
   1. Antacids
   2. Systemic antibiotics
   3. H_2-receptor antagonists
   4. Proton pump inhibitors
3. The nurse has completed a medication history on a client being considered for H_2-receptor antagonist therapy involving cimetidine. Which medication classification in the client's history poses a potential drug interaction concern? **Select all that apply.**
   1. Antacids
   2. Beta blocker
   3. Anticoagulant
   4. Tricyclic antidepressant
   5. Calcium channel blocker
4. The nurse should provide what information to a client being prescribed an H_2-receptor antagonist? **Select all that apply.**
   1. Administer the medication at bedtime
   2. Administer the medication with food
   3. Do not take within 1 hour of an antacid
   4. Avoid taking medication with dairy products
   5. Report any diarrhea to your primary health care provider
5. The nurse should provide what information to a client being prescribed a systemic antibiotic for the treatment of a gastric ulcer? **Select all that apply.**
   1. Avoid smoking
   2. Keep the head of the bed elevated
   3. Administer the medication with water
   4. Eat small meals that focus on bland foods and beverages
   5. Extended release pills may be crushed for ease of swallowing
6. A client with gastroesophageal reflux is to receive metoclopramide (Reglan) 15 mg orally before meals. The concentrated solution contains 10 mg/mL. How much solution should the nurse administer? **Record your answer using one decimal place.**
   Answer: _____ mL

See Answers on pages 456-458.

Other Antiulcer Drugs
- Used to promote healing of ulcers
- Examples include misoprostol, sucralfate
- Available in PO preparations

Mode of Action
- Misoprostol reduces gastric acid secretion and increases gastric mucous that protects against peptic ulcers; it is a prostaglandin analogue
- Sucralfate reacts with hydrochloric acid to form a thick substance that adheres to ulcers to protect from further exposure to gastric acid

Contraindications, Precautions, and Drug Interactions of Other Antiulcer Drugs*

Drug	Contraindications/Precautions	Drug Interaction
misoprostol	*Contraindications:* Hypersensitivity, prostaglandins *Precautions:* Breastfeeding, children, geriatric patients, fever, sepsis, cardiac/renal/inflammatory bowel disease *Pregnancy:* Absolute fetal abnormalities; not to be used at any time during pregnancy	Decreased when taken with food
sucralfate	*Contraindications:* Hypersensitivity *Precautions:* Breastfeeding, children, renal failure, hypoglycemia (diabetics) *Pregnancy:* No adverse effects in animals; no human studies available	Tetracyclines, phenytoin, digoxin, antacids

*Pregnancy categories have been revised. See http://www.fda.gov/Drugs/DevelopmentApprovalProcess/DevelopmentResources/Labeling/ucm093307.htm for more information.

Adverse Effects/Side Effects
- Diarrhea
- Abdominal pain
- Flatulence
- Indigestion
- Nausea
- Vomiting
- Spontaneous abortion
- Constipation
- Metallic taste
- Menstrual disorders

Nursing Care
- Administer sucralfate 1 hour before meals and at bedtime
- Administer misoprostol with food
- Elevate head of bed
- Ensure female patients are not pregnant
- Monitor hydration status
- Teach patient to avoid alcohol, cigarette smoking, chocolate, spicy foods
- Teach patient to avoid large meals 2 hours before bedtime

ANTIDIARRHEALS AND LAXATIVES

Antidiarrheals

Opioids
- Used to treat acute and chronic diarrhea
- Examples include diphenoxylate with atropine, loperamide
- Available in PO preparations

Mode of Action
- Slow GI motility by decreasing peristalsis in the small and large intestines; decrease colon contractions

Contraindications, Precautions, and Drug Interactions of Antidiarrheal Opioids*

Drug	Contraindications/Precautions	Drug Interaction
diphenoxylate with atropine	*Contraindications:* Hypersensitivity, children <2 yr, severe electrolyte imbalance *Precautions:* Breastfeeding, hepatic disease, ulcerative colitis, dehydration, substance abuse *Pregnancy:* Only given after risks to the fetus are considered; animal studies have shown adverse reactions; no human studies available	MAOIs, anticholinergics, CNS depressants

Contraindications, Precautions, and Drug Interactions of Antidiarrheal Opioids—cont'd

Drug	Contraindications/Precautions	Drug Interaction
loperamide	***Contraindications:*** Hypersensitivity, colitis, constipation, dysentery, GI bleeding/obstruction/perforation, ileus ***Precautions:*** Breastfeeding, children <2 yr, geriatric patients, dehydration, hepatic disease, severe ulcerative colitis ***Pregnancy:*** Only given after risks to the fetus are considered; animal studies have shown adverse reactions; no human studies available	Alcohol, antihistamines, analgesics, opioids, sedatives, hypnotics

*Pregnancy categories have been revised. See http://www.fda.gov/Drugs/DevelopmentApprovalProcess/DevelopmentResources/Labeling/ucm093307.htm for more information.

Adverse Effects/Side Effects

- Nausea
- Vomiting
- Abdominal cramps
- Respiratory depression
- Drowsiness
- Insomnia
- Confusion
- Blurred vision
- Tachycardia
- Fatigue
- Paralytic ileus

Nursing Care

- Correct underlying fluid and electrolyte imbalances before administering drug
- Monitor for respiratory depression
- Encourage intake of fluids
- Teach the patient not to consume alcohol
- Teach patient to avoid driving or hazardous activities
- Teach patient to notify prescriber if diarrhea persists for more than 2 days
- Teach patient medication may be habit forming

Laxatives

Chemical Stimulants

- Used to stimulate defecation
- Examples include bisacodyl, senna
- Available in PO, rectal preparations

Mode of Action

- Stimulate peristalsis, irritate intestinal mucosa, stimulate nerve endings of intestinal smooth muscle

Contraindications, Precautions, and Drug Interactions of Chemical Stimulant Laxatives*

Drug	Contraindications/Precautions	Drug Interaction
bisacodyl	***Contraindications:*** Hypersensitivity, nausea, abdominal pain, acute hepatitis, appendicitis, GI obstruction ***Precautions:*** Breastfeeding, rectal fissures, severe cardiovascular disease ***Pregnancy:*** Only given after risks to the fetus are considered; animal studies have shown adverse reactions; no human studies available	Antacids, H_2-blockers, gastric acid pump inhibitors, dairy products

Continued

Contraindications, Precautions, and Drug Interactions of Chemical Stimulant Laxatives—cont'd

Drug	Contraindications/Precautions	Drug Interaction
senna	*Contraindications:* Hypersensitivity, Crohn's disease, ulcerative colitis, heart disease *Precautions:* Breastfeeding *Pregnancy:* Only given after risks to the fetus are considered; animal studies have shown adverse reactions; no human studies available	Digoxin, diuretics, anticoagulants

*Pregnancy categories have been revised. See http://www.fda.gov/Drugs/DevelopmentApprovalProcess/DevelopmentResources/Labeling/ucm093307.htm for more information.

Adverse Effects/Side Effects
- Weakness
- Nausea
- Abdominal cramps
- Urine discoloration (senna, cascara sagrada)
- Mild rectum, anus inflammation

Nursing Care
- Administer laxative when convenient for patient
- Shake liquid suspension well
- If administering through NG tube, flush tube with water after administration
- Don't crush enteric-coated tablets
- Do not administer if patient complains of nausea, vomiting, acute abdominal pain
- Ensure patient has easy access to toilet or bedpan
- Teach patient to drink plenty of fluids, eat a high-fiber diet, and exercise

Bulk Stimulants
- Used in chronic constipation, ulcerative colitis, diarrhea, diverticulosis, irritable bowel syndrome, hypercholesterolemia
- Examples include methylcellulose, polycarbophil, psyllium hydrophilic mucilloid
- Available in PO preparations

Mode of Action
- Increase stool mass and water content, promoting peristalsis and defecation

Contraindications, Precautions, and Drug Interactions of Bulk Stimulant Laxatives*

Drug	Contraindications/Precautions	Drug Interaction
methylcellulose	*Contraindications:* Hypersensitivity, appendicitis, GI obstruction, rectal bleeding, phenylketonuria *Precautions:* Hemorrhoids, rectal bleeding *Pregnancy:* No risk demonstrated to the fetus in any trimester	Anticoagulants
polycarbophil	*Contraindications:* Hypersensitivity, GI obstruction, rectal bleeding *Precautions:* Hemorrhoids, rectal bleeding *Pregnancy:* No risk demonstrated to the fetus in any trimester	Anticoagulants
psyllium hydrophilic mucilloid	*Contraindications:* Hypersensitivity, GI obstruction, fecal impaction, nausea, vomiting, abdominal pain *Precautions:* Hemorrhoids, rectal bleeding *Pregnancy:* No risk demonstrated to the fetus in any trimester	Cardiac glycosides, anticoagulants, salicylates

*Pregnancy categories have been revised. See http://www.fda.gov/Drugs/DevelopmentApprovalProcess/DevelopmentResources/Labeling/ucm093307.htm for more information.

Adverse Effects/Side Effects

- Flatulence
- Feeling of abdominal fullness
- Intestinal obstruction
- Fecal impaction
- Severe diarrhea
- Nausea
- Vomiting
- Anorexia

Nursing Care

- Administer laxative when convenient for patient
- Mix with at least 8 oz of cold liquid
- Have patient drink mixture immediately
- Ensure patient has easy access to toilet or bedpan
- Teach patients with diabetes to check drug label and use brand that doesn't contain sugar

Lubricants

- Used to stimulate defecation
- Example includes mineral oil
- Available in PO preparations

Mode of Action

- Lubricates stool and intestinal mucosa; prevents water reabsorption from bowel lumen

Contraindications, Precautions, and Drug Interactions of Lubricant Laxatives*

Drug	Contraindications/Precautions	Drug Interaction
mineral oil	*Contraindications:* Hypersensitivity, GI obstruction, appendicitis *Precautions:* Diarrhea *Pregnancy:* No risk demonstrated to the fetus in any trimester	Anticoagulants, laxatives, stool softeners

*Pregnancy categories have been revised. See http://www.fda.gov/Drugs/DevelopmentApprovalProcess/DevelopmentResources/Labeling/ucm093307.htm for more information.

Adverse Effects/Side Effects

- Nausea
- Vomiting
- Diarrhea
- Abdominal cramping
- Rectal leaking

Nursing Care

- Administer laxative when convenient for patient
- Administer on empty stomach
- Follow facility protocol for rectal administration
- Ensure patient has easy access to toilet or bedpan

Emollients

- Used to soften stools in patients who should avoid straining during bowel movement
- Examples are docusate sodium, calcium, and potassium
- Available in PO and rectal preparations

Mode of Action

- Acts as bowel detergent that allows water and fats to penetrate stool, making it softer and easier to eliminate

Contraindications, Precautions, and Drug Interactions of Emollient Laxatives*

Drug	Contraindications	Drug Interaction
docusate	**Contraindications:** Hypersensitivity, GI obstruction, fecal impaction, nausea and vomiting **Precautions:** Breastfeeding **Pregnancy:** Only given after risks to the fetus are considered; animal studies have shown adverse reactions; no human studies available	Mineral oil, other laxatives

*Pregnancy categories have been revised. See http://www.fda.gov/Drugs/DevelopmentApprovalProcess/DevelopmentResources/Labeling/ucm093307.htm for more information.

Adverse Effects/Side Effects
- Diarrhea
- Throat irritation
- Bitter taste
- Abdominal cramping
- Rash
- Anorexia

Nursing Care
- Administer laxative when convenient for patient
- Teach patient not to crush or chew enteric coated tablets
- Ensure patient has easy access to toilet or bedpan

Hyperosmolars
- Used to treat constipation, ensure complete bowel evacuation, used in bowel retraining
- Examples are lactulose, sorbitol, sodium phosphate polyethylene
- Available in PO and rectal preparations

Mode of Action
- Draw water into the intestine, distending the bowel and promoting peristalsis; softens stool

Contraindications, Precautions, and Drug Interactions of Hyperosmolar Laxatives*

Drug	Contraindications/Precautions	Drug Interaction
lactulose	**Contraindications:** Hypersensitivity, low-galactose diet **Precautions:** Breastfeeding, geriatric patients, diabetes mellitus **Pregnancy:** No adverse effects in animals; no human studies available	Laxatives, antacids, antiinfectives
sorbitol	**Contraindications:** Hypersensitivity **Precautions:** Breastfeeding, geriatric patients, diabetes mellitus **Pregnancy:** No adverse effects in animals; no human studies available	Laxatives, antacids
sodium phosphate polyethylene	**Contraindications:** Hypersensitivity **Precautions:** Breastfeeding, geriatric patients, renal disease **Pregnancy:** No adverse effects in animals; no human studies available	Laxatives, antacids

*Pregnancy categories have been revised. See http://www.fda.gov/Drugs/DevelopmentApprovalProcess/DevelopmentResources/Labeling/ucm093307.htm for more information.

Adverse Effects/Side Effects

- Weakness
- Fatigue
- Abdominal cramps
- Nausea
- Vomiting

- Diarrhea
- Hypokalemia
- Hypovolemia
- Increased blood glucose levels (lactulose)

- Dehydration
- Cardiac arrhythmias (sodium phosphate polyethylene)

Nursing Care

- Administer laxative when convenient for patient
- Shake suspension thoroughly
- Teach patient not to crush or chew enteric coated tablets
- Ensure patient has easy access to toilet or bedpan

ANTIEMETIC AGENTS

Phenothiazines

- Alleviate nausea and vomiting, control motion sickness
- Examples include chlorpromazine hydrochloride, perphenazine, prochlorperazine maleate, promethazine hydrochloride, thiethylperazine maleate
- Available in oral, intramuscular (IM), intravenous (IV), rectal, transdermal preparations

Mode of Action

- Block dopaminergic receptors in chemoreceptor trigger zone in the brain

Contraindications, Precautions, and Drug Interactions of Phenothiazines*

Drug	Contraindications/Precautions	Drug Interaction
Chlorpromazine hydrochloride	**Contraindications:** Hypersensitivity, children <6 months, liver damage, coronary disease **Precautions:** Breastfeeding, geriatric patients, seizure disorders, hypo/hypertension, closed angle glaucoma **Pregnancy:** Only given after risks to the fetus are considered; animal studies have shown adverse reactions; no human studies available	CNS depressants, antihistamines, epinephrine
perphenazine	**Contraindications:** Hypersensitivity **Precautions:** Breastfeeding, geriatric patients, seizure disorders, glaucoma, hepatic disease **Pregnancy:** Only given after risks to the fetus are considered; animal studies have shown adverse reactions; no human studies available	CNS depressants, antihistamines
prochlorperazine maleate	**Contraindications:** Hypersensitivity, hypersensitivity to phenothiazines, infants/neonates/children <2 yr **Precautions:** Breastfeeding, geriatric patients, seizure disorders, glaucoma, hepatic disease **Pregnancy:** Only given after risks to the fetus are considered; animal studies have shown adverse reactions; no human studies available	CNS depressants, anticholinergics, antidepressants

Continued

Contraindications, Precautions, and Drug Interactions of Phenothiazines—cont'd

Drug	Contraindications/Precautions	Drug Interaction
promethazine hydrochloride	**Contraindications:** Hypersensitivity, breastfeeding, agranulocytosis, jaundice **Precautions:** Cardiac/renal/hepatic disease, asthma, glaucoma, diabetes, urinary retention **Pregnancy:** Only given after risks to the fetus are considered; animal studies have shown adverse reactions; no human studies available	CNS depressants, MAOIs, anticoagulants
thiethylperazine maleate	**Contraindications:** Hypersensitivity **Precautions:** Breastfeeding **Pregnancy:** Only given after risks to the fetus are considered; animal studies have shown adverse reactions; no human studies available	CNS depressants, anticoagulants

*Pregnancy categories have been revised. See http://www.fda.gov/Drugs/DevelopmentApprovalProcess/DevelopmentResources/Labeling/ucm093307.htm for more information.

Adverse Effects/Side Effects

- Drowsiness
- Confusion
- Anxiety
- Respiratory depression
- Extravasation (IV use)
- Euphoria
- Agitation
- Depression
- Headache
- Insomnia
- Restlessness
- Weakness
- Hypotension
- Fainting
- Tachycardia
- Dizziness
- EPSE symptoms
- Tardive dyskinesia (long-term use)

Nursing Care

- If giving IM, rotate injection sites
- If giving IV, ensure patency
- Do not give subcutaneously
- For motion sickness, administer drug 30 to 60 minutes before travel
- Eliminate noxious stimulants from diet and environment
- Provide oral hygiene to the patient who vomits
- Instruct patient to change positions slowly
- Teach patient to avoid alcohol and hazardous activities

Antihistamines

- Alleviate nausea and vomiting, control motion sickness
- Examples include dimenhydrinate, diphenhydramine hydrochloride, hydroxyzine hydrochloride, meclizine hydrochloride, trimethobenzamide hydrochloride
- Available in PO, IM preparations

Mode of Action

- Block H_1 receptors, which prevents acetylcholine from binding to receptors in the vestibular nuclei

Contraindications, Precautions, and Drug Interactions of Antihistamines*

Drug	Contraindications/Precautions	Drug Interaction
dimenhydrinate	*Contraindications:* Hypersensitivity, infants, neonates, tartrazine dye hypersensitivity *Precautions:* Breastfeeding, children, geriatric patients, cardiac dysrhythmias, asthma, closed-angle glaucoma *Pregnancy:* No adverse effects in animals; no human studies available	Alcohol, anticholinergics, MAOIs, tricyclics, CNS depressants
diphenhydramine hydrochloride	*Contraindications:* Hypersensitivity to H_1-receptor antagonists, neonates *Precautions:* Breastfeeding, children <2 yr, increased intraocular pressure, asthma, hypertension, cardiac/renal disease *Pregnancy:* No adverse effects in animals; no human studies available	CNS depressants, tricyclics, alcohol, MAOIs
Hydroxyzine hydrochloride	*Contraindications:* Hypersensitivity, hypersensitivity to cetirizine, pregnancy first trimester, breastfeeding *Precautions:* Geriatric patients, renal/hepatic disease, COPD, closed-angle glaucoma, asthma *Pregnancy:* Only given after risks to the fetus are considered; animal studies have shown adverse reactions; no human studies available	CNS depressants, phenothiazines, antidepressants, MAOIs
meclizine hydrochloride	*Contraindications:* Hypersensitivity to cyclizines *Precautions:* Breastfeeding, children, geriatric patients, closed-angle glaucoma, hepatic/renal disease, urinary retention, GI obstruction, contact lenses *Pregnancy:* No adverse effects in animals; no human studies available	Antidepressants, phenothiazines, atropine, CNS depressants
trimethobenzamide hydrochloride	*Contraindications:* Hypersensitivity, children, shock, sensitivity to opioids *Precautions:* Children, geriatric patients, cardiac dysrhythmias, encephalitis, electrolyte imbalance *Pregnancy:* Only given after risks to the fetus are considered; animal studies have shown adverse reactions; no human studies available	CNS depressants, alcohol

*Pregnancy categories have been revised. See http://www.fda.gov/Drugs/DevelopmentApprovalProcess/DevelopmentResources/Labeling/ucm093307.htm for more information.

Adverse Effects/Side Effects

- Drowsiness
- Restlessness
- Insomnia
- Confusion
- Dry mouth
- Blurred vision
- Constipation
- Rash
- Urinary retention

Nursing Care

- If giving IM, rotate injection sites
- Do not give subcutaneously
- For motion sickness, administer drug 30 to 60 minutes before travel
- Eliminate noxious stimulants from diet and environment
- Provide oral hygiene to the patient who vomits
- Instruct patient to change positions slowly
- Teach patient to avoid alcohol and hazardous activities

Serotonin Receptor (5-HT3) Antagonists

- Alleviate nausea and vomiting, control motion sickness
- Examples include ondansetron, dolasetron, granisetron, palonosetron
- Available in PO, rectal, IV, and IM preparations

Mode of Action

- Block serotonin stimulation in the chemoreceptor trigger zone and vagal nerve terminals

Contraindications, Precautions, and Drug Interactions of Serotonin Receptor Antagonists*

Drug	Contraindications/Precautions	Drug Interaction
ondansetron	*Contraindications:* Hypersensitivity, phenylketonuric hypersensitivity, torsades de pointes *Precautions:* Breastfeeding, children, geriatric patients, QT prolongation *Pregnancy:* No adverse effects in animals; no human studies available	Apomorphine, rifampin, phenytoin
dolasetron	*Contraindications:* Hypersensitivity *Precautions:* Breastfeeding, children, geriatric patients, hypokalemia, electrolyte imbalances, QT prolongation *Pregnancy:* No adverse effects in animals; no human studies available	Antidysrhythmics, cimetidine, rifampin
granisetron	*Contraindications:* Hypersensitivity, benzyl alcohol *Precautions:* Breastfeeding, children, geriatric patients, cardiac dysrhythmias, electrolyte imbalances, cardiac/hepatic/GI disease *Pregnancy:* No adverse effects in animals; no human studies available	Beta blockers, antidysrhythmics, local anesthetics
palonosetron	*Contraindications:* Hypersensitivity *Precautions:* Breastfeeding, children, geriatric patients, hypokalemia, hypomagnesia *Pregnancy:* No adverse effects in animals; no human studies available	Diuretics, antidysrhythmics, apomorphine

*Pregnancy categories have been revised. See http://www.fda.gov/Drugs/DevelopmentApprovalProcess/DevelopmentResources/Labeling/ucm093307.htm for more information.

Adverse Effects/Side Effects

- Confusion
- Anxiety
- Euphoria
- Agitation
- Depression
- Headache
- Insomnia
- Restlessness
- Weakness

Nursing Care
- If giving IM, rotate injection sites
- Do not give subcutaneously
- For motion sickness, administer drug 30 to 60 minutes before travel
- Eliminate noxious stimulants from diet and environment
- Provide oral hygiene to the patient who vomits
- Instruct patient to change positions slowly
- Teach patient to avoid alcohol and hazardous activities

Cannabinoids
- Alleviate nausea and vomiting, control motion sickness
- Examples include dronabinol, nabilone
- Available in PO preparations

Mode of Action
- Works on receptors in the brain to decrease nausea and vomiting

Contraindications, Precautions, and Drug Interactions of Cannabinoids*

Drug	Contraindications/Precautions	Drug Interaction
dronabinol	*Contraindications:* Hypersensitivity, mental illness *Precautions:* Breastfeeding *Pregnancy:* Only given after risks to the fetus are considered; animal studies have shown adverse reactions; no human studies available	CNS depressants
nabilone	*Contraindications:* Hypersensitivity, mental illness *Precautions:* Breastfeeding *Pregnancy:* Only given after risks to the fetus are considered; animal studies have shown adverse reactions; no human studies available	CNS depressants

*Pregnancy categories have been revised. See http://www.fda.gov/Drugs/DevelopmentApprovalProcess/DevelopmentResources/Labeling/ucm093307.htm for more information.

Adverse Effects/Side Effects
- Abdominal pain
- Confusion
- Euphoria
- Weakness
- Anxiety
- Somnolence

Nursing Care
- Teach patient to avoid alcohol and hazardous activities
- Teach patient that cannabinoid use can be habit-forming
- Teach patient signs and symptoms of cannabinoid withdrawal

Neurokinin Receptor Agonists
- Alleviate nausea and vomiting, control motion sickness
- Examples include aprepitant
- Available in PO and IV preparations

Mode of Action
- Decreases emetic reflex

Contraindications, Precautions, and Drug Interactions of Neurokinin Receptor Agonists*

Drug	Contraindications/Precautions	Drug Interaction
aprepitant	*Contraindications:* Hypersensitivity to aprepitant, polysorbate 80 *Precautions:* Breastfeeding, children, geriatric patients, hepatic disease *Pregnancy:* No adverse effects in animals; no human studies available	Anticoagulants, phenytoin, grapefruit juice

*Pregnancy categories have been revised. See http://www.fda.gov/Drugs/DevelopmentApprovalProcess/DevelopmentResources/Labeling/ucm093307.htm for more information.

Adverse Effects/Side Effects

- Headache
- Dizziness
- Insomnia
- Anxiety
- Bradycardia
- Pruritus
- Rash
- Urticaria

Nursing Care

- For cancer patients, administer first dose 1 hour before chemotherapy
- Teach patient that nonhormonal form of birth control is needed
- Teach patient to avoid alcohol and hazardous activities

ADSORBENT, ANTIFLATULENT, AND DIGESTIVE DRUGS

Adsorbent Drugs

- Neutralize toxins
- Example is charcoal
- Available in PO preparations

Mode of Action

- Attract and bind toxins in the intestine, inhibiting toxins from being absorbed from GI tract

Contraindications, Precautions, and Drug Interactions of Adsorbents*

Drug	Contraindications/Precautions	Drug Interaction
activated charcoal	*Contraindications:* Hypersensitivity, GI obstruction *Precautions:* GI bleeding *Pregnancy:* No risk demonstrated to fetus in any trimester	Alcohol, syrup of ipecac

*Pregnancy categories have been revised. See http://www.fda.gov/Drugs/DevelopmentApprovalProcess/DevelopmentResources/Labeling/ucm093307.htm for more information.

Adverse Effects/Side Effects

- Black stool
- Constipation
- Dehydration

Nursing Care

- Do not administer other medications within 2 hours of administering activated charcoal
- Do not administer to semiconscious or unconscious patient, unless airway and NG tube are in place
- Mix with tap water to form syrup
- Do not mix with dairy or sherbet
- Repeat dose if patient vomits shortly after administration
- Follow treatment with stool softener or laxative

Antiflatulent Drugs

- Used to treat gastric bloating, postoperative gaseous bloating, diverticular disease, spastic/irritable colon
- Example is simethicone
- Available in PO preparations

Mode of Action

- Produces film in intestines that disperses and prevents mucous-enclosed gas pockets

Contraindications, Precautions, and Drug Interactions of Antiflatulent Drugs*

Drug	Contraindications/Precautions	Drug Interaction
simethicone	*Contraindications:* Hypersensitivity *Precautions:* Breastfeeding, geriatric patients *Pregnancy:* Only given after risks to the fetus are considered; animal studies have shown adverse reactions; no human studies available	Aluminum, magnesium, lanthanum

*Pregnancy categories have been revised. See http://www.fda.gov/Drugs/DevelopmentApprovalProcess/DevelopmentResources/Labeling/ucm093307.htm for more information.

Adverse Effects/Side Effects

- Belching
- Flatus

Nursing Care

- Shake suspension form thoroughly
- Teach patient to chew tablet form thoroughly
- Teach patient to ambulate and change positions frequently to help pass flatus

Digestive Drugs

- Aid in digestion
- Examples are dehydrocholic acid and pancreatic enzymes (pancreatin, pancrelipase, lipase, protease, amylase)
- Available in PO preparations

Mode of Action

- Dehydrocholic acid increases bile output in the liver
- Pancreatic enzymes replace deficient or missing pancreatic enzymes by digesting proteins (trypsin), carbohydrates (amylase), and fats (lipase)

Contraindications, Precautions, and Drug Interactions of Digestive Drugs*

Drug	Contraindications/Precautions	Drug Interaction
dehydrocholic acid	*Contraindications:* Hypersensitivity *Precautions:* GI bleeding *Pregnancy:* No adverse effects in animals, no human studies available	Antacids, iron
pancreatic enzymes	*Contraindications:* Hypersensitivity *Precautions:* GI bleeding *Pregnancy:* No adverse effects in animals, no human studies available	Antacids, iron

*Pregnancy categories have been revised. See http://www.fda.gov/Drugs/DevelopmentApprovalProcess/DevelopmentResources/Labeling/ucm093307.htm for more information.

Adverse Effects/Side Effects
- Abdominal cramping
- Biliary colic
- Diarrhea
- Nausea

Nursing Care
- Administer before or with meals, as indicated
- Teach patient not to crush or chew enteric-coated pills

OBESITY DRUGS

Appetite Suppressants
- Used to decrease appetite in obese patients
- Examples are phentermine hydrochloride, lorcaserin hydrochloride
- Available in PO preparations

Mode of Action
- Phentermine hydrochloride increases norepinephrine and dopamine in the brain, suppressing appetite
- Lorcaserin hydrochloride activates 5-HTc receptors in the hypothalamus, suppressing appetite

Contraindications, Precautions, and Drug Interactions of Appetite Suppressants*

Drug	Contraindications/Precautions	Drug Interaction
phentermine hydrochloride	*Contraindications:* Hypersensitivity, alcohol, diabetes, CHF, glaucoma, hypertension, renal impairment *Precautions:* Breastfeeding *Pregnancy:* Absolute fetal abnormalities; not to be used at any time during pregnancy	Antidepressants, tramadol
lorcaserin hydrochloride	*Contraindications:* Hypersensitivity, pregnancy, breast-feeding, renal impairment *Precautions:* Children, bradycardia, AV block, dialysis, neutropenia, suicidal ideation *Pregnancy:* Absolute fetal abnormalities; not to be used at any time during pregnancy	SSRIs, MAOIs, bupropion, lithium, tramadol

*Pregnancy categories have been revised. See http://www.fda.gov/Drugs/DevelopmentApprovalProcess/DevelopmentResources/Labeling/ucm093307.htm for more information.

Adverse Effects/Side Effects

- Nervousness
- Dry mouth
- Constipation
- Hypertension

Nursing Care

- Monitor patient for agitation and anxiety
- Monitor blood pressure
- Do not administer to patients with cardiovascular disease, hypertension, history of drug abuse
- Teach patient that appetite suppressants are for short-term use only
- Teach patient importance of healthy diet and exercise

Fat Blockers

- Used to decrease weight in morbidly obese patients
- Example is orlistat
- Available in PO preparations

Mode of Action

- Binds to gastric and pancreatic lipases in GI tract preventing absorption of fat ingested in a meal

Contraindications, Precautions, and Drug Interactions of Fat Blockers*

Drug	Contraindications/Precautions	Drug Interaction
orlistat	**Contraindications:** Hypersensitivity, chronic malabsorption syndrome, cholestasis **Precautions:** Breastfeeding, children, hypothyroidism, anorexia nervosa, bulimia, diabetes **Pregnancy:** Absolute fetal abnormalities not to be used at any time during pregnancy	Warfarin, pravastatin

*Pregnancy categories have been revised. See http://www.fda.gov/Drugs/DevelopmentApprovalProcess/DevelopmentResources/Labeling/ucm093307.htm for more information.

Adverse Effects/Side Effects

- Abdominal pain
- Oily spotting
- Fecal urgency
- Flatulence
- Fatty stool
- Fecal incontinence
- Increased defecation

Nursing Care

- Administer multivitamin to replace lost vitamins and minerals
- Teach patient importance of healthy diet and exercise

APPLICATION AND REVIEW

7. A client is being considered for appetite suppression therapy. Assessment screenings for which medical diagnoses should the nurse plan to implement to assure client safety? **Select all that apply.**
   1. Cardiovascular disease
   2. Hypertension
   3. Gastric ulcers
   4. Drug abuse
   5. Pregnancy

8. A client is being considered for fat blocker, orlistat, therapy. An assessment screening for which condition should the nurse plan to implement to address client safety?
   1. Bulimia
   2. Asthma
   3. Eczema
   4. Insomnia

9. Which statement made by a client prescribed the fat blocker, orlistat, indicates an understanding of the medication's potential adverse effects?
   1. "I need to wear a sunscreen when I'm outside."
   2. "This medication may cause headaches."
   3. "I may have difficulty falling asleep."
   4. "Fecal incontinence may occur."

10. Which assessment finding is considered either a precaution or a contraindication for the prescription of an appetite suppressant?
    1. High alcohol consumption
    2. Currently breastfeeding
    3. History of glaucoma
    4. Suicidal ideations

See Answers on pages 456-458.

ANSWER KEY: REVIEW QUESTIONS

1. **Answer: 200** mL/hr.
   The rate on an infusion control device (ICD) is specified in mL/hr. Fifteen minutes is ¼ of an hour; the equivalent hourly rate is 4 times the volume. The nurse also programs the number of milliliters in the infusion as the volume to be infused (VTBI). The "Desire over Have" formula can be used to solve this problem.

$$\frac{\text{Desire}}{\text{Have}} \quad \frac{60 \text{ minutes}}{15 \text{ minutes}} = \frac{x \text{ mL}}{50 \text{ mL}}$$

$$15x = 60 \times 50$$
$$15x = 3000$$
$$x = 3000 \div 15$$
$$x = 200 \text{ mL/hr}$$

Client Need: Pharmacologic and Parenteral Therapies; **Cognitive Level:** Application; **Nursing Process:** Planning/Implementation

2. **2 Systemic antibiotics block acid production in the stomach; decreasing excess stomach acid allows the ulcer to heal.**
   1 Antacids neutralize gastric acid in the stomach, which reduces total amount of acid in GI tract. **3** H_2-receptor antagonists block histamine from stimulating the acid-secreting parietal cells of the stomach. **4** Proton pump inhibitors block gastric acid secretion by combining with hydrogen, potassium, and adenosine triphosphate in parietal cells of stomach
   Client Need: Pharmacologic and Parenteral Therapies; **Cognitive Level:** Analysis; **Nursing Process:** Assessment/Analysis

> **Study Tip:** Write this phrase on a piece of paper: **a**nti**b**iotics **b**lock **a**cid. Then fold the paper in half vertically and see if you can get the a's to overlap and the b's to overlap. Do this while reminding yourself that systemic antibiotics block acid production in the stomach until you have this fact committed to memory.

3. Answers: 1, 2, 3, 5

The H_2-receptor antagonist, cimetidine, poses a drug interaction risk when administered with an antacid, anticoagulant. Beta blocker and/or calcium channel blocker.

4 Tricyclic antidepressants are not known to pose a drug interaction risk when taken with cimetidine.

Client Need: Pharmacologic and Parenteral Therapies; **Cognitive Level:** Analysis; **Nursing Process:** Planning/Implementation

4. Answers: 1, 2, 3, 5

The H_2-receptor antagonists should be administered with food at bedtime, but not within 1 hour of taking an antacid. Diarrhea is an adverse effect of this drug classification and should be reported to your primary health care provider.

4 The H_2-receptor antagonists may be taken with dairy products.

Client Need: Pharmacologic and Parenteral Therapies; **Cognitive Level:** Analysis; **Integrated Process:** Teaching/Learning; **Nursing Process:** Planning/Implementation

5. Answers: 1, 2, 3, 4

Systemic antibiotics prescribed for gastric ulcers should be administered with water. The client should be instructed to keep the head of the bed elevated to help minimize gastric reflux and meals should be bland with several small meals being eaten during the course of the day. Smoking should also be avoided.

5 Clients should be taught not to crush, chew, or break extended release products.

Client Need: Pharmacologic and Parenteral Therapies; **Cognitive Level:** Analysis; **Integrated Process:** Teaching/Learning; **Nursing Process:** Planning/Implementation

6. Answer: 1.5 mL.

Use the "Desire over Have" formula of ratio and proportion to solve this problem.

$$\frac{\text{Desire}}{\text{Have}} \quad \frac{15\,\text{mg}}{10\,\text{mg}} = \frac{x\,\text{mL}}{1\,\text{mL}}$$

$$10\,x = 15$$

$$x = \frac{15}{10}$$

$$x = 1.5\,\text{mL}$$

Client Need: Pharmacologic and Parenteral Therapies; **Cognitive Level:** Application; **Nursing Process:** Planning/Implementation

7. Answers: 1, 2, 4, 5

Appetite suppression therapy should not be administered to patients with cardiovascular disease, hypertension, or a history of drug abuse. Pregnant clients should be prescribed an appetite suppressant because of the risk of fetal abnormalities.

3 Gastric ulcers are not associated with the contraindications or precautions for appetite suppression therapy.

Client Need: Pharmacologic and Parenteral Therapies; **Cognitive Level:** Analysis; **Nursing Process:** Planning/Implementation

8. 1 Bulimia is a precautionary condition for the prescription of orlistat and so clients should be screened before beginning such therapy.

2 Asthma is not associated with the contraindications or precautions for orlistat therapy. **3** Eczema is not associated with the contraindications or precautions for orlistat therapy. **4** Insomnia is not associated with the contraindications or precautions for orlistat therapy.

Client Need: Pharmacologic and Parenteral Therapies; **Cognitive Level:** Analysis; **Nursing Process:** Planning/Implementation

9. 4 The medication's effect on fat absorption may result in fetal incontinence.

1 Sun sensitivity is not associated with the adverse effects of the fat blocker, orlistat. **2** Headaches are not associated with the adverse effects of the fat blocker, orlistat. **3** Insomnia is not associated with the adverse effects of the fat blocker, orlistat.

Client Need: Pharmacologic and Parenteral Therapies; **Cognitive Level:** Analysis; **Integrated Process:** Teaching/Learning; **Nursing Process:** Evaluation/Outcomes

10. **2** Breastfeeding is considered a precaution or a contraindication for the prescription of an appetite suppressant.

1 Alcohol consumption is a contraindication for some appetite suppressants. **3** Glaucoma is a contraindication for some appetite suppressants. **4** Suicidal ideations are considered a precaution for the prescription of some appetite suppressants.

Client Need: Pharmacologic and Parenteral Therapies; **Cognitive Level:** Analysis; **Nursing Process:** Assessment/Analysis

---

Study Tip: *Notice how often breastfeeding is a precaution or contraindication in drug descriptions.* Think about the possible consequences of a drug taken by a breastfeeding mother being included in the milk for her infant. Not all drugs show up unchanged in breast milk, but just in case, consider it as you read questions like this one. Would you want to suppress the appetite of a breastfeeding infant? Not likely!

Burchum, J. R., Rosenthal, L. D. (2016). *Lehne's pharmacology for nursing* (9th ed.). St. Louis: Saunders.

Fulcher, E. M., Fulcher, R. M., Soto, C. D. (2012). *Pharmacology Principles and applications* (3rd ed.). Philadelphia: Saunders.

Huether, S. E., McCance, K. L., Brashers, V. L., Rote, N. S. (2012). *Understanding pathophysiology* (5th ed.). St. Louis: Mosby.

Lehne, R. A. (2013). *Pharmacology for nursing care* (8th ed.). St. Louis: Saunders.

Lilley, L. L., Collins, S. R., Snyder, J. S. (2017). *Pharmacology and the nursing process* (8th ed.). St. Louis: Elsevier.

McCuistion, L., Vuljoin-DiMaggio, K., Winton, M. B., Yeager, J. J. (2018). *Pharmacology: A patient-centered nursing process approach* (9th ed.). St. Louis: Elsevier.

Kee, J. L., Hayes, E. R., McCuistion, L. E. (2015). *Pharmacology: A patient-centered nursing process approach* (8th ed.). St. Louis: Saunders.

Kizior, R. J., Hodgson, B. B. (2017). *Saunders nursing drug handbook, 2017*. Philadelphia: Saunders.

Skidmore-Roth, L. (2015). *Mosby's drug guide for nursing students* (11th ed.). St. Louis: Mosby.

Skidmore-Roth, L. (2017). *Mosby's 2017 nursing drug reference* (13th ed.). St. Louis: Mosby.

U.S. Food & Drug Administration. (2017): *Drugs*. www.fda.gov/drugs. Silver Spring, MD: Author.

Darunavir, 366–368t
Dasatinib, 395–397t
Daunorubicin, 393t
Dawn phenomenon, management of, 226
Decongestants, 311
  adrenergic, 311–312, 312t
  anticholinergic, 313, 313t
  corticosteroid, 313–315, 314t
Deep vein thrombosis (DVT), 200–201
Deficient antidiuretic hormone, 250
Dehydrocholic acid, 454t
Delavirdine, 364–365t
Delayed-reaction allergies, definition of, 1
Delusional/paranoia disorders, 73–74
Demeclocycline, for syndrome of inappropriate
    antidiuretic hormone secretion (SIADH), 252–253,
    252–253t
Dementia, 121
  cause of, 121
  clinical findings of, 121
  mild to moderate, treatment of, 127–128
  therapeutic interventions for, 121
Dendritic cells, 387t
Denial, against anxiety, 68
Dependence, in sedative-hypnotics, 41t
Depressive episode, of bipolar disorder, 70
Desipramine, 23–24t
  for affective disorders, 81t
Desired effect, definition of, 1
Desmopressin, 218t
  for diabetes insipidus, 250, 251t
Desogestrel, 292–294t
Desvenlafaxine, for affective disorders, 87–88t
Dexamethasone, for Addison disease, 267, 268–269t
Dexlansoprazole, 439t
Dexmedetomidine, 110–112t
Dextromethorphan, 317t
Diabetes insipidus, antidiuretic hormone replacement
    for, 250–251
  adverse effects/side effects of, 251
  assessment/analysis of, 251
  evaluation/outcomes of, 252
  planning/implementation of, 251–252
  therapeutic interventions for, 250–251, 251t
  types of, 250
Diabetes mellitus, 222–226
  angina and, 157
  classification of, 222
  clinical findings in, 223–224
  etiology of, 222–223
  long-term complications of, 223, 223f
  pathophysiology of, 222–223

Diabetes mellitus (Continued)
  risk factors for, 222
  therapeutic interventions for, 224–226
Diabetic diet, 433
Diabetic ketoacidosis (DKA), 222, 224, 225
Diaphragm, 285
Diastolic blood pressure, 200
Diazepam, for affective disorders, 75–77t
Didanosine, 362–363t
Diet
  for diabetes mellitus, 224
  types of, 432–433
Digestive drugs, 453–454
Diltiazem, 167t, 194–195t
Dimenhydrinate, 449t
Dinutuximab, 401t
Dipeptidyl peptidase 4 inhibitors, 234–236t
Diphenhydramine, 315–316t
Diphenhydramine hydrochloride, 449t
Diphenoxylate, with atropine, 442t
Diplococci, bacteria, 334
Dipyridamole, 210t
Directed donation, 204
Disopyramide phosphate, 185t
Disorganized schizophrenia, 72
Displacement, against anxiety, 68
Disseminated intravascular coagulation (DIC), 203
Dissociation, against anxiety, 68
Diuretic drugs, 130–148
  application and review for, 136–144, 149–155
  carbonic anhydrase inhibitors, 151–153
  for heart failure, 134
  loop, 147–148
  osmotic, 150–151
  potassium-sparing, 149–150
  thiazide, 144–146
  thiazide-like, 146–147
Dobutamine, 110–112t
Docusate, 446t
Dofetilide, 192–193t
Dolasetron, 450t
Dolutegravir, 372t
Donepezil, 127t
Dopamine, 107–108t
Dopaminergic receptors, 105
Dopaminergics, for Parkinson's disease, 97–99
  adverse/side effects of, 99
  contraindications to, 97–98t
  drug interactions of, 97–98t
  mode of action of, 97–98
  nursing care and, 99
  precautions of, 97–98t